MOSBY'S
NURSING **LEADERSHIP**
MANAGEMENT
ONLINE

A WORK TEXT AND ONLINE COURSE

MOSBY'S NURSING LEADERSHIP & MANAGEMENT ONLINE

A WORK TEXT AND ONLINE COURSE

ROBERT L. ANDERS, DrPh, APRN, CNAA, CS

Associate Dean
College of Health Sciences
Professor and Director
School of Nursing
University of Texas–El Paso
El Paso, Texas

JAMES A. HAWKINS, EdD, MBA

Chairman and Chief Executive Officer
JHawk & Associates—Educational Consultants
Honolulu, Hawaii

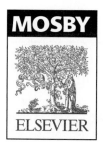

MOSBY

ELSEVIER

11830 Westline Industrial Drive
St. Louis, Missouri 63146

MOSBY'S NURSING LEADERSHIP & MANAGEMENT ONLINE: ISBN-13: 978-0-323-03991-8
A WORK TEXT AND ONLINE COURSE ISBN-10: 0-323-03991-X

Notice

ISBN-13: 978-0-323-03991-8
ISBN-10: 0-323-03991-X

Senior Editor: *Yvonne Alexopoulos*
Developmental Editor: *Kristin Hebberd*
Editorial Assistant: *Sarah Vales*
Publishing Services Manager: *Deborah L. Vogel*
Senior Project Manager: *Deon Lee*
Design Manager: *Teresa McBryan*

Printed in the United States of America

Last digit is the print number: 9 8 7 6 5 4 3 2

Reviewers for Online Course Modules

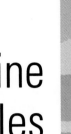

Rosalinda Alfaro-LeFevre, RN, MSN
President
Teaching Smart/Learning Easy
Stuart, Florida

Karen Brasfield, RN, MSN, CMSRN
Instructor
Department of Nursing
Everett Community College
Everett, Washington

Jacqueline Rosenjack Burchum, DNSc,
  APRN, BC
Assistant Professor
College of Nursing
University of Tennessee Health Science Center
Memphis, Tennessee

Diane E. Featherston, MSN, APRN, BC
Clinical Instructor
College of Nursing
Wayne State University
Detroit, Michigan

Nancy C. Grove, RN, BSN, MEd, MSN, PhD
Director and Associate Professor
Nursing Program
University of Pittsburgh at Johnstown
Johnstown, Pennsylvania

Ruth I. Hansten, RN, BSN, MBA, PhD, FACHE
Principal Consultant
Hansten Healthcare PLLC
Port Ludlow, Washington;
Adjunct Faculty
School of Nursing
University of Washington
Seattle University
Seattle, Washington

Andrea W. Koepke, BSN, MAN, DSN
Director
School of Nursing
Anderson University
Anderson, Indiana

Suzy Lockwood, BSN, MSN, PhD
Assistant Professor
Harris School of Nursing
Texas Christian University
Forth Worth, Texas

Sharie Metcalfe, PhD, RN
Associate Professor
School of Nursing
Illinois Wesleyan University
Bloomington, Illinois

Claudia Louth Mitchell, RN, BSN, MSN,
  Certificate in Gerontology
Instructor, Professor of Nursing
Associate Degree Nursing Program
Santa Barbara City College
Santa Barbara, California

Denise Top Rhine, RN, MEd, CEN
Professor
Associate Degree Nursing
Oakton Community College
Des Plaines, Illinois

Susan T. Sanders, MSN, RN, CNAA
Director
Patient Care
QHR Patient Services
Brentwood, Tennessee;
Adjunct Nursing Faculty
Middle Tennessee State University
Murfreesboro, Tennessee

Gail Scoates, RN, MS
Clinical Educator
OSF St. Joseph Medical Center
Visiting Faculty
School of Nursing
Illinois Wesleyan University
Bloomington, Illinois

Margaret Mary West, DNSc, RN
Associate Professor
Geisinger Site Coordinator
Nursing Education Center
Thomas Jefferson University
Danville, Pennsylvania

Preface

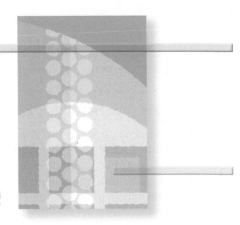

This work text and online course are collaborative endeavors far greater than the working efforts put forth by the authors. They are a melding of the best concepts of two different worlds: nursing science and free enterprise. The two authors—one an accomplished nursing professional and eminent educator and the other a business owner, entrepreneur, and educational consultant—believed that the combination of the finest qualities of both worlds, so often thought to be alien from one another, could, in fact, work together to enhance the nursing profession as a whole by broadening the scope of its next generation of managers.

Nursing is one of the most respected of professions, but it is also one that is in great need. Everywhere there are major challenges to be faced: labor relations, patient care quality, quality service, risk management issues, turnover, absenteeism, job satisfaction, employee morale, and cost efficiency. There are organizations that meet these issues head on and seem to win through them consistently, and there are others that never quite achieve their goals. What makes each different? Why does one stand out and another get by?

The answer is the quality of management and its ability to adapt to an ever-changing environment.

Management is more than the application of a set of skills. It is, in fact, a profession unto itself. It is a full-time, highly competitive, and extremely challenging vocation—one that is every bit as demanding, rewarding, and exciting as clinical nursing. It is a dynamic environment that operates most successfully when it is exercised with patience, concern, and understanding. The successful manager is an individual who cares about others above self, who communicates openly and encourages excellence in others. These factors are identical in both the world of health care and the world of business.

Hugely successful businesses rarely number their success by income alone. In fact, the most successful feel best when they think about how well individual employees succeed and in the manner that they affect the communities they serve. In developing their success, both business and health care have acquired a wealth of knowledge and a large number of skills that can be used to enhance each other's performance, success, and influence. It is the intent of this textbook to blend these qualities so closely that they become applicable in every management position, no matter in what field they are employed.

This course of instruction is about the melding of excellence from two very different, but still very similar, industries. It is learning that management is about people—leading, encouraging, and inspiring them toward achievement. It is about using the position of management to administer what is right, just, and fair. It is about understanding that the management of others is a privilege to be honored through personal sacrifice, commitment, and integrity. It is about discovering the value in helping others achieve by encouraging excellence, creativity, and imagination.

The work text and online course are about the development of excellence—that of both yourself and those that you will eventually lead. They are about understanding that responsibility and accountability are individual qualities that are nurtured and encouraged in others through positive demonstration. Management is about overcoming challenge by creating an environment of trust, cooperation, and teamwork, where all contribution is valued and all capability is encouraged.

This course of instruction originated because two men, from two very different backgrounds, shared the belief that management is universal, and that the skills that achieve excellence in the Fortune 500 boardroom are exactly the same ones needed to achieve success as a nurse manager; only the application is different.

USING THE WORK TEXT

The work text is intended to be used in conjunction with the online course. The first 16 chapters discuss issues related to undergraduate courses of study in nursing leadership and management. Each of these chapters corresponds to an online course module of the same name. Users are advised to read through each work text chapter before attempting to work through the online module to maximize learning.

Information presented within the work text chapter will be used and applied to the case-based online module. Text references within the module (specifically on the *Focused Reading Assignment* and *Review of Key Concepts, Principles, and Terms* screens in each module) direct users back to discussions within this work text and provide questions that help ensure that they have mastered the principles of that area of leadership and management necessary to work through the online module. Within the module, learning activities constantly quiz the user to determine his or her level of understanding in applying these concepts.

The remaining 10 chapters of this work text are devoted to graduate-level topics in nursing leadership and management that go above and beyond the scope of the online course. These can be used as supplemental learning materials for users who want to take their education one step further.

ADDITIONAL RESOURCES

Accessible through the online course (http://evolve.elsevier.com/AndersHawkins/nursingLM/) are a number of additional learning tools for instructors, as follows:

- A Test Bank containing nearly 250 NCLEX®-style examination questions with rationales for correct and incorrect responses and approximately 285 additional true/false questions
- A collection of approximately 450 PowerPoint lecture slides to facilitate a traditional classroom presentation and discussion or for customized use in online learning courses
- Module-specific and in-class Assignments for both individuals and groups
- Open-ended Discussion Board questions designed to facilitate online discussion
- A customizable Sample Syllabus to provide an example of how this work text and online course can be put to use in a semester course

ROBERT L. ANDERS
JAMES A. HAWKINS

Acknowledgments

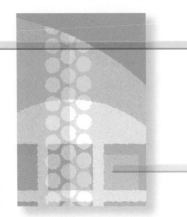

There are no words to express how much we owe to the hundreds of people who contributed to the success of this book. We can't begin to express our appreciation, and we will always be humbled by your excellence.

Special Thanks to:
Yvonne Alexopoulos
Tab Bates
Crissy Halterman
Kristin Hebberd
Deon Lee
Warren Phillips
Tracy Bayne
Sarah Vales

Thank you seems far too small an accolade to acknowledge your contributions.

Contents

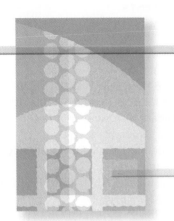

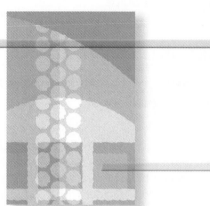

USER GUIDE
for Mosby's Nursing Leadership & Management Online: A Work Text and Online Course

GETTING STARTED

If your course is being led by an instructor:

1. SYSTEM

Your instructor will provide information about the system on which your course is being hosted. Evolve® courses can be run on a variety of systems, and your instructor will decide which one is right for this course.

2. USERNAME AND PASSWORD

Your instructor will also provide you with the username and password needed to access the system where this course is located.

3. LOGIN INSTRUCTIONS

If your instructor's course is being hosted on the Evolve Learning System, please go to page xxvi for instructions about how to log in. If your course is on a different system, your instructor will provide information about how to log in.

4. ACCESS CODE

The first time you access this course, you will need the access code located inside the front cover of this book, regardless of which system is hosting the course. When you are prompted, enter the code **exactly** as it appears inside the front cover.

If you plan to take the course on your own:

(**Note:** By taking the course independently, you will not have any instructor to help you with the course. You will have 12 months from the date you are enrolled to complete the course.)

1. SYSTEM

All independent learners are enrolled into a course hosted on the Evolve Learning System.

2. SELF-ENROLLMENT

Please go to page xxvi for instructions about how to self-enroll in the course.

3. USERNAME AND PASSWORD

If you do not have an existing Evolve account, you will be able to create one during the self-enrollment process.

4. LOGIN INSTRUCTIONS

Please go to page xxvi for instructions about how to log in to the Evolve Learning System.

5. ACCESS CODE

The first time you access this course, you will need the access code located inside the front cover of this User Guide. When you are prompted, enter the code **exactly** as it appears in this guide.

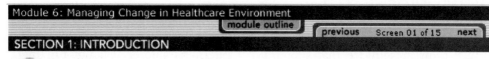

Module 6: Managing Change in Healthcare Environment

module outline

previous   Screen 01 of 15   next

SECTION 1: INTRODUCTION

Introduction

This module focuses on the fundamentals of managing change within the healthcare environment, and how a nurse manager can skillfully apply them within a given work situation.

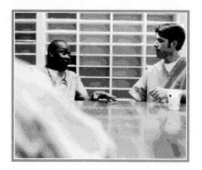

The module is organized into five Sections:

1. **Introduction** - provides an overview of the entire module.

2. **Fundamentals of Managing Change** - provides a review of the key concepts.

3. **You are the Manager** - provides information you will need to know to complete the scenarios in Section 4.

4. **Getting to Work** - provides real world scenarios where you can apply what has been learned in Chapter 6.

WHAT *IS* MOSBY'S NURSING LEADERSHIP & MANAGEMENT ONLINE?

Mosby's Nursing Leadership & Management Online is a revolutionary online course and accompanying work text that blends theory, research, and practical experiences into fundamental leadership and management skills. This course delivers an innovative approach, merging successful business applications into nursing leadership and management practice for optimal and effective results. *Mosby's Nursing Leadership & Management Online* combines dynamic content, practice, and assessment into one resource that can be used in the classroom, home, or anywhere else you can access the Internet.

Mosby's Nursing Leadership & Management Online immerses you in a true-to-life leadership and management environment through . . .

- **16 ready-to-use online modules** that cover the most pertinent and emerging leadership and management topics within nursing today—from the fundamentals of leadership and management to delegation, cultural issues, legal/ethical issues, team building, communication, quality assurance, technology and health care management, and many more!

- A **case-based approach** that provides a case scenario or situation that sets the stage as you work through the module, utilizing the information gathered from the work text and additional data sources presented within the module.

- **Numerous learning activities** such as multiple-select questions and matching exercises that allow you to interact online and master the concepts learned in the text. Immediate feedback and rationales are provided to help you keep track of your performance.

- **Photographs** demonstrating various dialogues between managers and staff members, various methods of communication, body language, and much more.

- **Pop-up screens,** such as definition boxes, sample electronic messages, and other important case-related documents, to minimize text overload and help keep you engaged in the modules.

TECHNICAL REQUIREMENTS

To use an Evolve Online Course, you will need access to a computer that is connected to the Internet and equipped with web browser software that supports frames. For optimal performance, it is recommended that you have speakers and use a high-speed Internet connection. However, slower dial-up modems (56K minimum) are acceptable.

Screen Settings

For best results, the resolution of your computer monitor should be set at a minimum of 800 × 600. The number of colors displayed should be set to "thousands or higher" (High Color or 16 bit) or "millions of colors" (True Color or 24 bit). To set the resolution:

WINDOWS

1. From the **Start** menu, select **Settings** and **Control Panel**.
2. Double-click on the **Display** icon.
3. Click on the **Settings** tab.
4. In the **Screen area** use the slider bar to select **800 by 600 pixels**.
5. In the **Colors** drop down menu, click on the arrow to show more settings.
6. Click on **High Color (16 bit)** or **True Color (24 bit)**.
7. Click on **Apply**.
8. Click on **OK**.
9. You may be asked to verify the setting changes. Click **Yes**.
10. You may be asked to restart your computer to accept the setting changes. Click **Yes**.

MACINTOSH

1. Select the **Monitors** control panel.
2. Select **800 × 600** (or similar) from the **Resolution** area.
3. Select **Thousands** or **Millions** from the **Color Depth** area.

Web Browsers

Supported web browsers include Microsoft Internet Explorer (IE) version 6.0 or higher, Netscape version 7.1 or higher, and Mozilla version 1.4 or higher.

If you use America Online (AOL) for Web access, you will need AOL version 4.0 or higher **and** one of the browsers listed above. Earlier versions of AOL and Internet Explorer will not run the course properly, and you will have difficulty accessing many features.

For best results with AOL:

- Connect to the Internet using AOL version 4.0 or higher.
- Open a private chat within AOL. (This allows the AOL client to remain open, without asking if you wish to disconnect while minimized.)
- Minimize AOL.
- Launch one of the recommended browsers.

Whichever browser you use, the browser preferences must be set to enable cookies as well as Java/JavaScript, and the cache must be set to reload every time.

Enable Cookies

Browser	Steps
Internet Explorer 6.0 or higher	1. Select **Tools**. 2. Select **Internet Options**. 3. Select **Privacy** tab. 4. Use the slider (slide down) to **Accept All Cookies**. 5. Click **OK**. **OR** 4. Click the **Advanced** button. 5. Click the check box next to **Override Automatic Cookie Handling**. 6. Click the **Accept** radio buttons under **First-party Cookies** and **Third-party Cookies**. 7. Click **OK**.
Netscape 7.1 or higher	1. Select **Edit**. 2. Select **Preferences**. 3. Select **Privacy & Security**. 4. Select **Cookies**. 5. Select **Enable All Cookies**.
Mozilla 1.4 or higher	1. Select **Tools**. 2. Select **Privacy**. 3. Expand the **Cookies** section and check the following box: **Allow sites to set cookies**.

Enable Java

Browser	Steps
Internet Explorer 6.0 or higher	1. Select **Tools → Internet Options.** 2. Select the **Advanced** tab. 3. Scroll down the list until you see the **Java (Sun)** section and select the box that appears below it.
Netscape 7.1 or higher	1. Select **Edit → Preferences.** 2. Select **Advanced.** 3. Select **Scripts & Plugins.** 4. Make sure the **Navigator** box is checked to **Enable JavaScript.** 5. Click **OK.**
Mozilla 1.4 or higher	1. Select **Tools.** 2. Select **Web Features.** 3. Select the boxes next to **Enable Java** and **Enable JavaScript.**

Set Cache to Always Reload a Page

Browser	Steps
Internet Explorer 6.0 or higher	1. Select **Tools → Internet Options.** 2. Select the **General** tab. 3. Go to the **Temporary Internet Files** section and click on the **Settings** button. Select the radio button for **Every visit to the page** and click **OK** when complete. 4. Select the radio button for **Every visit to the page.** 5. Click **OK.**
Netscape 7.1 or higher	1. Select **Edit → Preferences.** 2. Select **Advanced.** 3. Select **Cache.** 4. Select the **Every time I view the page** radio button. 5. Click **OK.**
Mozilla 1.4 or higher	1. Select **Tools.** 2. Select **Privacy.** 3. Expand the **Cache** section and designate a disk space number if one is not already in place.

Plug-Ins

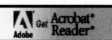

Adobe Acrobat Reader—With the free Acrobat Reader software you can view and print Adobe PDF files. Many Evolve products offer documents in this format, including student and instructor manuals, checklists, and more.

Download at: http://www.adobe.com.

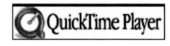

Apple QuickTime— Install this to hear word pronunciations, heart and lung sounds, and many other interesting audio clips within Evolve Online Courses.

Download at: http://www.apple.com.

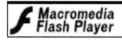

Macromedia Flash Player—This player will enhance your viewing of many Evolve web pages as well as educational short-form to long-form animation within the Evolve Learning System.

Download at: http://www.macromedia. com.

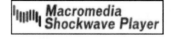

Macromedia Shockwave Player— Shockwave is best for viewing the many interactive learning activities within Evolve Online Courses.

Download at: http://www.macromedia. com.

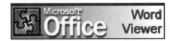

Microsoft Word Viewer—With this viewer, Microsoft Word users can share documents with others who do not have Word software. Users without Word can then open and view Word documents. Many Evolve products have test banks, student and instructor manuals, and other documents available for download and viewing on your local computer.

Download at: http://www.microsoft.com.

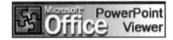

Microsoft PowerPoint Viewer—This viewer makes it possible for you to view PowerPoint 97, 2000, and 2002 presentations even if you do not have PowerPoint software. Many Evolve products have slides available for download and viewing on your local computer.

Download at: http://www.microsoft.com.

LOGIN INSTRUCTIONS

IMPORTANT NOTE: These instructions apply only to users whose course is running on the Evolve Learning System. If you are taking an instructor-led course, please ask your instructor which system is hosting your course and where to find applicable instructions. Evolve courses can be run on a variety of systems, and your instructor will decide which one is right for a particular course.

1. Go to: http://evolve.elsevier.com/student.
2. Enter your username and password in the **Login to My Evolve** area and click the **Login** button.

3. You will be taken to your personalized **My Evolve** page where your course will be listed in the **My Courses** module.

SELF-ENROLLMENT INSTRUCTIONS

IMPORTANT NOTE: These instructions apply only to individuals who will be taking the course on their own. By taking the course independently, you will not have any instructor to help you with the course. You will have 12 months from the date you are enrolled to complete the course.

1. Go to http://evolve.elsevier.com/AndersHawkins/nursingLM/.
2. Under the **Online Course** heading, click on the **Self-Study Student? Enroll Here** option. This will launch the enrollment wizard for your course.
3. Complete the enrollment wizard. During this process you will create an Evolve username and password. You will also be asked to provide identifying information about yourself and will need to provide the access code from inside the front cover of this guide.
4. Once the wizard has been completed you will be able to log in to your Evolve account and begin your Online Course immediately.

SUPPORT INFORMATION

Technical support is available to customers in the United States and Canada from 7:30 am to 7:00 pm, Central Time, Monday through Friday by calling, toll-free: **1-800-401-9962**. You can also send an email to evolve-support@elsevier.com.

There is also **24/7 Support Information** available on the Evolve Portal (http://evolve.elsevier.com) including:

- Guided Tours
- Tutorials
- Frequently Asked Questions (FAQs)
- Online Copies of Course User Guides
- And much more!

PART I

UNDERGRADUATE CURRICULUM

Introduction to Management

OUTLINE

LEARNING SYNOPSIS

Upon successful completion of this chapter, readers will possess a fundamental understanding of the topics that will be discussed in this textbook and will have a broad overview of the nursing management profession.

OBJECTIVES

1. Identify selected challenges that are facing the nursing management profession in today's business-oriented world
2. Identify some of the historical aspects of the nursing profession that have required nursing management to evolve
3. Identify the challenges faced by nurse managers as they perform their required work within the bureaucracy of the normal healthcare organization
4. Describe the influences of the nurse manager on the healthcare unit
5. Describe the quality of accountability as it applies to the nurse manager and his or her role as the leader of the nursing unit
6. Identify methods used by the nurse manager to fulfill his or her responsibility to provide quality patient health care
7. Describe how the advent of nursing management research is affecting the nursing profession

Nurse managers simultaneously function as subordinates, superiors, and customer service representatives. Contemplate this statement: As subordinates, nurse managers are held responsible for the overall performance of their units by senior members of the nursing staff and hospital and office administrators. They are accountable to patients and their families, and responsible for the establishment and maintenance of professional standards and environments. The challenge faced by nurse managers is to fulfill their responsibilities to the organization, patients and their families, and the nursing profession, while they depend on the efforts of their subordinates to make this performance possible. This text has been designed to help nurse managers meet the requirements of this challenge and of the nursing profession in general.

Nurse managers face additional challenges, such as the following:

- Increasing their competency in today's demanding healthcare environment
- Responding effectively to the many changes in their environment and profession that are brought about by internal and external forces
- Making ethical decisions in a wide variety of increasingly complicated circumstances
- Assisting staff members who are chemically dependent

This chapter includes information that can assist nurse managers in effectively meeting these and a myriad of other challenges that occur daily in the individual nursing unit and in the profession as a whole.

Productivity is a definitive measure of the amount of work performed and the quality of the work accomplished, with the effective use of available resources considered a key factor. (A complete discussion of productivity is included in another chapter of this textbook.) The composition of the organization in which the work is performed; the individual structures of the working groups within the organization; the quality, training level, and commitment of the available staff; and the nurse manager all have an impact on the productivity of the work group. Nurse managers directly influence the productivity of the individual performers and the various work groups that they supervise. They are also responsible for integrating the overall performance of these work groups so that they contribute to the goals and objectives established by the organization as a whole. Only when such integration occurs can high productivity be achieved.

Managing change and managing the transitions that take place during the process of change are also issues that are becoming increasingly important to nurse managers and the nursing profession as a whole. Over the past several decades, the healthcare profession has been in a nearly constant state of evolution that shows no sign of abatement in the foreseeable future. Among the significant changes that have occurred are the following:

- The placement of restrictions on the profession by third-party reimbursement organizations
- An ever-increasing sense of competition, both real and imagined, among healthcare institutions
- An acute and rapidly accelerating shortage of qualified, professionally trained nurses
- The increased predominance of the multihospital group structured as a for-profit corporation

These major changes, and an almost countless array of others occurring at a rapid rate in today's healthcare industry, ensure an ever-changing environment for nurse managers, their staff, and patients. To be effective and truly realize their potential, nurse managers must be prepared to deal effectively with these changes and work within a constantly evolving work environment. The status quo—the desire to keep things as they have always been, or as one would like them to be—can no longer be the basis for professional decision-making. Furthermore, tomorrow's effective nurse managers will need a far more global view of the nursing profession and the circumstances in which it operates in order to forecast and plan for the many new challenges that will require their constant attention.

The evolving nursing profession and professional environment, along with the inevitably increasing emphasis that will be placed on improved productivity, requires that education in ethical decision-making be a fundamental part of the training of the next generation of nursing professionals. Nurse managers, as the leaders of the profession, will find themselves ever more frequently in the mire of ethical dilemmas in their attempts to make logical decisions. As the performance-related factors of increased productivity requirements, staff and resource shortages, and the need to provide the patient with the best possible care all crash into one another, the pressure for individual and team excellence will mount.

The nursing profession perhaps has not been as aggressive in the past as it should have been in recognizing chemical dependency in its ranks and has only recently come to grips with the reality of this problem. Concern for a colleague in need challenges every nursing professional to help, and this desire to assist enmeshes the nurse in profound legal and ethical issues. As the nurse manager moves to assist the colleague in trouble and, at the same time, ensure patient safety, these issues become more and more profound. As increased and more reliable information concerning substance abuse becomes available, the interventional skills required to meet this critical situation effectively must be learned and applied. The issue of substance abuse is only one of the many ethical dilemmas that will be faced by tomorrow's nurse manager.

The nursing profession no longer provides the safe working environment that historically has been its hallmark. This is especially true for those nurses desiring to become nurse managers. To ensure that he or she can function professionally within this increasingly dangerous environment, the nurse manager must step outside the traditional box and concentrate on the following:

1. Development of effective management skills
2. Advancement of his or her own professional nursing skills as well as the skills of every member of the nurse manager's team and even the skills of those people with whom the nurse manager has frequent contact in the working environment
3. Never-relenting pursuit of new skills suited to an unpredictable environment

A process of continual learning is the only real solution to the dilemmas that will face the nursing profession in the future. Nursing as a whole, and the nurse managers who provide the leadership for the profession, must be willing to step forward and commit to accepting this challenge.

THE FOUNDATION OF NURSING MANAGEMENT

Ever since humans began banding together to accomplish goals that could not be achieved by any one person, the skills of effective management have been essential to ensure coordination of individual efforts. The purpose of this textbook is to study management in general and nursing management specifically.

High-quality nurse leadership is fundamental in ensuring high-quality nursing care. This simple truth applies to the entire nursing profession, beginning with the position of nurse manager—the leadership position most directly associated with the delivery of quality nursing care.

Nurse managers have the dual responsibilities of representing the institution to the patient and the patient to the institution. To discharge these responsibilities effectively, not only must they be proficient in clinical practice but they must also be able to complete their assigned tasks related to the operations and objectives of the institution. Accomplishing these fundamental responsibilities is a very difficult assignment.

The Managerial Environment

Institutions that provide health care are unique and complex social organizations that generally function as bureaucracies. These institutions often afford a work environment that makes performing simultaneously as both a professional practitioner and an employee very difficult for the nurse manager. Bureaucracies, by definition, place the needs of individuals below the needs of the institution, a practice that frequently creates serious contradictions for professionals attempting to provide high-quality nursing care. In addition, the nurse frequently finds that he or she is required to serve and satisfy three different authority groups: administration, physicians, and patients. This trilevel authority situation contributes significantly to the challenges encountered by nurse managers as they function within the hospital framework. Because it is nurse managers who carry the responsibility of helping their staff work effectively in this environment, they must be advocates for both patients and staff, and must be able to convince the administration of the need for and value of individualized care.

Working within a bureaucracy is not always unpleasant, however. In fact, there are many advantages that help to offset the disadvantages. For example, employees frequently discover that the rules and policies established by a bureaucratic institution provide increased structure within the system and a greater sense of security. Although many employees find the rules and policies to be confining and restrictive, other employees derive a greater sense of authority and a feeling of impartiality and fairness from these same well-defined policies and rules. For the most part, the primary difference in how the rules and policies of a bureaucracy are interpreted by members of the staff lies in the attitudes held by the individual employees.

Nurse managers must be capable of demonstrating to the staff as well as the administration, both in fact and through example, that strict adherence to rules and policies is necessary and, at the same time, that flexibility can be exercised when the provision of high-quality nursing care demands it. Any flexible adjustment made to the rules should be clearly defined and carried out only when professional judgment indicates a need to alter a rule or policy for a specific patient or a specific circumstance to ensure the patient's recovery. It is both a logical and reasonable expectation that nurse managers assume the role of patient advocate in dealing with the hospital administration (remember that they also represent the administration to the staff and patients). They are the managers charged with direct patient care and, as such, their dual role as patient care advocate and administrator assists them in providing the best possible environment for the delivery of such care.

Most nurses begin assuming their administrative and management roles with very high ideals and personal goals. They may want to enhance the patient care provided within their units by structuring the environment, realigning the staff, providing continuing educational opportunities, or performing other activities that will result in an environment more conducive to patient recovery. However, it is quite common for nurses in administration to lose track of their initial goals and to begin to identify with the bureaucrats rather than with the care givers. This change of orientation occurs more frequently among senior administrators than it does among nurse managers, but it is still seen often enough in junior managers to be of concern. To avoid this "turn toward bureaucracy," nurse managers must maintain a commitment to nursing care and nurses, and must continue to see their role as that of an advocate for staff and patients. Only then will nurse managers become effective leaders of their nursing units.

The management and leadership skills necessary for this important and complex position are the primary topics in this text. Along with these topics, this chapter discusses other functions of management, some of which are less definitive:

- Determining the character of the nursing unit
- Ensuring that patient care is the major performance priority within the unit
- Establishing positive relationships with other levels of the nursing hierarchy

Other Management Functions

DETERMINING THE CHARACTER OF THE NURSING UNIT

Determining the character of the nursing unit is a somewhat obscure function but is probably the most important of the three just listed. The nurse manager establishes the beliefs and values of the unit and, through the staff, reflects them to the patients. How frequently are the differences among nursing staff groups noted? Even within the shift groups on the same unit a phenomenon such as this can be witnessed: one group is proficient but appears cold and aloof, seemingly unable or unwilling to deliver the service required to establish the proper relationship with patients and their families, whereas another appears courteous, professional, and nurturing. The cause of the difference in performance, both real and perceived, is the nurse manager. The expectations established by the first-level manager mold the attitudes and behaviors of the staff and set the tone of the unit.

Nurse managers also determine the quality of the relationship that exists between the unit nursing team and those with whom it has contact—both professionals and staff. If the unit leader interacts with physicians, housekeeping personnel, and the other hospital groups in a professional manner, the unit staff will as well. The opposite is also true; if the nurse manager does not relate to others in a professional and cooperative manner, the staff, even if they don't agree, will all too frequently emulate the actions of their leader.

The general atmosphere within the unit reflects another aspect of its character. A low-keyed unit in which the staff move from one task to another with a minimum of disturbance radiates a sense of competence and efficiency. This perception is far better than that evoked by a nurses' station at which a number of people are continually sitting around entertaining each other while patients or families wait for information or assistance. Even if the staff in this last situation are as competent or efficient as those in the first situation, they will not be perceived as such by the casual observer. Patients and families are normally under a great deal of stress, and they need to perceive professionalism in the staff to trust them enough to gain support and confidence from them.

ENSURING PATIENT CARE AS A PRIORITY

Nurse managers are responsible for ensuring that patient care is the fundamental priority of their units. This fact should be understood by all, but reality demands that this most fundamental of nursing responsibilities be continually reinforced to nursing staff. Each nurse must be constantly reminded that care is critical to the patient's recovery and that ensuring an environment in which the patient can receive proper care is the foremost reason the patient has been hospitalized. Medical care may be delivered in a variety of other settings without the presence of nursing care. In the hospital environment, however, excellent nursing care is obligatory. Nurse managers must keep this fact before their staffs and continually reinforce its importance. Nurses must be continually encouraged to take pride in the valuable contribution they are making to the welfare of the patient, and nurse managers provide much of that reinforcement as they recognize excellence, encourage improvement, and demand quality performance. If nurse managers allow their staffs to lose sight of the contribution they make, the morale of the entire unit can suffer.

ESTABLISHING RELATIONSHIPS

The third major function of the nurse manager is to establish a positive relationship with those at the other levels of the nursing hierarchy and the organizational team. A large segment of the organization's personnel look to the nursing staff for assistance and guidance, and those at the supervisory and senior management levels of nursing expect the unit staff to implement the overall objectives of the nursing division. Both sets of expectations are critical to the quality of work provided by the nursing staff of every unit. Once again, it is nurse managers who establish the relationship between their units and all other associated, supported, and supporting units within the organization. If nurse managers are able to work effectively with personnel at all levels, then their staffs will most likely be integrated into the organization in a similar professional and cohesive manner.

In this as well as in the other two major functions described previously, it is apparent that nurse managers are the pivotal performers within nursing units. There is absolutely no questioning the fact that the quality of patient care provided by every nursing unit is directly related to the quality of the leadership provided by the individual nurse manager.

ACCOUNTABILITY

Accountability is defined as being responsible for one's actions and accepting the consequences for one's behavior. Because the nursing profession's fundamental goal is to provide high-quality care to the patient, accountability within the profession means *acceptance of the obligation for providing excellent patient care and the willingness to accept the responsibility for the outcomes realized through the actions used to provide it*. The challenge for nurse managers becomes apparent when their decisions regarding what is best for the patient conflict with others' opinions, needs, and/or goals. In some cases, nursing has allowed the majority of patient care decisions to be made by others (i.e., physicians and administrators). However, the evolution of nurses' roles and changes in the nursing profession have encouraged many nurses to become more assertive in presenting their ideas, which increases their accountability.

Accountability can be considered in several contexts, as shown in Box 1-1. At the level of the individual performer, accountability is normally expressed through the ethical decision-making processes used and the individual's competence, commitment, and integrity. The American Nurses Association (ANA) has established a code for nurses and has presented it as a guide to help individual nurses make ethical decisions. At the institutional level, accountability is seen in the nursing department's mission, philosophy, and objectives, and through peer reviews conducted in association with patient audits. Professional account-

ability is based on standards of practice, such as those developed by the ANA.

Society affirms the accountability of its members by enacting legislation that does the following:
- Establishes rules and regulations for the protection of the rights, health, and safety of the individual
- Provides for an agency or group to monitor and enforce applicable rules and regulations
- Establishes a mechanism (usually access to a court of law) to protect members whose rights, health, or safety are infringed upon by other members of society

Following are a few examples of the protective legislation that affects the nursing profession:
- Civil rights legislation
- Laws regulating the practice of nursing
- Laws governing occupational safety and health
- Laws requiring and implementing state boards of nursing
- Legal precedents founded in court decisions involving medical negligence and/or malpractice

Society also protects its members by overseeing its allocation of resources (tax money) and by establishing requirements and standards that institutions and individuals must meet to qualify for certain types of allocations (funds, grants, etc.). It is usually the responsibility of accrediting agencies, such as the Joint Commission on Accreditation of Healthcare Organizations (JCAHO), to establish performance standards and to verify each institution's compliance with these standards. Healthcare organizations that are accredited by JCAHO do not have to obtain federal approval to receive government funds. Agencies that do not have JCAHO accreditation must meet the requirements of the U.S. Government's Centers for Medicare and Medicaid Services (formerly the Health Care Finance Administration) to receive medical payments from federal health insurance programs. Another method that society uses to maintain accountability in healthcare institutions is the stipulation of levels of reimbursement, such as the use of diagnosis-related groups (DRGs) as the basis for Medicare payments.

THE NURSE MANAGER AND PATIENTS

Nurse managers relate to and interact with patients both directly and indirectly. Although nurse managers may only occasionally give direct patient care, they have contact with patients while conducting rounds, reviewing patient records, receiving and preparing reports on patient status, and responding to questions and requests from staff, patients, and families. Nurse managers may want to feel as if they have moved away from patient care, but their jobs actually entail far greater responsibility for patients than they had as staff nurses. In fact, nurse managers have the opportunity to make a substantial contribution to the well-being of patients and staff by ensuring that quality care is an unconditional performance requirement in their units. This is a tremendous responsibility. An example of a job description for a nurse manager is provided in Fig. 1-1.

THE EDUCATION OF NURSE MANAGERS

Only in the recent past have healthcare professionals acknowledged the necessity for formal preparation of those assuming supervisory and management nursing roles in hospitals. In fact, only within the past two decades have nurse managers been expected to be qualified in terms of both education and experience sufficient to promote, develop, and maintain a professional environment that advances quality nursing practice and effectively manages the nursing resource. Today, many universities offer graduate majors in nursing administration. The American Association of Colleges of Nursing (AACN) and the American Organization of Nurse Executives (AONE) have issued a joint position statement on graduate education in nursing administration, shown in Box 1-2 (see p. 11).

RESEARCH AND NURSING MANAGEMENT

Research into nursing management is in its very early stages of growth. Those professionals who have an interest in this area are usually found practicing nursing administration. This situation has recently started to change dramatically as schools of nursing begin to supply a steady stream of graduates from masters and doctoral programs in nursing management.

Congressional legislation passed in 1985 led to the establishment of the National Center for Nursing Research (NCNR) within the National Institutes of Health, and since that day, nursing research has moved into the mainstream of scientific efforts in the United States. In 1993, the NCNR was elevated to the status of an institute and is now known as the National Institute of Nursing Research (NINR). The NINR's mission is to support clinical and basic research to establish a scientific basis for the care of individuals across the life span, including the following:

- Care of patients during illness and recovery
- Reduction of risk for disease and disability
- Promotion of healthy lifestyles
- Promotion of quality of life for those with chronic illnesses
- Care for individuals at the end of life

The fundamental goal of the NINR is to support the evolution of nursing research and training in several areas, including the following:

- Health promotion and disease prevention
- Acute and chronic illness
- Development of nursing systems for care delivery in institutions where nursing management research is being funded

The nurse manager's most important obligation with regard to nursing research is to critically evaluate management research findings with an eye toward their practical application. However, the following factors interfere with fulfillment of this responsibility:

Lack of qualifications: Many nurse managers practicing today still do not have the educational preparation necessary to evaluate research. Although their numbers are few, some are graduates of associate degree or diploma programs, which do not include research evaluation in the curriculum. Most graduates of baccalaureate programs have been given at least a fundamental appreciation of research and have been exposed to the process of research evaluation. However, the development of clinical skills remains the primary goal of these undergraduate programs, and it is highly unlikely that critical evaluation of

The Nurse Manager's Job Description

An Example of Responsibilities

Position Purpose: Serves as the official supervisor of an assigned division and functions to plan, direct, coordinate, implement, control, evaluate, and improve the quality of patient care delivered.

Specific Responsibilities

1. Interviews, selects, formally evaluates, and terminates assistant nurse manager/clinical nurses, registered professional nurses, licensed practical nurses, nurse assistants/technicians, and unit clerks in the division.

2. Establishes division *standards, goals, objectives, priorities,* and *facilities change* based on the needs of patients and their families, physicians, and staff and on the results and recommendations of various division audits. Generally plans and executes administrative programs within the framework of the total nursing service program and follows up with a written annual report on division activities and future plans.

3. Ensures competent, well-trained nursing personnel by identifying skill needs and subsequently recommending formal educational and developmental activities or personally instructing subordinates.

4. Directs or personally engages in patient/family teaching for optimal recovery and health.

5. Maintains timely documentation and anecdotal records on staff to be used in the preparation of performance appraisals.

6. Holds regularly scheduled staff meetings, which provide opportunities for discussion of division problems, orientation to new projects, procedures, changes in care approaches, etc.

7. Contributes to creating a work climate that encourages positive staff morale, motivation, and commitment through frequent contact with the staff (high visibility and accessibility); through the implementation of a leadership style appropriate to the demands of the situation; through consistent enforcement of division policy; through intensive evaluation of subordinates and provision for timely feedback; through interdepartmental and interpersonal mediation, troubleshooting, and problem solving; and through rendering expert service and role modeling.

8. Develops the role of assistant nurse manager according to division needs and arranges for the assistant to function effectively in the absence of the nurse manager.

9. Plans for future staffing, supply, and equipment requirements for maintaining or improving the quality of patient care and of the environment of the division. In conjunction with the unit manager, establishes supply standards and recommends capital expenditures.

10. Supervises the allocation of division resources, remaining accountable to an established budget.

11. Controls work time schedules for entire staff and makes scheduling adjustments when necessary.

12. Equitably delegates patient care/division maintenance assignments and authority according to perceived strengths and limitations of subordinates, maintaining accountability.

13. Directs the appropriate orientation of new staff into the division.

14. Acts as a clinical resource, rendering expert services, and is prepared to assist with direct patient care when needed.

15. Arranges educational in-service programs when the need and opportunity arise.

16. Creates an open and accurate line of communication—upward, downward, and laterally—with particular respect to confidentiality.

17. Initiates and/or delegates writing of patient care plans.

Fig. 1-1 ■ Sample job description for a nurse manager. (Data from Vancouver General Hospital, Vancouver, British Columbia.)

Continued

18. Establishes an effective working relationship with the medical staff, admissions, dietary, housekeeping, laboratory, radiology, respiratory therapy, and other service areas related to the specialty of the division. In particular, makes daily rounds of the patients and ensures that patients' medical plans and directives from the physicians are properly executed; surveys the environment and condition of each patient to ascertain the quality of every service being provided.

19. Expeditiously handles staff, physician, patient, and interdepartmental complaints and problems, providing accurate and timely follow-up.

20. Responds quickly and intervenes in crises or conflicts of any nature that occur in the division.

21. Remains responsible for the implementation of appropriate procedures in the event of emergencies, disasters, etc.

22. Coordinates interpersonal relations among nursing staff and physicians, department heads, and patients/families through problem identification and decision-making.

23. Attends to the various environmental cues suggestive of potential problems to quickly remedy them (e.g., monitors physician/staff relations and patient/family perceptions of care received, interprets subtle messages conveyed by informal leaders).

24. Enforces hospital and nursing service policy and procedure.

25. Counsels and provides remedial action for staff infraction of established professional guidelines.

26. Supervises the documentation of pertinent and current patient information.

27. Ensures that incident reports are prepared on unusual circumstances or events that occur.

28. Ensures that contact is made with visiting nurses or social workers concerning posthospital patient care.

29. Reviews and responds to division mail and telephone calls/messages of varied nature.

30. Evidences involvement in the institution and its policies by providing service on committees that recommend policies, procedures, and standards of patient care delivery, such as the total head nurse group, the policy and procedures committee, the nursing audit committee, and ad hoc committees as appointed.

Fig. 1-1—cont'd ■ Sample job description for a nurse manager.

nursing research is a major focus in these basic courses of instruction. It is at the master's program level that the nursing professional is provided with a fundamental working knowledge of the research process and with the skills necessary to evaluate the importance of research results. Today, however, many institutions still do not require that nurse managers have a master's degree. Yet this, too, is changing, especially in larger institutions and those located near universities that have masters-level nursing programs.

Lack of proper mindset: To contribute effectively to research activities, nurse managers must adopt an inquisitive frame of mind—a perspective not always compatible with the fast-paced decision-making environments typical of institutional nurse management. Such a frame of mind involves questioning the status quo and considering whether changes would improve the outcome of any given situation; once again, these are skills that are not normally found in the nursing manager intent on compliance.

Failure to appreciate the value of research: Many nurse managers still do not recognize the value of research to their practice. However, in today's cost-conscious environment, critical assessment of the data produced by research is an essential part of nursing management. Research that addresses how the profession can provide quality services to patients in the most efficient manner must be evaluated, replicated to validate findings, and applied appropriately. The research evaluation process is not examined in this textbook, but many nursing research texts are available.

SUMMARY

■ Nurse managers simultaneously function as subordinates, superiors, and customer service representatives.

■ Productivity is a conclusive measure of the amount of work performed and the quality of the work accomplished, with the effective use of available resources considered a key factor.

BOX 1-2

Graduate Education: A Joint Statement

The American Association of Colleges of Nursing (AACN) and the American Organization of Nurse Executives (AONE) believe that graduate education in nursing administration must be comprehensive, relevant, appropriate, and responsive to present and future healthcare environments and nursing practice settings. The AACN and AONE believe that the nurse executive is responsible for leadership and management of the nursing organization, is accountable for the clinical practice of nursing, and functions as a member of the executive management team. The nurse executive is expected to facilitate effective, efficient patient care.

Educational preparation for nursing administration should take place in university schools of nursing offering specialized graduate programs in nursing administration. These programs should incorporate those academic disciplines essential to the practice of organizational management. This preparation integrates concepts from the disciplines of nursing, business, and management, which results in a unique and specialized configuration of knowledge. This knowledge provides the theoretical foundation for nursing administrative practice. The synthesis and application of this knowledge are essential to the development of nurse executive leadership for professional nursing practice.

Data from American Association of Colleges of Nursing/ American Association of Nurse Executives: *Joint position statement on education for nurses in administrative roles,* Washington, DC, 1997, AACN/AONE.

- Managing change and managing the transitions that take place during the process of change are also issues that are becoming increasingly important to nurse managers and the nursing profession as a whole.
- The major changes, and an almost countless array of others occurring at a rapid rate in today's healthcare industry, ensure an ever-changing environment for nurse managers, their staff, and patients.
- The evolving nursing profession and professional environment, along with the inevitably increasing emphasis that will be placed on improved and increased productivity, requires that education in ethical decision-making be a fundamental part of the training of the next generation of nursing professionals.

- The nursing profession no longer provides the safe working environment that historically has been its hallmark. This is especially true for those nurses desiring to become nurse managers.
- Ever since humans began banding together to accomplish goals that could not be achieved by any one person, the skills of effective management have been essential to ensure coordination of individual efforts.
- Nurse managers have the dual responsibilities of representing the institution to the patient and the patient to the institution.
- The general atmosphere within the unit reflects another aspect of its character.
- Nurse managers are responsible for ensuring that patient care is the fundamental priority of their units.
- *Accountability* is defined as being responsible for one's actions and accepting the consequences for one's behavior. Because the nursing profession's fundamental goal is to provide high-quality care to the patient, accountability within the profession means *acceptance of the obligation for providing excellent patient care and the willingness to accept the responsibility for the outcomes realized through the actions used to provide it.*
- Difficulty often occurs when a nurse manager's beliefs about what is best for the patient conflict with the beliefs of another (physician, administrator).
- Only in the recent past have healthcare professionals acknowledged the necessity for formal preparation of those assuming supervisory and management nursing roles in hospitals.

FINAL THOUGHTS

The position of nurse manager is varied and demanding and includes the dual roles of being both a leader and a follower. To fulfill these roles effectively, the new nurse manager must possess the following:

1. A belief that every person on the staff has a responsibility to share in addressing and developing solutions for the challenges that occur in the workplace
2. A management philosophy that places the needs of others ahead of his or her own
3. A commitment to patient-focused, quality care outcomes that have customer satisfaction as a primary concern
4. A desire to continually strive to advance his or her abilities by keeping pace with healthcare changes and their effects on role and function

5. A commitment to lifelong learning
6. A belief that others' trust, and trust in others, are fundamental to leadership
7. An understanding that being a manager is a responsibility, not a position, and that doing the job requires dedication, hard work, and an unswerving belief in the value of others

THE NURSE MANAGER SPEAKS

Nurse managers should evaluate the following factors in making their decisions regarding nursing coverage:

Acuity level of the patient's condition: If the patient's condition is unstable, a transfer can be made to the surgical intensive care unit; if the patient's condition is stable, he or she should be kept in the postanesthesia care unit. A major consideration is the patient who has had a craniotomy, whose condition may be stable by observation but then may suddenly deteriorate rapidly.

Competency of staff: Can one or two registered nurses manage the patients, or is an unlicensed assistant needed? Cultural differences among the staff should remain a subconscious concern.

Availability of staff: Who is available to assist in case of an emergency? a physician? a nursing supervisor?

Safety: This is not negotiable! This challenge will not be resolved without clinical thinking.

Management Fundamentals for the Healthcare Industry

OUTLINE

LEARNING SYNOPSIS

Upon successful completion of this chapter, readers will possess a fundamental understanding of how the nurse manager must operate in the most common circumstances found in nursing, including an understanding of the organizational and environmental characteristics and constraints posed by the working environment and the typical types of organizational structure in the institutions where nursing management takes place.

OBJECTIVES

1. Identify the characteristics and major elements of basic organizational theory
2. Identify the key functions, challenges, and products of a modern healthcare organization
3. Describe the basic features of each of the four schools of organizational theory presented
4. Identify the components of the major types of organizational structure used in the healthcare industry today
5. Describe the different types of organizational structure seen in nursing departments
6. Identify methods that can be used to accurately define organizational effectiveness in the nursing profession and the healthcare industry

The vast majority of the world's population live in an organizational society, spending most of their time and productive energies working toward the satisfaction of established goals and objectives. This style of life is both sensible and economical, for it has been proven that a properly organized and coordinated joint effort can develop more knowledge and information, create more technology, and produce more goods, services, opportunities, and security than all individual efforts combined.

To generate exceptional capability and production, however, an organization must rely on individual behavior that is consistent with its objectives. This means that an individual working within the organization must perform in prescribed ways, relinquishing a portion of individual freedom and autonomy. For many people, the loss of personal freedom is no small sacrifice and is continually weighed against the economic and personal benefits received in exchange for their services. By itself, financial remuneration rarely provides adequate or long-term motivation for the sacrifice of one's autonomy. Therefore, the working environment and the relationship that exists between organizations and the people who labor in them must receive constant attention. The person normally assigned the responsibility for this mediating role is the front-line manager, and the activity performed is referred to as *supervision.*

This chapter deals with the responsibilities of a unique type of administrator—the nurse manager—and the contributions he or she can make to the development and delivery of quality health services within the medical profession. The manager's functions are indispensable, complicated, often arduous, and always challenging. Performance of these functions requires sensitivity as well as the ability to effectively balance the needs of the healthcare organization, patients, physicians, subordinates, and self. The professional nurse manager must possess knowledge and skills different from those required for nursing practice, yet few nurses have been adequately prepared through their education or training to assume managerial duties or to function in a supervisory position. It is most often the case that these professional practitioners must depend on what they have learned from their experiences with former supervisors who themselves learned supervisory techniques "in the trenches." The only other alternative is to believe that the necessary skills are acquired through some sort of personal instinct or common sense reasoning, a prospect that can leave the individual with significant apprehension. This chapter is designed to provide a formal background in the theory, processes, and requirements relevant to the professional nurse manager. Successful comple-

tion of this chapter will provide the management-bound nurse practitioner with a formal educational foundation that can be used to develop managerial potential.

The points to be discussed here must be considered in light of the realities of the environment in which nursing management takes place. Therefore, the role of nurse manager is discussed in terms of the most common circumstances encountered in nursing. Organizational and environmental characteristics and constraints are evaluated under conditions as close as possible to those under which the nurse manager works. To provide a comprehensive understanding of the nature of nursing management, this chapter also examines the typical structure of the medical institution in which nursing is practiced and the environments in which the nurse manager and the institution must perform.

BASIC ORGANIZATIONAL THEORY

An organization is an assortment of individuals working together under an established hierarchy of authority, and with an appropriate division of labor, to satisfy a preestablished goal. Such a situation implies the existence of management. The individual activities of people rarely become effective or coordinated by themselves. Within an organization, coordination and effectiveness are the result of the effective management of individual efforts.

Many types and styles of organization can be identified, based on output, size, ownership, composition, and/or purpose. The definition of an organization provided earlier included a division of labor and a hierarchy of authority, which are subcomponents of every organizational structure.[1] To examine the structure of a healthcare organization, one must characterize it along the following three dimensions:

1. *Complexity:* the intricacies involved in the technical aspects of the nursing profession, the normal division of labor and responsibilities within the healthcare institution, the distinct lines drawn between the different levels of the organizational hierarchy, and the geographical dispersion of organizational units
2. *Formalization:* the degree to which the organization relies on rules and procedures to direct its members' behavior; formalization is independent of size
3. *Centralization:* the location of decision-making authority

Organizational theory is the study of structure within an institution or establishment. All science has as its goal the comprehension, prediction, and/or direction of an event or process; thus, organizational theory seeks to develop a thorough understanding of structure so that organizations can be planned in such a way that maximal predictability and control is built into the design—or, more simply, so that organizations can be designed in such a way that they facilitate the achievement of goals.

The prevailing method used by modern organizational theorists to analyze business is the "systems perspective." This approach is nothing more than identification of a set of interrelated parts arranged in a unified whole.[1] All manner of things are, or are composed of, "systems." For example, societies, computers, human bodies—and, yes, even hospitals—are systems. Systems can be either open or closed. By definition, a closed system is always self-contained, and such systems can most frequently be found in the physical and mechanical worlds. The study of closed systems has little applicability to the analysis of organizations, which are considered to be open systems (Fig. 2-1). This categorization is based the fact that an open system must interact with its environment, a situation that truly characterizes a healthcare facility. Researchers have identified the following 10 fundamental elements common to all open systems.[2] A comprehensive understanding of these characteristics will assist in developing a conceptual understanding of how organizations operate.

1. *Input, or importation of energy:* Open systems receive a variety of different types of energy from the environments in which they operate. In a manner not entirely unlike the way the human cell receives oxygen and nourishment from the blood stream (its environment), an organization receives capital, human resources, materials, and energy (e.g., electricity) from its environment.

2. *Throughput:* Open systems transform the energy and materials available to them into usable materials required to satisfy their function. Just as the human cell transforms nourishment into structure, an organization creates a new product, processes materials, trains people, or provides a service by transforming capital, resources, materials, and energy into its product or service.

3. *Output:* As a result of its performance, an open system delivers some type of product (e.g., a manufactured substance, an inquiring mind, or a well body) back into the environment from which it receives its capital, resources, materials, and energy.

4. *System of cyclic events:* An organization functions through an integrated system of cyclic events. Organizational activities occur over and over again in a self-closing cycle, as the resources received from the environment (input) pass through the various functions of the organization (throughput) and are transformed into product (output).

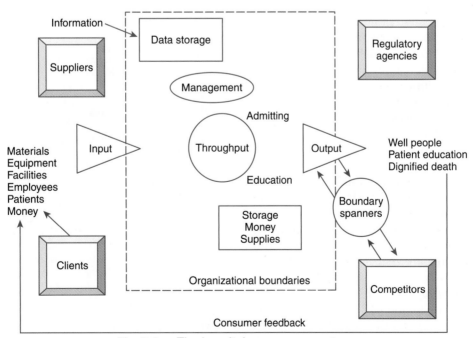

Fig. 2-1 ■ The hospital as an open system.

5. *Negative* **entropy**: An effective and smoothly operating system keeps some of its input material in a "ready reserve" so that it will be available for future use. For example, the human body stores fat that it can supply to generate operating energy when no fresh fuel (food) is available. An organization operates in a similar manner by placing part of its resources in reserve (money in the bank) or employing extra personnel for availability in times of need. This process reduces the possibility of degradation of the organization's effectiveness and the degree of uncertainty within the system during normal operation.

6. *Information input:* Information input is the feedback and coding process. Every organization must be able to receive new information and feedback from the environment, encode it, and then store it so it can be used at appropriate times to predict changes in the environment. This process enables the organization to plan for a large variety of influences and for the effects of change that would, if left unchecked, create chaos within the organization.

7. *Steady state:* Sometimes referred to as **homeostasis**, *steady state* refers to the maintenance of a relatively stable relationship between the input it receives and the output it produces, or its "energy exchange." Just as the human body is predisposed to stay in a steady state (barring negative outside influences), resisting significant change in its proportions and mass over time, so does an organization attempt to stay in a steady state by predicting changes in the environment and regulating its input as information about output (market analysis) is generated. The fundamental principle in maintaining a steady state is preserving the character of the organization.

8. **Differentiation**: Organizational elements tend to develop into specialized subsystems based on specialized tasks; for example, in humans, multiple processes cause apparently indifferent (undifferentiated) cells, tissues, and structures to attain their mature form and function. This growth and metamorphosis is widespread throughout the typical organization as different subsystems evolve into complex and intricate operations. Examples of differentiation within an organization are mechanization and computerization.

9. *Integration and coordination:* The two different processes of integration and coordination combine to form the ninth characteristic of an organization. As differentiation moves forward, processes that bring the system together counter it. Management is the integration-coordination subsystem that operates within an organization, just as the cerebral cortex is the integration-coordination subsystem within the human body. Management's function is to facilitate growth and harmonious coordination within the organization; in other words, it is supposed to ensure that the organization operates smoothly, efficiently, and economically.

10. **Equifinality**: There is real truth in the statement that any established goal can be achieved using a variety of means. This principle was first introduced formally by S. P. Robbins in his 1983 work, *Organizational Theory*.[1] What it means is that, as an open system operates and develops within its environment, it establishes different goals at different times and chooses different methods to achieve them. The open system does this to attain its ultimate goal, which is survival. The adaptability of humans for survival, for instance, represents a form of equifinality. Organizations behave in much the same manner. For example, when the National Foundation for Infantile Paralysis realized its original goal, it found another cause to champion so that it could survive as an organization.

Nursing can be considered as a product line if the open systems perspective of Katz and Kahn[2] is adopted. This approach has recently found strong advocates within the nursing profession.[3,4] Originally, Procter and Gamble developed product-line manage-

---

Entropy is a measure of the degree of disorder or uncertainty in a system. Negative entropy is the ability of a system to maintain certainty and order in its operation.

Homeostasis is a relatively stable state of equilibrium or a tendency toward such a state between the different but interdependent elements or groups of elements in an organism, population, organization, or group. (Source: *Merriam-Webster Online Dictionary*.)

Differentiation is the development from the one to the many, the simple to the complex, or the homogeneous to the heterogeneous. (Source: *Merriam-Webster's Collegiate Dictionary* as shown on QuickClick, a service of NBCi.com.)

Equifinality is not listed in the dictionary but is a concept identified and labeled in the book *Organizational Theory* by S. P. Robbins (Upper Saddle River, NJ, 1983, Prentice Hall). This book is a major source of information for this chapter. The term is used here to mean the principle that any final goal or end can be reached by a variety of means.

ment as a business technique in the late 1920s. The technique evolved from the decision to allow production and marketing decisions to be made at the lowest possible level to maximize efficiency and profits (decentralization). In this process, the one person who is closest to the product is given authority over it and is referred to as the product-line manager (PLM). The PLM can respond far more quickly to the changing environmental pressures or shifts in the marketplace that affect a single product than can a senior executive or director of the company. Because of this ability to respond immediately, the PLM is given the responsibility for all forecasting, planning, production, and marketing for his or her specific product. Viewed from an open systems perspective, the PLM is responsible for all of the functions (input, throughput, and output) that are related to his or her specific product.

In contrast to the PLM are the specialists and specialized departments, each of which is given the responsibility for a single function (input, throughput, or output) for all products. When this analysis is applied to the nursing profession, the breakdown is as follows: (1) As individuals, nurses, records staff, physicians, and purchasing staff are responsible for their respective *inputs*. (2) Individual nursing sections, dietetics, and other specialty departments are responsible for *throughput*. (3) Nursing as a total entity within the organization and the department of education and training are responsible for *output*.

Traditionally, healthcare organizations have neither defined their product nor managed it in a product-line manner. From a marketing perspective, a product exists solely to satisfy a customer need. Time and money savings, convenience, enhancement of life, improved appearance, ego, and vanity are customer needs that businesses produce products to satisfy. The "products" of healthcare organizations are improved health, a better quality of life, enhanced awareness (health education), and wellness. These products are not always easily defined or packaged, a fact that creates a major dilemma for healthcare organizations. But a healthcare product can be identified, and input, throughput, and output for that product can be managed. The major question is, Will nursing manage one or more of these products by itself or allow others to do this for nursing? There is no question as to whether product-line management will become part and parcel of the nursing profession. It will, and that is a fact. Why? Because product-line management makes good business sense, especially during tight economic times. Whether or not this prospect is fashionable, or even palatable, is not the question. The reality is that nursing, as a profession, is a business, responsible to the organization for the efficient, profitable, and quality operation of its area of responsibility.

A business must have an accurate method of accounting for both the revenue it consumes (input) and the revenue it generates (output) during the production of a product so that it can determine the efficiency of production (throughput). At its most fundamental and most complex levels, nursing is a production process. Because this is so, it is possible for the healthcare organization to determine profit or loss and relate it to its "product line." Traditionally, health care has been able freely to pass on its costs directly to the customer in the form of increased charges. This process of cost-plus billing was changed dramatically, however, by the federal government's introduction of the prospective payment system, which uses diagnosis-related groups (DRGs) to determine payments for health care, and by the corresponding responses by cost-conscious insurers that it generated. The federal government (which pays almost 40% of U.S. healthcare costs) and the business community (which pays another 30%) have grown resistant to the seemingly continual and dramatic escalation of healthcare costs. Consequently, the healthcare industry is facing a critical and life-threatening challenge for the first time, and to meet it, the industry must develop a means to determine costs and generate revenue that can be linked to the specific products and services it provides.

The result of these changes is that product-line management will receive increased attention from the nursing profession, largely because nursing is a major expense focus for every healthcare organization and its line of products. The fact that the industry has failed to adequately define these products will also change, because marketing departments are becoming a viable part of the effective and cost-conscious healthcare organization. A business (and health care is most assuredly a business) cannot market effectively without first identifying its customers' needs and then defining a product that will satisfy those needs.

Another reality of the business world that is invading the hallowed halls of the medical profession is that the price of a product and the quality of that product are directly affected by the department that produces it—in this case, the nursing department. Power and influence can be gained from this fact; however, far more important to remember is that it also implies a tremendous responsibility on the part of nursing for the survival of the institution. Thus, the efficiency of throughput, T_E (largely accomplished by nursing, but also by medical and other staff), is related to the quality of output, O_Q, which to a large extent determines critical inputs, I_C; or, put mathematically, $I_C = T_E + O_Q$. To restate in laymen's terms, the amount of money that is available to pay salaries and provide facilities (I_C) is directly proportional to the efficiency (T_E) and quality (O_Q) of the nursing department and the rest of the healthcare organization.

! CRITICAL POINT

The price of a product and the quality of that product are directly affected by the department that produces it. Although it is true that power and influence can be gained from this fact, it is far more important to remember is that a tremendous responsibility for the viability and survival of the institution comes along with it.

As a final point in this analysis, let us take a moment to investigate the possible products of the nursing profession, as follows:

Education: Training professional staff and enhancing awareness for patients and their families. This is an area that has traditionally enjoyed significant attention.

Wellness: Improving the health conditions of potential patients and the general population. This is another area that has been easy for the healthcare industry to identify and emphasize.

Health care: This is an obvious product and now can be organized by DRG—467 product lines.

Industrial wellness: Helping employers keep their employees healthy through the reduction of industrial hazards.

Physical fitness: Helping people stay in excellent physical condition through the use of exercise, diet, and supervision.

Health education: Making the population aware of potential health problems and assisting in the development of programs and information that will help individuals avoid illness.

In the future, each healthcare organization will become more efficient in the management of one or several specific product lines than in the management of others, and each will begin to specialize in its efficient product lines to maximize input (profit). The nursing profession's largest role in the throughput of a product line is in the management of production. Overall, the value of adopting an open systems perspective and developing high-quality product-line management in accordance with its principles will not be realized through the introduction of new products. The value will come from understanding that nurse managers direct an expense center which exercises great control over the throughput of its product line(s). If one follows this last thought through, it is easy to see how nurse managers can significantly influence the potential of the organizations to which they belong.

HEALTHCARE SERVICE ORGANIZATIONS

Healthcare service organizations turn product-line inputs (resources) such as money, people, supplies, and technology into healthcare services. These organizations produce as outputs the improved physical, mental, or emotional health of their patients. This transformation can occur only when there are sufficient amounts of inputs to allow the process to take place. Therefore, anything that affects inputs is a real concern for those responsible for the overall health and well-being of the institution.

Consider for just a moment the tremendous influence physicians have on a healthcare facility's existence. Because they control to a significant extent the number of patients who are admitted to a hospital (input) and the length of time each stays (flow-through), physicians are responsible for controlling the input of money necessary to operate the facility. Physicians, being intelligent individuals, are very much aware of their importance to the organization, and as a result of their input, the organization is sensitive to physicians' wants, needs, and expectations.

Physicians, however, are by no means the only ones who influence the purpose and operation of a healthcare institution. For example, hospital social workers, as well as the patient and the patient's family, exercise influence over the selection of the long-term care facility to which a patient is discharged. As another example, personnel in parallel social service agencies may influence the selection of a specific community health center.

Changes in patient flow to any institution can, in turn, affect the funding decisions made by governmental and other agencies granting financial support, such as organized charities (United Way, Red Cross, and/or private benefactors).

Insurance companies or governmental agencies (Medicare) acting as third-party payment authorities can also change the mission of an organization by manipulating the payments for certain covered services. In fact, the federal government did precisely that when it enacted Public Law 98-21, which called for the use of DRGs to facilitate the payment of Medicare benefits through a system based on anticipated performance rather than through the system based on reimbursement for past performance that had been used previously by the Medicare program. But this is only one of the many influences having a dramatic effect on the operation of healthcare facilities. The following are some others:

Availability of qualified nurses: The current, and increasingly critical, shortage of professional nurses has forced hospitals to adopt drastic measures, such as closing units, mandating overtime, or risking patient care with low staff-to-patient ratio. Adding to the serious situation is the problem of increasing patient use of hospital facilities.

Competition: Competition has become the reality in healthcare delivery systems. Advertising freestanding clinics and health services is but one of the ways organizations are attempting to capture the healthcare market. The implications of competition are much debated, but there seems little doubt that the extraordinary changes taking place in the healthcare field will result in the demise of many institutions.

Marketing: Marketing is a challenge that only recently has been addressed by the healthcare industry. Today, healthcare institutions are realizing that, to be perceived properly, they must continually inform their communities about their capabilities (i.e., market their skills).

The healthcare facilities that succeed in filling their beds to, or near to, capacity are quite likely to put others out of business. Competition creates two distinct sets of performers—winners and losers—and the fact is that many more businesses fail than succeed. The healthcare industry can no longer avoid this reality. To meet the challenge of increased and more capable competition, healthcare facilities are now aggressively developing new marketing strategies. These strategies will have a very definite impact on the purpose of the institutions, because organizations, like their human memberships, will fight hard to survive. To successfully achieve this goal, healthcare institutions must continually adapt themselves to a constantly changing environment. Many institutions are beginning to realize the importance of the relationships between the organization and its environment in defining the organization's purpose.

In summary, an organization's purpose is the product of the environment(s) in which it functions, and in the long run, it is society as a whole that creates that environment. It has been suggested that certain discernible people and groups within society determine or shape an organization's purpose and influence its structure and operations.[5] These people and groups have been termed the *task environment* and include the following four elements or clusters (see Fig. 2-1):

1. *Clients:* people who use the services of the organization
2. *Suppliers:* those who provide essential labor, capital, supplies, equipment, and property
3. *Competitors:* those who compete against the organization for patients and/or supplies
4. *Regulatory agencies:* federal governmental agencies, standard-setting professional organizations, collective bargaining units, and all others who might act to restructure or restrain the operation of the organization

The relationship between the healthcare organization and its task environment becomes one of exchange, with one area earning resources that it may export to acquire the needed inputs from other areas. The greater the need of one organization for the exports of another, the greater the control, assuming that the entity has the ability to produce at the desired level.

Within the inner core of the organization are the central activities or functions of the health service institution as supplied by those people who actually deliver the health care. This core, which depends totally on a steady and predictable stream of inputs from the task environment, operates most effectively and efficiently when it is sheltered from the disturbances and uncertainties of the task environment. In other words, the central activities of the health service organization must somehow be buffered from the uncertainty and instability of the environment in which they occur.

In the optimal environment, patients come to the healthcare facility in a steady and predictable stream to receive delivery of hands-on care, and the resources required to deliver these services in a high-quality manner are always available in bountiful supply. In what has been called *boundary spanning,*[5] external influences serve to safeguard the central activities (technical core) of the organization from the inconsistencies of the business environment. Boundary spanners within a healthcare facility include personnel in purchasing or medical records departments, those responsible for liaison with the Joint Commission on Accreditation of Healthcare Organizations, and nurse managers, all of whom cushion the direct care providers from the business environment and ensure to the greatest degree possible the availability of inputs (patients, money, other resources).

The closer an individual works to the actual level at which care is rendered, the more focused the individual performer's role becomes and the more specific the information that is used. Conversely, the farther away an individual is from the actual delivery of the services being provided (the higher up the hierarchy) the more broadly scoped the role and the wider the breadth of information needed. For this reason, many people working at the point of delivery feel that their senior management is "out of touch" or "disinterested." That is seldom the case, however. The truth is that the effective coordination and control of the process of patient care, the accurate anticipation and prediction of problems, and the provision of necessary supplies that must occur at the top of the hierarchical ladder are dependent on the information supplied by the people working at the bottom or front-line service delivery points. The challenges to effective management are (1) for senior managers to remember what it was like working on the front line, (2) for managers to find time to spend down on the front line keeping themselves acquainted with the difficulties being faced, and (3) for people working at the point of delivery to remember that they may be seeing only a small portion of the total picture.

THEORIES OF ORGANIZATION

The ancient Sumerians recorded the earliest example of systematic organizational thinking around 5000 BC. The topic was also part of the thinking of the exceptional early civilizations of the Egyptians, Babylonians, Greeks, and Romans. After the fall of the Roman Empire, however, organizational theory remained almost totally forgotten until the Industrial Revolution of the early 1800s. There were exceptions to this, of course: the process was examined by a number of Renaissance thinkers, such as Machiavelli in the 1500s. Adam Smith, who described the management principles we know today as specialization and the division of labor, could also be considered an exception, as his work was extremely early in the Industrial Revolution, when it was still largely confined to Britain.[6]

The theory of organization received a boost when the Industrial Revolution spread in earnest in the late 1800s and early 1900s. The demand for labor created by new industry caused many people to start to think creatively about how to organize new companies to optimize efficiency, streamline costs, and divide the responsibilities of labor. The results of this early work are apparent today in a number of different schools of thought regarding the design and management of organizations. These different approaches are commonly identified as the classic, neoclassic, technologic, and modern systems theories.

Classic Theory

The traditional approach to organizational theory, sometimes referred to as *classical theory,* centers almost exclusively on the formal structure of an organization. The primary focus is on achieving efficiency through design. In this theory, the workforce is seen as operating at its highest productivity when it is working within a rational and explicit task and organizational design. Therefore, this theory believes that the best method to follow when designing an organization is to subdivide work, specify the tasks to be done, and then

place people into the plan. Classic theory focuses on the following four elements:
1. Division and specialization of labor
2. Hierarchy of authority or chain of command
3. Structure or organization
4. Extent or span of control

Several theorists have contributed to the development of classic organizational theory. In 1911, Frederick Taylor wrote *The Principles of Scientific Management.*[7] This work formed the early foundation of management theory. In it, Taylor described the following four fundamental principles of scientific management he believed would maximize individual productivity[8]:
1. *Develop the "science" of every job* by studying the motions required to perform the job, standardizing the necessary actions (work), and improving the conditions in which the work is accomplished.
2. *Select workers carefully* by matching people who possess the proper skills with the correct job.
3. *Train and motivate* the workers to perform the job carefully and thoroughly and then offer them incentives to produce.
4. *Provide visible support* to the workers by planning their work and by removing obstacles that limit their performance.

Frank Gilbreth and Lillian Moller Gilbreth[9] added the scientific management approach to the classic theory by suggesting that time and motion study (the science of reducing a job to its basic physical motions) be included in the process. When this addition is used, wasted movement in the performance process is eliminated and new incentives are created based on the newly designed job. Much of such scientific management forms the basis for the job simplification, work standards establishment, and incentive wage plans in use today.

In 1916, Henri Fayol wrote the book *Administration Industrielle et Générale,*[10] in which he proposed the following five rules of management:
1. *Foresight:* Plan for the future, specify goals.
2. *Organization:* Provide resources for the plan.
3. *Command:* Select and lead people in implementing the plan.
4. *Coordination:* Ensure that all employees' efforts fit together to achieve the goal.
5. *Control:* Verify progress toward the goal.

These rules form the basis for the classic management functions: planning, organizing, controlling, and decision-making. Fayol also specified 14 principles of management (Table 2-1), which he advocated be used to implement his five rules of management. These rules and principles are discussed at length in another section of this text.

TABLE 2-1

Fayol's General Principles of Management

Principle	*Description*
1. Division of work	The object of division of work is to produce more and better work with the same level of effort. It is accomplished through reduction in the number of tasks to which attention and effort must be directed.
2. Authority and responsibility	Authority is the right to give orders, and responsibility is its essential counterpart. Whenever authority is exercised, responsibility arises.
3. Discipline	Discipline implies obedience and respect for the agreements between the firm and its employees. Establishment of these agreements binding a firm and its employees, from which disciplinary formalities emanate, should remain one of the chief preoccupations of industrial heads. Discipline also involves sanctions judiciously applied.
4. Unity of command	An employee should receive orders from one superior only.
5. Unity of direction	Each group of activities having one objective should be unified by having one plan and one head.
6. Subordination of individual interest to general interest	The interests of one employee or group of employees should not prevail over that of the company or broader organization.
7. Remuneration of personnel	If the loyalty and support of workers is to be maintained, they must receive a fair wage for services rendered.
8. Centralization	Like division of work, centralization belongs to the natural order of things. However, the appropriate degree of centralization will vary with the particular concern, so it becomes a question of the proper proportion. The problem is to find the measure that will give the best overall yield.
9. Scalar chain	The scalar chain is the chain of superiors ranging from the ultimate authority to the lowest ranks. It is an error to depart needlessly from the line of authority, but it is an even greater one to keep to it to the detriment of the business.
10. Order	A place for everything and everything in its place.
11. Equity	Equity is a combination of kindliness and justice.
12. Stability of tenure of personnel	High turnover increases inefficiency. A mediocre manager who stays is infinitely preferable to an outstanding manager who comes and goes.
13. Initiative	Initiative involves thinking out a plan and ensuring its success. This gives zeal and energy to an organization.
14. Esprit de corps	Union is strength, and it comes from the harmony among the personnel.

Data from Fayol H: *General and industrial administration*, New York, 1949, Pitman, pp 20-21.

The classic approach was further augmented by Max Weber,[11] who used the term *bureaucracy* to designate the ideal, intentionally rational, most efficient form of organization (today, this word has come to suggest long waits, inefficiency, waste, etc.). Many of Weber's recommendations for developing the most rational, fair, and efficient organization parallel the ideas of Fayol and his contemporaries.

Although the work of the scientific management theorists has formed the core of the classic theory, the theory itself is widely criticized today. This criticism is based on the fact that, unless factors such as technology, labor pool, and organizational climate and environment are considered, there is no one best way to design an organization. Some critics suggest that

many of the classic prescriptions offered as cures are not as explicit as they seem.[12] For example, one might ask how far specialization should proceed. If specialization is carried to the extreme, it becomes a ridiculous process—the entire workforce will be made up of extremely apathetic workers, each of whom performs a single routine, mundane, and repetitive 1-minute task. Logic dictates that specialization should be taken only as far as human judgment deems appropriate and should be stopped before the application of this "objective" principle turns out to be highly subjective. Failure to fully define such concepts as specialization is not, however, the only criticism that has been directed at the classic approach. Many more critics are concerned with such major flaws as (1) the lack of similarity between the formal or planned organization or task and the actual organization, (2) the dehumanization of the worker, and (3) the inflexibility of operation that it implies.

Neoclassic Theory

The widespread criticism of and dissatisfaction with classic theory led to the development of *neoclassic theory*. Neoclassic theory accepts the basic structures of classic theory as explicated but modifies them by considering the effective use of people. This approach was widely adopted by the human relations movement of the 1930s and today has come to be identified with that movement. A major assumption of this type of organizational thinking is that people seek social relationships, act and react to group pressures, and pursue personal gratification. An early advocate of study of the social aspects of organizations and the originator of the theory regarding coordination of effort through participative management was Mary Parker Follett. In fact, she actually proposed her theory long before the beginnings of the human relations movement.[13]

The Western Electric Company, between 1924 and 1932, initiated a succession of studies at its Hawthorne plant in Chicago. The *Hawthorne studies,* as they came to be known, were originally intended to evaluate the principles of scientific management. The first study analyzed the effects of lighting on productivity.[14] The results of the study were inconclusive because productivity throughout the groups varied randomly, including in one group in which production increased when the lights were turned down. The researchers, seeking an explanation for what they viewed as inconsistent behavior, concluded that unexpected "psychologic factors" were responsible. Further studies were conducted to examine the effects of physical working conditions and factors such as the length and frequency of rest breaks and the length of the basic work week.[14] Again, no relationship was found between these isolated factors and productivity. The researchers concluded that the social setting created by the research itself accounted for the variation in productivity that had been witnessed. The researchers believed that the workers may have felt special because of the attention given to them as part of the research and that the workers may have simply worked harder. These studies led to identification of what is known today as the *Hawthorne effect,* or the tendency for individuals to perform better than expected when special attention is provided. The Hawthorne tests also prompted organizational theorists to focus more on the social aspects of work and organizational design.

In 1938, Chester Barnard wrote *The Functions of the Executive,*[15] in which he maintained that it was extremely difficult to compel or even to provide incentives for individuals to perform any task that they considered unreasonable. He also argued that formal authority could not work without willing participants. The Hawthorne studies and the human relations movement also influenced later theorists such as Abraham Maslow and Douglas McGregor. These researchers proposed motivational theories to explain the link between organizational design and productivity. This text discusses the work and conclusions of these theorists in later chapters.

The neoclassic theorists shared a desire to humanize classic organizational theory without totally rejecting its ideas regarding structural design. Each of these theorists acknowledged the necessity for designing a rational organizational structure but believed that this could, or at least should, be accomplished through a process involving cooperation, participation, and motivation of the individual employee. In a manner of speaking, these researchers closed the gap between classic and systems theory.* Their presentations used the classic structure but also considered the effects of the individual performer.

Technologic Theory

During the 1960s, a large number of researchers focused their attention on the connection between technology and organizational processes. For example, in 1965, the researcher Joan Woodward[16] surveyed 100 British manufacturing firms in an effort to determine precisely what management practices contributed the most to a successful business. Her studies concluded that the conditions imposed by differing technologies tend to determine the type of organizational structure that develops. Woodward classified businesses into the following three basic types of production technology:

1. *Unit production:* creation of custom-made products on an individual basis
2. *Mass production:* large-volume manufacturing
3. *Process production:* continuous-process manufacturing

The most successful firms in her survey tended to have organizational structures that were similar to the typical pattern for each production type.

Woodward's work, along with the efforts of a variety of other researchers in similar areas, helped structure the final shift to what is now recognized as

---

*The systems theorists view productivity as a function of structure, people, technology, and environment.

modern systems theory. In this approach, organizational structure, technology, the environment, and the individual all combine to determine the organization's overall effectiveness.

Modern Systems Theory

In modern systems theory, an organization is defined as a complex sociotechnical system. The organization is perceived as an entity whose operation is based on specific inputs received in a defined environment (i.e., as an open system). In developing modern organizational theory, its proponents have relied at various times on conceptual analysis, experimental research, and an integrative approach. Examples of their diverse thinking are the open systems approach as defined by researchers Daniel Katz and Robert L. Kahn,[2] the decision system approach outlined by James G. March and Herbert A. Simon,[17] and the information-processing approach designed by Jay R. Galbraith.[18]

Some fundamental and critical questions posed by modern systems theorists are as follows[19]:
- What are the critical parts of the system?
- What is the nature of their mutual dependency?
- What are the primary elements within the system that link the parts together and facilitate their adjustment to each other?
- What are the goals sought by the system?

The fundamental element of the organizational system is the individual participant and the role he or she plays. Next is the formal arrangement of the functions and elements of the organization. These are grouped into an interdependent pattern that is referred to as the *formal* organization. Also identified and considered equally important is the *informal* organization. In this approach, both the formal role requirements of the organization and the informal expectations of the work group, along with the physical environment, are considered to have an impact on overall production. The systems approach to organizational study examines the following:
- Role playing (the different functions performed by the participants)
- Communications
- Leadership
- Balance (between organizational subparts, control and regulatory processes, and feedback methods)
- Group processes
- Motivation
- Decision-making
- Goals (such as organizational effectiveness, stability, productivity, and survival)

Modern systems theorists believe that their work provides a framework for understanding organizational behavior and its effectiveness. Although this approach may be an excellent method of describing the general components of organizational functioning, the concepts provided do not always generate precise, verifiable hypotheses. Because this is true, it is best to think of the systems approach to organizational theory as a functionally broad method of analyzing organizations; the specifics of organizational behavior must still be examined. At best, the systems approach provides only the "big picture" of an organization.

Katz and Kahn, in their 1978 work,[2] viewed an organization as a continuous cycle of input, transformation, and output. They believed that physical structure is not an inherent part of an organizational system as it is of the system of the human body. One can destroy the physical structure, they declared, but as long as the articles of incorporation, mission, employees (who may come and go), and job descriptions (definitions of roles and authority) are maintained, the organization will survive. Even if the original purpose the organization was created to fulfill changes, the organization will survive by developing new inputs, throughput, outputs, and goals. The March of Dimes organization provides a good example. Its original goal was to provide funds for the care of polio victims and for research to eliminate the debilitating disease itself, but when Jonas Salk created a successful polio vaccine, the original goal was no longer relevant. To maintain itself as an organization, it established new goals based on helping the handicapped. The patterns and events of organizational activity are the elements important to survival. Katz and Kahn focused on role-taking and role-maintaining processes in conducting their analysis and arriving at their conclusions.

Another pair of researchers, March and Simon,[17] viewed the organization as an information-processing network containing a variety of different decision points for both the individual members of the organization and the group as a whole. If one can determine the various decision points and understand the myriad variables (forces acting on the decision-maker) related to each, one can comprehend the most critical behaviors within the system. March and Simon suggested that the classic concept of rational decision-making has limited application within organizations. They felt that in most circumstances the entity tasked with solving a problem does not know or recognize all of the available options and therefore may not have all of the information necessary to properly evaluate the question. Because having the proper information and the ability to understand it are the basic requirements for rational decision-making, decision-making within organizations can be rational only within certain limits. March and Simon called this limited decision-making process "bounded rationality." Rather than use rational decision processes to maximize economic return, many organizations, and the individual members who compose them, set their goals at a lower level. That is, they will establish an arbitrary form, or minimally acceptable level of return, and pick the first alternative that promises to exceed this level.

Furthermore, March and Simon suggested, instead of continually making decisions, members and organizations create programs, or sets of intricate, systematic behaviors that can be used to react to ordinary environmental stimuli. The establishment of these programs provides a logical reason why so much of human behavior is predictable. In March and Simon's view, therefore, organizational theory is simply a process of identifying the basic behavioral programs created by organizational members and the various stimuli that affect the decision-making process.

Galbraith[18] provided yet another approach to organizational theory. He viewed the organization as one would picture a large communications system. According to his theory, as the level of uncertainty within an organization increases, so does the amount of communication (information) necessary to keep the organization secure. To carry this idea a step further, the organization is simply a system in which the ultimate goal is the reduction of uncertainty. Because all communication channels are limited in what and how much they can effectively carry (without increasing uncertainty), overloading the communication lines will eventually exceed their capacity to reduce uncertainty. In other words, too much communication saturates the organization so that communication is no longer an effective tool for dispelling uncertainty and becomes a negative influence that actually creates it. This is especially true in an unpredictable environment such as the one faced by the nursing profession over the last few decades with the advent of DRG-based payment and rapidly increasing competition. When such saturation occurs, it becomes necessary to (1) increase capacity or (2) reduce the quantity of communication. Galbraith's research not only identifies strategies for increasing communication capacity, it provides methods for decreasing uncertainty and describes different system types that are associated with it. One of these is referred to as the "matrix organization." This type of establishment employs two distinct but overlapping management systems: (1) a departmental structure, and (2) a project or product structure. In this type of organization, the individual employee may report to several different people, in a direct contravention of classic rules. Yet the matrix type of organization is repeatedly found in engineering and research firms because of its high information-processing capacity.

Even with all of its flaws, modern systems theory remains a useful tool for improving awareness of the structure of organizations and the influences that act on them. Although accurate assessment of many of the hypotheses generated by modern systems theory has frequently proven difficult, it must be kept in mind that the aim of this approach is not to define the ideal organizational plan but, instead, simply to recognize the vast complexity of the typical organization and the interactive effects of a wide range of influences. This theoretical approach has provided significant benefit because it allows the identification of important organizational influences and considers how the human variables affect the organization.

ORGANIZATIONAL STRUCTURE IN HEALTH CARE

The vast majority of today's health service organizations are characterized by a bureaucratic structure similar to that shown in Fig. 2-2. This type of configuration is designed to provide several essential elements of a smoothly functioning organization, as follows:

- It provides a command* (management) structure and reinforces authority
- It provides for a formal system of communication up, down, and across the facility
- It shields the care givers from the task environment

The typical bureaucratic structure is flawed, however, because it is most often rigid (inflexible), formal, uncongenial, and normally not comfortable for any of the individuals working within it. Formal communication downward in the hierarchy often takes on a despotic and repressive tone. Even more critical, however, is that the structure is very rigid and often severely limits the ability of those working within it to respond rapidly to changes occurring in the environment around them or to the marketplace outside of their surroundings.

---

*The word *command* is used in this context only to reinforce the requirement that the structure provide for a hierarchy of authority within the management arrangement of an organization. The process of command is most often used in situations in which those in senior positions maintain life-and-death influence over subordinates and in which response to orders is absolute and a failure to obey may result in severe discipline up to and including death. A classic example of command is a military organization. The medical profession commonly uses a rigid management type of structure.

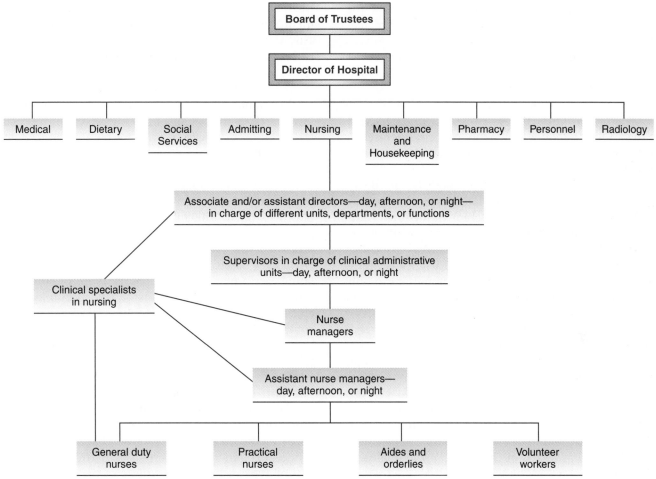

Fig. 2-2 ■ Typical bureaucratic structure, with special focus on the nursing department.

Health service organizations are, first and foremost, structured (designed) to increase the likelihood of the success and survival of the organization. Although this fact is critical, significant challenges occur when the administrators creating the organization omit from their design the consideration of such vital factors as differing social, political, economic, and resource climates. Such a situation is further exacerbated by the imposition of personal perspectives onto the organization (i.e., creators structure it to work as they want it to, or for their benefit). Because of these breakdowns in design, the actual structure of an individual healthcare institution can vary greatly from one organization to another.

There are some characteristics that are similar, however; for example, the structures of most healthcare institutions are based on a set of dissimilar but interdependent functions. These functions are broad and are typically broken down into the responsibilities performed by persons operating in a variety of formal performance groups. Exactly how these groups report to and interact with one another is usually deter-mined by the preliminary organizational chart compiled by the bureaucracy that creates the groups.

The vertical dimension in Fig. 2-2 reflects the organization's hierarchy; that is, the lines of authority and responsibility. To function properly, an organization must be able to exercise control over the actions of its membership, and the system of hierarchy provides the authority for this control. A look at the vertical dimension of the chart provides some understanding of how healthcare organizations use differentiation to pursue their goals and how this same differentiation can result in an organizational prescription for the nurse manager. The horizontal dimension on the chart relates to the division and specialization of the labor performed within the organization.

The Vertical Dimension

The organizational chart shown in Fig. 2-2 is shaped much like a pyramid that has been separated into several vertical levels. These levels are based on the administrative necessity for proper dispersal of the authority and responsibility required to ensure reasonable control. The greatest degree of authority exists at the top of the pyramid, and authority decreases as the layers descend down through the bureaucracy. Individuals carrying out the responsibilities shown at the tops of organizational structures are usually referred to as executives—people who have very broad responsibilities and who concern themselves primarily with the general well-being and direction of the organization.

To many people occupying positions farther down in the structure, and this includes many nurses, the executives often appear indifferent to the "real" purposes of a healthcare institution because they are typically focused on issues that are not as associated with patient care as the clinical staff believe is necessary and appropriate. However, it is important to fully understand that today's economic system is built on the reality of competition, and health service organizations are being compelled to operate within that system on the same basis as many other service-oriented institutions. Therefore, it is imperative that these executives perceive and evaluate their organizations as a business and keep their eyes on the environment. This requirement will cause them to perceive the institution differently than do the purely medical staff, but that difference in perception should not be construed as a lack of caring about the quality of patient care.

For example, executives may be confronted with a question such as, Should the hospital open an outpatient clinic in a shopping mall to maintain its share of the healthcare market, keep beds filled through the resulting referrals, and provide additional income? The survival of the entire organization may well depend on what decisions are made by executives as they attempt to answer questions of this nature and how well they coordinate the extremely diversified activities required to accomplish the work associated with the answers. The attention that administrative executives devote to the actual operation of the facility is focused far differently than is that of the nursing staff. Executives focus most often on the operation of the entire institution, not on that of any single part of it, such as patient care. Given this much broader scope, it is no small wonder that executives seem indifferent to the staff nurse who attends principally to the specific internal functions of the organization.

The authority level immediately below that of the executives is typically referred to as *middle management*. The role of this level is to coordinate and direct the activity of functional work groups so that they can efficiently accomplish directives issued by the executives. The position of associate/assistant nursing director is an example of a middle management position. This person exercises control over a clinical area that is composed of a large number of individual performers who may be working within a variety of separate units.

Although the position of nurse manager is lower in the managerial hierarchy and is more internally focused than that of the next higher organizational level, nurse managers usually respond indirectly to the patients served by their staff. The responsibilities for which nurse managers are accountable force them to be more concerned with *what* work has to be accomplished rather than *how* the work is actually performed. The majority of their time is spent planning for future performance and establishing processes that will allow their units to meet the challenges posed by the future, such as meeting escalating performance requirements with diminishing nursing resources. The efforts of this specific hierarchical level are boundary spanning, coordinating, and controlling.

The Horizontal Dimension

The horizontal dimension in Fig. 2-2 relates to the specialization of labor. In healthcare institutions this dimension usually consists of an arrangement of departments similar to that shown. Each department, service, or program represents a particular portion and/or type of human contribution necessary to the total care-giving process. The requirement of management is to fit these individual contributions together to produce a high quality, as well as the necessary quantity, of care.

Discord between the horizontal units of a typical health service organization is normally unavoidable, because many of the functions performed by these units are delivered by specific disciplines (nursing, medicine, or social work), and each group of professionals has its own set of values, attitudes, and perspectives. Conflict between the groups is most often caused by the fact that each typically considers its contribution to be more critical than that of the next group or even of the whole. Another major factor is the competition between groups for the limited resources available. This already difficult situation is intensified by the fact that professionals tend to communicate most frequently, and with greater ease, within their own peer groups. This acts to reinforce peer decisions and control, which compounds the difficulty each group experiences when interacting with other units.

Yet the increasingly complex and intensive technology associated with health care makes it essential that each individual group coordinate its efforts with those of the rest of the organization. Health services are administered on the basis of patient need, and to optimize the process, it is imperative that a large number of individuals, each with his or her own expertise, work together in delivering care. The degree to which services are provided in a smooth and appropriate flow determines every institution's "continuity of care," a primary concern and function of all healthcare organizations.

TYPES OF HEALTHCARE ORGANIZATIONS

Healthcare organizations can be grouped into five different care categories:

1. Acute
2. Long-term
3. Ambulatory
4. Home health
5. Temporary health

In addition, each may be private (owned by an individual, group, or corporation) or public (owned by a governmental entity), and for profit and nonprofit. Traditionally, most healthcare institutions and agencies have been nonprofit, but the trend has been changing with the recent development of proprietary, or for-profit, hospitals and hospital chains. Institutions may also specialize in one area of health care, such as alcohol treatment, but most continue to function as "general" hospitals.

The largest number of healthcare organizations today are acute care hospitals. Many of these organizations are privately owned, but others are considered public and are owned and operated by local, state, or federal governmental agencies.

Many of these healthcare institutions, regardless of their other characteristics, also serve as teaching institutions for physicians, nurses, and other healthcare professionals. However, the term *teaching hospital* most often indicates that the organization maintains a resident staff on duty 24 hours a day. In contrast to the teaching hospital is the community hospital, which operates with only private practice physicians on its staff. Private physicians are typically far less accessible than a staff resident, so the medical supervision of patient care differs. This difference carries over to the staff and supervisory nurses and the patient care they are responsible for delivering.

The number of long-term care institutions has risen in parallel with the increase in the elderly population. Today, more people are living longer under conditions of poorer health, which has increased the demand for long-term care. This is believed to be the area in which maximum growth will be seen in the first three decades of the new millennium.

Health care is also delivered in ambulatory care settings, in the home, and by agencies that provide temporary service personnel. Ambulatory care providers are similar to hospitals in that they may be private (emergency aid facility) or public (county health department clinic), and proprietary (physician's office) or nonprofit (screening clinics).

Home health care is a trend that has grown rapidly in recent years. Rising medical costs and the need for cost containment have forced hospitals and many third-party payers (insurance companies) to critically examine the length of patient stays in care facilities. These investigations have resulted in an across-the-board change in policy that has led to earlier discharge of patients and the return home of much of the more acutely ill patient population. This situation is further complicated by the fact that more people are surviving life-threatening illness and trauma and require longer care. To answer this need for home health care, visiting nurse associations (nonprofit, private), local health departments (nonprofit, public), temporary service agencies (proprietary, private), and a variety of departments within acute care hospitals provide home health care. The largest growth in this area has occurred in private (for-profit and not-for-profit) home care agencies. Services provided by these agencies are primarily nursing, but some of the larger firms also offer professional services such as physical therapy or social services.

One of the main reasons for the growth of temporary service agencies is the current acute shortage of qualified nurses. A primary function of these agencies is to supply nurses and other healthcare workers to hospitals that are temporarily short-staffed. In addition, they provide private-duty nurses to patients on an individual basis. Many hospitals, both large and small, rely heavily on these organizations to fill specialized staffing needs when shortages and fluctuations in the number of patients make scheduling of in-house staff difficult and inefficient.

Multifaceted hospital systems also are becoming increasingly more common. These organizations often combine the traditional functions of the nursing home, psychiatric facility, health maintenance organization (HMO), and home care agency.

Multiinstitutional arrangements can take many forms, as follows[20]:

Formal agreement: Two or more institutions adopt a cooperative agenda while maintaining individual responsibility for the delivery of unique actions or services.

Shared services: Two or more independent organizations combine their clinical and/or administrative capabilities.

Consortia on planning or education: Groups of institutions meet jointly with local health system agencies to determine which institutions will provide specific services to the community.

Contract management: An organization enters into an agreement with an outside management firm to subcontract the responsibility for day-to-day management of the organization without changing the ownership of the organization.

Leasing: An organization contracts with an outside firm as in contract management, but in this case the subcontracting firm not only regulates day-to-day operations but also establishes and enforces policy.

Corporate ownership with separate management: A corporation owns several institutions and contracts for their administration with independent firms.

Complete corporate ownership: A corporation owns and manages several institutions.

These multiinstitutional arrangements can be integrated either horizontally or vertically. A *horizontally* integrated system is one in which the units comprising the system each provide the same or similar services. In contrast, a *vertically* integrated system is one in which individual units provide unique services. An example of a vertically integrated system is one that incorporates an HMO, a psychiatric hospital, an acute care hospital, and a nursing home. Although these types of arrangement have been highly promoted, researchers point out that their overall effect on performance and efficiency will have to be determined by the test of time and experimental study.[20] The benefits and limitations of these types of healthcare organization are shown in Box 2-1.

It is very likely that a nurse manager, over the span of a career, will be responsible for supervising patient

---

BOX 2-1

Benefits and Limitations for Nursing of Multiinstitutional Systems

BENEFITS

Economics

Access to capital to finance new programs, services, and continuing education

Availability of financial support to otherwise failing institutions

Spreading of program startup costs over a larger base

Technology

Corporate production of patient education and training aids

Corporate-wide computerized cost accounting, patient care information, and patient classification systems

Availability of new and more sophisticated patient care equipment

Diversification

Market analysis for special projects

Availability of new programs and services involving nursing (surgical centers, home healthcare programs, wellness centers, child day care, and hospice programs) that bring enhanced career mobility within the same corporate structure

Alliances with nonhealth lines of business, such as uniform companies, that allow staff purchases at lower than market prices

Fringe Benefits

Stock options allowing purchases at reduced rates

End-of-year stock bonuses

Vested retirement accounts that are transferable if employees relocate outside the system

Continuing education for nursing staff and management

Educational leave programs

Financial rewards for writing and publishing

Awards (with monetary value) for community service and excellence

Attractive insurance and tax-deferrable benefits

Transfer of benefits (seniority, etc.) if personnel relocate within the system

Professional Benefits

Improved registered nurse–to–patient ratio

Increased number of clinical specialists and nurse researchers

Decentralized nursing organizations

Ability to attract specialists to rural areas

Upward mobility for nursing staff

Systemwide mobility

LIMITATIONS

Autonomy

Reduction in nurse executive autonomy, especially with regard to institutional governance and diversification

Failure of nurse executives to recognize their corporate responsibility and tendency to focus only on their own institutions

Quality

Short-term staff overloads and reductions in initial quality when rapid expansion occurs without the necessary resources and personnel in place

Reduction of registered nurse mix due to regional determination of standard

Lack of ongoing influence of consultants in a given institution

Data from Freund CM, Mitchell J: Multi-institutional systems: the new arrangement, *Nurs Econ* 3(1):24, 1985.

care in every type of healthcare organization discussed. Therefore, the management principles presented in this chapter have been made applicable to any and all healthcare settings. Because the highest percentage of professional nurses are employed by hospitals, however, the examples used focus primarily on nursing management as it relates to that environment. Nevertheless, when it is appropriate and applicable, other healthcare settings are also discussed.

THE DEPARTMENT OF NURSING

The nursing department is almost always the largest single unit in any hospital. Directing its operation is the nursing service administrator. This position is also known by a variety of other similar names such as nursing administrator, director of nursing, and vice president for nursing. In this text, this position will be referred to as nursing director. Reporting to this manager as his or her immediate juniors will be at least one assistant for every work shift of the day, because the nursing department is staffed on a 24-hour basis. In addition, the nursing department will have clinical specialists in areas such as obstetrics, pediatrics, geriatrics, oncology, and the operating room. Every clinical service will usually have more than one nursing

unit, each with a nurse manager in charge. There may also be staff positions in such areas as in-service education and recruiting. Special nursing units include medical, surgical, pediatric, obstetric, psychiatric, operating room, recovery room, emergency department, and intensive care.

Fig. 2-3 presents an organizational chart for a typical centralized department of nursing, structured into a hierarchical authority pattern. Fig. 2-4 illustrates a decentralized nursing service.

A recent phenomenon that affects the structuring of nursing departments is the effort to make the decision-making process in healthcare institutions, especially decision-making among the nursing staff, more democratic. Such innovations may take forms of varying complexity. One is a relatively simple participative type of decision-making, or the collective voicing of all of the nurses. Another is establishment of a "congress," which is typically composed of one council (human resources) responsible for staffing levels, recruitment, and retention, and another council (nursing care) focused primarily on care standards, audit criteria, research, and staff education.

Shared governance is a process that affords the staff nurse an equal opportunity to contribute to the major decisions made regarding nursing practice. This type

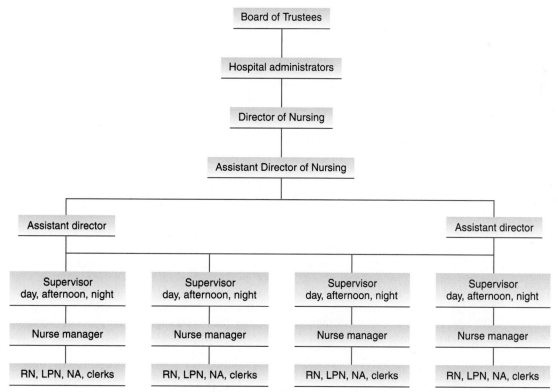

Fig. 2-3 ■ Traditional centralized nursing service. *LPN,* Licensed practical nurse; *NA,* nurse's aide; *RN,* registered nurse. (Data from Rowland HS, Rowland BL: *Administration handbook,* Germantown, Md, 1980, Aspen.)

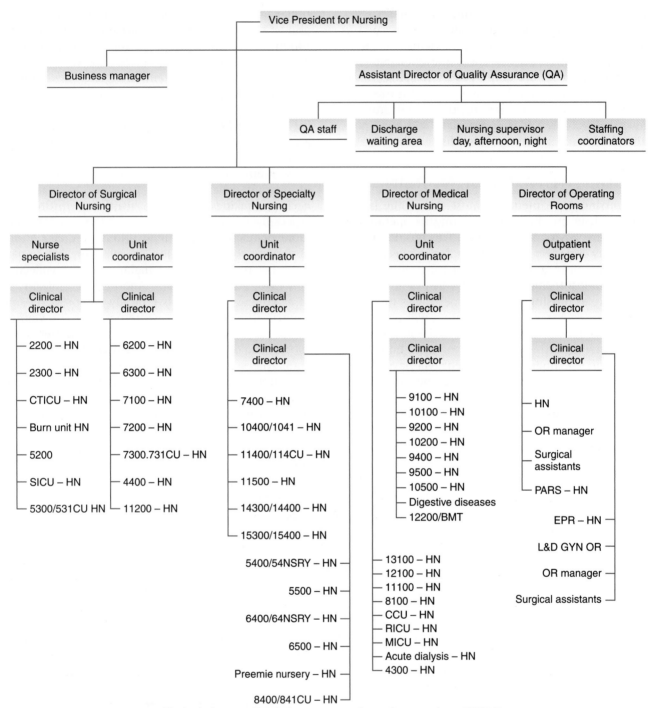

Fig. 2-4 ■ Typical decentralized department of nursing service. *BMT,* Bone marrow transplant; *CCU,* critical care unit; *CTICU,* cardiothoracic intensive care unit; *CU,* critical care unit; *EPR,* electronic paramagnetic resonance; *HN,* head nurse; *L&D GYN,* labor and delivery, gynecology; *MICU,* medical intensive care unit; *NSRY,* nursery; *OR,* operating room; *PAR,* postanesthesia room; *RICU,* respiratory intensive care unit; *SICU,* surgical intensive care unit.

of decision-making program is usually built on a foundation of primary nursing and peer review and includes some requirement for clinical advancement. Most shared governance systems follow an academic or medical governance model; that is, nurses elect members to a congress or delegation that represents them in the shared governance process. Such systems have only recently begun to develop.

Some shared governance systems are much more elaborate and include democratically elected advisory boards that are tasked with controlling the participants' own practice within the healthcare system. In these systems, nursing staffs, like medical staffs, determine the clinical skills required of staff nurses and regulate the work of each through a process of peer review, whereas other practice issues are decided by elected forums.

The intent of these innovative management systems is to increase job satisfaction and lower turnover among those nurses who are frustrated by the lack of opportunity to help guide the direction of their practice within the typical healthcare institution. However, it is also possible that these new approaches may lower satisfaction for the minority of nurses who do not wish to participate in democratic forums or spend time in the meetings and other group work required in a shared governance system. Nevertheless, overall efficiency may be enhanced by these systems as nurses assume more of the responsibility for their units, divisions, and practice and move away from the historical reliance on float, pool, or agency nurses to fill the gaps. The feeling is also strong that the quality of patient care will improve dramatically when nurses are placed in control of their own practice. Many hospitals have extensively examined these types of systems, and a number have run pilot programs or simply instituted these systems after carefully weighing the costs and benefits. These practices represent a revolutionary method for managing the nursing personnel within an organization, and only time will provide the answers to the economic questions that are currently being posed. Overall, however, it is the consensus of the nursing profession that such programs are good for nursing, regardless of the economic outcomes. Through these systems, nurses can broaden their capabilities and enhance their professional potential by gaining an equal voice in nursing practice and in health care in general.

ORGANIZATIONAL EFFECTIVENESS AND TODAY'S HEALTHCARE PROFESSION

Accurately defining organizational effectiveness is very difficult, especially in a service industry such as

health care. Where does one look to determine outcome? Is it the number of patients processed? In teaching hospitals, is it more important to cure patients or to provide a learning environment for interns and nurses? Open systems frequently have multiple functions and exist within environments that create uncertainty. In situations such as this, effectiveness may be measured by the organization's ability to adapt, maintain itself, survive, and, ultimately, grow. When viewed from a systems perspective, effectiveness can be defined by how well the organization copes with its environment. Few things are more important or meaningful than this for today's healthcare industry.

A wide variety of factors make it extremely difficult for the bureaucratically structured organization to be effective today. This is due primarily to the fact that the strength of a bureaucracy lies in its capacity to manage conventional activities in a predictable environment through the guidance of a well-developed and rigid chain of command supported by inflexible and strict rules. The bureaucratic nature of many organizations, especially in the healthcare industry, makes it almost impossible for them to deal effectively with the rapid and continuous environmental change that occurs today. In addition, growth is a factor that introduces complexity into the bureaucratic pyramid. Complexity is usually manifested as increased administrative overhead, tighter controls, rigid rules, and greater impersonality and represents the downside of growth. On the positive side, however, increased diversity can also be a product of growth.

Today's environment demands diverse, highly specialized competencies that are often incompatible with the normally rigid bureaucratic hierarchy. The demands of today's nursing profession require fundamental changes in managerial philosophy. New management concepts are needed regarding people and their values, needs, and reactions to the uses of power. Finally, the integration of innovative, non–status quo thinking into organizational decision-making is an absolute necessity. No organization designed to deal with a stable environment, in which organizational processes are rigid or are based on historical performance, can react to environmental pressures in an effective manner. In fact, the inability of the traditional bureaucratic hierarchy to do just that is the reason that so many healthcare organizations have failed to survive.

Nevertheless, bureaucracies can still be found in abundance in the healthcare industry, and many remain viable and are very successful. Most of these organizations, however, exist in stable environments that are not growing rapidly. Furthermore, many are still being operated under a system of centralized control directed by rigid sets of regulations, which remains the management style of choice in the dominant organizational coalition. Only when technology and competition remain stable, however, will such a power structure not stifle an organization.

It is difficult, if not impossible, to view health care as it operates today as a stable, predictable environment. In today's environment, organizational effectiveness for healthcare institutions entails the following[21]:

Adaptability: the ability to solve unique problems quickly in anticipation of and reaction to changes occurring in the environment

A sense of organizational purpose: knowledge and insight regarding the exact mission of the organization (where it is headed and why); this is something that must be shared by all members of the organization to be truly effective

Ability to test reality: the ability to identify, accurately predict, and correctly interpret the environment and its implications for the organization

Integration: the ability to ensure that all organizational subparts are operating cohesively and are not working at cross purposes

From the open systems perspective, such organizational effectiveness means the following:

- Perceiving changes in the environment
- Supplying and understanding relevant information
- Basing the decision-making process on that same relevant information rather than on historical performance
- Changing throughput to reflect these decisions
- Effectively managing undesired side effects
- Outputting new products or services in line with perceived environmental demands
- Obtaining feedback on the changes made

If these processes are examined from another perspective, it is easy to see that there are many points at which management can break down and reduce the effectiveness of the organization. The following list of 14 positive management reactions can assist nurse managers in ensuring that this does not happen in the organizations they help manage. An organization will be successful if every member of the management team does the following:

- Perceives environmental changes in a timely manner
- Accurately defines the type and impact of needed environmental changes
- Ensures that aggressive competitive steps are taken to obtain market share in innovations
- Shares relevant information with all organization decision-makers
- Provides an atmosphere that stimulates and encourages creative decision-making

- Recognizes the assumptions inherent in decisions made internally or by external change agents or consultants
- Ensures that the entire production system is converted and committed to change
- Recognizes that simply announcing change will not make it occur
- Encourages participation in every aspect of a change by organizational members tasked with its implementation
- Recognizes and effectively manages both the natural resistance to change and the personal transitions brought about by the change
- Ensures that all systems and their corresponding subsystems adapt to change as required
- Communicates to the environment that change is occurring so that the product or service can be exported in a timely manner
- Obtains and responds to feedback
- Uses the feedback received to implement modifications in the change

These positive actions are only part of an overall performance strategy that can be used in a changing environment and that is fully integrated. It is absolutely critical that an organization fully integrate its performance. For example, it is of little value to have an outstanding market research department if the organization fails to influence its production system to change in response to that department's findings. Likewise, it does not help to have a flexible production system if the organization has difficulty perceiving changes in the environment in which it operates.

Furthermore, to be innovative in today's environment, organizations must have the following three kinds of people[22]:

1. *Creative idea generators:* entrepreneurial risk takers who champion innovative solutions
2. *Sponsors:* middle managers who recognize the business significance of new ideas, can carry ideas through to implementation, and can balance the operating and innovating needs of the organization
3. *Orchestrators:* those with the political skills to ensure the survival of innovation, which almost always creates disharmony due to change

There are many ways to accomplish the coping strategy that has been advocated here. One sure way is to ensure that new ideas are not integrated with the operations section of the organization—especially, staff controls—until they have been confirmed. Innovation and operation are natural opposites, much as are creative and status quo decision-making.

Another method is to create a research and development department whose entire function is to originate and vigorously evaluate new ideas. On a larger scale, a project management approach and a matrix organizational structure are extremely beneficial.

In designing and operating their organizations, nurse managers are no longer held captive by the bureaucratic model. Improved productivity, continued growth, and even survival in today's healthcare environment require innovative organizational design and management. Because this chapter is designed for the nurse manager rather than the administrator, we have focused on management. However, productivity enhancement and innovation are themes that affect both administration and day-to-day operations. They are also absolute requirements in today's healthcare industry.

SUMMARY

- The nursing profession operates today in an organized society in which individuals must effectively balance a lack of personal freedom in furthering organizational goals with the economic and personal benefits of increased productivity.
- Managers mediate the process in which individuals surrender autonomy for other benefits.
- Today's healthcare organizations are open systems that operate much like the human body. Their ultimate goal is to survive, and they change various resources (people, capital, supplies) into services.
- Organizations produce goods and services that are exchanged for the resources required to survive.
- Many factors influence the organization's performance (e.g., patients, suppliers, competitors, governmental regulatory bodies, physicians, third-party payers, and the labor market).
- Organizations can be perceived as social systems consisting of people working in a predetermined pattern of relationships toward a common goal.
- The goal of most healthcare organizations is to provide a preestablished mix of health services.
- There are four differing schools of organizational theory: classic, neoclassic, technologic, and modern systems.
- Within the organization, an authority structure is created that determines the formal communication system and guides the organizational activities. This structure can be examined on two dimensions: horizontal and vertical.
- There are five basic types of healthcare institution: acute care, long-term care, ambulatory care, home health care, and temporary health care. Each type may be private or public, proprietary or nonprofit.
- Nursing is normally the largest department in a healthcare organization and includes many units that can be organized in either a centralized or decentralized manner.

- The nurse manager relates mutually with patients and staff to manage a nursing unit effectively.
- Organizational effectiveness is a difficult concept in health care today. Innovation and creative problem solving are needed and must be fostered.

FINAL THOUGHTS

Peter Drucker, in his book *Management: Tasks, Responsibilities, Practices,* said, "Management is a generic function that includes basic tasks in every discipline and every society" (p. 19).[23] He identified the following five fundamental functions of a manager:

1. *Establish goals and objectives* for each area of responsibility and communicate them to the employees who are responsible for accomplishing them
2. *Organize and analyze* the activities, situations, and relations necessary to realize the objectives and divide them into manageable tasks
3. *Motivate and communicate* with the employees responsible for accomplishing the objectives through teamwork
4. *Analyze, appraise, and interpret* performance requirements and communicate the meaning of measurement tools and the results they obtain to both the staff and senior managers.
5. *Develop* the staff and self continually.

THE NURSE MANAGER SPEAKS

The following are considered basic nurse manager functions:

1. Delineate objectives and goals for the area of responsibility (unit) and communicate them to the staff members who are expected to accomplish them
2. Assess and evaluate the activities within the nursing unit; make sound decisions regarding the division of labor within the unit
3. Set the example of a good team player by treating others with respect and regard, maintaining a positive outlook, and providing positive reinforcement
4. Complete the performance appraisal process on a day-by-day basis and communicate the results to the staff on an irregular but frequent basis; communicate to senior management annually
5. Develop the capabilities of the staff continually through programs such as mentoring, in-house training, and preceptorships
6. Advance personal capability by attending seminars, workshops, and educational programs and by obtaining specialty certification

REFERENCES

1. Robbins SP: *Organizational behavior,* ed 11, Upper Saddle River, NJ, 2004, Prentice Hall.
2. Katz D, Kahn R: *The social psychology of organizations,* New York, 1978, Wiley.
3. Stanton LJ: Nursing care and nursing products: revenue or expenses? *J Nurs Adm* 16(9):29, 1986.
4. Anderson RA: Products and product-line management in nursing, *J Nurs Q* 10(1):65, 1985.
5. Thompson JD: *Organizations in action,* New York, 1967, McGraw-Hill.
6. Smith A: *An inquiry into the nature and causes of the wealth of nations,* London, 1925, Methuen (Edited by E. Cannan; originally published in 1776).
7. Taylor FW: *The principles of scientific management,* New York, 1911, Harper.
8. Schermerhorn JR Jr: *Management for productivity,* ed 3, New York, 1989, Wiley.
9. Gilbreth F, Gilbreth L: *Time and motion study as fundamental factors in planning and control,* Mountainside, NJ, 1921, Mountainside Press.
10. Fayol H: General and industrial administration, London, 1949, Pitman.
11. Weber M: *From Max Weber: Essays in sociology,* London, 1958, Oxford University Press.
12. Howell WC, Dipboye RL: *Essentials of management and organizational psychology,* ed 3, Cincinnati, 1986, Thomson Brooks/Cole.
13. Fox EM, Urwick LF, editors: *Dynamic administration: the collected papers of Mary Parker Follett,* New York, 1982, Buccaneer Books.
14. Gillespie R: *Manufacturing knowledge: a history of the Hawthorne Experiments,* Cambridge, Mass, 1991, Press Syndicate of the University of Cambridge.
15. Barnard CI: *The functions of the executive,* ed 13, Cambridge, Mass, 1998, Harvard University Press.
16. Woodward J: *Industrial organization: theory and practice,* London, 1965, Oxford University Press.
17. March JG, Simon H: *Organizations,* New York, 1958, Wiley.
18. Galbraith JR: *Organizational design,* Reading, Mass, 1977, Addison-Wesley.
19. Scott WG: Organizational theory, *J Acad Manage* 4:6, 1961.
20. Freund CM, Mitchell J: Multi-institutional systems: the new arrangement, *Nurs Econ* 3(1):24, 1985.
21. Schein EH: *Organizational psychology,* Upper Saddle River, NJ, 1980, Prentice-Hall.
22. Galbraith JR: Designing the innovative institution, *Organ Dyn* 10:5, 1982.
23. Drucker PF: *Management: tasks, responsibilities, practices,* New York, 1985, Harper and Row.

SUGGESTED READINGS

Hardy ME, Conway ME: *Perspectives for health professionals,* New York, 1978, Appleton-Century-Crofts.

Huber DL, editor: *Leadership and nursing care management,* ed 3, Philadelphia, 2006, Saunders.

Marquis BL, Huston CJ: *Leadership roles and management functions in nursing,* Philadelphia, 1996, Lippincott.

McCoy BH: The parable of the Sadhu, *Harv Bus Rev* 75:2(May-June) 1997.

Simons GF, Vasquez C, Harris PR: *Leadership: empowering the workforce,* Houston, 1993, Gulf Publishing.

Fundamentals of Leadership and Management

OUTLINE

LEARNING SYNOPSIS

Upon successful completion of this chapter, readers will possess a fundamental understanding of leadership and management: what they are, how they apply to the nursing profession, and how they interact with one another.

OBJECTIVES

1. Be able to identify different management styles
2. Be able to identify different challenges faced by individuals who become managers
3. Describe why management is an incredibly difficult job for the average performer

4. Define *managerial leadership*
5. Identify the major myths concerning managerial leadership
6. Be able to identify one's own individual potential for leadership
7. Understand exactly what it is that managers and leaders do
8. Understand that leadership is the emotional side of management
9. Understand why leadership is so hard to identify within the ranks of average management
10. Understand the basic relationship between management and leadership
11. Comprehend why leadership is always a temporary condition
12. Identify and understand the three major types of leadership: situational, transitional, and hierarchical

Congratulations! This chapter is an exercise in your willingness to extend yourself through the acceptance of new and innovative material as you experience a completely fresh approach to the topic of management. As a student in advanced education, you have no doubt been subjected to a wide variety of different philosophies regarding the profession of management, and if you are truly astute, you will have noticed that most of these presentations fall into one of two distinct categories:

1. *The deadly boring epic:* The best part of this approach to teaching management is that when you have finished the course, the textbook will provide you with a great doorstop for your office.
2. *The recycled and sugar-coated platitude:* The standard old required reading is full of clichés and psychobabble that sound absolutely terrific in the classroom but fails miserably in the performance environment.

You may find this chapter to be very different from other writings on the subject because (1) it shows management as a challenge, not a burden; (2) it shows management as an opportunity, not an ordeal; and (3) it shows management as a skill and leadership as an art. First, this text takes a somewhat lighthearted look at a traditionally difficult process. The pages reflect a strong belief that even management can be fun and entertaining. There is absolutely no reason for managers to be dour, withdrawn, and boring individuals. In today's world it is perfectly logical, and even makes good business sense, for front-line managers to get their jobs done while they are enjoying themselves. In fact, it is felt to be essential that all managers develop a strong sense of humor to help them overcome the seemingly insurmountable challenges that they will face from time to time. All nurses who assume a management position will have days when they will be challenged—perhaps to the very limits of their ability and beyond. But most of the time, these professionals will experience the absolute joy of managing (teaching a new skill to an employee, helping a subordinate nurse provide for the needs of a new patient, reaching an important goal, and so on) and will experience a sense of fulfillment that they otherwise might never have imagined possible.

Second, popular management books are generated by the thousands annually. The theories they promote come and go, and not many last for more than an instant. Like it or not, many managers, and the companies they work for, seem to be ruled by the business fad of the month or the latest theory of performance. This chapter is not based on fad, however. Instead, it is focused on presenting tried and true solutions to common management problems and providing information on the fundamental relationship between the *skill* of management and the *art* of leadership—information and solutions that will stand up over time, regardless of the specific circumstances, location, or environment in which the nurse manager is employed. You will find only things that are practical in these pages, ideas and concepts that can help you through the normal business day or support you in those turbulent "Maalox moments" known to all managers.

This chapter endeavors to break some of the rules and reinforce some others. It provides a comprehensive overview of management principles that can help relieve some of the stress caused by the world's most intimidating job. It also sheds some light on the often-confused terms *management* and *leadership* and clarifies how to use each effectively.

First, however, let us make a few assumptions:

You are a nurse manager who wants to advance your capability.

OR

You are an individual aspiring to become a nurse manager.

OR

You are an individual who is uncontrollably attracted to the process of advanced learning.

No matter what your reason for studying this subject—if, for instance, you are curious and want to learn the intimate details of the management and leadership techniques that can help you get the best from people now and throughout your career, or you are just trying to get through this course—you are about to enter the most exciting aspect of business imaginable, management and the persuasion of leadership.

Management is a profession. If anyone ever tries to tell you otherwise, then that person (1) has never been a manager, or (2) has lost touch with reality. Management is a profession—one that most of the world's most successful people have chosen. There is virtually no other profession in which an individual can have such a direct, dramatic, and positive impact on the lives of others and on the ultimate success of his or her enterprise.

Leadership is an art. It is the careful application of a few basic skills that are suited to the specific time and place that brings out the best out in people who choose to follow it. It is inspiration, motivation, and exhilaration. Leadership is not, however, a technical skill. Although it is definitely something that can be learned, it is more a persuasion than an application.

DIFFERENT MANAGEMENT STYLES

One popular definition of management is "getting things done through others." Another definition more specifically describes it as "making something happen within a specific area through the use of available resources." Seems simple enough! If there is one thing that management is not, however, it is simple. If it were, why would so many bright, well-educated nursing professionals have such difficulty doing it well? And why do so many healthcare companies across the world continually search for people with management capability when their institutions literally abound in educated and highly motivated personnel? Why do some of the world's most successful healthcare companies spend billions of dollars annually trying to develop the skill level of their managers?

Why? Because good management in the healthcare community, and in any other industry for that matter, is an incredibly scarce commodity, at once both precious and fleeting. Despite the years of evolution of management theory and the hundreds of thousands of people who hold PhDs, MDs, and MBAs from the world's most prestigious universities, many workers—and in fact many managers—have developed a somewhat distorted view of management and its practice, primarily because so many managers so frequently execute it so poorly.

There is an old Anglo-Saxon adage that says, "If it's foggy in the pulpit, it will be cloudy in the pew." To adapt this maxim to the average medical work environment, we can say that if management doesn't understand what to do, then the care-providing nurse can't possibly be expected to perform correctly.

Have you ever heard any of the following comments in your office or working environment?

- "We don't have the authority to make that decision."
- "She's in charge of the department—fixing the problem is her responsibility, not mine."
- "Why do they keep asking me what I think when they never pay attention to anything I say?"
- "I'm sorry, but that is our policy. We are not allowed to make exceptions."
- "If my manager doesn't care, why should I?"
- "Working hard in this job doesn't get you anywhere faster."
- "You can't trust employees; turn your back for a second and they will be goofing off."

When managers hear comments like these in the hallway, in the restroom, after a rather difficult meeting, or at the end of a demanding day, red flags should be waving in front of their eyes, and alarm bells should be ringing in their ears. Statements like these indicate that management and staff are not communicating effectively and that the staff lack confidence in their managers. Nurse managers who have employees who report these kinds of problems are very, very lucky as long as the employees report them early enough so that managers have time to do something about the problems presented. Most managers, however, are not fortunate enough to have employees who will tell them that these sorts of problems exist, and thus most managers continually have the opportunity to commit the same mistakes over and over.

The expectations and commitments that employees carry with them on the job are, in large part, a product of the way they are treated by their managers. The following sections describe the most commonly practiced styles of management. Do you recognize your management style or perhaps the one used most often by your boss?

Tough and Demanding: The "Hard as Nails" Approach

What is the best way to make something that has been well planned actually happen? Everyone seems to have a different answer to this question. Some people view management as something that you do *to* people, not *with* them. If you've been around the business part of a healthcare profession for more than a day, you have probably heard the battle cry of this type of manager: "I don't care if you like it or not; that is the way it's going to be done. Do you understand?" Or perhaps you have heard the ever-popular threat, "It had better be on my desk by the end of the day—or else!" If worse comes to worst, this type of manager will unveil the ultimate weapon: "Mess up just once more and I'll fire you!"

This style of management is most often known as *theory X management*, and its basic premise is that all people are inherently lazy and must be forced to perform. This form of management operates through intimidation and always, *always*, gets a response. The question is, Will it be the type of response desired? Of course, there is only one answer to this question, and that is, *No*, the response will not be what is desired. When a manager closely scrutinizes his or her employees' work, what is achieved is almost always very short-term compliance. In other words, a manager will never receive the best that people are capable of by "building a fire *under* them." If someone wants to be successful as a nurse manager, it is far better to find a way to "build a fire *inside* of them."

There is no doubt that certain occasions call for a nurse manager to take command of the situation. If the building is on fire, for example, it is bad form to call a meeting to decide who will put it out. By the time you find an opening in everyone's schedule, the building will be a burned-out shell. Similarly, if a proposal has to be mailed to the customer via an overnight delivery service because it absolutely has to be there tomorrow and there are still some last-minute changes your customer would like to see, then it is imperative that the manager take charge and ensure that the right people are on the job.

Soft and Easy: The "Mr. Nice Guy" Approach

On the other end of the spectrum is the manager who perceives that a *nice guy* must fill the manager's role. This is known as *theory Y management*, and it assumes that all people want to do a good job. In the extreme interpretation of this theory, managers are supposed to be sensitive to the feelings of their employees and be careful not to do anything that might disturb their tranquility and sense of self-worth. An example might be the manager who approaches an employee as follows:

> Uh, there is this small problem with your charting; none of the entries are correct. Now please don't take this personally, but we need to consider our alternatives for taking a more careful look at how you note the doctor's orders in the future.

Who is to say that nurse managers won't get a response with this approach, but will it be the best possible response? What is more likely is that employees will perceive this type of conduct as weakness, and many will eventually take advantage of the situation. Or perhaps those nurse managers will not mind having to do all of the charting, all of the time ... by themselves!

It is a sad commentary, but all too often in our world, being a nice guy is perceived as being easy—or worse yet, simpleminded.

The Ideal Compromise: The "Professional" Approach

Good nurse managers realize that they don't have to be tough all of the time—and that being nice will often help them finish far ahead of the competition. If employees are diligently performing their assigned tasks and no business emergency requires a manager's immediate intervention, the best approach is often to stay out of the employees' way and let them do their jobs. Not only will this method teach the staff to be responsible but it will also allow managers to concentrate their efforts on the things that are most important to the bottom-line success of their organizations. (If nurse managers spend all of their time doing their employees' work, who will do theirs?)

The real job of a nurse manager is to inspire employees to perform at their best possible level by establishing a working environment that encourages them to excel. In fact, the best nurse managers focus their energy toward removing the organizational obstacles that prevent good employees from doing their jobs and on obtaining the resources and training that employees need to perform effectively. All other goals, no matter how lofty or urgent, must take a back seat to these fundamentals.

Bad systems, bad policies, bad procedures, and poor treatment of others are organizational weaknesses that nurse managers must develop a talent for identifying and either repairing or replacing. Good managers spend their time building a strong organizational foundation for their employees. *Support your staff, and they will support you.* Time and time again, when given the opportunity to achieve, workers in all kinds of businesses—from hospitals to venture capital firms—have proven this rule to be true. If you haven't experienced it in your place of business, it's a good bet that either you or your boss is mistaking your employees for the problem. Quit forcing them and start forcing the organization. The result will be employees who want to succeed and a business that flourishes right along with them.

Squeezing (forcing) employees may be easier than fighting a convoluted system and cutting through the bureaucratic barnacles that have grown around the organization. Managers may be tempted to point and yell at their staff, "It's your fault that we didn't achieve our goals." Although blaming the employees for the shortcomings of the organization may be tempting, it will never solve the real problems. Sure, there will be a quick, short-lived response when the staff is forced to work, but ultimately that "A"-style exercise will cause a failure in the fundamental role of the nurse manager, which is to effectively eliminate the organization's real problems.

Band-Aids Don't Really Cure

Despite what many people would have you believe, good management is not achieved through simple solutions or quick fixes. Like placing a Band-Aid over a cut artery, the job just won't get done with that approach. Being a nurse manager is not a simple job. Even though the best management solutions tend to be found through the application of common sense, turning common *sense* into common *practice* is never simple.

Management is all about attitude. It is a way of life. It is a very real desire to work with people and help them succeed, as well as a desire to help the organization succeed. Management is a lifelong learning process that doesn't end when you walk out of a 1-hour seminar or even after you graduate from Harvard or Stanford with an MBA, MD, or PhD. It's like the old story about the unhappy homeowner who was shocked to receive a bill for $100 for fixing an electric light switch. When he asked the electrician to explain why the bill was so high, the electrician simply stated, "$5 is what I charge for tightening the loose connection on your switch, and $95 is what I charge for knowing which connection to tighten."

Management is a *people* job. If you would prefer not to work with people—helping them, listening to them, encouraging them, and guiding them—then you shouldn't attempt to become a nurse manager.

THE CHALLENGE OF MANAGEMENT

When individuals with the capability to become managers are assigned to a job or asked to complete a task, most find it relatively easy to complete the activity without outside assistance. The quality of the results achieved is typically attributable to the level of effort the individual puts forth. To accomplish the task, the assignee first reviews it, then makes a mental judgment to determine the best approach to ensure completion, and then establishes some sort of guideline to keep himself or herself on track while the task is finished, perhaps a set of milestones or intermediate objectives. Provided the individual is given the proper

tools and resources to complete the assignment, there is every reason to believe that the results achieved will be satisfactory. Why is this assumption made? Because people who enter the ranks of management generally are considered the best "doers" within their work groups. Executive managers, when they look for nurse managers, almost always select the top performers from among those who are eligible for promotion. Therefore, this textbook assumes that you were, or would have been, a top-performing nurse.

When an individual wants to accomplish a task using the assistance of another person, it is frequently necessary to employ an entirely different set of skills than those that might have been used if the task were accomplished individually. Once the decision has been made to pass the responsibility for completion of a task on to someone else, an impersonal element is introduced into the relationship between the person delegating and the person performing the work (Box 3-1).

BOX 3-1

True Story

Before Barbara was appointed nurse supervisor, she was a member of a nursing staff assigned to a pediatric unit on the second (afternoon) shift. In that position, she updated charts, passed medications, and assisted in the day-to-day patient care on the floor. She was considered to be a member of the team, and everything was fine. She came to work dressed appropriately—just like her contemporaries—and often spent social time with the other nurses before or after the shift. The bond that the team shared, however, changed after Barbara was promoted to nurse manager of the unit.

In her new role as the nurse manager, Barbara first physically changed her office. Instead of working behind the unit desk with the other nurses, she moved into a small office up the hall that was designated for the nurse manager. A secretary was assigned to guard her door and shield her from the day-to-day activity on the floor. Stylish and expensive business suits replaced the relaxed nurse's apparel. Instead of working with the patients and enjoying the conversation of the other nurses, Barbara now had to concern herself with more high-level issues such as cost overruns, scheduling, and the quality of health care provided. As her role changed, so did Barbara, and as a result, so did her relationship with her former co-workers. To achieve the goals assigned to her, Barbara was forced to quickly make a transition from a "doer" to a "manager of doers."

Once an individual becomes a nurse manager, simply being a great performer is no longer enough, no matter how good that person's technical nursing skills are. Nurse managers have to augment their nursing skills with others, such as planning, organizational leadership, and follow-up skills.

In other words, once the individual puts on the mantle of nurse manager, being a good performer is no longer enough. Now the person must also be a good manager of performers.

The Traditional Approach

If the challenge of making the transition from a performer to a manager were not enough, today's nurse managers face another significant challenge—one that has shaken the very foundation of the modern healthcare system. The new reality is the partnering relationship that must exist between managers and workers in the workplace.

In the traditional business model there were managers and workers, period; this made management a fairly direct proposition. In the traditional model managers divided the organization's work into a series of small, discrete tasks and assigned them to the individual workers (performers) within their charge. After individual assignments were made, managers closely supervised each worker's performance and issued directives and corrections as necessary to ensure that each individual completed his or her assigned task on time and within budget. This traditional style of management relied heavily on fear, intimidation, and the exercise of power over people to accomplish goals. If things didn't develop in accordance with the plan, then management would *command* its way out of the problem: "I don't care what you have to do to get it done! Just get it done—now!" Under this traditional form of management, the line between performer and manager was drawn very clearly, and much too often.

The Modern Approach

Today, things are very different in the nursing profession. For one thing, management has finally realized that what is occurring *inside* is a reflection of what is occurring *outside* the organization. The changes that have occurred outside the nursing environment over the past two decades have had a profound influence on the internal nursing environment. These changes include the following:

- The **flattening** of organizational hierarchies
- The development of new technology and rapid innovation
- The proliferation of small, closely held businesses
- Widespread **downsizing** or **reengineering**

- A change in the values of labor in general and of the individual worker in particular
- Demands by the customer for ever-better customer service
- A nearly overwhelming increase in global competition in almost every field of endeavor

Today, nurse managers still have to divide and assign work, but more and more of this responsibility is being assumed by the actual performers themselves. What is really important, however, is that management has finally learned that it cannot *command* employees to deliver their best work; instead, it must create an environment that fosters a *desire* within employees to deliver their best work. In short, today's reality is the partnership that exists between managers and workers in the workplace.

! CRITICAL POINT

In the world of medicine and nursing, the advent of and current reliance on information technology has turned the old way of doing business on its side. With the appearance of computer networks, email, and voice mail, the walls that have traditionally separated individuals, departments, organizations, and even entire industries are crashing down. It used to be that if you wanted information, you had to work your way up, over, and down through the organization. Today you just tap in with your computer. Today, everyone can know as much about an organization as the chairman of the board.

The landscape of business in general and nursing in particular has changed dramatically over the past several decades. Those companies, professions, and individuals that have looked forward and accepted the changes are leaving far behind those that have failed to evolve alongside these changes. There is no longer room for the old mindset of management that treated employees as an "asset" or, worse yet, as children. And why not? you may ask. Because competition is teaching managers how to unleash the power within their employees. Competition is pushing managers past the point of simply talking about these changes;

Flattening is the removal of layers of jobs that traditionally existed between executive management and the front-line performer within a business or organizational structure.

Downsizing and **reengineering** are terms associated with the restructuring of organizations. These occur through the careful analysis of product versus cost and consumer trends, and they are designed to reduce the overhead costs of the organization. Rarely, however, do these modifications reduce the amount of work required to be performed within an organization. The focus is not normally on reduction of performance but instead on reducing the number of people who remain to accomplish that work.

they are making them! Everywhere, in every market, and around the world—and no one is being left out, not in Europe, not in Asia, and not in the Western Hemisphere. Groups like the World Trade Organization, the European Union, the countries participating in the North American Free Trade Agreement, Asian-Pacific Economic Cooperation members, the World Bank, and the International Monetary Fund are making it a rather small world in every aspect of business. Consider for a moment what three leaders have to say:

1. *Multinational business:* The Chrysler Corporation believes that its ability to increase its annual earnings by 246% within a single year is directly attributable to *empowerment*. Today, when decisions are necessary, they are made by someone close to the issue and who has an intimate understanding of the requirements.[1]

2. *Medicine:* Harvard University's dean of the medical faculty, Dr. Joseph B. Martin, has long attributed the school's remarkable success and sterling reputation to its focus on people. He believes that every member of the medical school faculty is given the opportunity to be what they dream of being and that it is his and the medical school's job to make sure people understand that.[2]

3. *Service:* Darryl Hartley-Leonard, former president of the Hyatt Hotels Corporation, was known to put his philosophy regarding empowerment into very simple terms by telling everyone who would listen that employees were not as dumb as many employers thought they were.[3]

It's a New Future

The world of nursing is changing to a degree that was unexpected but was as unavoidable as death and taxes. The nursing profession can no longer place itself in a vacuum and escape these changes, even though individuals and groups will avoid them as long as they can. If individuals really want to be successful nurse managers, however, they will not avoid change but welcome it, savor it, and use it to their advantage, because continual change is a fact of life of tomorrow's nursing.

Things are going to become even more chaotic in this new millennium than they were over the last three decades of the last one. New technologies will continue to advance at lightning speed to provide the nursing profession with quantities of information that no one would have thought possible even 10 years ago.

Smart nursing management programs, recognizing this trend, are infusing their curricula with a man-agerial mindset heavily laced with entrepreneurial enthusiasm, because the survival of the individual nurse manager demands it. In 1987, management guru Tom Peters predicted the dynamic change we are experiencing today in his book *Thriving on Chaos*.[4] He said, "The excellent organizations and individuals of tomorrow will cherish impermanence—and thrive on chaos" (p. 42). The reason is that out of impermanence and chaos come the opportunities that will keep the nursing profession revitalized and growing.

MANAGEMENT IS HARD WORK

No one ever said that managing employees in the healthcare industry would be easy. Those who believe this to be true should probably reevaluate their decision to become nurse managers. The truth is that managing is one of the most difficult—yet potentially most rewarding—jobs that anyone can undertake within an organization.

People are incredibly complex, and to get their best work, day in and day out, nurse managers have to understand what motivates them and what makes them think. As the pace of nursing care has gotten faster, and as restructuring, reengineering, and downsizing have flattened the hierarchies and created a need for nurse managers to share more and more of their traditional duties with the front-line nurse, nurse managers have found their profession to be more complicated than ever before.

Until recently, management was a fairly simple proposition. According to most university MBA programs, all one had to do to become an effective manager was to master the following four classic tasks of management:

1. Planning
2. Organizing
3. Leading
4. Controlling

Become proficient in these four, and no one could deny success. Today, however, the profession of nursing management is undergoing tremendous change. Nurse managers are finding that more and more emphasis is being placed on the ability to lead, and it is becoming apparent that this aspect of the job does not always complement the other three.

Understanding What Managers Do

The definition of *management* (getting work done through others) is deceivingly simple. But, as every nurse manager knows, management can be a very complicated, stressful, and sometimes even traumatic and exhausting job.

Although most of the employees whom the average nurse manager will direct are highly educated technical specialists (those who are able to focus on a fairly narrow range of responsibilities), the healthcare industry expects its nurse managers to be generalists. Instead of knowing a lot about a few topics, nurse managers need to know a little bit about almost everything that falls within the boundaries of their profession and the business environment in which they work.

For example, a nurse might spend all day ministering to the needs of the patients under his or her charge. However, the nurse manager in charge of the unit not only must understand what the particular nurse is doing and why he or she is doing it, but also must understand the jobs of the employees that oversee housekeeping, admissions, human resources, radiologic services, laboratory work, physical therapy, budgeting, auditing, and more. Having technical knowledge or even expertise in this many different areas is not enough for the nurse manager; he or she also needs to understand how to get the best performance possible out of these different employees, day in and day out.

No matter how little actual human contact nurse managers might have during the course of the workday, working with people is the absolute foundation of their job.

In traditional organizations, management is split into the following three basic levels, each with its own unique set of responsibilities and functions:

1. *Executive management:* This group includes such notables as the chairman of the board, chief of staff, chief executive officer, chief operating officer, chief information officer, chief financial officer, vice president for patient services (sometimes known as the chief nursing officer), and other vice presidents and executives. Together, they comprise the organization's highest-ranking management team. This level of management is usually responsible for creating an organization's vision and key goals, for communicating these to other managers and employees, and for monitoring the organization's progress toward meeting them.

2. *Middle management:* Nursing directors, assistant nursing directors, specialty directors, unit coordinators, and many other kinds of managers who report directly to executive management comprise the middle management level. Whereas the job of executive management is to develop an organization's vision and key goals, middle management is tasked with creating the plans, systems, and organizations to achieve them. Middle managers generally report directly to

executive managers but may be individual specialists like auditors.

3. *Supervisors:* Known by an amazing number of specific titles, supervisors are the part of management that works closest with front-line performers. In the nursing profession, this is most often the nurse manager. Because these individuals are closest to the front line, they are also management's link to the organization's customers and patients. Supervisors are responsible for executing the plans developed by middle managers and for monitoring worker performance on a day-to-day basis. Supervisors generally report to middle managers.

The good news is that this traditional model makes seeing where you reside on the corporate ladder easy. The bad news is that the model creates a very clear boundary—a wall, really—separating managers from workers and different levels of managers from one another. As is explained later, however, these traditional walls are starting to crumble in many organizations. Today each junior-level manager is routinely performing roles previously reserved solely for senior managers. The shift away from the traditional roles and their confining boundaries has led to an incredible productivity gain in organizations that have evolved enough to benefit from it.

! **CRITICAL POINT**

As all MBA students learn during the course of their studies, there are four traditional functions of management. In today's fast and furious world of business, these traditional roles are undergoing significant change, and successful managers are learning to adapt to this new environment. These changes are occurring within the nursing profession as rapidly as anywhere else, and intelligent nurse managers develop flexibility, insight, and a positive and cooperative manner when accomplishing their jobs or supervising their employees.

Planning

Organizations need goals. Goals reflect what is most important to an organization, and they make it easier for a manager to prioritize work and to allocate resources such as people, money, and capital equipment. Management's key jobs include developing organizational goals and then planning the strategies and tactics that the organization will use to reach these goals.

For example, to carry out the planning function, the hospital's executive management team may meet in seclusion at a destination removed from the physical site of the hospital. These trips usually last for a full week, and the work goes on nearly around the clock. The goal is to create the organization's 5-year (long-range) plan. It is from this plan that the direction of the organization will be established and the major goals and objectives defined.

WARNING !

*Research has found that in most growing companies, and this includes most healthcare organizations, regular planning is set aside, or at least not considered a critical management function, to allow managers sufficient time to deal with the stresses and demands of day-to-day operations. As a result, individual managers spend most of their time running from one critical situation to another with no yardstick by which to measure their progress. Actions like these cause the organization to drift, like a ship without a rudder. In fact, it is not uncommon to see different members of the same management team possessing **and operating by** completely different goals and objectives, none of which match the key milestones established by executive management.*

It is highly recommended that your organization not allow this complacent attitude to evolve in its management team.

Organizing

Organizing is the allocation of the resources (i.e., people, money, and capital equipment) necessary to achieve the organization's goals. Managers accomplish this task using tools such as organizational charts, assessment of personnel levels, staffing plans, and budgets.

When a management team returns from an offsite planning meeting, for example, team members usually start to coordinate their efforts by drawing up a new organizational chart to implement the plans that they developed during their meetings.

Today's organizations must be faster to adapt and more flexible than ever before. The days of the old-fashioned, rigid organizational chart—with its built-in bureaucracy and hierarchy—are fast disappearing from most organizations. In place are organizations with self-managing work teams, cross-trained workers, virtual employees, flexible work schedules, hot groups, and more. The key to success in the fast-paced world of modern business is the ability to adapt to a rapidly changing marketplace—and to do so completely and without reservation.

Leading

Leading employees means providing a motivating environment and guiding efforts. Today's nurse managers have a wide variety of positive motivational tools at their disposal to accomplish this, including the following:

- Communicating the vision
- Establishing recognition and reward programs
- Providing encouragement
- Personally extending oneself

Of course, the traditional negative motivational tools are still available and, sadly, still in use in many organizations. These include discipline, threats, intimidation, and coercion. But these are rarely resorted to in a leadership environment.

Once the new organization has been designed and implemented, the time comes for the managers to lead the employees by obtaining their buy-in to the new plans, goals, and objectives. In most quality organizations, a good deal of time is spent by executive management visiting with various departments within the organization to discuss the plan and solicit support. Although executive managers may encounter some initial resistance, their willingness to build consensus will eventually bring the most dedicated naysayer into the fold.

Today just being a good manager is not enough; organizations need their managers to be good leaders, to inspire employees, and to encourage them to give their very best every day of the week.

WHAT REALLY *IS* MANAGERIAL LEADERSHIP?

Leadership is a quality to which every manager and would-be manager should aspire and which most are capable of exercising. Napoleon Bonaparte believed that every soldier in his army had the potential to become a general and lead the army in his absence under the right set of circumstances. You may or may not subscribe to this view. However, the practical truth is expressed by the following statements:

- People are not born with natural managerial skill or leadership ability.
- Leadership is not an inherent part of management. It is quite separate and must be developed as part of the total package of skills a manager must deploy.
- No one has ever truly possessed a "divine" right to rule or lead others. This means that managerial ability or leadership skill does not come with, nor is it inherent in, any management position to which you may be assigned, no matter how senior a position you might hold.
- Inculcating leadership skills or managerial skills and developing proficiency in their use is not an intrinsic part of education. Having an advanced degree does not make a manager more capable, simply more educated. Although it is true that many managerial positions are open only to people with degrees, or even advanced degrees, simply possessing one is no guarantee that a person will be successful in a managerial role or

leadership situation. Don't make the mistake of believing that because you have an advanced degree you are a more capable or proficient manager or leader than those who do not.

Managerial leadership is nothing more than a set of qualities that, when demonstrated in the proper context, can cause others to follow. Although this may be a circular definition of the skill, it does indicate that managerial leadership requires two participants: (1) a leader, and (2) a follower. Although it has been hotly debated for generations what, exactly, causes a group to follow one person and not another, the fact is that the average person selects one person to follow for only a few basic reasons.

Throughout history, individuals aspiring to become leaders have had to demonstrate two characteristics over and over again: (1) the ability to inspire others to go beyond what they think they are capable of doing, and (2) the ability to motivate others to accomplish goals previously thought to be unattainable. These two characteristics emerged because the managers worked hard to bring their followers along by doing the following:

- Inspiring trust
- Demonstrating consistency
- Motivating through words and deeds

These characteristics describe what a manager or leader *does*; however, they don't really define what leadership *is*. That is thoroughly explained in the following statement: *Leadership is a willingness to accept responsibility and the accountability that is associated with it, the ability to elicit the assistance of others, the willingness to listen, and the selflessness to put the welfare of others before one's own.* When an individual puts these skills together in the proper combination, people will begin to turn to that person when they require direction. To help in understanding how these things establish the quality of leadership, let's look at each one in depth.

! CRITICAL POINT

*Leadership is a willingness to accept **responsibility** and the **accountability** that is associated with it, the ability to elicit the assistance of others, the willingness to listen, and the selflessness to put the welfare of others before one's own.*

Accepting Responsibility and Accountability

Managerial leadership begins when an individual is willing to embrace responsibility. Simply accepting the responsibilities that come with a management position or the responsibilities that someone else assigns is not enough to demonstrate leadership. To show a capability to lead, the individual must be the one who takes the risk to step forward and say, "I want to do that." No one can be a leader if he or she waits for someone else to assign responsibility.

Beyond that, no one can be a leader if he or she is afraid of responsibility and the accountability that comes with it. History provides a great many examples of this principle; for example, the late U.S. president Harry S. Truman kept a small sign on his desk that said, "The buck stops here!" President Truman knew that, no matter what your role in life, you can never hope to demonstrate leadership unless you accept responsibility. His sign made a bold statement. It said, "If something goes wrong, I am the reason why. Failure is my responsibility and no one else's."

To become a leader, every nurse manager must have the confidence to accept the responsibility for failure. If a nurse manager does not want to accept this aspect of the job, the nurse manager will have an incredibly difficult time getting anyone to accept him or her as leader. In the definition of leadership provided earlier, the point was included that a leader must put the welfare of others above his or her own. No one can demonstrate this quality if he or she assigns blame to others. If a nurse manager is the type of individual who looks outward for an excuse instead of inward for a reason, it is doubtful that he or she will ever be able to inspire trust. If a nurse manager cannot inspire trust, it becomes extremely difficult to solicit the assistance of, or exercise influence over, other people. It doesn't matter what the individual's specific job title is, or what responsibilities the person may have been given with his or her current position.

It is also true that the nurse manager will always receive the lion's share of the credit when things go correctly. No matter how much the nurse manager might tell others that it was his or her subordinates who created the success, it will always be the nurse manager's name that will be remembered longest. Why? Because it is the nurse manager who always shoulders the responsibility and it is the nurse manager who is continually at risk. The willingness to accept responsibility and to assume risk without attempting to seek glory for oneself makes an indelible impression on others. This is the one great benefit of being a nurse manager. Review the following stories and see if you can identify the manager-leader.

TWO HOUSEWIVES

In the early 1970s, two Irish housewives, one Catholic and one Protestant, were appalled by the violence in Northern Ireland. The pair, Betty Williams and Mairead Corrigan, took it upon themselves to do something about it. They sought out the responsibility and assumed the risk by forming an organization known as the Community of Peace People. Their purpose was to open a dialogue between women and children of the warring factions. They reasoned that if hatred could be overcome in the individual home, it could also be overcome in the streets. Their actions were instrumental in bringing to a close one of the most bitter conflicts in history, and for their efforts these two women received the Nobel Peace Prize in 1976.

THE VICE PRESIDENT AND DIRECTOR

In the late 1980s, an up-and-coming individual (we'll call him David) was named vice president and director of nursing operations at a large regional hospital. In this position, he was to direct the operation of the hospital's entire nursing department and was responsible for the quality of health care and service provided to the hospital's patients. David believed that his new position made his wishes law within the nursing department, and he directed his operation on the premise that what he wanted was good for the department and mandatory performance for all who worked for him. It was *his* wishes, implemented in the manner *he* desired, that were acceptable. Any outside ideas were treated as inferior, and those people who had the audacity to possess them were labeled as malcontents and rabble-rousers. If things were not implemented in the exact manner David envisioned, then they were wrong, and those employees who had different approaches and expressed creativity were dealt with ruthlessly. The result was that the hospital David represented lost business to its competition at an unprecedented rate. When these losses occurred, several assistant nursing directors reporting directly to David were assigned blame for the failures and were unceremoniously fired. Ultimately, hundreds of millions of dollars of potential revenue was lost in the 5 years David guided the helm, but far more tragic than the loss of revenue was the loss of image the hospital suffered within the community. When the board of directors finally realized just how bad the situation truly was, it was too late to correct the damage. The hospital, to stem the loss of revenue and with the knowledge that it would cost millions more to recover its image, withdrew from the community. Hundreds of individuals lost their jobs, and the community lost an irreplaceable asset.

It is *never* the position that creates a good manager. The true stories of Betty Williams and Mairead Corrigan clearly demonstrate that anyone can become a leader, and the tragic but also very true story of David shows that it is not position and power that create managerial skill. These cases—and thousands more could be cited—show that the willingness to accept responsibility and accountability is what demonstrates leadership and makes a quality manager.

The willingness to accept responsibility is the foundation of management, and the willingness to be held accountable is the cornerstone of leadership. Without these two characteristics, no one can be a quality manager or be perceived as a leader—*regardless of the position he or she holds.*

Eliciting the Assistance of Others

To be perceived as a leader, a manager must be able to get others to cooperate and go along with what the manager designates as the correct performance. If a manager can cause others to see the future as he or she sees it and agree on the course of action that will be followed to achieve it, then, and only then, will those others cooperate in realizing the manager's vision. A manager will be perceived as a leader only when other people willingly agree to do things the way that the *would-be* leader prescribes.

To accomplish this, the manager must not only have a clear vision of the future (such as the accomplishment of a specific job, the attainment of a certain goal) but must also have the ability to articulate that vision in such a manner that it is easily understood by others, many of whom may be less capable than the "leader."

Listening

As a general rule, people follow others who possess more knowledge about a subject than they do. Do not confuse knowledge with education. Education is the result of formal study; knowledge is the collective wisdom one possesses and can disseminate effectively.

Knowledge is acquired by listening effectively. All great leaders were effective listeners. They were able to gather information from others by listening to what was said and what was not said, and by noticing body language, tone of voice, inflections, and even the movement of a speaker's eyes. If an individual wants to be perceived as a leader, that individual must hone his or her listening skills.

Placing the Needs of Others Above One's Own

Leadership requires that managers be willing to sacrifice their personal goals and desires so that a greater goal can be achieved. This may mean that managers must put their own goals on hold, sometimes for long periods, and work feverishly to help others achieve *their* goals, even if this means a personal loss or setback for the manager.

Leaders help others achieve, and through that achievement gain status for themselves. Being a leader means sacrificing oneself for the benefit of others and allowing others to witness that sacrifice.

Sadly, it is never enough simply to give of oneself unselfishly; one must be able to subtly allow others to know that the sacrifice has taken place. Many times this requires no effort at all on the manager's part, because those for whom sacrifices are being made are a willing audience and will gladly spread the word. However, there are times when the sacrifice is not going to be a matter of public knowledge. At those times, the manager brings forth the achievement quietly and without fanfare, letting the audience hear about the sacrifice as from another.

There is a very fine line between letting others realize that you are sacrificing for them and ingratiating yourself, or, to put it even more simply, blowing your own horn. Horn blowers are seldom viewed as leaders; to the contrary, they are typically perceived as selfish and controlling. So if managers must bring their sacrifices to another's attention, it is imperative that they exercise restraint and caution when doing so.

Practicing Leadership Skills Consistently

To be perceived as a leader, you must be able to elicit assistance from others, listen to the needs of others, and put other people's needs ahead of your own with *consistency*. It is not enough to do these things when it is convenient, or when you feel that it will enhance a gain; even the smallest child can accomplish all three when they wish something from their parents. Only a complete egomaniac does not occasionally listen to the needs of others, and putting the needs of others ahead of your own for a short while is not terribly difficult, especially if it will get you something you desire. When displayed in this self-based manner, however, these skills will not mark you as a leader but rather as a selfish, self-centered individual bent on personal gain.

The key to leadership is to exercise all of these separate skills on a consistent basis so that you, the manager, will be perceived as a reliable practitioner of leadership skills. It is the consistency of effort that people respect (Box 3-2).

MYTHS OF MANAGERIAL LEADERSHIP

Understanding what leadership *isn't* is almost as important a lesson as understanding what it *is*. As with most intangibles, many stories are circulated about leadership, and a good many of them are false. This is especially true when people start to discuss the two very separate subjects of *leadership* and *power*. Because these two concepts are often confused and seem to be inextricably linked, many misconceptions

---

BOX 3-2

Leadership Is Demonstrating Consistency

Consistency makes all the difference in showing leadership. You don't have to occupy high office or be in a position of authority to be a leader. You must do the following three things:
1. Elicit the assistance of others
2. Listen effectively
3. Place the needs of others ahead of your own

You must do these things all of the time, especially when it hurts. That means you don't take credit, you allow it to be shared. You never assume you are right, you allow others to tell you if and when you are, and when you are not you accept the responsibility for failure.

Being a leader is never easy. What makes it especially difficult is that if your attempts to do the three basic things listed earlier are perceived incorrectly by others, you may be marked as having qualities that are completely the opposite of those desired in a leader. The key to being perceived as a leader is demonstrating these three things *consistently*.

---

and untruths have arisen about leadership. There are all kinds of reasons why myths arise about a subject, but in the case of leadership, the one reason that is encountered most often is *to validate an existing power structure's domination over another group*. It is worthwhile to investigate some of these many myths and put them to rest before continuing farther into this subject.

Myth of the Born Leader

In ancient times, and even in some quite modern eras, certain individuals were considered to rule by "divine right"; that is, they obtained their right to rule over a specific group of people from some sort of Supreme Being. The myth of the born leader, sometimes called the "sword in the stone" doctrine, is just as questionable as the concept of divine right. One example of this myth (and the one that gives rise to the term *"sword in the stone" doctrine*) is the legend of King Arthur. According to this legend, only a person of pure heart and purpose would be able to withdraw a certain sword embedded in a stone and thereby win the right be named King of England. Arthur removed the sword and became king. The modern form of the legend was recounted in *The Once and Future King* by T. H. White, who took the theme of the natural leader from the mythology that supports Western civilization.

The myth that leadership is a "right of birth"—for it is indeed a myth—has been used for generations to close out large segments of the population from leadership roles. For example, for centuries the population of the Roman Empire believed that their gods chose their emperors and thereby invested them with the divine right of rule. We, of course, scoff at that belief in today's sophisticated world of modern technology. But then why was a black man not allowed to play quarterback in the National Football League until 1988, when Doug Williams led his team to victory in Super Bowl XXII? And why was it not until 1960 that a Catholic was believed fit to run for the office of President of the United States?

Believers in the myth of the born leader held that these two characteristics, and perhaps thousands more, could not be overcome; that the color of a person's skin or a person's religious persuasion could indicate that the person was of such inferior quality that he or she could never ascend to a leadership position. How wrong we now know these beliefs to have been. The truth is that the myth of the born leader has been used for centuries as an excuse to tolerate a variety of social ills—nearly all of which have some form of prejudice at their roots. This myth has been a significant contributor to the leadership crisis that exists today in the nursing profession and nearly every other field of endeavor, from business management to high political office.

Myth of the Biggest or Fastest

Because children begin to demonstrate leadership qualities at a very early age, many people wrongly believe that successful leadership begins in the school yard. An example of this belief can be found in words often attributed to Arthur Wellesley, first Duke of Wellington, who led the troops that defeated Napoleon at the Battle of Waterloo: "The Battle of Waterloo was won on the playing fields of Eton."[5] At that time people believed that the greatest military officers were graduates of Eton College in England. Because Napoleon was a graduate not of Eton but of France's famed St. Cyr Military Academy, whereas the Duke of Wellington was an Eton graduate, it was a common belief that Napoleon's defeat was foretold before either leader had completed military school.

People want to believe that the swiftest, strongest child—the one who can throw the ball the farthest or fastest—automatically becomes the group leader. It then follows that the children who do not have these skills become the followers, which places them on a lifelong path of supporting roles. On might think this belief would be put to rest forever by the existence of a man like Bill Gates, founder and current CEO of Microsoft, the Seattle-based multibillion-dollar software manufacturer, who is certainly not a physically endowed individual but who is clearly a man who dominates the world of electronic media. However, the myth continues to hold strong in many parts of the world. Obtaining an equitable level of support for women's athletics first required overcoming the belief that leadership skills begin with physical dominance and are demonstrated, possibly even determined, at a very early age. It took an act of the U. S. Congress to establish women's rights in this area (Title IX of the U.S. Code).

Myth That All Managers Are Leaders

One of the most common myths about leadership is that *leadership* and *management* are one and the same. Nothing could be further from the truth. *Management provides the authority to lead. It is not, by itself, leadership.* Leadership is often a dynamic part of management, but the two qualities are very different. Most organizations, including those in the healthcare industry, both for-profit and nonprofit, are structured as a hierarchy. If the organizational chart of such an enterprise is examined, a definite chain of command (management structure) can easily be identified. This document establishes within the organization a system of authority that all decision-making must follow and that all employees, including managers, must acknowledge. This structure gives rise to a principle that says, *if an individual desires to be a leader, he or she must already be in a management position.* It is extremely difficult to demonstrate leadership ability in a nonmanagerial position in such a hierarchically structured organization, and the requirement that an individual be part of the managerial structure before being given the opportunity to demonstrate leadership gives birth to the myth that management is interchangeable with leadership.

MANAGERS MAY BE UNFIT

The difficulty with command (organizational management) structures is that such structures often place people in positions of leadership based on nonleadership criteria. In most segments of the healthcare industry and throughout much of the international business world, for example, a college education is a prerequisite for achieving a position of authority, even though there is no direct correlation between education and intelligence, or education and capability (Box 3-3). The simple assumption that drives this requirement is that individuals who have completed college are sufficiently smart and disciplined to have completed schoolwork voluntarily. What this has to

Important Lesson from History

A classic example of the damage that can be caused by confusing command with leadership occurred during the United States' involvement in the Vietnam conflict. In the decade or so that the United States was involved in that war, countless college-educated men were commissioned as junior officers (lieutenants) and given command over men with more experience and, in many cases, more ability. The truly smart lieutenants deferred to their more experienced noncommissioned officers (sergeants) when decisions were necessary to get them through the dangers of jungle warfare. However, many more made the mistake of thinking that their position within the command structure required that they *make* the decisions and that others *follow* them—no matter how dangerous the consequences may be. These not-so-intelligent officers thought that the command authority they held conferred on them the wisdom of leadership and did not listen—even when faced with a critical situation. This confusion caused many of these young officers to make decisions that imperiled their lives and the lives of the men who served with them.

do with being able to motivate others toward performance excellence is a mystery for the ages.

Another normally accepted prerequisite for a management position is that the individual be thoroughly indoctrinated with the values of the organization. Organizations in the healthcare industry, along with nearly every other type of business, spend endless amounts of training time attempting to instill a "company way" of doing things in their managers and then wonder why the people they have chosen and in whom they have invested so heavily fail in critical leadership situations that require ingenuity, inventiveness, and creativity.

SUCCESS DEPENDS ON LEADERS

Many of the positive changes that have taken place in the healthcare industry over the past two decades have occurred because business in general has realized the dangers inherent in confusing management with leadership. For example, one of the reasons that entrepreneurial companies grow faster than more traditional companies is that they tend to be less formal in their structure. Because these companies do not have "assigned" leadership positions, they are forced to allow leadership to develop within the organization

through the actions of their best performers and most gifted employees. The absence of "key" personnel forces individual employees to exhibit creativity, initiative, and leadership skills as a normal part of their job performance.

MANAGEMENT FOCUSES ON TASKS, NOT PEOPLE

Companies that operate through a well-defined management structure normally provide well-defined tasks and standards of performance to the people operating within that structure and then evaluate the participants according to how well they perform against the standards. Often performance is evaluated using management's established idea of how things should be done, and when real creativity and initiative are shown, performance is graded as poor because it does not reflect the established company standard (Box 3-4).

Traditional organizations also tend to believe that the quantity of work an individual is capable of performing is directly related to the quality of the individual. Assignment of multiple tasks is commonplace, often to the point of smothering the individual performer. The heavy workload and short delivery deadlines that often accompany the assignments limit the performer's ability to exercise his or her imagination and creativity. The driving force within the individual shifts from achieving creative excellence to

Efficiency Does Not Always Equal Quality or Success

A large Midwestern healthcare organization focused its nursing staff on the efficient use of resources instead of applying itself to meeting the needs of specific patients. Nurses who spent more time assisting patients with their needs than the hospital's administration deemed necessary, even if it was a difficult situation, were severely criticized for not supporting the "mission" of the hospital, even when their efforts produced higher patient satisfaction. The result was that the hospital's most profitable and loyal business relationships were severely damaged as the front-line personnel shifted their time to "acceptable" pursuits. Private practitioners had their patients admitted to other facilities located nearby that were known to provide higher quality patient care, even if it meant inconveniencing the patients and their families because of the longer travel distances involved.

"getting it out the door." The trend toward leaner organizations has dramatically intensified this situation.

One of the methods that creative organizations have implemented to remove some of the negative performance factors from their evaluation process is the requirement that supervisory employees share responsibility for the failure of any individual given a task to perform. This is a Band-Aid approach, however, and does not solve the problems inherent in the traditional organizational structure.

Too many organizations rely on their "command" structure to move their businesses forward. The challenge here is that possessing a well-developed command structure has little to do with effective management, let alone with quality leadership. These structures are about authority and keeping the enterprise moving in the direction it is already going. They are rarely about exploring new directions, no matter how desperately the latter may be needed.

The critical factor here is that *authority* is not *management,* nor is it *leadership.* Moving individuals into managerial roles without adequately training them in the proper methods of administering their authority or in the process of leading other people is an injustice to the organization, to the managers, and, most certainly, to the subordinate employees who must answer to them.

UNDERSTANDING LEADERSHIP POTENTIAL

Leadership is an integral part of human interaction. Even in a world in which work is performed by consensus, the qualities of leadership—listening well, evoking assistance from others, and placing the needs of others or of the group above one's own—are essential to human progress. It is a very real truth that few things get done unless the individual members of an organization pull together, and little teamwork is developed without the presence of leadership. Therefore, every organization must have a clear picture of who its leaders really are and how these individuals emerge from within the organization's structure. It is important, then, that every organization remember the following basic principles regarding the creation of leaders:

Every person has the potential to become a leader. The qualities of leadership enumerated earlier are qualities that any person can choose to make his or her own. This is what is meant when it is said that any person can become an effective leader. The challenge is that each person must *choose* to do so. Anyone can be placed into a managerial position, but whether or not leadership flows from the position afterward is completely up to the individual who occupies it. Individual choice, not occupancy, identifies leaders in their positions of authority.

Leadership is the result of motivation—not birth or circumstance. Leaders arise because individuals possess a rare combination of talent and zeal and are capable of channeling their enthusiasm into enhancing the performance of others. No one is a born leader, and the challenge of circumstance does not create greatness. Although outside influences such as the environment during childhood or the level of education can certainly contribute to one's ability to lead, they are incapable of producing leadership by themselves. It is only because the environment and/or education taught the importance of sacrifice and the willingness to accept the excellence in others that the quality of leadership emerges.

In addition, although it is certainly true that critical circumstances can vault an individual to notoriety, circumstances rarely cause an individual to perform well. Napoleon, arguably one of history's great leaders, was a child of poverty who pushed himself to greatness because he possessed an incredible ability to persuade others to do his bidding. John F. Kennedy overcame tremendous bigotry to lead America during one of its most critical periods.

Leadership is a quality that comes from within each individual, and every individual has the ability to bring it forth. The difference is that some *choose* to do so, and others simply do not. Humans have proven time and time again that any adversity can be overcome if one possesses the will and the motivation to do so.

Effective management and the quality of leadership cannot exist without responsibility and accountability. The reason that people feel that effective management and leadership are products of circumstances is that significant events cause people to stand up and accept the responsibility for dealing with them.

The acceptance of responsibility is the fundamental step every manager must take if he or she wishes to be perceived as a leader, regardless of his or her position within the management structure. Without the willingness to step forward and say, "I want to do that," no manager can become a leader. This is what was meant earlier when it was said that people have to "want" to do something, not just be content with having responsibilities assigned to them. The decision to seek responsibility should never be a hasty one. Acceptance of responsibility involves risk—personal risk—and any manager seeking responsibility should understand that by doing so he or she also risks being held accountable.

Being held accountable is the part of responsibility that scares off most people who occupy management positions. Being held accountable means that, if things go wrong, it is the manager who will be found deficient or at fault, or who will be chastised for the failure. Leaders willingly take on this risk and then apply themselves effectively through the use of their motivational skills to ensure that the responsibility is discharged successfully. When something does go wrong, the leader does not attempt to place blame on another person. Leadership means that the responsibility for failure is the leader's alone. Success can and should be shared with all that participate, but failure is solely the leader's burden.

Managers who accept the cloak of leadership know that there is no real reason to fear failure. Even at its worst, failure is nothing more than a learning opportunity, and many times, it is the most effective way a lesson can be taught. It is not failure that destroys, but the inability to use it as the opportunity it presents that results in lasting damage. The late Malcolm Forbes was a dominant leader in the business world because he understood, and took great pleasure in telling others, that "failure is success if we learn from it." These words echo those of the great industrialist Henry Ford, who said, "One who fears failure limits his activities. Failure is only opportunity, more intelligently presented, that allows us to begin again." Finally, Sir Winston Churchill declared, "The price of greatness is responsibility."

Leadership improves human dignity. Although most people would consider this aspect more a result of leadership than one of its distinguishing traits, it is mentioned here because it is so important to the welfare of the group. Good leadership, as displayed through the practice of quality management, improves the level of human dignity enjoyed by every individual affected by it and has a profound influence on the capabilities, attitudes, and performance of any group. Leadership, by its mere presence, encourages others to do more, take greater pride in their work, and generally enjoy their productive efforts.

Almost all managers will be called upon to be leaders at some point in their careers, at least for a little while, even if they do not realize it. For example, every person who has filled the role of nurse has been perceived, at least initially, as a leader. Taking on this role means accepting the responsibilities that ensure the well-being and survival of another life. If you have ever volunteered to serve on a committee, even in a subordinate role, the very act of stepping forward and volunteering, of putting yourself at risk for the good of the group, has made you a leader.

Leadership is something that most people actually practice throughout their lives and are only afraid of when they are confronted with the prospect of failure. As this chapter has indicated, however, failure is nothing more than a learning opportunity when it is put to good use. The fear of facing an opportunity to grow should never hold back any nurse from accepting additional responsibility.

NEEDS OF MANAGERS AND LEADERS

Some people within the healthcare industry will never believe that any person can be a leader. The reaction of this group of naysayers is, "If it's so easy, why doesn't everyone do it?" A further truth about leadership answers this question: although leadership *is* something than anyone can achieve, it is seldom easy, never happens naturally, and rarely occurs without significant effort. Leadership is the result of putting someone who possesses the desire, training, and circumstances to lead together with a group of people who require leadership. The development of quality management as demonstrated through the exercise of leadership is often a result of trial and error, exposure, and personal risk. Not everyone is willing to pay the price that this process can extract. Even for those who are willing to pay this price, however, leadership is rarely something that can be attained without help. Let us take a look at what someone needs to become a leader.

Leaders Need Training

There are many leaders in the nursing profession; most of these people simply need some encouragement and training to bring out their leadership qualities. Leaders require training. Even after being elected, a new president of the United States of America or a new chairman of the People's Republic of China receives a thorough education in the roles and responsibilities that come with this position. Napoleon, as has been noted previously, undertook long, demanding years of training before entering the French army. Mao Tse-tung received a wide variety of lessons that included both formal education and tremendous hardship before rising to greatness. John F. Kennedy trained at Harvard, was an officer in the U.S. Navy, and served for over 10 years in the U.S. Congress before being elected president. The list of recognized leaders could go on for pages, and every one of them would share a similar characteristic: all had to receive some form of training before they rose to leadership.

All leaders go through periods of training before taking on additional responsibilities, and no leader rises to the top without the assistance of others. One does not just come to **greatness**. Achieving it is a long process filled with exposure to small events that join together to become experience and ability. The path of leadership, even after it is attained, is one of constant training and retraining, of open-mindedness and a desire to enhance one's skills. Training is an everyday and lifelong event for the leader.

Leaders Need Goals

A classic reason that emerging as a leader is such a tough process for the average manager is that leadership requires a goal that cannot be attained without the leader's help. If a group of people are capable of dealing with their own problems on a day-to-day basis, they do not require leadership. It is only when the group members require direction and guidance to attain a goal that leadership is necessary. The goal then is a fundamental part of leadership.

Many people have ascended to positions of great power but have not been regarded as significant leaders. A recent example is former U.S. president Bill Clinton. On his campaign trail, his advisors told him and the nation, "It's the economy, stupid." What this meant when loosely translated was, "It's not leadership, stupid." As a student of history, Clinton realized that the best thing to do in times of economic certainty was to get out of the way and help the economy build on itself by loosening regulation and lowering interest rates. This was not a leadership decision, however, but rather calculated thinking that rightly viewed the economy as something that had a life of its own. Because Clinton the candidate was smart enough to stay out of the way of market capitalism, he created for himself a smooth road to the White House.

Conversely, after being elected, *President* Clinton was expected to lead, even though there were few real opportunities for him to demonstrate his capacity for the art. What resulted was perhaps President Clinton's greatest failure: he could not identify a leadership role for himself. Without the focus created through the exercise of leadership, his administration became embroiled in scandal.

Leaders Need Followers

Leadership depends on reaction. When managers are listening carefully to the needs of others and what is heard is that their groups do not require anything from them, then what is really being said is that there is no opportunity to demonstrate leadership. If managers persist in trying to lead when no leadership is required, the very people they are attempting to help will regard them as pests or, worse yet, as bores.

Furthermore, the managers are likely to become identified as insignificant individuals, and then when people *do* need help in reaching a goal, they will not be inclined to listen to those managers' views.

People have to be *willing* to follow another person. Managers create this desire in others by providing them with an example to emulate, not by attempting to direct efforts that they themselves are capable of performing. If a manager sets a good example, is willing to take responsibility, accepts accountability, and makes a sincere effort to help others enhance their own capabilities, people will recognize that manager as having leadership capability. When circumstances permit, and the manager steps forward to accept it, the manager will be rewarded for his or her patience with a leadership role.

Managers—*all* managers—want to be involved in leadership. The challenge that many of them face is that they are not patient enough to develop the foundations that create willingness in others to follow: trust, consistency, and example in deeds and words.

LEADERSHIP IS THE EMOTIONAL SIDE OF MANAGEMENT

To do the things necessary to be perceived as a leader—elicit assistance, listen well, and place the needs of others above their own—managers must demonstrate emotional maturity, wisdom, and humility. Psychologist Daniel Goleman described the ability to embrace responsibility as *emotional intelligence*. He defined this quality as a combination of the right proportions of self-awareness, self-regulation, motivation, empathy, and social skill. Goleman also believed that the higher up the ladder of responsibility one goes, the more critical leadership skills become and the higher the level of emotional intelligence that must be displayed if success is to be achieved.[6]

Emotional intelligence as described by Goleman depends on one or more of the critical skills necessary for good leaders. Let us examine how three of the leadership skills discussed earlier correlate with and complement the qualities associated with emotional intelligence.

Greatness is defined for the purposes of this text as the quality of having earned the admiration of others through a positive demonstration of one's capabilities. Under this definition, John Kennedy, Mao Tse-tung, Syngman Rhee, Florence Nightingale, and Dr. Jonas Salk, for example, would be considered "great."

Ability to Elicit Assistance

The ability to motivate a group depends on the ability to elicit assistance from individuals: first from oneself, and then from others.

The idea of assisting oneself may seem slightly humorous, but it is essential to success. The process is best demonstrated when an individual takes on an unpleasant task and excels at it. The accomplishment of such a task often requires an act of conscious will. That is self-assistance. The fact is that anyone can do a job when little is being risked and nothing personal can be lost. It is when you would prefer not to do the job, but do a great job anyway, that you become a professional.

People are much more likely to assist their manager if they feel that their assistance is welcome and will be appreciated. One of the best ways to gather the support needed when the chips are down is to be grateful for what is received when the risk is minimal.

Ability to Listen

Self-awareness, self-regulation, and empathy all begin with the ability to listen, both to one's inner voice and then to the voices of others. Listening to oneself helps one understand one's own drive and motivation, whereas listening to others helps reveal what drives and motivates them.

Ability to Place the Needs of Others Above One's Own

Self-regulation depends on the ability to do for others before doing for oneself. This is necessary because things often will not go a manager's way, and when adversity arises it is important that managers not show disappointment or hostility, or seek to place the blame elsewhere. Managers are always held accountable for their actions, and maintaining control in situations of adversity demonstrates dependability, reliability, and understanding.

It is absolutely imperative that managers be able to maintain control over their emotions and continually demonstrate a high degree of emotional intelligence in the day-to-day discharge of their responsibilities. Goleman deduced from his studies that the demonstration of emotional intelligence accounted for 90% of the difference between average performers and recognized leaders.[6] If managers lose control of their emotions when they carry out their normal work or when they are under mild stress, there is every reason to believe that they will not be allowed to assume a leadership role when greater responsibility is required.

Let us now take a look at the five key attributes of emotional intelligence over which managers must maintain control if they are to be perceived as leaders.

Self-Awareness

Self-awareness is the ability to recognize and understand one's moods, emotions, and drives, but beyond that, it is the ability to recognize the effect these things have on others. How managers project themselves has a big impact on the willingness of others to recognize them as leaders and to follow the instructions they receive.

Managers who demonstrate a high level of self-awareness are almost universally harder on themselves than are other people. They demand far more in their performance than they expect from others and deliver results by focusing their energies on the task at hand.

On the job, how managers accept their responsibilities and roles is a critical measure of self-awareness. Do they simply accomplish the tasks they are given, or do they embrace these responsibilities and look for the value in their work? Do they allow the trivial events of the day keep them from performing at their highest capacity or can they brush aside these minor events and stay focused on accomplishing their goals? Do they deal effectively with disappointments and failures, possibilities always faced by leaders?

Self-Regulation

Self-regulation describes the actions necessary to control or redirect disruptive impulses such as anger, prejudice, stubbornness, and mood shifts. It also includes the abilities to suspend judgment and to think carefully before acting.

To effectively manage oneself is not an easy process. Human beings are emotional and reactive by nature. When exposed to outside stimuli, all have the tendency to be territorial and protective of the things that have become comfortable to them. Add to this the fact that no two individuals are exactly the same and most likely will not react to the same stimulus in an identical manner, and one can see that the opportunity for conflict and confrontation is always but a breath away. It takes real control to hesitate, take a deep breath, and ask oneself, "Could it be different than what I am seeing?" Most of the time the answer will be, "Yes, it could be a great deal different." Self-management means taking that second to entertain the possibility of difference and being smart enough to realize that being different does not necessarily mean being wrong.

As reported by Schneider,[7] Leonard Michelson, MD, PhD, of the University of Michigan Medical School stated that the normal reaction to an outside stimulus is a three-step process: (1) perception, (2) thought, and (3) action. He also noted, however, that in many instances response to an outside stimulus is an automatic process that has been learned through previous encounters with the stimulus, perhaps even by preceding generations. For example, when we touch something hot, we immediately pull away from it. We don't stop to perceive that the item is hot, nor do we think about how we will react—we just jerk our hand away. The same holds true for actions people may take when they work under stress or when their opinions are challenged. They simply respond—many times without thinking or concerning themselves with the possible outcomes such a response can create.

A manager who demonstrates self-control is less likely to respond emotionally to a situation. Self-control has the tendency to slow down the action, instead of speeding it up. When managers use self-control, they buy themselves time to assess the situation and try to figure out the right thing to say or do that will result in positive movement toward a goal or agreement on a subject.

Motivation

Motivation is the passion a person has for the work in which he or she is involved. It can be seen when an individual pursues a goal with energy and persistence. It is the drive that compels a person to go beyond the expectations of others. It is the joy that is experienced by someone who enjoys accomplishing.

Motivation also involves the ability to communicate one's individually held passion to others. Merely approaching work with enthusiasm and gusto is not enough. Managers who want to be perceived as leaders must radiate their commitment so that their emotions are contagious to those about them. This is a critical part of developing the means of evoking assistance from others.

A motivated manager serves as an example for others and through that example gains the ability to obtain help when necessary.

Empathy

Emotional intelligence involves not *sympathy*, but *empathy*. Many managers get these two responses mixed up. Sympathy is the willingness to feel compassion toward another. Empathy is the ability to understand another's emotional makeup and the skill to treat a person according to his or her ability; that is, to deal emotionally with another's efforts. Empathy is not a touchy-feely experience; it involves the ability to listen and the willingness to put someone else's needs above one's own.

When managers handle a situation by adopting the other person's perspective, when they look for reasons other than those that are obvious to explain why something occurred, and when they are willing to put aside their own priorities to help others accomplish theirs, they are acting empathetically.

Social Skill

Social skill is the willingness to manage relationships, to build support networks, to find common ground, and to build rapport.

The ability to find common ground between themselves and others is instrumental in helping managers create relationships. When managers can communicate their desires in terms that every person addressed can understand, they have greatly enhanced their ability to move people toward finding a resolution to shared problems. To accomplish this and to build trust within their groups, managers who want to be perceived as leaders operate in a friendly and open manner, and project enthusiasm and optimism. Leaders know that people *share* trust; it is not something that can be asked for or demanded. Highly motivated managers work hard to develop trust within their group, and once they have obtained it they guard it carefully.

WHY LEADERSHIP WITHIN MANAGEMENT RANKS IS SO HARD TO IDENTIFY

If becoming a leader is something that anyone can do, then why do a great many people bemoan the shortage of leaders? If you read any noteworthy publication, from the *Harvard Medical Review* to *Fortune* magazine, you will come across articles contending that a critical shortage of leaders exists at every level. "Where are the eloquent, inspirational people like Mao, Roosevelt, Churchill, Gandhi, John Kennedy, and Ho Chi Minh?" complain the writers of today.

In reality, leadership is nothing more than a comprehensive set of skills that can be learned by anyone and then honed to enhance one's capability, but the general perception in the healthcare industry, and in business in general, is that good leadership is a scarce commodity. The following sections help to explain just why this perception is so prevalent today.

Leaders May Appear in Response to Circumstances

Managers who possess leadership ability are usually all around us, working at normal jobs, at junior levels, awaiting the circumstances that will propel them into the spotlight. If it is true that leadership potential exists in nearly everyone, then one must conclude that there is not a shortage of leaders, but a shortage of circumstances that allow their individual leadership skills to come to the forefront.

This point can be proved by examining two of history's most complex U.S. presidents: Herbert Hoover and Franklin Delano Roosevelt (FDR). President Hoover led the nation through World War I and afterward worked diligently to develop a league of nations that should have helped to prevent the catastrophe of World War II. The Great Depression struck America in 1929, however. Hoover failed to respond adequately and because of this inability lost the recognition that should have been his as a great humanitarian. FDR, on the other hand, was thought of in most circles as a weak-kneed patrician and a pale image of his cousin Teddy Roosevelt. But after his election to the presidency, FDR set upon a program of listening to the miseries of the common person and working toward easing them. His ability to listen and to act on what he heard turned Roosevelt's reputation toward greatness.

Another example is Harry Truman, a tailor from Missouri and a scoffed-at lackey of the Pendergast political machine who was forced on a reluctant FDR as a running mate in the waning days of World War II. When Roosevelt died shortly after winning his unprecedented fourth term, the mantle of leadership fell on the poorly prepared Truman. To his credit, and to the total surprise of many, he rose to the occasion, bringing the war to a swift and decisive conclusion and extending the benefits of FDR's economic reforms to most of rural America.

The simple fact is that neither FDR nor Truman may ever have been recognized for his leadership if the circumstances had been different. Although both of them certainly possessed the qualities of leadership, without the circumstances of depression and death forcing each of them into a leadership role, it is unlikely that either would have had the opportunity to demonstrate his total capability nor to win the respect of his followers.

Leadership May Not Necessarily Be a Desired Quality

If one takes a cynical look at why leadership is often thought of as scarce, one might come to the realization that many organizations simply don't want around people who demonstrate the positive and often forceful traits of leadership *until* circumstances demand them. Possibly the very qualities that allow people to step forward and meet the most demanding of challenges are the same ones that will keep them out of high-visibility roles unless circumstances demand it.

Consider the case of Sir Winston Churchill. He was a shrill, unwanted voice in the darkness of the 1930s as Europe placated Hitler. When his predecessor,

Prime Minister Neville Chamberlain, talked of "peace in our time" and was greeted with cheers in the streets of London, it would have been difficult to find 10 people who knew anything positive at all about Churchill. A short time later, however, as British troops were being pushed into the sea at Dunkirk, the British voters jumped to Churchill's cries of war. Yet the zeal born out of desperation did not sustain him; within months of the war's end, British voters ousted what many now consider their greatest statesman ever, because they grew tired of his style of leadership.

MANAGEMENT AND LEADERSHIP: THE BASIC RELATIONSHIP

Up to this point, this initial chapter on basic management and leadership has focused on developing a fundamental understanding of how the skill of management and the art of leadership operate and complement each other in a business situation.* There is one more aspect of this topic that needs to be discussed before we move on, and that is the relationship between management and leadership. Many people operate under the misguided perception that these two are one and the same, but this chapter has repeatedly argued that they are not and has presented evidence that supports this contention. Leadership asks the *what* and *why* questions, whereas management tends to focus on the *how*. Managers who exercise good leadership tend to carry out their responsibilities by empowering their subordinates, whereas traditional managers tend to hold close their authority to enact change. Under an empowerment structure, responsibility is not stolen from employees but openly shared with them. In a classic structure, management holds responsibility within itself and does not share the opportunity or the credit that is associated with the possession of authority. The following two important distinctions separate classic management from leadership-directed management:

1. *Things are managed; people are led.* Admiral Grace Hopper, a professional nurse and the first woman to obtain flag rank in the United States Navy, understood that a major difference between management and leadership was the object of the actions taken. She believed that managers work with processes, models, and

---

*Throughout this text the authors consider the nursing profession as a business. Although few professional nurses think of their vocation as part of a business, it is. As competition among healthcare organizations intensifies, more and more emphasis will be placed on this aspect of nursing.

systems—things. Leaders, on the other hand, work with people.[8]

2. *Management focuses on doing things right; leadership focuses on the right thing.* Warren Bennis, a professor at the University of Southern California, has made a career of studying the habits of leaders (particularly corporate executives). He has pointed out that when an individual thinks about doing things right, control mechanisms and the how-to of things are brought to mind. This process is referred to as management. When the individual considers the future, however, the mind immediately thinks about doing the right things—about dreams, missions, strategic intent, and purpose. This approach is often referred to as leadership.[9]

! *CRITICAL POINT*

Doing the right thing is never enough if you do not do it correctly, and doing things correctly will not work if you are not doing them for the right reason. Excellent leadership is best demonstrated when it is coupled with effective management, and excellent management is never achieved without demonstrated leadership at its core.

LEADERSHIP AS A TEMPORARY MANAGEMENT CONDITION

It is totally improper to believe that because an individual takes the lead he or she will remain there, because the conditions that cause leadership to occur are *always* temporary. Leadership, or the act of leading, takes place because three things have intersected: (1) a goal, (2) a need, and (3) a person who is willing to accept responsibility. Because this is true, the very act of providing leadership is something that depends on being in the right place at the right time.

The situation is even more complex than that. Different situations and different times require different types of leadership. If the circumstances call for leadership and the appropriate person is available to provide that leadership, the best type of leadership, *situational* leadership, is available. At other times, the match-up is not correct—either the leader available doesn't suit the conditions, or the leader is appropriate but the timing is wrong. When leadership occurs under these two types of conditions, different kinds of leadership are seen: *transitional* and *hierarchical* leadership, respectively.

This part of the chapter focuses on the various forms of leadership and provides you with methods to detect which type exists, under what combination of time and circumstances. The goal is to help you understand that you, as a potential leader, must approach the demonstration of leadership with flexibility and an open mind. The effective and high-quality leadership you delivered yesterday may be totally inappropriate for the combination of conditions and time that exists when you next have the opportunity to show leadership.

Leadership is not something that repeats itself exactly every time it is exercised. You, as a potential leader, cannot learn a single system or form of leadership and use it over and over again. You must learn the principles of leadership and use them in varying combinations to match the specific conditions and time.

Leadership is transient, and a manager is allowed just so many chances to succeed before followers start to look elsewhere for another leader. Most people are willing to follow, but nearly everyone will pass judgment on the competence of the leadership provided and will question the ability of the individual each time a new set of circumstances appears. It is a rare individual who is so blindly loyal to another that he or she never questions that person's ability to provide leadership in a given situation. The following story illustrates this principle:

> After Joseph Stalin passed away, a power struggle ensued for control over the communist party within the Politburo of the Union of Soviet Socialist Republics (USSR). Nikita Khrushchev eventually rose to the forefront, but his hold on the reins of government was shaky at best. One day, while cleaning out Uncle Joe's old desk and settling in, the newly appointed premier came across a well-battered but elegant box. Prying open the tiny lock that held it closed, the Premier found that the box contained three letters, each tied with a red ribbon, and a note that read, "To my successor." On the first envelope were printed the words, "To be opened during your first crisis." Since Khrushchev was having difficulty extricating himself from the power struggle that continued around him, he opened the envelope. A single card of the finest linen paper had two simple words written on it: "Blame me." Khrushchev immediately called together what would later be named the Third Party Congress, denounced Stalin, won widespread support, and averted the crisis of leadership.
>
> Several years later, Khrushchev, faced with open revolt in several of the Soviet states, felt that the conditions were right to call this period his "second crisis." He again opened the elegant but battered box and took out the second note. Thereupon were printed the following four words, "Do as I did!" Khrushchev applied the wisdom with terrible efficiency, brutally crushing revolts in Hungary, Poland, and East Germany. Once again he averted chaos, but only temporarily.
>
> By the mid-1960s, with the Soviet State in the midst of widespread famine and his sixth 5-year plan

failing miserably, Khrushchev opened the last of the three letters. This time the note read, "Choose a new leader and write him three letters."

Leadership is a temporary condition for the following two very good reasons:

1. *The circumstances may end.* Leading is about helping another person satisfy a need or attain a goal. It is easy to understand that, once the goal is reached or the need is satisfied, the need for leadership is also fulfilled. This can be easily understood by examining the following question: What does the dog do with the car he was chasing once he has caught it?

2. *Times and requirements change.* The respected, even revered leader of today, unless he or she changes to keep pace, will find himself or herself out of touch with the requirements posed by tomorrow's needs. The circumstances that called forth the leader's excellence may change, and the skills and energies used yesterday may not be sufficient to satisfy the new requirements. In fact, tomorrow's struggle may be directly opposed to every quality leaders used to satisfy yesterday.

Fig. 3-1 illustrates the way in which timing and circumstances work together to give rise to different types of leadership—or, for that matter, to no leadership at all.

SITUATIONAL LEADERSHIP

Situational leadership—the right person in the right place at the right time—is obviously the most effective type of leadership. One of the best ways to witness this type of leadership is to read the daily newspaper. There you will find literally hundreds of news reports that depict the right people responding to a set of circumstances at the right time to fulfill a leadership role—a *situational* leadership role.

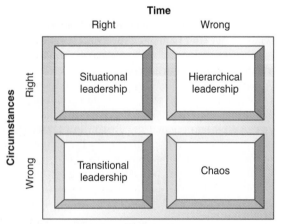

Fig. 3-1 ■ The type of leadership that arises depends on the specific combination of time and circumstances.

To validate his belief in the commonality of situational leadership, Marshall Loeb, former managing editor of *Fortune* and *Money* magazines, once performed a lengthy exercise as part of his research for a book he was preparing on the subject of leadership. Using an average local newspaper, Loeb searched articles for examples of where leadership had been displayed. He excluded both sports articles, which commonly show leadership examples, and obituaries. Surprisingly, he found more than 80 articles displaying leadership. This experiment can be performed using any hometown newspaper and is a good way to develop a better understanding of what situational leadership is and how often it occurs in life.

In situational leadership, a chain of events creates the need for someone to step forward out of the crowd and provide direction. Each example in the news accounts that you will read later in this chapter describes specific conditions that called for someone to take a stand or make a decision exactly at that time— before the moment was lost. As you will see as we explain the circumstances surrounding each news story, all of the individuals who stepped forward became leaders as they rose to meet the needs of the moment.

We have tried to show a variety of different situations, often dramatic ones. This has been done because the situations in which leadership occurs are not always obvious. Sometimes leadership will emerge in the midst of a great crisis, and at other times it will appear because of an argument or disagreement that requires resolution. In still other cases the leader stands up for a principle or defends someone less capable than himself or herself. Regardless of the details, each case describes a moment in time when someone was needed to step forward and advance a cause or a goal, or simply to take charge of a situation so that the outcome would be improved.

Situational leadership is going on everywhere, at every moment of every day. Each person living on earth is capable of becoming a situational leader. When the right set of circumstances presents itself, you will be able to become a situational leader if you practice the leadership skills described earlier in the chapter.

The following leadership examples are organized by the type of decisions made by the leader to assess the situation and assume the role of leader in the given situation.

Safety and Welfare Decision

This first news story deals with a yacht race that ended in tragedy. High winds and giant ocean swells swamped many of the boats involved in the race, and, despite

Yachtsmen Reluctant to Leave Race

Larry Ellison, founder and chief executive officer of software giant Oracle Corp., and his 80-foot yacht Sayonara *crossed the finish line Tuesday to win the famed race from Sidney, Australia, to Hobart, Tasmania, for a second time. "It wasn't a race," he said. "We were focused on getting the boat here in one piece and every member of the crew with it."*

the best efforts of well-trained search and rescue teams, several of the racing enthusiasts drowned. On board the yacht *Sayonara*, skipper and industrialist Larry Ellison faced a critical decision when the rescue teams wanted to take his crew to safety. Should he give the order to abandon his yacht to the Pacific Ocean and allow his team to board the waiting helicopters and fly to safety, or should he attempt to bring the yacht through the storm with its entire crew still on board?

The decision (and the process Ellison used to arrive at that decision) was a classic case of situational leadership. As an extremely wealthy man, Ellison could have afforded to make either decision. Losing the expensive yacht would probably not have resulted in an irremediable economic loss, and paying the cost of helicopters to come out and pick up himself and his crew and carry them to safety was an expense that he could easily bear. Putting these two things aside, Ellison was really confronted only with the needs of the situation. Assuming his role as leader, he talked with the crew and solicited their ideas and cooperation, and together they assessed the situation. Together, they decided to finish the race and not abandon the boat, a decision that Ellison made easier by pointing out that, if the situation worsened, he would call for evacuation.

Moral Decision

The second story deals with the personal decision of a nurse who strongly believed himself to be a conscientious objector to military service. It depicts the dilemma that can be created when one's beliefs conflict with laws. In this case, the nurse stuck to his beliefs, even in the face of personal hardship, and did not give in to a law that he felt was unjust. The nurse involved knew that the decision to stand up for his

Nurse Gets Hard Time

An American nurse said in an open letter from his prison cell that he would not appeal his 10-year sentence. His decision came from his firm resolve to eliminate the mandatory service section for medical personnel, which is part of the selective service law. The letter ended in the words "penned with continued resolve."

beliefs could cost him as much as 10 years in prison. He reasoned that he could have escaped this fate if he would only renounce his beliefs and allow himself to be inducted into the army. If he did, he would be able to live a "normal" life. But if he chose to stand up for his beliefs, he would truly demonstrate that his beliefs were genuine and not contrived to eliminate the possibility of service in the armed forces. He felt that his actions would demonstrate that the law requiring medical service in time of national emergency was unconstitutional and should be abolished, and by accepting the alternative of jail, he hoped to rally other professionals to oppose this law.

This nurse had to exercise an entirely different kind of situational leadership. If we believe that the bottom line of leadership is to help a group of people move toward the accomplishment of a goal, then the act of selfless commitment in the hope of inspiring others takes the simplicity of leadership to levels approaching heroism. The nurse, who ultimately was not successful in getting the obligatory service statute repealed, was repeatedly asked by the court to abandon his quest and return to a normal life. Each time he was asked, he politely—but firmly—refused.

By refusing to make an appeal, the dissident nurse believed himself to be questioning the very authority (the U.S. Selective Service Act) that had caused him to be sentenced to confinement. Whether you agree with this nurse's actions or not, it is important to see that, at great personal sacrifice, he used the situation to assert his leadership and bring the issue of a human being's right to self-determination to national attention.

Inspirational Decision

This news item concerns a man who understood that only in extremely rare situations does a leader have the opportunity to please all of the people with his or her decision. Actually, as you seek to be a leader, it will not be uncommon for the people asking for a decision from you to have views diametrically opposed to your own. How will you handle situations like this? How will you demonstrate situational leadership when the group you wish to lead does not believe as you do?

Are Computers Godless?

A leading Orthodox rabbi ruled this week that the word God *may be erased from a computer screen or disk, because the pixels do not constitute real letters. Rabbi Moshe Shaul Klein published his ruling this week in a computer magazine aimed at Orthodox Jews. According to Jewish law, all printed matter with the word* God—Elohim *in Hebrew—and its manifestations in any other language must be stored or ritually buried.*

As was mentioned earlier, many people believe that, to be an effective leader, you must possess the wisdom of King Solomon, and that, if you don't, you must make your decision using the same type of deductive reasoning that Solomon employed. In the story of Solomon, two women brought a child to the king to decide which of the women had a more legitimate claim to the child. Each woman declared that she was the baby's mother. After hearing their stories, Solomon drew his sword and said that, because it was impossible for him to determine the true mother, he would cut the child in half and give each woman a part. The woman who was the baby's real mother immediately gave up her claim because she could not bear to see the child hurt. King Solomon viewed this selfless act as proof of her claim and gave that woman the child.

The New York Rabbi, Moshe Shaul Klein, was not faced with as dramatic a decision as the great king of the ancient Hebrews, but he did have a challenge in front of him that he viewed as having biblical proportions. He knew that Orthodox Jews were facing a serious challenge in determining how they should exercise their ancient Hebrew laws in the face of new technology. He listened to several opinions and weighed them carefully, because he believed that a wrong decision would make it impossible for Jews to use computers and cost them the benefit of employing the most advanced technology available.

By rendering the verdict he did, Rabbi Klein actually followed in the footsteps of the ancient Hebrew king. In making his decision, our modern-age Solomon looked for a common ground between his beliefs and the desires of the group and, at the same time, left room for just a smattering of vagueness. His ruling is one for the ages; it could never have presented itself until the advent of computers and will not change until some more powerful group refuses to accept Rabbi Klein's decision.

Decision for the Greater Good

As the full news article relates, Madelyn Freundlich had taken a stand regarding a case involving the separation of siblings in a proposed adoption. By doing so, Freundlich was exercising leadership in the abstract. Freundlich had no legal standing in this particular case but maintained a high degree of involvement based on an interest in the procedures that were used to qualify spe-

cific adoption processes. Her beliefs were based on a lengthy research study and a concern for what she viewed as the potential psychologic harm that can occur when children are separated from the love of a sibling. This case just happened to occur at a time of heightened awareness and concern over adoption issues in the United States.

The precedent that Freundlich felt provided the foundation for her participation in the case was first established during the latter part of the 1960s. At that time, the Sierra Club, an international environmental group headquartered in San Francisco, California, filed an *amicus curiae* brief (a brief filed by a "friend of the court"—a group with no legal standing in the lawsuit) on behalf of a group of ancient redwood trees in California. The suit was filed because the Sierra Club believed it had a constitutional right to represent something that obviously could not represent its own rights.

Freundlich labored long and hard in her assumed leadership role on behalf of the two children and won the right to keep the brother and sister together as wards of the court. Today, she continues her fight to broaden the parameters that guide the court in determining such custody issues and to improve adoption processes in general.

Many people refer to the style of leadership shown by Freundlich as the "Joan of Arc" form of situational leadership. As everyone knows, Joan was a young peasant woman who led the armies of France during a war against Britain. It is historically reported that she had a vision that a certain prince was the rightful heir to the throne and that she should fight for him. Joan raised an army and was victorious, securing the throne of France for her prince. This story provides the inspiration for people today who may not be a direct part of something but who are aroused enough by the situation to take a leadership role on behalf of that cause. This form of leadership is actually one of the most frequent causes of change in the world.

Mediation Decision

It has been noted previously that leadership involves moving a group of people toward the resolution of a goal or need, and although most often that is the situation, there is always an exception to the rule. Such is the case when circumstances require a leader to devote his

> **What Limits Sibling Rights?**
>
> "The time has come to examine how much we value children and their interests," said Madelyn Freundlich, executive director of the Adoption Institute, a New York think tank.

> **Shooting of Teenager Is Unprovoked**
>
> Police Chief Jerry Carroll met with black community leaders Monday after relatives who saw Tyisha Shenee Miller die said she was unconscious and couldn't have raised a gun at officers, as police claimed.

or her energy to getting the group to refrain from acting while a conflict remains unresolved. This type of leadership is shown when an individual steps between two opposing groups and uses his or her influence to get the parties to calm down and to initiate a process of communication aimed at resolving the conflict.

The current example illustrates this type of leadership. Jerry Carroll, police chief of Riverside, California, stepped between two conflicting factions to prevent further violence from erupting after the shooting of a young minority child by police. His position was extremely difficult because he had to keep one part of his community from exploding into riots and protest and, at the same time, not give in to another portion of the community that was acting defensive and angry.

This kind of leadership requires that the individual first win the trust of both sides in the conflict and then carry out a multitude of leadership responsibilities. In the example given, the chief of police had to maintain order within the community, conduct an impartial investigation on behalf of the victim's family, and, finally, maintain the trust and morale of the Riverside Police Department while he was conducting the investigation.

This is a situation for a strong leader, one who listens well and is determined to win the trust of all of the parties involved. Such a leader must listen very carefully to all points of view, actively and continually solicit the support of the groups involved, and effectively place the needs of each group above his or her own—all in the interest of arriving at a resolution that will satisfy all parties.

Philanthropic Decision

One of the things that can inspire people to assume the responsibilities of leadership is the desire to improve the lives of others. One can use one's leadership skill to help a single person, a group, or, for that matter, an entire community. Many times, people do not have the time it takes to demonstrate leadership but can support the leadership process in other ways, such as through contributions of money. In this way, many philanthropic orga-

> ### Space Suit Helps Boy Live Dream
> A NASA space suit fulfilled 9-year-old Jonathon Pierce's Christmas wish to play outside like other children. Jonathon suffers from erythropoietic protoporphyria (EPP), a rare skin disorder that causes skin to swell, redden, and blister when exposed to the sun's ultraviolet light. Kiwanis International Foundation bought Jonathon the $2500 pants, jacket, gloves, mask, goggles, and gel-filled "cool suit," which he wears underneath to keep from overheating.

nizations that contribute to the success of nonprofit service groups also support the leadership of those groups. People who raise funds to help organizations are also demonstrating this type of situational leadership.

Kiwanis International is an organization that often demonstrates philanthropic leadership. In this example, the organization focused its leadership on helping a single individual fulfill a lifelong dream.

The type of leadership being provided in this situation is obvious. Organizations like Kiwanis International are continually contributing to individuals, groups, and communities to assist them in moving toward the accomplishment of a goal or fulfillment of a need. This is leadership at its finest. To sacrifice one's own position or, as in this case, financial means for the welfare of another not only is an act of leadership but is an inspiration to everyone. This type of leadership does not always involve money. A person can exercise philanthropic leadership by contributing time or a special skill.

Healthcare Institutional Decision

Many people believe that healthcare institutions, as a general rule, do not do a very good job of providing situational leadership. The bureaucratic processes that hinder most of these organizations make it very difficult for them to move decisively. In reality, however, these organizations provide situational leadership on an almost continual basis. A look at almost any healthcare institution will reveal examples of how it provides leadership. Healthcare institutions help their clients (patients) attain goals or, at a minimum, solicit their cooperation in attaining goals. Through the provision of often selfless service, healthcare institutions win the trust of the communities to which they minister on a daily basis. These institutions take a significant leadership role in the community by continually striving to place the needs of others above their own.

Consider the present example. This news item could very well be talking about one of the programs operated by any healthcare institution. The fact that it mentions this specific organization only indicates that this organization happened to be making news the day the writers of this text conducted their research.

In the example given, the Arizona State Department of Aging is seen to be listening to the needs of a specific group and then working with others to pro-

> ### Elderly Abuse Hotline Launched
> The Arizona State Department of Aging is launching television and radio ads to promote a new, confidential, toll-free elder abuse hotline, 1-800-490-8505.

vide a solution. This is a classic example of situational leadership.

TRANSITIONAL LEADERSHIP

Transitional leadership exists when the time is right, but the circumstances are wrong. In other words, the moment is right, but the individual who is designated as the leader is incapable of delivering the leadership needed. The French expression *faux pas,* which literally means "false step," is the perfect description of transitional leadership. A faux pas occurs in social situations on a frequent basis, and everyone realizes how an individual who delivers a "false step" in such an environment can be affected. It follows, then, that someone exercising transitional leadership is more than likely just a few short steps away from a hasty exit from the position that requires his or her leadership.

An example of transitional leadership can be seen in recent events at Apple Computer. In 1996, Apple was suffering from flat sales, significant operating losses, and a lack of vision and focus. The board of directors looked around the industry to find an individual to lead the organization out of its downward slide and restore Apple to its former position as an industry leader. Their eyes fell upon Gil Amelio, a former executive of National Semiconductor Corporation (NSC) and a leader with demonstrated experience in saving large corporations from financial ruin. He had engineered a recovery at NSC that included a fourfold improvement in the price of its stock and the creation of more than $3 billion in stockholder equity. It seemed that Amelio was the right man for the job, at the right time.

Although Amelio was an individual with significant talent, he was not infallible. His efforts met with significant interference from Steve Jobs, co-founder of Apple, a major stockholder, and a past chairman of the board. As the length of time that Amelio served as CEO increased and the company remained fixed in its flat performance, it became clear that Amelio might not be the man for the job. Because his relationship with Steve Jobs was extremely difficult, Amelio's focus shifted from extricating the company from financial ruin to the very personal act of salvaging his own career. Jobs finally replaced Amelio as the CEO, introduced a new line of computer (the iMac), and engineered a recovery for the corporation.

Amelio, despite his previously outstanding performance, became an endangered species at Apple, Inc.—*the transitional leader.* Although the time was right for a leader of Amelio's background, experience, and capabilities, the situation was wrong. Apple desperately needed leadership, but Amelio did not fit into the company's extremely loose and relaxed culture, as was illustrated when he first met Steve Jobs and the desire to loosen his tie became his first thought. Amelio concentrated his energy on the appearance of leadership, not on the more difficult resolution of the problems and on the tasks associated with it.

The transitional leader may be highly competent, may possess all of the skills of an effective leader, and may even have actually delivered inspired leadership in the past, but if that person's ability, talent, and desire do not match the conditions in which leadership must currently be displayed, there is little chance that individual's leadership will succeed. This is an important lesson in the fact that leadership is a *temporary* condition. The qualities and capabilities that help someone attain success today may be totally wrong for the circumstances of tomorrow. Managers must recognize the temporal condition of leadership and resolve to remain flexible in how they approach each set of conditions, or they will find themselves on the path of transitional leadership and ultimately failure.

One of the biggest challenges that faces the classic transitional leader is the fear of risk. Somewhere along the line, even great leaders can switch from being situational leaders to being transitional ones if they become risk adverse and refuse to pursue their point of view. In his recent book *The Success Profile,* author Lester Korn provides a table titled "Factors Involved in a Career Turning Point" (p. 53).[10] The two factors listed as most important are "right place" and "right time." The third is "high-risk project." According to Korn, all of these elements must occur together in proper context or there is a risk for failure. The transitional leader creates failure by becoming unwilling to confront risk—even if that is the single thing that is necessary for success.

William Glavin, a former chief executive at Xerox Corporation, believed that people should have enough confidence that they aren't worried about being fired for saying or doing the wrong thing. He believed that people should not allow anyone to scare them. Instead, everyone should maintain enough confidence to say, "I can always get another job." If you do this, chances are you will do the right thing.

HIERARCHICAL LEADERSHIP

Transitional leadership is the type of leadership that takes place when the time is right but the circumstances are wrong. *Hierarchical* leadership is demonstrated when these two conditions are exactly the opposite; that is, the circumstances are right but the time is wrong. The person who most often demonstrates hierarchical leadership is someone who has assumed a leadership role because it is "his or her turn," because of right of promotion or length of time on the job, or, in the case of a monarch, because of the death of a predecessor and birth order.

The challenge faced by hierarchical leaders is that they are the designated person in charge, regardless of whether they want the role or are qualified for it. For example, King George III of England was totally unqualified to lead the English in the fight against France in the Seven Years War (one phase of which was the French and Indian War). However, his father, King George II, died in the middle of the war and George III was thrust into this pivotal leadership role. Although England won the war, the new king's leadership ability was so lacking that his policies caused England to lose the peace. His programs of heavy taxation and denial of colonial rights, even when his chief advisor, Sir William Pitt, championed those rights, led to the American colonies' eventual secession. In 1776 when the cause of colonial rights was peaking, the incapable hierarchical leader, who could not step aside, forced the colonists' hand by sending troops to quell a difference of opinion. This action led to the American Revolution, and the rest, as we say, is history.

Hierarchical leaders often miss the timing required to turn themselves into great leaders because they traditionally do not listen well. They turn a deaf ear to the circumstances surrounding the need or miss the underlying meanings of what is being said because they are almost always tone deaf to the critical elements of leadership. Hierarchical leaders are in positions of leadership because circumstances have put them there and only the most radical of processes can force them out. Examples of this type of leadership, and the resulting failures, abound throughout history: in czarist Russia, a weak leader met conditions with force instead of compassion and was overthrown; in Japan, the emperor, who was believed to be a god but was himself the victim of unscrupulous warlords, was followed blindly into the devastation of World War II; in France, a timid and slightly addled Louis XVI lost his head because of the quality of his decisions. Think about these situations, and the meaning of hierarchical leadership and its potential dangers for the healthcare industry will become very clear.

Not all hierarchical leaders fail. In a few cases these individuals turn the corner and become masters of situational leadership. One example is King George VI of England. He led the British government and people through the perils of World War II after being forced into the role of king when his brother, King Edward VIII, abdicated just prior to Hitler's occupation of the Sudetenland. Although the new king did not want the job, he discharged the responsibilities of his position well enough to provide inspirational leadership to his countrymen during a time of great peril. Many historians claim that it was the fiery oratory of Sir Winston Churchill that braced the spine of England against the German onslaught. But ask almost any Englishman who lived through the terrible ordeal of World War II and you will most likely hear another story: it was the king, moving among his subjects at hospitals, orphanages, bomb sites, and war factories and rallying the people with his calm voice and words of encouragement that made the real difference.

SUMMARY

- Leadership—and this is the point of this chapter—is not something that simply occurs. It takes the proper combination of time, circumstances, and individual to create success.
- The one thing that all managers who aspire to be perceived as leaders must remember is that one critical key to leadership is flexibility.
- A leader must evaluate carefully before taking action.
- Simple reliance on the success of previous operations will never guarantee success in a new one. The skills that made a person a leader yesterday must be evaluated and exercised in a manner that others are willing to perceive as leadership today, or they simply will not work.
- The criteria that people establish for following another person change with conditions, time, and need. So must the actions of the potential leader, or these critical elements will not agree.
- *Management is a profession*—one that most of the world's most successful people have chosen. There is virtually no other profession in which an individual can have such a direct, dramatic, and positive impact on the lives of others and on the ultimate success of his or her enterprise.
- *Leadership is an art.* It is the careful application of a few basic skills that are suited to the specific time and place that brings out the best out in people who choose to follow it. It is inspiration, motivation, and exhilaration. Leadership is not, however, a technical skill.
- Good nurse managers realize that they don't have to be tough all of the time—and that being nice will often help them finish far ahead of the competition.
- Despite what many people would have you believe, good management is not achieved through simple solutions or quick fixes.
- Managing is one of the most difficult—yet potentially most rewarding—jobs that anyone can undertake within an organization.

- Managerial leadership is nothing more than a set of qualities that, when demonstrated in the proper context, can cause others to follow.
- Managerial leadership begins when an individual is willing to embrace responsibility. Simply accepting the responsibilities that come with a management position or the responsibilities that someone else assigns is not enough to demonstrate leadership.
- It is *never* the position that creates a good manager.
- To be perceived as a leader, a manager must be able to get others to cooperate and go along with what the manager designates as the correct performance.
- Leadership requires that managers be willing to sacrifice their personal goals and desires so that a greater goal can be achieved.
- *Authority* is not *management*, nor is it *leadership*.
- Doing the right thing is never enough if you do not do it correctly, and doing things correctly will not work if you are not doing them for the right reason. Excellent leadership is best demonstrated when it is coupled with effective management, and excellent management is never achieved without demonstrated leadership at its core.
- It is totally improper to believe that because an individual takes the lead he or she will remain there, because the conditions that cause leadership to occur are *always* temporary.
- The three skills necessary for a nurse manager to become an effective leader are (1) the ability to put the needs of others ahead of one's own, (2) the ability to listen, and (3) the ability to elicit the support of others.

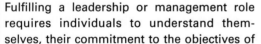

FINAL THOUGHTS

Fulfilling a leadership or management role requires individuals to understand themselves, their commitment to the objectives of the organization and patient care, their special skills, their knowledge of the organization, their ability to establish a vision, their personal values, their desire and ability to make timely decisions, their personal ability to identify and solve challenges within the nursing unit before these become a problem, and human behavior.

Traditional leaders must also alter their personal styles so that they can accommodate the needs of a rapidly changing workforce, the necessity for effective decision-making, and the concept of the patient as a customer of the nursing unit. Professional nurses will greatly enhance their ability to contribute to the success of the nursing unit if they develop their leadership potential.

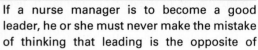

THE NURSE MANAGER SPEAKS

If a nurse manager is to become a good leader, he or she must never make the mistake of thinking that leading is the opposite of following. Following requires an active presence and full engagement with the leader, whereas a leader need not even see the follower to be effective in his or her effort.

Not all nurse managers are leaders. Simply occupying a position of authority does not automatically make anyone a leader. Authority is not leadership and neither is management.

The concept of leadership as relying on teamwork and the building of consensus to achieve success is substantially different from the concept of leadership that was taught a mere generation ago. In today's healthcare industry, exercising leadership means that nurse managers must be able to get others to want to do the things that need to be done, rather than simply ordering people to do them. To accomplish this, today's nurse managers and executives must be willing to place the needs of their staffs ahead of their own. The organizational mission, from its creation through its realization, must be a partnership between the nurse manager who leads and the staff members who perform. If the organization's mission is strictly goal driven, devoid of concern for the welfare of the staff, the only thing it will provide for the organization is a recipe for failure.

Do not confuse leadership with management. One is focused on motivating people, the other on getting things accomplished.

REFERENCES

1. *Fortune*, March 20, 1995.
2. Martin JB: *Letter to enrolling students*, retrieved 2002 from http://www.harvard.edu.
3. *The Wall Street Journal*, March 5, 1999.
4. Peters T: *Thriving on chaos: handbook for a management revolution*, New York, 1987, Knopf.
5. Lichfield J: Waterloo's significance to the French and the British, *The Independent (London)*, Nov 17, 2004; available online at http://hnn.us/roundup/comments/8630.html.
6. Goleman D: *Emotional intelligence*, New York, 1998, Wiley.
7. Schneider M: *Productive conflict skills*, Ann Arbor, Mich, 1999, University of Michigan.
8. Nielsen JL: *Lady admiral: the story of Grace Hopper*, New York, 1984, Harper and Row, p 83.
9. Bennis W, Nanus B: *Leaders*, New York, 1983, Dell.
10. Korn L: *The success profile: a leading headhunter tells you how to get to the top*, Vancouver, BC, Canada, 1990, Fireside.

SUGGESTED READINGS

Allee V: *The knowledge evolution: expanding organizational intelligence,* Woburn, Mass, 1997, Butterworth-Heinemann.

Baskin K: *Corporate DNA: learning from life,* Woburn, Mass, 1998, Butterworth-Heinemann.

Bennis W, Nanus B: *Leaders: strategies for taking charge,* New York, 2003, HarperCollins.

Blanchard K: *The heart of a leader: insights on the art of influence,* Tulsa, Okla, 2004, Honor Books.

Brown JS: *Seeing differently: insights on innovation,* Harvard Business Review book series, Cambridge, Mass, 1997, Harvard Business School Press.

Davis M: *A practical guide to organizational design,* Menlo Park, Calif, 1996, Crisp Publishers.

Dettmer W: *Breaking the constraints to world-class performance,* Milwaukee, 1998, ASQ Quality Press.

Economy P: *Business negotiating basics,* Chicago, 1993, IDG Books.

Economy P: *Negotiating to win,* Glenview, Ill, 1991, Scott Foresman Books.

Greenberg J: *Behavior in organizations: understanding and managing the human side of work,* ed 8, Upper Saddle River, NJ, 2002, Prentice Hall.

Helgesen S: *Web of inclusion: a new architecture for building great institutions,* Milwaukee, 1995, ASQ Quality Press.

Hersey P: *Management of organizational behavior: leading human resources,* ed 8, Upper Saddle River, NJ, 2000, Prentice Hall.

Hill N: *Napoleon Hill's key to success: the 17 principles of personal achievement,* New York, 1997, Plume.

Hirschhorn L: *The workplace within: psychodynamics of organizational life,* Boston, 1990, MIT Press.

Maister D: *True professionalism: the courage to care about your people, your clients, and your career,* New York, 1997, Free Press.

McCormack M: *What they don't teach you at the Harvard Business School,* New York, 1986, Bantam Doubleday.

Muirhead BK: *High velocity leadership: the Mars Pathfinder approach to faster, better, cheaper,* New York, 1999, HarperCollins.

Nelson R: *Fundamental management practices: people, projects and teams,* Chicago, 1996, IDG Books.

Nelson R: *Decision point,* Upper Saddle River, NJ, 2000, Prentice Hall.

Nelson RB: *Empowering employees through delegation,* New York, 1993, McGraw-Hill

Reinman J: *Thinking for a living: creating ideas that revitalize your business, career and life,* Athens, Ga, 1991, Longstreet Press.

Schon D: *The reflective practitioner: how professionals think in action,* Aldershot, Hampshire, United Kingdom, 1985, Ashgate.

Stone D: *Difficult conversations,* New York, 1999, Viking.

Fundamental Performance of the Nurse Manager

LEARNING SYNOPSIS

Upon successful completion of this chapter, readers will possess a fundamental understanding of the functions of management in general and of nursing management in particular and will be familiar with the traditional views of management responsibilities as well as some of the more-up-to-date theories and practices of human resource management.

OBJECTIVES

1. Identify the basic elements of the traditional management concept
2. Describe the various factors that influence the nurse manager and affect his or her performance
3. Identify six major factors that influence the nurse manager's environment
4. Describe the basic functions of traditional management
5. Identify first-level management functions and compare them with traditional management and senior management functions

This chapter discusses the fundamental duties of the nurse manager (supervisor) in a healthcare setting with special emphasis on the traditional responsibilities of management. In addition, it provides an introduction to some of the more up-to-date theories regarding human resource management and highlights some of the functions that are particularly characteristic of healthcare settings.

Fig. 4-1 shows many of the environmental, organizational, social, and other factors that determine the milieu in which the nurse manager must function. Table 4-1 lists the management functions that the nurse manager must perform.

THE FUNCTIONS OF MANAGEMENT

Management can be defined as the process of accomplishing the required work through the performance of others—accurately, on time, and within the established budget. Throughout this chapter the terms *supervision* and *management* are used almost interchangeably, although traditionally management has been viewed as encompassing a broader role, one that goes well beyond the direct supervision of people to include a variety of other functions involving the allocation of resources to accomplish organizational goals. The functions of management as they pertain to the nurse manager are shown in Table 4-1.

This chapter focuses on the traditional management functions of *planning*, *organizing*, and *controlling* as they apply to the nurse manager. Although the

TABLE 4-1

Management Functions of the Nurse Manager

Function	Description
Planning	Determining long- and short-term goals of the institution and the individual objectives that must be achieved to realize them
Staffing	Selecting personnel to carrying out the goals and objectives and placing them in positions appropriate to their skills and knowledge
Organizing	Structuring the resources of the institution so that the goals and objectives can be achieved
Directing	Providing guidance and motivational leadership so that assigned personnel are capable of carrying out the actions needed to achieve the goals and objectives
Controlling	Analyzing results in terms of predetermined standards of performance and implementing the actions necessary to ensure that the unit accomplishes the goals and objectives satisfactorily
Decision-making	Identifying a problem, searching for alternative solutions, and selecting the alternative that best achieves the decision-maker's objectives

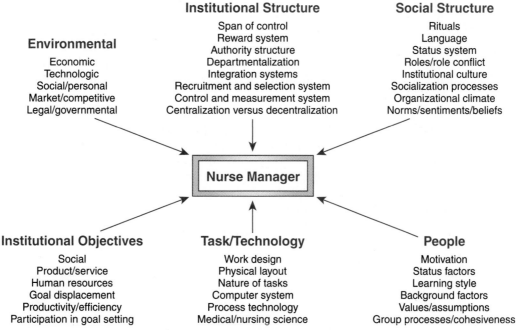

Institutional Structure
Span of control
Reward system
Authority structure
Departmentalization
Integration systems
Recruitment and selection system
Control and measurement system
Centralization versus decentralization

Social Structure
Rituals
Language
Status system
Roles/role conflict
Institutional culture
Socialization processes
Organizational climate
Norms/sentiments/beliefs

Environmental
Economic
Technologic
Social/personal
Market/competitive
Legal/governmental

Nurse Manager

Institutional Objectives
Social
Product/service
Human resources
Goal displacement
Productivity/efficiency
Participation in goal setting

Task/Technology
Work design
Physical layout
Nature of tasks
Computer system
Process technology
Medical/nursing science

People
Motivation
Status factors
Learning style
Background factors
Values/assumptions
Group processes/cohesiveness

Fig. 4-1 ■ Factors influencing the nurse manager.

functions of staffing, directing, and decision-making will be touched on, they are given less attention because they are covered in depth in other chapters.

Planning

The ability to plan effectively is extremely important to nurse managers because the future is always unpredictable. This is especially true in dynamic professions such as healthcare, where environmental factors are changing constantly and at an ever-increasing pace. Planning is basically a five-step procedure, as follows:

1. *Establishment:* Development of the goals and objectives
2. *Evaluation:* Analysis of the present situation
3. *Prediction:* Analytical evaluation of anticipated trends and events
4. *Formulation:* Development of an operational plan, which is sometimes referred to as a *planning statement*
5. *Conversion:* Transformation of the plan into the actions necessary to accomplish the goal; this process starts with the creation of an action statement

There are two types of planning: *strategic* and *contingency*. It is generally easy to differentiate between the two different types, although both are developed using a similar process. *Strategic* planning is the process used to determine the long-term goals and objectives of the organization and the policies that will be followed in the accomplishment of those objectives. In a healthcare organization, this form of planning is generally conducted by the executive management group in conjunction with the board of directors. Although other management levels may not be directly involved in the strategic planning process, they are directly affected by the strategic plan itself. This is because the plan contains the objectives they will be asked to achieve and because it outlines the procedures they will be asked to follow in their efforts. The organization's effectiveness is determined by its management's collective knowledge and implementation of the organization's strategy and its application in the unit for which each specific manager is responsible.

Contingency planning is identifying and dealing with the many challenges that can arise while accomplishing the goals of the organization. Quality performance in the organization is assured only when each department and unit manager

- Fully understands specific objectives of the department or unit
- Is aware of the potential circumstances that may delay or prevent the achievement of those objectives

- Organizes and assigns tasks to prevent the occurrences of these challenges, or, at the very minimum, understands what must be done to prevent the challenges from limiting performance

To effectively carry out contingency planning, nurse managers must accomplish specific tasks. The most important contingency planning functions are conducted at the unit or department level and involve the tasks described in the following sections.

SETTING OBJECTIVES

The unit's and department's contingency planning processes begin with and support the strategic plan provided to them by the executive management team. Because the process of strategic planning involves establishing objectives as well as the policies to achieve them, nurse managers must understand their organization's objectives and the processes used to create them. In a healthcare organization, objectives address the following four general areas:

1. *Products and services:* For healthcare organizations this is the most critical area of goal and objective development because it directly affects the process of patient care. These goals and objectives identify what patient care needs will be satisfied directly by the organization and what types of patient care facilities will be required to teach and/or perform research. The relative importance of these goals depends on a variety of factors, such as (1) whether the organization is a private or public facility, (2) whether it is affiliated with a teaching university or some other organization, and (3) what its size and geographical location are.

2. *Efficiency:* In the present context, efficiency refers to the level of performance of the work necessary to accomplish the organization's objectives. What variety of resources are required per unit of care? That is: (a) How many nurses are required per patient-day*? (b) How much time is expended for each procedure? (c) How many square feet of facility space should be allocated per service? (d) How will the efficiency of the unit be measured (e.g., average hospital stay, occupancy rates, expenditures compared with budgeted amounts, or hours of nursing care required for a specific combination of patients)? In view of the rapid growth in healthcare costs over the last three decades, outside groups such as third-party payers (insurance companies) and

---

Patient-day is a work structure identifier defined as one patient for one 24-hour day.

governmental agencies have become obsessively concerned with hospital efficiency.

3. *Social responsibilities:* Objectives in this area relate to satisfying the obligations that have been established by the community or society that the organization serves. Will the organization aggressively seek to be a good citizen or will it merely meet its minimal obligations by obeying the letter of the laws governing its behavior? Many healthcare organizations have considerable political influence and may be in a position to influence the laws under which they are regulated. This influence has been attained, to a large degree, through the efforts of major lobbying organizations such as the American Nurses Association and American Medical Association.

4. *Human resources:* Objectives in this area concern the efforts that will be made to satisfy employee needs and desires to gain and maintain their commitment to the goals of the organization. Specific objectives are typically formulated in the areas of nurse manager development and employee attitude and satisfaction.

Box 4-1 presents a statement of nursing service philosophy developed by one university-affiliated private hospital. Note that the statement describes the nature of the organization and the direction in which its management has determined it will go in the future. Box 4-2 provides the organization's mission statement, and Box 4-3 lists the organization's annual corporate goals and nursing service objectives. Also included are some specific objectives needed to achieve the broader-based goals. Obviously, goal statements for other types of organizations such as a non–university-affiliated or community hospital may differ significantly and would perhaps reflect a significantly different view of secondary care. Regardless of what type of organization develops them, goal statements need to be reviewed periodically to keep them realistic and consistent with the environment in which the organization operates.

Statements of goals, such as those shown in Box 4-3, focus the entire unit's thinking on the future, on what is expected to happen in the future, and on how the unit's current activities assist the organization in achieving its goals. Organizations that employ this process of specific goal development are regarded as *proactive;* their administrators spend a lot of their time contemplating future events and preparing the organization to deal with them effectively. Those organizations that do not develop clear goals are generally considered to be *reactive.* These are organizations that generally operate on a day-by-day basis and spend a great deal of their time and attention on problem solving instead of problem prevention.

BOX 4-1

Example of a Hospital Nursing Service Statement of Philosophy

Nursing is an individualized process of providing high-quality care to patients as they progress through their treatment and return to a productive life.

We are committed to the provision of high-quality patient care and to the accountability of our professional nursing staff for the specific level of quality they provide each patient in their charge. Our accountability process includes assessing patients' healthcare needs; developing individual diagnoses; planning for and delivering well-managed, risk-adverse nursing activities; and ensuring that the care that is delivered is critically evaluated on a continual basis.

Our staff is committed to delivering respectful and professional care that ensures the rights and dignity of each patient, as that patient views them. We serve as advocates for the patient, and we accomplish this by effectively communicating the level of quality and the individual services we provide. We continually strive to collaborate with other professionals within the medical field to ensure that we deliver only the finest quality service to our patients. To the greatest degree possible, we involve our patients and their family members in the development and evaluation of the individual care they receive before it is delivered.

We accept the responsibility to share relevant knowledge and information to the communities we serve in both anticipation of and response to their needs. We recognize our responsibilities for delivering only the highest quality patient care possible and see it as our primary role in supporting the communities we serve.

Data from Barnes Jewish Hospital, St Louis.

The fundamental principles of planning can also be applied by first-level nurse managers. For example, a number of famous and prestigious hospitals have developed nursing service strategic planning models that align with the hospital's strategic planning process. These models incorporate the corporate strategy as well as the results of an in-depth assessment of the nursing department, planning sessions with the clinical service division managers, and assessments of new services that may have been originated during the previous year. The key areas analyzed in these internal assessments include patients, families, physicians, staff, and internal hospital departments, as well as local, national, and international nursing issues.

Example of a Mission Statement for a Teaching Hospital

To be dedicated to the provision of healthcare leadership and the delivery of outstanding medical practice through the creation of an exceptional medical school

To provide only the highest quality medical education at all levels

To provide only the highest level of patient care, through a full range of medical services, including primary, secondary, triage, and acute care

To ensure that cost-effective, compassionate, and high-quality healthcare is made available to every patient we serve

To provide an environment that encourages the medical staff to use their initiative, creativity, and professionalism in delivering their practice to the extent of their qualifications and in accordance with the directives provided by the Hospital Board of Directors and within the spirit and intent of the codes of ethics provided by the American Medical Association and the American Nurses Association

To provide employees with superior compensation and benefits and the opportunity to perform at their full potential as individuals and as members of their individual professions within a working environment that promotes high-quality service and well-managed risk

Data from Mt. Sinai Hospital, Los Angeles.

In assessing the external environment, nursing services have two primary areas of focus. The first is the analysis of organizational directives and the evaluation of related issues to determine departmental applicability. Examples of issues examined include the aging of the population, clinical service strengths, and physician relations. The second component of these external environment assessments is market analysis. These reviews typically focus on the following broad areas:

- Future direction(s) for consumer relations
- Patient satisfaction and complaint surveys
- Public expectations of nursing care
- Staffing availability
- National trends in nursing service recruitment for the previous 3 or 4 years
- Entry-into-practice issues
- Quality direction(s) for the hospital as a whole
- Evaluation of the nursing services by a physician or group of physicians

When the nursing department is assessed as a whole, the nursing services involved typically examine several areas, including the following:

- Current employee attitudes
- Actions taken to correct identified deficiencies
- Salary and benefits (i.e., surveys were taken at surrounding area hospitals and reviewed to determine the position of the nursing service in relation to peer positions elsewhere)
- Recommendations of the Joint Commission on Accreditation of Healthcare Organizations and the organization's plans for and/or progress in meeting any identified deficiencies
- Other active nursing programs that might have been employed throughout the year

During the organizational assessment component of each study, the nursing department's relationships with other hospital departments and with the local and national nursing communities in the areas of education, research, and publishing are also reviewed.

These surveys are designed to acquire information that can be used to develop 3-year departmental plans. Such a departmental plan is used to establish objectives for nurse managers that identify key issues to be addressed during the covered 3 years. To accomplish these objectives, nurse managers are provided with information about the organizational strategy, the nursing department goals and objectives, and any clinical service activities that affect their areas of responsibility.

When a division-level assessment is performed, the following areas should be reviewed critically:

- Patient care delivery systems available
- Quality scores
- Staff development
- Patient, family, and physician satisfaction
- Staff satisfaction
- Support and peer department evaluations
- Physical plant assessments (facilities available)
- Equipment needs
- Impending clinical practice changes that could affect the service quality or performance of the units

The most effective planning processes are participative and involve both management and staff in the discussion and development of unit goals and objectives. Once developed, the goals and objectives are prioritized, and action plans are created. It is essential that division-level planning efforts align with both the departmental and hospital plans. For the most part, nurse managers are responsible for this type of planning for their units, and the very best involve their staffs as completely as possible.

A common problem seen in healthcare organizations that do not have clear-cut planning programs

BOX 4-3

Example of Nursing Service Goals and Objectives

PATIENT CARE DELIVERY

Goal A: To develop a coordinated care continuum

Objective 1: To expand the heart transplant program by implementation of a mechanical assist program

Objective 2: To explore the feasibility of developing a comprehensive critical cardiology service

Objective 3: To develop a geriatric psychiatric program

Objective 4: To develop a systematic process for organ retrieval in support of the organ transplant program

Objective 5: To further develop the epilepsy program in the Neurosurgery Department

Objective 6: To explore the development of a cooperative care unit

Objective 7: To assist in the development of a plan to create a center of excellence in pulmonary medicine

Objective 8: To develop an outpatient psychiatric day hospital

Objective 9: To develop an outpatient center for cardiac assessment and screening

Objective 10: To develop an outpatient diabetic center

Objective 11: To develop a plan for a centralized outpatient facility for medical therapies or diagnostic procedures

Objective 12: To investigate the feasibility of developing a comprehensive outpatient treatment facility for dermatologic patients

Goal B: To improve the efficiencies and effectiveness of operations

Objective 1: To develop, where appropriate, intermediate care units for patients who do not need intensive care but need more than general unit care, and to evaluate the effectiveness of these units

Objective 2: To design cost-effective nursing care delivery practices and systems

Objective 3: To determine nursing care cost information per diagnosis-related group (DRG)

Objective 4: To implement a nursing portion of the computerized pharmacy information system

Objective 5: To ensure quality patient care through the establishment of standards, revision of documentation, and establishment of quality monitoring systems

Goal C: To identify new markets and improve the awareness, utilization, and value exchange of services

Objective 1: To promote Cardiology Department services.

PERSONNEL

Goal A: To bring about increased sensitivity to consumers

Objective 1: To participate in revising the consumer relations program and implement changes applicable to the Nursing Department

Goal B: To implement career development programming

Objective 1: To continue development of a registered nurse career ladder program

Goal C: To manage compensation systems

Goal D: To ensure recruitment and retention

Goal E: To improve benefit systems

Goal F: To improve communication

Objective 1: To establish a framework for communication that ensures staff involvement in problem identification and resolution

FINANCIAL VIABILITY

Goal A: To achieve targets for operating and non-operating net excesses of revenues over expenses

Objective 1: To review pricing structure for all areas and recommend changes where indicated

Goal B: To increase donor contributions

Goal C: To maintain an "AA" rating for capital access

Goal D: To provide the financial support necessary to meet the community responsibility for the care of indigents

Goal E: To maximize participation in viable alternate delivery systems

Goal F: To develop financial systems that are responsive to the changing environment

EXTERNAL ENVIRONMENT

Goal A: To influence the development of clinical services management and medical staff relations

Goal B: To participate in medical, nursing, and allied health education and research programs

Goal C: To pursue opportunities in the hospital's relationships in the medical center

Goal D: To develop an ongoing rapport with political and healthcare leaders

Goal E: To establish a long-range strategy in relation to competition and new business opportunities

is a phenomenon known as *goal displacement*. This is a process in which individual units in the organization pursue their own narrowly defined goals rather than ensuring that they work to satisfy the overall goals of the organization. Goal displacement often manifests itself as excessive enforcement of rules or excessive concern over the success of the unit, rather than the accomplishment of the goals established by the organization. This phenomenon is seen most often in bureaucratically organized organizations and in those in which the broad goals of the organization are written in general and ambiguous terms. When goals are overgeneralized and unclear, individual units are unable to agree on how they should support the organization's mission and vision, and, left without proper direction, each unit simply pursues its own short-term ambitions.

Not only must an organization establish objectives, but as many people as possible at all levels of the organization must be involved in the process. One technique for attaining this involvement is a process called *management by objective* (MBO).[1,2] MBO is a formal process that involves the following stages:

Determination of the overall objectives of the organization: Once these objectives are developed, they are shared with subordinate units, so that the latter can use them to formulate objectives for their specific areas of responsibility. These subordinate objectives are discussed by the employees and the individual unit managers to ensure that they are consistent with the organization's broad goals.

Development of a plan: Once the individual unit's objectives have been developed, a plan is formulated to achieve them. This plan specifies the measures of achievement to be used, a feedback process that will help the unit determine whether or not the objectives have been accomplished, and an evaluation process to verify the results.

Periodic review: Periodic review of the MBO plan is useful so that corrective action may be taken as quickly as possible. The review may indicate that adjustment of the objectives (up or down) is necessary or that changes must be made in the means used to achieve them.

Both academicians and management practitioners have expressed concerns regarding the effectiveness of programs like the MBO process, because historically such programs have been more successful in improving employee satisfaction and morale than in increasing productivity. Even considering their many shortcomings, however, these processes can serve as an effective planning and control technique. The MBO method tends to work best in situations where the following apply:

- Clear and concise organizational objectives are present.
- Senior managers and administrators are committed to participation by lower-level personnel in the goal-setting process.
- Individual and measurable tasks are identified and included.
- Performance feedback and managerial follow-up is required.
- There is a high level of trust between managers and performers.
- Full participation in formulation of objectives is encouraged.
- Employees are highly motivated to achieve.

Many professionals argue that the aforementioned situation represents a nearly ideal work environment and that MBO-type programs are likely to work best where they are needed the least. Nevertheless, objective setting remains a very important supervisory function, and these programs can be effective tools for the organization.

EVALUATING AND PREDICTING

The second stage in the planning process is the assessment of the organization's current situation and prediction of future events, sometimes referred to as a SWOT analysis. SWOT is an acronym for *S*trengths, *W*eaknesses, *O*pportunities, and *T*hreats. The SWOT analysis requires that the internal and external environment of the organization be evaluated from a strategic planning point of view. An internal evaluation is the process of assessing the present strengths and weaknesses of the organization (i.e., which activities are performed well and which are accomplished poorly). Present activities and the policies relating to them might be grouped into the following categories:

- Patient care, teaching, and research
- Human resources
- Organizational system
- Auxiliary services
- Management and administration reputation
- Physical facilities
- Budgets (financial development)
- Technologic capabilities
- Finance and accounting

After the factors affecting the internal environment of the organization have been evaluated, specific policies can be formulated. This process is best expressed in the double-column format shown in Table 4-2, with questions on the left and possible answers, choices, or observations on the right. SWOT analysis is discussed further in Chapter 17.

The specific allocations of resources necessary to achieve the organizational goals are developed from

TABLE 4-2

Specific Policy Formulation

Policy Questions	Examples
What services will be offered by the organization?	Various types of patient care Teaching Research
What kinds of patients will be served?	Children, the aged, those with special conditions
How will these services be delivered?	Freestanding treatment facilities such as emergency aid clinics, surgical centers, and outreach programs
How will these potential patients be informed about the services offered?	Advertising by organizations providing alcoholism treatment, billboards advertising emergency aid facilities
How will these services be priced?	Based on percentage of indigent patients served; relationships with insurers such as Blue Cross, Medicare, Medicaid, etc.
How will the organization be financed?	Private donation, patient billing, insurance compensation, and governmental support
What kind of care will be provided?	General care, specialty care, trauma care, referral, pediatrics
What will be the patient mix in terms of acuity levels?	All levels

these general policies. Procedures, rules and regulations, schedules, and budgets are established as part of the overall organizational plan.

Organizing

Once a strategic plan has been developed, the organizational structure necessary to carry out that plan must be established. Table 4-3 shows some of the factors that influence the organization's structure.

The plan determines what tasks need to be performed to achieve the goals. These tasks are then subdivided into subtasks. It is from this division of labor or specialization of tasks (e.g., one person to give the medications, another to transport patients off the unit) that the organization will acquire its efficiency.

The individual tasks need to be coordinated, however. The best way to achieve this coordination of effort is to group like tasks and assign them to the same department, such as nursing or housekeeping. This process, often referred to as *departmentalization*, can be based on the following:

Product or service (e.g., maternity, psychiatric, pediatric)
Type of client (e.g., elderly, children)
Function (e.g., accounting, finance, housekeeping)
Process (e.g., operating room, radiology)
Time (day, evening, night)
Geographic location (e.g., emergency services)

AUTHORITY AND INFLUENCE

An organization's structure of authority provides one of its most important means of coordination. Authority involves the control over specific types of rights that are vested in identifiable members of the organization. There are two general types of authority rights:

1. The right to apportion organizational responsibilities
2. The right to evaluate the performance of these responsibilities to establish the rewards and restrictions received by the individuals who perform the work associated with them

These rights may be held by many different people in the organization. Whether or not a person has these rights can be determined by the answers to the following two questions:

1. Would the person allocating organizational tasks and/or evaluating the performance of these tasks be evaluated negatively by his or her supervisors for doing so?
2. Would the person to whom the tasks have been assigned be evaluated negatively for noncompliance?

If the answer to the first question is No and the answer to the second question is Yes, then the person concerned has authority rights.

Authority rights can be exercised either by direction or by delegation. *Direction* includes the specification of how a task is to be performed; *delegation* leaves the decision as to how the task is to be performed up to the subordinate. *Delegation* is the most common form of allocation in organizations that employ professionals.

Authority rights are generally exercised in three stages: (1) criteria setting, (2) sampling, and (3) evaluation. In organizations that employ a large number of professionals, such as health care, the profession itself usually establishes the criteria by which an individual should be evaluated, but it is normally the individual manager's right to sample work behavior and compare this behavior against the established standard.

TABLE 4-3

Effects of External Environmental Factors on Healthcare Organizations

Environment Factor	Selected Effects
ECONOMIC	
Inflation	Increased cost of equipment
State of the economy, business cycle	Decrease in elective surgery and fewer beds filled during recessions
Fiscal and monetary policies	Increased or decreased availability of government funds to support health care
LEGAL AND GOVERNMENTAL	
Healthcare regulation	Requirements for professional standards review
	Need for compliance with organizational law
	State review of rates
	Requirement for state certificate of need to open new facilities
	Determination of reimbursement mechanisms
Healthcare support	Changes in fiscal policies (support for teaching and research)
Legal liabilities	Increased malpractice suits
Accreditation agencies	Need to meet JCAHO or state division of health criteria or lose governmental support
MARKET AND COMPETITIVE	
Nonhealthcare competitors	Emergence of new services or elimination of unneeded serviced
Changes in patient needs	Modification of practices
Changes in population (e.g., aging)	Increased demand for long-term healthcare facilities
Substitute products	Provision of emergency aid facilities
TECHNOLOGIC	
Changes in technology	Need for retraining
Cost of new technology	Increased cost of hospitalization
SOCIAL AND PERSONNEL	
Availability and cost of personnel	Nursing shortage or surplus
New opportunities for women	Demand by nurses for more participation in decision-making
Changing attitudes toward health care, death, physical fitness	Increase in sports injuries, increase in holistic health care, appearance of "right to life" movement

---

One approach to authority is presented in the "zone of indifference" theory, which was originally developed by Barnard[3] and elaborated on by Simon.[4] This theory places less emphasis on the organization as a source of authority and focuses more on the relationship that exists between the supervisor and subordinate and on the sources of the influence that one exerts over the other.

The following major sources of influence have been identified[5]:

Reward and *coercion:* The supervisor has the ability to negotiate positive or negative rewards on behalf of the subordinate in areas such as salary, recognition, work schedule, specific duties, and continued employment.

Legitimacy: The subordinate believes that the supervisor has the right to provide direction and issue instructions; this belief is frequently based on acceptance of the social system.

Expertise: The subordinate believes that the supervisor has a greater knowledge in the given area.

Reference: To one degree or another, the subordinate identifies with the supervisor and therefore patterns his or her behavior accordingly.

Nurse managers, depending on the guidelines established by their organizations, generally possess both reward and coercive influence over their subordinates. In addition, they generally possess legitimacy influence because most of their junior staff nurses tend to believe that their managers have the right to issue instructions. Expert and referent influences, however, are present only after a nurse manager and a staff nurse have worked together in the senior-subordinate roles for a period. The nurse manager might also share expert and referent influence over newer staff nurses with more experienced nurses. The more types of influence supervisors exercise over their subordinates, the greater the control they will have. This makes it extremely important for individuals to be selected as nurse managers based on a combination of technical expertise and personal leadership qualities, including their ability to serve as role models.

BUREAUCRACY

Although authority is the most common means used to link together the tasks, people, and technology of the organization, other coordination techniques are also used. For example, the bureaucratic organization relies heavily on rules and regulations as a means of integration. In this type of organization, the structure consists of a number of formal positions arranged in a hierarchical manner. Position holders are assigned formal duties with a high degree of specialization, and a formally established system of rules and regulations governs their decisions and actions. Generally, individuals are employed on the basis of professional or other predetermined qualifications rather than political, family, or other connections. Normally, people who seek this type of position do so as part of their individual career advancement plans. In the ideal organization, bureaucratic officers hold their positions because of their levels of expertise and apply the organization's rules and regulations in an impartial manner (without favoritism) in an effort to make rational decisions and achieve administrative efficiency.

Bureaucracy is a word that is often used disparagingly to indicate an organization in which excessive enforcement of rules leads to inefficiency. The reason is that most of these organizations face a major problem in the form of goal displacement. Inside such an organization, the energies of the individual unit participants are generally focused more on enforcing or following the rules than on providing services to the clients. This type of situation is all too common in healthcare organizations because most continue to operate in the bureaucratic mode (at least to some degree), especially in their support and administrative departments.

OTHER METHODS OF COORDINATION AND INTEGRATION

Other means commonly used to achieve coordination and integration, especially between different units in the organization, are direct contact, liaison positions, task forces (temporary committees), teams (permanent committees), integrating personnel, integrating departments, and a matrix organizational structure.

For example, nursing committees are usually considered to be integrating forces.[6,7]

Controlling

Control in an organization involves the following:
- Establishment of performance standards
- Determination of the measurement means used to compare actual performance against the standards
- Evaluation of performance
- Feedback to supply performance data to the individual performer so that behavior can be modified

Programs like MBO, presented earlier as a planning device, can also be considered control mechanisms because they encompass all four of the basic requirements. First, they involve the determination of objectives (standards) against which performance can be measured. Second, specific measures are established to determine whether these objectives are met. Third, the actual accomplishment of the objectives is measured in relation to the standard. Finally, this information is relayed back to the individual, and this feedback can be used to implement corrective action as necessary.

MBO-like processes are generally monotonous systems that are applicable only to a limited range of tasks and situations. They usually involve a significant amount of self-control. For this reason, they suit many healthcare organizations, because most rely heavily on internalized control. Achieving this type of self-control, however, requires that the organization properly select and train its individual performers to ensure that they have the capability and desire to behave in the manner required to accomplish the organization's tasks. Especially important to self-control are the socialization processes that cause individuals to internalize the values of their profession and accept a code of behavior. Socialization as a means of control is useful in healthcare organizations because continuous monitoring of behavior is both difficult and performance suppressing.

SOCIALIZATION

There are five important stages in the socialization process[8]:
1. *Anticipatory socialization:* During this stage individuals acquire what they believe to be the attitudes, values, and beliefs of the group to which they hope to belong. Some of this learning, unfortunately, incorporates the many myths propagated by outside elements and encountered in contacts with individuals in the occupations themselves. Consider, for instance, how many times hospitals and the individual professions operating within them have been

portrayed incorrectly by television and have thereby caused would-be nurses to develop erroneous impressions about nursing as a profession.

2. *Learning in a presocializing organization* such as a university or a formal school of nursing: During this period, which culminates for most nursing professionals in graduation and passage of a licensing examination, the individual becomes more aware of the real norms of the profession.

3. *Recruitment:* The organization seeks to select individuals who already possess the skills and values desired by the organization. Proper selection makes the job of the nurse manager in the healthcare facility easier.

4. *Organizational socialization:* This type of socialization introduces individuals to the norms and values of the particular organization in which they are employed. "Reality shock" often occurs when individuals find that the norms and values of the actual work environment are different from those learned in the first two stages and anticipated during the third stage. This cold dose of reality often results in feelings of helplessness, powerlessness, frustration, and dissatisfaction.[9]

5. *The "rite of passage":* The final stage of socialization occurs when a person is finally accepted into full membership status and is committed to the actual norms and values of the organization in which they work. Four phases have been identified in the role transformation from student to staff nurse: (1) honeymoon, (2) shock, (3) recovery, and (4) resolution. The primary reason such phases are seen is that the subcultures of school and work have different values and norms. In nursing schools, the dominant values transmitted are a commitment to comprehensive patient care and an emphasis on individualization and family involvement. Use of judgment, autonomy, cognitive skills, and decision-making are stressed in this system. In the work subculture, however, the emphasis is different. Here the primary focus is on providing *high-quality* and *safe* care for all patients. Organization, efficiency, cooperation, and responsibility are highly valued.[9]

   - *Honeymoon:* The new graduate is pleased with his or her first job as a "real nurse" and focuses on learning the routines of the hospital, perfecting his or her skills, and becoming accepted by other members of the staff.
   - *Shock:* The second stage begins when the novice nurse finds out that some of the values taught in school are not as highly esteemed in the work environment.

   - *Recovery:* The third stage occurs as the new nurse begins to accept some of the aspects of the work environment that before seemed insufferable.
   - *Resolution:* The final adjustment takes place when the new nurse is able to constructively separate work and school values.

Effective and understanding nurse managers can help novice nurses through this socialization process by facilitating the exchange of experiences that can assist in resolving the conflict. It is incredibly important to help newly graduated nurses understand that the adjustment process they are undergoing is universal and to allow them to express and explore their feelings with others as they move through the various stages of assimilation.

MANAGERIAL SURVEILLANCE

Another type of control system is managerial surveillance. This process involves both direct observation (supervision) and indirect observation (maintenance of records) of the subordinate's behavior. The amount of control that can be derived from each observation source is related to the type of authority structure in the organization. In some managerial situations in a healthcare facility, such as in emergency departments and in units with a large number of beginning nurses, control through direct observation may be very important. In highly technical areas, managerial surveillance through direct observation may play a less important role.

One of the factors relating to managerial surveillance is the "span of control" of the supervisor, or the number of individuals for whom the supervisor is directly responsible. Narrow spans of control (those involving fewer than five subordinates) generally allow for a greater degree of control, whereas spans of control involving more employees make it difficult for nurse managers to control each subordinate through direct observation.

Nurse managers should implement wider spans of control when the work is of a routine nature, staff members are well trained and proficient, procedures are well established, tasks are tightly structured, or subordinates are well spread out within the unit. It is far more realistic to indirectly observe others when they are physically isolated or dispersed.

A number of sources of information can be used for indirect observation, including the following:
- Budgets
- Activity reports
- Patient surveys
- Schedules
- Statistical reports
- Narcotics reports

- Time sheets
- Patient charts

The types of information available differ from one organization to the next, just as do the standards used to evaluate the information.

As noted earlier, the more sources of influence a supervisor has over a subordinate, such as reward, coercion, legitimacy, reference, and expertise, the more likely that the supervisor will be able to direct the subordinate's behavior and guide it toward the accomplishment of organizational objectives. Rules and regulations also serve as a source of control, especially when these rules and regulations have been internalized. Reliance on this means of control is most common in those parts of the organization that have a bureaucratic structure.

PRINCIPLES OF CONTROL

No matter what specific method of control nurse managers use to influence the performance of others, to be effective they must be cognizant of the following fundamental principles of control:

Avoid "setting the fox to watch the henhouse." In this situation (first referred to by this phrase by Klein and Ritti[8]) individual performers provide their supervisors with the information that will be used to evaluate their performance. Obviously, this process is extremely easy for the unscrupulous performer to manipulate, because the information provided is generally subjective or open to judgment and not easily verifiable. When such self-reported data are used for evaluation, verification of content is *strongly advised* and *extreme caution is warranted*. This is not a recommended evaluation process in most cases.

Focus on desired behavior: Another important principle is that "measured behavior" eliminates "unmeasured behavior." If nurse managers focus on specific, measurable aspects of the job when giving feedback to the individuals under their supervision, unmeasured and undesired behavior is almost always reduced. This is a recommended evaluation process.

Understand the paradox of control: In attempting to control the efforts of subordinates, managers may unknowingly impose new requirements. This often leads to countermeasures being employed by subordinates, to avoid the control, to modify the information, or even to seek substitution of the desired action. This, in turn, leads to countermeasures by the manager, and so on, creating a vicious cycle. The "paradox" of control actually says that influence over the behavior of others can most often be achieved by perceptively giving up control. In other words, the more freedom people are given, the more they can be trusted to do what is right.[10]

Decision-Making

Decision-making is the foundation of every aspect of the manager's job and includes the following five elements:

1. Identification of a problem
2. Establishment of the criteria that will be used to evaluate potential solutions to the problem
3. Search for alternative solutions or actions (with recognition that not every action has an alternative)
4. Evaluation of the alternatives (if available)
5. Selection of a particular alternative

This process can take place in a very brief time (e.g., deciding to whom to assign a certain task) or may occur over months or even years (e.g., choosing a career, a spouse, or a new job). There is a huge difference between taking the time necessary to make an intelligent decision and procrastinating. One is an important aspect of management; the other signals ineffectiveness.

Researchers have pointed out that, when making decisions, good managers tend to use a simplified model of the real situation and focus on seeking satisfactory rather than "optimal" solutions. Most skillful managers establish some minimal criteria for an acceptable decision and then search until a solution is found that meets these criteria.[4]

FIRST-LEVEL MANAGEMENT FUNCTIONS

The functions of planning, organizing, and controlling are particularly relevant to the position of first-level manager. For the person serving as the front-line supervisor, these functions, at least most of the time, involve dealing effectively with contingencies. Because the nurse manager's fundamental responsibilities are varied (i.e., to maintain the highest possible level of patient care and, at the same time, to satisfy other, sometimes conflicting goals such as staying within budget and keeping staff satisfied), the factors that work against the accomplishment of these primary goals must be considered. These "other factors" are typically referred to as contingencies and for the purposes of this chapter are defined as those unplanned interruptions, unanticipated events, and inconvenient or awkward circumstances that prevent the work from being accomplished as originally planned.[11] Much of the discussion presented here regarding planning, organizing, and controlling by the nurse manager is based on the following ideas:

> Planning, for a supervisor, means identifying the most probable sources of contingencies in advance . . . and ensuring that his or her subordinates are ready for them. This means that the subordinates are properly equipped and in the right places at the right times; and above all that they are properly trained. Control means making sure the contingencies are properly dealt with, and, when necessary, intervening in the subordinate's work to prevent a contingency from getting out of hand (p. 106).[11]

The basic functions of the nursing process (i.e., assessing, planning, implementing, and evaluating) are very similar to the management functions of planning, organizing, and controlling, as shown in Table 4-4.

Planning

Contingency planning is very difficult for the nurse manager because of the crisis nature of hospital work and the many unknowns involved in patient care. Nevertheless, the nurse manager must make every attempt to be continually aware of the contingencies that may prevent work from being accomplished. These include, for example, (1) new, inexperienced, part-time, or temporary staff who do not know the policies and procedures of the organization thoroughly and may not be very committed to them; (2) tardiness or unexpected absenteeism, which leaves the unit short of personnel (especially on holidays, weekends, or vacations); (3) staff tardiness in returning from lunch or breaks; (4) excessive demand for space when the division is at full capacity; (5) new residents who need to be oriented; (6) unexpectedly high number of critical care patients; (7) physician requests for special services; (8) scheduling of patients to be in two or more places at the same time; (9) unavailability of sufficient staff, especially for evening and night shifts; (10) unavailability of medications, supplies, or equipment at the right time; and finally, (11) resignation of staff members without giving notice.

Once nurse managers are aware of the presence of contingencies, they must be ready to act to reduce their impact before the situation progresses so that the contingency cannot be managed effectively. This may involve the establishment of nursing rounds at the beginning of each shift and at as many other times thereafter as circumstances dictate. In addition, good nurse managers will attempt to make themselves available to their staffs through unscheduled and frequent but brief contacts designed to determine inconspicuously whether the work of the unit is progressing satisfactorily.

There are three key words in this last sentence: (1) *unscheduled,* (2) *inconspicuously,* and (3) *brief.*

"Unscheduled" means that no advance notice is given. "Inconspicuously," in this context, means that the manager's actions should be encouraging, not prying; energetic, not condemning; and enthusiastic, not superior. Conversations should be short but not cryptic, because the latter communications appear dictatorial, and they should be work related—personal discussions should be left to breaks, lunch hours, or other social occasions.

Good nurse managers do not allow themselves to slide back into a performance role when discussing an interesting task with subordinates. They understand that they are *not* performers but producers of performance. If a subordinate is adequately handling a particular situation, then the good nurse manager will quickly recognize the performance and move on to something else. This helps to ensure that a problem does not start up at another location.

Making rounds also enables nurse managers to assess the quality of patient care and the performance of the staff in the unit. During this time, managers assess the quality of care being provided, staff members' organizing abilities and interpersonal skills, team cohesion, and individual patient status. "Paper patrolling," such as reviewing records, budgets, and performance data, can also ensure that work is being performed satisfactorily. High-quality nurse managers develop a system of red flags, things that indicate at a glance that work is not being done correctly, on time, or within budget. Things that are useful indicators of poor performance are patterns of absenteeism or lateness, low ratio of time spent in the delivery of direct nursing care to time spent performing overhead functions, patient-days volume, overuse or underuse of medical-surgical supplies or pharmacy items, and failure to annotate reports (including patient charts) with situations that could indicate a potential problem. Reviews should be done periodically and without prior notice to enable early identification of potential problem situations. It is never a good idea to perform the same component of review at the same time over and over. This "practiced" approach, although probably easier to schedule, also allows the staff to know what the nurse manager will be looking for and when. It is always best to keep a little uncertainty in the review process, because it prevents staff from hiding things. Consider the following story.

> A nursing department vice president (VP) took her role as supervisor of patient care seriously and always selected a couple of charts from one of the units she supervised and reviewed them for accuracy at the beginning of her shift each day. While she did this, she would casually observe the nurses on the unit. She did this at the same time each day.
>
> It was not long before the nursing staff expected the VP to come through their unit, so immediately

TABLE 4-4

Comparison of Tasks of Clinical Nurses and Nurse Managers

Clinical Nurse	*Nurse Manager*
ASSESSMENT	
Observing the patient and his or her environment	Observing staff reactions to policies and objectives
	Observing the needs of the community (priorities in health care), personnel trends, and availability of resources
Practicing communication skills (art of listening and interviewing)	Practicing communication skills (art of listening and interviewing)
Collecting facts, identifying priorities	Collecting facts, identifying priorities
PLANNING	
Interpreting in light of clinical knowledge and the facts	Interpreting in light of managerial knowledge and the facts
Setting short- and long-term goals for the patient and family	Deciding what to do to solve problems, keeping in mind quality of care and safety, and revising policies if necessary
Involving the patient and family in the plan of care and involving healthcare personnel in other disciplines as required to ensure coordination and progress toward similar goals	Involving staff and those in other disciplines to ensure coordination of planning and progress toward similar goals
IMPLEMENTATION (ORGANIZATION)	
Setting the plan into action, taking into account the following:	Setting the plan into action, taking into account the following:
■ The patient's ability to help himself or herself	■ The amount of delegation that can be safely performed
■ Professional resources	■ Professional resources
■ Equipment available	■ Time available
Meeting teaching needs (of the patient, family, and nursing and other students)	Meeting teaching needs (for the development of staff and the orientation of new staff to fulfill their respective roles)
Organizing for continuity of care	Organizing for continuity in providing a service
Providing team leadership and an environment in which good work can be done	Providing leadership in the area of responsibility and creating an environment in which good work can be done
	Organizing the budget
	Engaging in consumer relations
EVALUATION (CONTROL)	
Analyzing results of the implementation of the care plan for the patient and family	Analyzing results of the implementation of the plan in consultation with those delivering nursing care
Considering changes that have taken place and necessitate reassessment	Considering changes that are necessary and the case for replanning or adjustment of the plan
Considering the quality of care provided and the standards and policies that have been agreed upon	Considering the quality of care provided and the standards and policies that have been agreed upon
Identifying areas of nursing practice that require revision of research	Taking action where needed
Communicating the need together with a suggestion for action to the appropriate level	Helping clinical nurses and managers to undertake research projects and critiquing practice
Communicating changes in planning that may be required to keep the patient, colleagues, and other professionals informed	Communicating changes in planning that may be required to keep staff and other professionals informed

Data from Schurr M: Getting it together, *Nurs Times* 75(35):1472, 1979.

following the beginning of the shift, every nurse in every unit found something to gainfully occupy his or her time. Everyone visited a patient, annotated charts, or busied themselves with other "important" work. As soon as the VP went back to her office, however, the work slowed and performance returned to normal. The VP prided herself on having the most industrious section in the hospital.[12]

Finally, nurse managers must consider what activities are necessary to prevent problems from happening and what the plans are for dealing with problems once they have occurred. For example, does the unit have plans for dealing with certain kinds of disasters—such as external disasters that increase the demand for unit space, or snow or floods that prevent employees from getting to work, or internal disasters such as fire or loss of power?

Organizing

Organizing means having available the properly trained staff and the proper materials, information, and equipment to deal with contingencies. These elements are normally specific to an organization and the type of services it provides but can vary slightly from unit to unit within a given organization. The nurse manager must know what these elements are and make sure that they are always available. Backup materials and equipment are especially important. It is also critical for the nurse manager to be aware of the state of the unit's equipment.

Ensuring that proper resources are available at the right time and place to take care of the unit's work is one of the most important responsibilities of nurse managers. They must make sure that unit personnel have both the knowledge and the ability to do their jobs and that they are familiar with the policies and procedures of the specific unit. This is achieved through a process of continual training that is focused on ensuring high-quality patient care. Refresher (or developmental) training should also be included so that seldom used but important skills such as cardiopulmonary resuscitation are retained. Just as ballplayers have spring training and firefighters hold fire drills, so must nurses and nursing support staff engage in periodic rehearsals of appropriate behavior for specialized situations. They should also understand the reasons behind the organization's policies, procedures, rules, and regulations that affect their work. Many times, new or inexperienced personnel do not understand many of these rules, and it is the nurse manager's role to clarify them. Helping staff nurses to understand the reasons behind the rules will frequently lead to greater compliance with these organizational requirements. This is especially important when dealing with highly educated professionals.

Another important aspect of organizing is scheduling; that is, making sure that individuals with the appropriate skills are available on each shift. Obviously, scheduling is greatly affected by the organization's employment and compensation policies. In many organizations scheduling is centralized, but in others nurse managers are individually responsible for scheduling. When scheduling is centralized, nurse managers must work closely with the central scheduling office to ensure that adequate personnel are available. If nurse managers are given scheduling responsibility themselves, they must develop comprehensive, fair, and conforming scheduling skills, which is definitely not an easy task.

Proper scheduling includes knowing in advance the capabilities of each member of the nursing team, the team member's individual availability, the special needs of the unit, and the patients receiving care. These factors affect decisions regarding when and if additional personnel will be needed as well as the development of backup staffing plans. The more nurse managers know about each member of the team (e.g., the individual's knowledge and skills, home situation, and even biologic clock), the more effective they can be at ensuring the availability of adequate personnel to meet most contingencies. Working out potential substitutions in advance can help to reduce conflicts in crisis situations.

In addition to performing the aforementioned personnel duties, nurse managers must be able to help each staff nurse organize his or her time and activities. Time management is an important aspect of a manager's job. Techniques for improving time management are as important to the staff nurse as they are to the nurse manager. The best way nurse managers can demonstrate the benefits of effective time management is by providing a good example.

Patient care is most often organized according to the type of delivery system used in the unit. There are three common means of organizing the tasks of nursing: functional nursing, team nursing, and primary nursing. These three methods, which can be described as follows, often lead to very different problems for the nurse manager[13]:

1. *Functional nursing:* In this method, the provision of nursing care is divided into separate tasks. Each task is then performed by a different set of nurses depending on the complexity of the task (in terms of judgment and technical knowledge required), and the capability and experience of the individual staff members. Each staff member is responsible for only the tasks he or she is assigned during a given tour of duty.
2. *Team nursing:* In this method, a heterogeneous team of nursing personnel delivers nursing care to a group of patients. The leader of the team is

an experienced registered nurse. The team leader is given responsibility for the planning, continuity, and assessment of the nursing care regimens of all patients cared for by the team; for supervising the team members in the implementation of nursing actions; and for evaluating the results of these actions.

3. *Primary nursing* (in a hospital setting)[14]: In this method of delivering nursing care, registered professional nurses are given total responsibility and authority for assessing, planning, implementing, and evaluating the nursing care regimens of a specified number of patients in the healthcare facility.

   The primary nurse is responsible for the care of a patient 24 hours a day, from the time of admission to the nursing unit until discharge. Associate professional nurses carry out the nursing orders when the primary nurse is not on duty.[13]

In functional nursing, nurse managers are actively involved in planning patient care. They make specific assignments, are personally responsible for coordination between staff and shifts, and are the people to whom staff members refer their questions. Nurse managers have total responsibility for the unit and must act as first-level supervisors. In team nursing, some of the supervisory functions, especially planning patient care, assigning tasks, and coordinating these tasks, are taken over by the team leader. In primary nursing, the individual nurse is responsible for planning the nursing care provided and ensuring that the plan is adhered to, even when not personally on duty.

In team nursing, nurse managers also become senior managers in the sense that they are responsible for managing performance through other supervisors (i.e., the team leaders). To be effective in team nursing, the nurse manager must (1) be a good delegator, (2) work cooperatively with the team leaders, and (3) act as a resource person for each team leader.

In primary nursing, the nurse manager is often responsible for assigning primary nurses to patients, coordinating the activities of the primary nurses on all shifts, and creating comprehensive schedules that ensure that qualified associates are available when the primary nurse is not on duty.

Controlling

To exercise control, nurse managers must observe the performance of their subordinates and take constructive corrective action when their subordinates' efforts vary from established standards. This simply means that it is the nurse manager who intervenes when contingencies appear to be becoming uncontrollable or have already gotten out of control.

The following are two major and very specific concerns regarding the exercise of control:

1. *When to take corrective action or intervene:* Highly capable nurse managers step in and exercise authority only when a specific policy, procedure, rule, or regulation has been or is likely to be violated; when there is danger to a patient or personnel; when a subordinate appears to be overwhelmed or does not possess the necessary skill, information, or authority to act properly; or when there is a threat to the property of the organization. For example, nurse managers will exercise control if they observe a staff nurse using an improper procedure that can negatively affect a patient's health or safety. They will also exercise control by stepping in and offering help in emergency situations in which the staff nurse appears to be overwhelmed or in danger of becoming so. It is important to note here that exercising control does not necessarily mean that the nurse manager will perform the corrective action himself or herself. The nurse manager has the prerogative to delegate the handling of certain contingencies by assigning specific duties to other individuals. The ability to delegate responsibility effectively is extremely important to the success of the nurse manager and the nursing unit.

   The act of controlling, intervening, or correcting the behavior of junior personnel can be a frustrating experience for both the nurse manager and the subordinate. If it is done too frequently, managerial intervention may create a situation in which subordinates lose confidence in themselves, temper their desire to act, or become unwilling to take risks and thereby stop improving their abilities. On the other hand, if the nurse manager fails to take action when it is appropriate, serious problems can result, such as increased risk to patients. It is a tightrope that must be walked carefully every day.

2. *How to intervene:* Both nurse managers and subordinates should know in advance the situations or "trigger points" that call for management intervention. Equally important is the fact that subordinates should know the conditions under which the nurse manager will be willing to provide assistance to ensure that a situation remains under control. It is imperative that nurse managers understand the importance of maintaining frequent and close contact with subordinates. It does not matter whether the contact is established during nursing rounds or through a process of casual but semiofficial stops at the nursing unit, a practice that was previously referred to as "paper patrolling." The

critical factor is that nurse managers should focus their energy and time on the prevention of problems rather than on ensuring that corrective action has been taken.

SUMMARY

- Management is the process of getting work done through others—properly, on time, and within budget. Traditional management includes the functions of planning, staffing, organizing, directing, controlling, and making decisions.
- Planning is a four-stage process that consists of the following: (1) establishment of objectives, (2) evaluation of the present situation and prediction of future needs and trends, (3) formulation of a plan, and (4) conversion of the plan into action.
- Organizational objectives address four general areas: (1) product or service, (2) efficiency, (3) social responsibilities, and (4) human resources. Trends must be predicted both inside and outside of the organization. The MBO system is an example of an approach that can be used to guide these objectives into action.
- Once a plan is established, an organizational structure must be created to carry out the plan. This process is referred to as organizing. Healthcare organizations are typically structured on the basis of product or service, type of patient, function, process, time period, and/or geographic location of care.
- One of the most important means of coordination in an organization is its authority structure. Authority involves two general types of rights: (1) the right to allocate tasks, and (2) the right to evaluate performance. The authority of the manager over the subordinate also comes from other sources of influence of the former over the latter, such as reward and coercion, legitimacy, expertise, and reference (identification with the supervisor).
- Roles and their definitions help define the authority structure of an organization.
- Socialization is the process of fitting people into the required roles and informing them of the rules inherent in any authority structure. Socialization includes five stages: (1) anticipatory socialization (acquisition of beliefs), (2) learning in a presocializing organization (school), (3) recruitment, (4) organizational socialization, and (5) the "rite of passage." It is important for nurse managers to facilitate the socialization process.
- Managerial surveillance (through observation of behavior or records) is important to the process of exercising intelligent control. The nurse manager's span of control may determine the amount of time available for observation.
- Measured behavior tends to drive out unmeasured behavior. The staff will do what is important to the manager and/or what is recognized and rewarded.
- The fundamental management functions performed by nurse managers are planning, organizing, and controlling.

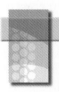

FINAL THOUGHTS

Rate the following statements on a scale of 1 to 5 (1 = strongly disagree; 2 = disagree; 3 = not sure or no strong feelings; 4 = agree; 5 = strongly agree):

1. I am responsible for my professional development.
2. I am confident about my ability to learn the skills I need to be an effective manager.
3. I am able to balance multiple priorities and responsibilities.
4. I am capable of developing a personal network of support.
5. I have a strong desire to influence others.

There is no magic score that indicates the ability to manage others. A person who answers "Not sure" in every category will score 15 points. Therefore, it is safe to say that a person scoring 20 or higher probably is confident enough to assume the responsibilities of management, and a person scoring 10 or lower is not. If you have a mentor or someone whom you respect, have that person rate you on these questions and compare scores. Are you being objective in assessing yourself?

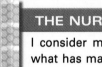

THE NURSE MANAGER SPEAKS

I consider my personal characteristics to be what has made me ready to assume my role as a nurse manager. I have always had a lot of self-confidence, and I was always good with other people. I have always found it exciting to meet and interact with other people, and I had learned a lot from my mentors over the years. The relationships I had developed with nurses at all levels helped me prepare mentally for the challenges of management. I knew I was ready to take the risk.

After I became a nurse manager, I learned that, when I visit a site to discuss a problem, I have to pay close attention to the personalities involved in the incident. Focusing totally on resolution can often be a major drawback to finding a solution and creating synergy in the unit. I make it a habit to take my time collecting data and have come to realize that sometimes the best solution is to do nothing dramatic. Many things can be dealt with by direct and frank discussion.

The thing I have learned about management is that it is a dynamic skill unto itself. It is not about being a great clinician, it is about being a great human being. My view of myself as a nurse manager is as a guide and facilitator. Control and retribution as in the bad old days do not work anymore.

REFERENCES

1. De Fee DT: *Management by objectives: when and how does it work?* Reading, Mass, 1971, Addison-Wesley.
2. Rue L, Byars L: *Management skills and applications*, ed 9, Burr Ridge, Ill, 2000, McGraw-Hill.
3. Barnard CI: *The functions of the executive*, ed 13, Cambridge, Mass, 1998, Harvard University Press.
4. Simon HA, March JG: *Organizations*, ed 2, Oxford, United Kingdom, 1993, Blackwell.
5. McClelland DC: *Power: the inner experience*, New York, 1976, Wiley.
6. Galbraith JR: *Organizational design: an executive guide to strategy, structure and design*, revised, ed 2, Hoboken, NJ, 2001, Jossey-Bass.
7. Jelenik M, Letterer JA, Miles RE: *Organizations by design: theory and practice*, ed 2, Plano, Tex, 1986, Business Publications.
8. Klein SM, Ritti RR: *Understanding organizational behavior*, ed 2, New York, 1984, Kent Publications.
9. Kramer M, Schalmemberg C: *Coping with reality shock*, Wakefield, Mass, 1989, Nursing Resources.
10. Dalton GW: *Motivation and control in organizations*, Homewood, Ill, 1971, Richard D. Irwin.
11. Gellerman S: *Effective supervision: planning, organizing and controlling*, ed 10, Rockville, Mass, 1995, BNA Communications.
12. Hawkins JA: *American business dynamics*, ed 2, Honolulu, 2004, Directions Corporation.
13. Kron T, Gray A: *The management of patient care: putting leadership skills to work*, ed 6, Philadelphia, 1967, Saunders.
14. Manthey M: *The practice of primary nursing*, ed 2, London, 1992, Kings Fund Publisher.

SUGGESTED READINGS

Belasco JA, Stayer RC: *The flight of the buffalo*, Los Angeles, 1994, Warner Books.
Douglas IM: *The effective nurse: leader and manager*, St Louis, 1984, Mosby.
Gillies DA: *Nursing management: a systems approach*, Philadelphia, 1982, Saunders.
Huber DL, editor: *Leadership and nursing care management*, ed 3, Philadelphia, 2006, Saunders.
Marcus LJ: *Renegotiating healthcare*, San Francisco, 1996, Jossey-Bass.
Marriner Tomey A: *Guide to nursing management and leadership*, ed 7, St Louis, 2004, Mosby.
Rowland BL, Rowland HS: *Nursing administration handbook*, Germantown, Md, 1985, Aspen.
Ryan DK, Oestreich DK, Orr GA: *The courageous messenger*, San Francisco, 1996, Jossey-Bass.
Simons GF, Vazquez C, Harris PR: *Transcultural leadership*, Houston, 1993, Gulf Publishing.

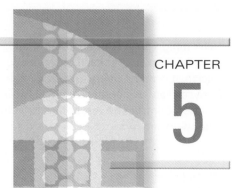

Developing and Managing Healthcare Productivity

OUTLINE

LEARNING SYNOPSIS

Upon successful completion of this chapter, readers will possess a fundamental understanding of how productivity is viewed, computed, and evaluated in the nursing department or unit.

OBJECTIVES

1. Be able to define productivity correctly as it applies to industry and to the healthcare field
2. Identify hospital products, or output
3. Define productivity using an open systems model
4. Identify effective methods for measuring productivity in the nursing environment
5. Describe methods for improving nursing productivity

Each year the countries of the world invest a good percentage of their combined total gross national product in the provision of health care to their citizens. In return for their investment, these nations expect their respective healthcare providers to be able to give an accounting of how the money was spent and what results were obtained with it. Because healthcare costs have risen faster than the rate of inflation over the past two decades, both consumers and policy makers have cried loud and long for reductions in healthcare costs, decreases in waste, prudent allocations of scarce resources, and evidence that the care provided is of high quality.

In recent years externally imposed economic limitations have required that healthcare facilities become far more attentive to productivity and its effect on cost. Nursing is one of the healthcare services that has been subjected to almost continual productivity evaluation. Nursing comprises the largest single department in most healthcare organizations and typically accounts for 50% or more of the average operating budget of institutions such as hospitals and nursing homes. Because of its typical size, and because reductions in the number of nurses hired can appear small in relation to the typical reductions implemented in other smaller departments, nursing services are often the targets of those who seek to further reduce the operating budget of a healthcare facility. As a result, the definition and measurement of nursing productivity has become a high priority for the professional nurse manager.

Unfortunately, the historical measurement of nursing productivity is a concept that is not well defined. This chapter investigates the concept of productivity and describes methods of measuring nursing productivity. It also outlines strategies that can be used by the nurse manager to enhance productivity within the nursing unit or department.

DEFINING PRODUCTIVITY

Economic and Industrial Definitions

Productivity, as an economic concept, is the relationship between the output of an industry and the resources required to produce that output or, as it is expressed in production circles, *output per input* or *O/I*. Output per unit is measured using a variety of methods, but the most common one is the *labor productivity statistic*. Labor productivity is measured as the dollar value of the output produced per worker-hour and provides a simple means to estimate the degree to which industries are becoming more or less efficient in their production methods. However, labor productivity, because it considers only a single input (the cost of labor), does not take into account other influences acting on the production process that might provide reasons for any increases or declines in efficiency, and it only marginally considers how hard employees actually work. The following are some of the other input-related factors that affect efficiency:

- Introduction of new technology
- Changes in the cost of raw materials
- Substitution of equipment
- Availability of resources or supplies

Such influences are extremely important, and their contribution should be carefully considered when attempting to estimate the efficiency of production. To compute the productivity of labor accurately, a measure should be used that takes into account all of the available productivity factors (total labor factor).

Healthcare Definitions

Defining productivity in the healthcare field is far more complex than simply determining whether only labor statistics or a total labor factor should be used to determine input. The process is extremely difficult because the fundamental question of what should be considered as inputs has yet to be definitively addressed; moreover, few professionals agree on precisely how outputs should be measured.

THE NATURE OF HEALTHCARE INPUTS

Typically, inputs present fewer measurement problems than do outputs. Inputs are such things as the labor, materials, and equipment used in the actual production of the services delivered. Inputs are normally measured in units such as the following:

- Number of hours of labor performed
- Hard dollars spent on equipment, remodeling, or building expenses
- Type and quantity of supplies used

The measurement of some of the inputs in the healthcare industry, however, is not as easy as one might think. For example, the nursing department, and the nurses who comprise it, do not form a homogeneous group, because virtually all nurses who are part of the team vary from one another in terms of level and quality of education, depth and breadth of experience, and individual talents, skills, and professional dedication. Initially, some of the differences in educational level and experience may be reflected in the individual compensation (pay) rates of the members of the nursing team. Education and experience do not always tell the entire story, however, because any two nurses who have achieved identical educational levels and years of experience can, and very frequently do, differ considerably in their efficiency and ability to perform a specific quantity and type of work. Methods for quantifying differences in skill level, then, are fundamental to determining a specific nurse's proficiency.

THE NATURE OF THE HOSPITAL'S PRODUCT

As has been shown, arriving at an exact definition of input is not an easy process; but even more challenging is determining exactly what healthcare *output* is. Two basic approaches are currently used to define output: patient-days and case mix.

Patient-Days. Until recently, hospital output was most frequently defined as patient-days; that is, the total number of days all patients were hospitalized in a facility over a period of time.[1] Further study revealed the obvious fact that some patient-days require the use of many more of the healthcare organization's resources than do others. For example, a day of care provided for a heart patient in the cardiac care unit is far more costly than a day of postpartum care in the maternity ward. Therefore, if output is to be defined accurately, the traditional method of simply counting patient-days is woefully inadequate.

Case Mix. A more modern concept of hospital output, and one often considered more realistic, assumes that the organization has more than one product. In this approach, patients are categorized into groupings, or clusters, based on similarities in their use of hospital resources. The following list shows various dimensions that have been used to *cluster* patients[2]:

- Diagnosis
- Prognosis
- Utilization
- Organ system involved
- Hospital department
- Patient demographics

In the United States, the most frequently used and best known application of the case-mix approach is the diagnosis-related group (DRG) system. This system categorizes patients into 468 separate resource-use groups. Each group is based on standardized patient information such as (1) diagnosis, (2) age, and (3) use of specific procedures. If a hospital uses the DRG case-mix approach, it can generate a large number of distinct products that differ from one another with regard to individual structure and cost of production. Each DRG can then be weighted to reflect the average cost of providing care to patients in that specific category. Although the DRG method is not without its challenges and many arguments have been made about the legitimacy of the individual resource clusters within the DRG system, this system or some case-mix system similar to it is likely to remain in use for the foreseeable future, simply because it provides far greater accuracy in measuring

hospital output than does the traditional *patient-day* method.

OUTPUT OR OUTCOME

Although case-mix measures have advanced the processes hospitals use to measure output *quantity,* they do not, by themselves, address the equally important subject of output *quality.* Determining the quality of services produced is another remarkably difficult challenge facing healthcare organizations. This challenge has been addressed in many different commercial product markets, such as those for household appliances and automobiles. Here, the consumer is usually able to evaluate the quality of a specific product through careful inspection or reference to a consumers' guide produced after thorough research of that product. If a manufacturer consistently delivers an inferior product, consumers express their dissatisfaction and desire for improved quality by not purchasing that manufacturer's products.

When consumers are required to *purchase* healthcare services, however, the options available to them are fundamentally different. Service delivery differs from the traditional conveyance of a product because the service is routinely developed and delivered in the immediate presence of the consumer. Because the delivery of health care is the provision of a service, its production and consumption are most often simultaneous events. Although consumers can and frequently do return defective products, it is far more difficult for consumers to reverse the effects of poor service, especially when the service is healthcare related. The consumer is handicapped even further because there is no existing consumers' guide to healthcare services and most consumers are incapable of evaluating the quality of healthcare services—or at least do not have the time to learn how to do so. Instead, the consumer (patient) must rely on the skill and ethical obligation of the healthcare professional to exercise sound judgment when making decisions about the type, quantity, and quality of health care required.

To protect the interests of the patient, it has increasingly become necessary to define healthcare output in terms of the quality as well as the quantity of delivered services. The ultimate goal of the healthcare industry is to describe its service production in terms of a quality-adjusted output or an *outcome.*

Adjustments to take into account the quality of the output can be based on either one of the following:

1. The soundness of the care process used to produce the output
2. The quality of the output itself

Generally, it is most convenient to measure the soundness of the care process itself, but a measurement such as this assumes that a verifiable relationship exists between the healthcare activities performed and the outcome attained by the patient. One question might be, for example, "Does a verifiable cause-and-effect relationship exist between preoperative instruction and enhanced recovery following surgery?" If a link between process and outcome can be demonstrated, then the existence of evidence showing that the best process was used also represents evidence of the quality of the service delivered. Although researchers have made considerable progress in demonstrating that these relationships do exist in nursing care, much work remains to be done, and progress continues to be agonizingly slow.

The alternative to measuring the care process is to directly assess the quality of the output (i.e., the outcome of care). This process, however, has traditionally proven to be both difficult and expensive. It is difficult because the ultimate outcome of many episodes of illness (care and treatment encounters) may not be known for some time after the care has been terminated. It is expensive because it often entails locating the patient after the care and treatment end to perform specific, nonroutine assessments. Finding significant indicators of quality that are easily measured has been an ongoing task for the last four decades and more than likely will continue to remain a key task far into the twenty-first century.

DEFINING NURSING PRODUCTIVITY

The preceding paragraphs discussed the fact that there are basically two approaches to measuring productivity in use today with in the healthcare field. The economic/industrial concept tells us that productivity is the ratio of work output to work input (i.e., units of output/units of input). This approach is derived from the scientific management tradition of the early twentieth century, when the question "How can we design processes and procedures to produce the product most efficiently?" was first asked. One example of the application of scientific management principles to the nursing profession is the patient classification systems (PCSs) that have been used for measuring nursing workloads.

Although the principles of scientific management have been applied to the area of nursing productivity, a second, more comprehensive model of nursing productivity continues to be advocated by the healthcare industry and the nursing literature. This second model attempts to include both effectiveness and efficiency by placing productivity in a systems framework. This model,[3] which was first applied to the U.S. nursing profession in 1976, incorporates an *open systems* framework such as that shown in Fig. 5-1 to describe the relationship between inputs, processes, and outputs. In addition, the model suggests that the influence of the environment must also be considered to develop usable data. These elements can be defined as follows:

Input includes the amount of nursing personnel and the various types of skills they exercise, the equipment and supplies used, and the monetary costs involved in providing the required care.

Process includes all of the activities and resources that are required to convert input into output.

Output represents the product(s) that result from the use of the processes and inputs.

Environment represents those influences that operate external to the organization or unit and over which the typical nursing manager has little or no control. These factors include (but are not limited to) labor laws, healthcare financing, policies, and personnel licensing laws.

It is imperative that one place all of the elements related to *effectiveness* into the operational definition of the output when discussing the efficiency of healthcare organizations.[4]

Effectiveness: That part of a hospital's output that refers to the safety, suitability, and quality of the care it delivers and that includes health status changes, patient outcomes, and patient satisfaction.

Efficiency: The condition in which the inputs and methods used to create a product or service result in the maximum possible output.

The two different approaches to defining productivity that have been outlined here offer practicing nurses a choice. On the one hand, nurses may be attracted by the simplicity and ease of measurement offered by typical industrial definitions of productivity

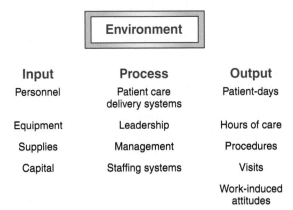

Fig. 5-1 ■ Framework of nursing productivity. (Data from Jelinek RC, Dennis LC: *A review and evaluation of nursing productivity,* DHEW No HRA 77-15, Bethesda, Md, 1976, Health Resources Administration.)

and yet be put off when they consider how the average industrial model reduces the complicated process of patient care to simple output-input ratios. On the other hand, the nursing profession is instinctively drawn to the comprehensive definitions of productivity that incorporate estimates of effectiveness, but this enthusiasm must be tempered by the fact that applying these definitions in the real world may be extremely difficult because of the limited time and money available to support the development of a comprehensive evaluation.

MEASURING NURSING PRODUCTIVITY

Currently, a variety of performance measures are used to evaluate the productivity of nursing services. Although some of these measures do not meet the strict definition of productivity as a ratio of output to input, most provide the individual nursing manager with important information about the efficiency of the nursing care delivered in the unit. The following discussion highlights a few of these measures.

Resources per Patient-Day

One of the simplest and most frequently used indicators of labor productivity is nursing hours per patient-day. This method of evaluation provides a simple and easily understood process for the nurse manager. As shown in Box 5-1, labor productivity is calculated by totaling the number of hours for which nursing personnel are paid during a specific time period and then dividing that figure by the total number of patient-days for the same period. To accurately reflect the cost of nursing care, the total paid hours must include the following three elements:

1. *Fringe benefit hours paid:* vacation, holiday, and sick hours used that were paid during the period in question
2. *Collateral hours paid:* any hours for which nursing administrators are paid
3. *Service delivery hours paid:* paid hours spent in direct patient care

Although nursing hours per patient-day was one of the first performance measures developed and remains one of the most frequently used, it is limited in that it attributes productivity and all changes in productivity from one time period to another to a single input: *the number of hours of nursing care provided.* This approach has several major flaws, because it does not consider any changes in the following critical areas:

- The care process
- The supplies and equipment used

BOX 5-1

Calculation of Resources Used per Patient-Day

NURSING HOURS PER PATIENT-DAY (C)

$$\frac{\text{Total number of paid hours for nursing personnel for period (A)}}{\text{Total number of patient-days for period (B)}}$$

or

$$\frac{A}{B} = C$$

or

DIRECT NURSING HOURS PER PATIENT-DAY (F)

$$\frac{\text{Total number of paid hours for nursing personnel providing direct care for period (D)}}{\text{Total number of patient-days for period (E)}}$$

or

$$\frac{D}{E} = F$$

NURSING SALARY COSTS PER PATIENT-DAY (I)

$$\frac{\text{Total payroll expenses for nursing personnel for period (G)}}{\text{Total number of patient-days for period (H)}}$$

or

$$\frac{G}{H} = I$$

DIRECT NURSING CARE SALARY COSTS PER PATIENT-DAY (L)

$$\frac{\text{Total payroll expenses for nursing personnel providing direct care for period (J)}}{\text{Total number of patient-days for period (K)}}$$

or

$$\frac{J}{K} = L$$

- Any factor that may have increased or decreased the actual efficiency or effectiveness of the care provided
- The skill level of the staff providing the care
- The type and intensity of the actual patient-days being considered
- The quality of the patient-days being produced

Another very similar performance measure used is *nursing salary costs per patient-day.* This is a slightly more refined measure, because the use of salary expenses does, to some extent, take into account the skill mix of the staff. Nursing salary cost per patient-day is calculated simply by totaling the actual salaries paid for nursing personnel and dividing that figure by the total patient-days for the same time period.

Standardization of Patient-Day

Both nursing hours per patient-day and salary costs per patient-day are computations that have proven useful as measures of labor productivity (i.e., personnel costs per unit of output). However, this holds true only if the nature of the patient-day is constant. If the characteristics of the patients cared for on a nursing unit change, it becomes very difficult using this method to know whether nursing productivity has also changed unless an adjustment is made that compensates for any change in the nature of the care given. To illustrate this difficulty, let us consider a nursing unit that provides the same number of hours of care during two different periods of time. If the number of patients and the level of patient dependency is exactly the same during the two time periods, actual labor productivity will also remain the same. However, if the overall level of patient dependency on nursing care increases during the second time period, the labor productivity for that period will also increase proportionally.

One way to consider the effect of patient dependency levels on productivity is to standardize what actually constitutes a patient-day by using information from a PCS, a system that is designed to measure nursing workload. Including this new factor allows productivity measurements to be standardized by replacing patient-days with the required hours of care as calculated by the PCS. Performance ratios can then be calculated as shown in Box 5-2. If desired, the required hours of care can be divided by 24 to produce required days of care. Such standardization of patient-days improves the validity of comparisons between nursing hours and nursing salary costs per patient-day or other monitoring period.

BOX 5-2

Calculation of Resources Used per Standardized Patient-Day

NURSING HOURS PER STANDARDIZED PATIENT-DAY (A)

$$\frac{\text{Total number of paid hours (or days) for nursing personnel for period (B)}}{\text{Total number of required hours (or days) of care for period (C)}}$$

or

$$\frac{B}{C} = A$$

NURSING SALARY COSTS PER STANDARDIZED PATIENT-DAY (D)

$$\frac{\text{Total payroll expenses for nursing personnel for period (E)}}{\text{Total number of required hours (or days) of care for period (F)}}$$

or

$$\frac{E}{F} = D$$

Degree of Occupation

The degree to which the nursing staff is occupied is another commonly used productivity indicator. The *degree of occupation* is regularly measured by nursing managers on a very informal basis using a "busyness scale." Nursing managers employ this "scale" as they observe unit staff in the normal performance of their duties. This involves making an educated judgment as to whether the number of staff members available is sufficient to handle the workload.

On the surface, this procedure appears too subjective and informal to be valid; however, many observers strongly believe that a skilled and experienced nurse manager can, in fact, act as a very finely tuned measurement instrument when it comes to assessing staffing adequacy. This assumption has led to the development of methods to help nurse managers more systematically assess the degree of occupation or staffing adequacy. One method requires the nurse manager to answer a series of questions about the activity level on the unit that day, such as the number of admissions made and surgeries conducted, and to make an educated judgment as to the adequacy of the number of staff assigned and the quality of care provided.

Many researchers have serious concerns regarding the validity of degree of occupation as a satisfactory productivity measure. For example, many argue that poor organization or a lack of support services and equipment can cause the staff to perform inefficiently. Because of the lack of these external factors, the staff may be appear to be extremely busy and the unit understaffed when current practice models are used, but that does not preclude the possibility that the quantity and quality of care given can be improved considerably without increasing the cost of nursing services.[5]

Utilization Rates

One of the most frequently applied and best understood performance measures in the nursing field is the ratio of required to actual staffing levels. This performance measure is also the one most frequently used by nurse staffing systems, and in the vast majority of situations it is based on patient classifications.

The institution's PCS is used by nurse managers to forecast the number of hours of care that each patient will require in the immediate future, normally one or two shifts in advance. Nurse managers use the information contained in the PCS as one of the major components for calculating utilization rates for nurse staffing in their units.

When calculating the amount of nursing assistance that will be needed in the unit, nurse managers first determine what is known as the "required hours of care." This figure simply details the amount of nursing time that will be required to care for all of the patients being assisted by a particular unit in a specified period of time based on the information in the PCS. To take account of additional requirements that exceed the "required hours of care," the nurse manager carefully considers special needs and marks this time as hours spent in "indirect care activities." This normally includes time for activities such as charting, making referrals, and performing unit maintenance activities, as well as time used by the assigned nurses for breaks and meals. The actual hours utilized (paid) are calculated at the end of a particular shift. From these two values, the utilization rate (productivity) can then be calculated as follows:

$$\text{Required hours of care} = \frac{\text{Utilization rate}}{\text{Nursing hours paid}}$$

Table 5-1 illustrates how utilization rate would be reported in a nursing management information system. The actual hours of patient care provided are subtracted from the number of hours that were predicted to be required, and the result is the difference. The utilization rate is then calculated by dividing the required hours of care by the number of hours actually provided and multiplying the result by 100. A rate of 100% indicates that the actual hours provided were equal to the number of hours required; a value lower than 100% means that the number of hours spent was higher than predicted; and a value higher than 100% indicates that fewer hours of care were provided than were required. Most healthcare organizations believe that an acceptable utilization rate is one that falls between 85% and 115%.

Although the calculation described probably represents the single best day-to-day monitoring measure available to nursing managers, it is not a true indicator of actual nursing productivity. Unless certain assumptions are made concerning the required hours of care,

it is more accurate to refer to such a calculation as a *utilization rate* (as has been done here) than as a productivity indicator. The reason is that, unlike standard economic definitions of productivity, the ratio of required to actual hours of care contains only an input measurement (actual hours) and does not incorporate an output measurement as required by the classic definition.

Required Hours of Care as an Output

The ratio of required to actual hours of care discussed in the preceding section is useful as a productivity measure only if the nursing service assumes or has demonstrated that the designated required number of nursing hours can provide the quantity and quality of care the hospital wishes to provide. In other words, the use of staff utilization ratios to determine productivity is based on one extremely important, but frequently and often conveniently overlooked, assumption: that the standard hours of care defined in the PCS and used to calculate the required nursing hours are sufficient to provide the level of service desired and therefore can legitimately serve as a substitute measure for output.

If the required hours of care is to be used as an output indicator, then this value should be thought of as *targeted hours of care*, or the minimum number of hours of care that are required to produce the quality of care desired. To ensure that targeted hours is an adequate substitute measure of desired output, the nursing department must validate the specific values used either by finding research studies by others which show that this amount of care produces the desired results or by carrying out its own evaluation studies. Such validation is required if an organization is to ensure that a given quantity and quality of care can be produced by a given number of nursing care hours.

TABLE 5-1

Typical Productivity Monitoring System

| Cost Identifier | FTE Hours | | | |
	Required Hours	Actual Hours	Difference	Productivity
432	45	45	0	100%
433	45	42	3	107%
434	45	48	−3	94%

FTE, Full-time equivalent. This is an expression usually given in labor days and is calculated as the number of hours required divided by the number of labor hours in 1 full day (usually 8 hours). FTEs may be substituted for hours.

An example taken from a typical maternity service can be used to illustrate this important fact. Let us assume that the service has determined that 5 hours of professional and 2 hours of nonprofessional nursing care meet the outcome standards set by the service for the postpartum period (Box 5-3). By a careful evaluation of outcomes, the providers of this service have determined that, when patients are discharged after a reasonable number of hospitalization days, they are generally satisfied with their treatment and are able to care for themselves and their infants properly. The complication rate is also judged to be acceptable.

If a nursing service provides the type of evidence that meets the institution's own standards, then targeted hours of the appropriate quantity and quality of care have been established properly.[5]

Box 5-3 shows the process for calculating the productivity of the unit. According to these calculations, when the actual hours of care provided match the targeted hours, productivity is said to be at 100%, but when actual hours performed exceed the targeted

amount, the unit's productivity will fall to a level below 100%. Calculating productivity in this manner causes a problem when the actual hours expended to deliver the service are less than the targeted amount. Although many institutions would calculate and report the unit's productivity as 106%, as shown in Box 5-3, many people doubt the validity of such a figure, arguing that productivity can never really exceed 100% in a legitimate calculation. A drop in actual usage of staff below the targeted level suggests that the standards originally used to establish the target were set too high or that the organization is willing to, and perhaps did, compromise its established standards without fully appreciating the potential consequences. For these reasons, some have suggested that productivity levels should never exceed 100% unless the clinical service can demonstrate that the care process has been made more efficient by using either new methods or new equipment *and* that the quality of the outcome has not been reduced.

IMPROVING NURSING PRODUCTIVITY

So far this chapter has reviewed and critiqued some of the more commonly used indicators of nursing performance and suggested ways to improve them. From this point forward, the chapter looks at how the nurse manager can improve nursing productivity. As can be seen from Fig. 5-1, there are two ways of improving productivity:

1. Changing the inputs
2. Changing the care process

Changes in the nursing environment, at least in most circumstances, are largely beyond the control of the typical nursing manager.

Changing the Inputs

Inputs are those things such as raw materials, personnel, supplies, and equipment that are used to provide a service or produce a product. Traditionally, very little attention has been given to the raw materials of nursing services because patients and families are difficult to think of in this manner.

The typical nursing staff has little control over the type of patients served. Recent hospital activities to identify specific areas of excellence and to market those professional services to the communities the institution serves may provide more control. So will the fact that many nursing departments and individual nursing practitioners are also marketing their special service capabilities. Such activities may increase the amount of influence that modern nursing staffs have over the type of patients for whom they care.

BOX 5-3

Targeted Hours of Care as an Output Indicator

OUTCOME STANDARDS
Average length of stay = 2.9 days
Knowledge and skill
- 90% of patients score above 80% on a postteaching test of knowledge
- 98% of patients give satisfactory return baby bath demonstration

Satisfaction
- 90% of patients satisfied or very satisfied as indicated by questionnaire

Complications
- 2% postpartum and newborn infection rate
- 50% of mothers continue to breast-feed for at least 1 month

CALCULATION OF PRODUCTIVITY
These standards can be met by providing 7 hours of nursing care per patient-day. Therefore, productivity can be calculated as follows, using hypothetical actual hours of care provided:

$$\frac{\text{Target}}{\text{Actual}} = \frac{7}{7} = 100\%$$

$$\frac{\text{Target}}{\text{Actual}} = \frac{7}{7.9} = 89\%$$

$$\frac{\text{Target}}{\text{Actual}} = \frac{7}{6.6} = 106\%$$

MATCHING SUPPLY WITH DEMAND

The most expensive single input in the provision of nursing care is obvious: labor. Therefore, it follows that the greatest productivity gains should be achieved through the careful selection and use of personnel. One of the easiest methods of controlling labor input is to base the requirements for care on patient classification data and then to schedule the appropriate nursing personnel to meet the expected demand.

Before the development of PCSs, the number of nursing staff scheduled for a specific shift or a specific unit was determined by preestablished global staff-patient ratios (i.e., so many nurses per so many patients). These global standards did not consider the individual requirements of the patients who were to be assisted; some patients, for example, required more and more specialized care than that made available through fixed staff-patient ratios, and some patients required less.[6]

PCSs are designed to correct this inadequate distribution of skill with regard to need by grouping patients into specific categories based on similarity in nursing care requirements. Using concepts derived from scientific management theory, PCSs first assume that nursing care can be subdivided into specific functions that vary in the length of time and specific skills required to perform them. Once the specific nursing functions are identified, then the actual time required to assist patients whose care requires different combinations of skills must be measured. PCSs use one of the following two basic approaches in characterizing required hours of care:

1. *Large number of tasks:* PCSs of this type use a long and comprehensive list of specific tasks, each of which has an identified time requirement. In this approach, patients are categorized into one of several groups (usually four or five) based on the time required for staff to complete all of the tasks identified for them.

2. *Small number of tasks:* Some PCSs base their categorization on only a few tasks, such as bathing, feeding, and ambulation, that have been shown to be critical indicators or predictors of the amount of care required.[7] In this type of PCS, patients are categorized into one of four or five groups based on how many of these critical indicators apply. Then the average amount of time required to care for the patients in each category is measured.

Regardless of the type of PCS used, the most important characteristic is that its categorizations be valid and reliable. Use of an invalid or unreliable PCS not only will lead to the inappropriate allocation of nursing personnel but can also cause dissatisfaction among the nursing staff. It is likely that individual staff members will attempt to undermine a system that they perceive to be inaccurate. The validity and reliability of a PCS can be maintained only through a process of regular monitoring that allows adjustments to be made in response to changes in conditions.

Once the nurse manager is convinced that the PCS produces accurate data, the system can be used many times each day. The actual classification tools are descriptions or checklists of a number of variables. How often patients are reclassified is a decision that is made by the nursing division and is based on a number of considerations, including the degree of change in a specific patient's condition from shift to shift and the ability of the staffing system to make changes in allocation.

After the nursing care requirements of each patient have been determined, the total amount of nursing time that will be required by all patients in the unit is calculated using the methods specified by the PCS. This *total time* is then used to predict the amount of care time that will be required for that specific set of patients for the next one or two shifts.

To determine the number of staff members needed to care for patients in those future shifts, nursing managers simply divide the *total time* by the number of hours worked by each nurse per shift (usually eight). The number of staff members required is then compared with the number of nurses who have been scheduled to work that shift minus any known absences.

The key to efficient resource use is to effectively match the types of skill that will be required with the staff that are available. If more nurses are needed than are scheduled, or if specific skills are required that cannot be provided by the scheduled nurses, the nurse manager will need to identify other nurses who can work that shift. The nurse manager does this by referring to a *float pool* of unscheduled employees or contacting a substitute nursing service. If more nurses are scheduled than are needed, the nursing manager may need to ask some of the staff to *float* to other units in the hospital that have a greater need, or simply not to come to work.

MAKING STAFF SUBSTITUTIONS

Because of the variation in education, skill, and experience among the nursing staff, nursing labor input usually does not exist in homogeneous units. These differences among staff are typically reflected in variations in salary that are linked to the level of expertise. Many experts believe that it is logical to take advantage of these salary differences. At first glance, and to the casual observer, it might seem that employing a larger number of lower-paid, nonprofessional staff would reduce personnel costs. For example, if the number of licensed practical nurses and nursing assistants were increased in relation to the number of registered nurses (RNs), more hours of labor per patient-day would be available without a corresponding direct increase in cost.

Strong theoretical arguments exist both for and against the use of staff substitution as a method of improving nursing productivity, however. Those who advocate the scientific management approach feel that productivity is greatest when the work of providing care to individual patients is divided into its component parts and the tasks are assigned to staff members according to their individual abilities. Under this philosophy, tasks are assigned to the least costly personnel capable of performing those tasks; the most qualified individuals are assigned only those tasks requiring their special expertise.[8] The advocates of the human relations theoretical framework represent the other side of the coin. This group disagrees with the lowest-capability-first method of assignment. According to this view, highly skilled workers such as registered nurses are more satisfied, and therefore more productive, when they are allowed to complete whole tasks, that is, to provide total patient care for a caseload of patients. This viewpoint does not support dividing the work into its component parts and assigning isolated tasks to individual performers.

Not only are there conflicting theoretical predictions as to what division of labor will be more productive, but the experimental studies performed to provide support for the various viewpoints have produced inconclusive results. Unfortunately, in some experiments in which the proportion of professional to nonprofessional staff was increased, primary nursing was also introduced.[9-12] As in any research study, the use of two experimental treatments simultaneously makes it nearly impossible to sort out which of the reported changes is attributable to which element of the overall experiment. This inability to differentiate between variables makes the data all but unusable as substantiating evidence to support a specific viewpoint. Other investigations of all-RN or predominantly RN staffing have been uncontrolled case studies rather than experiments and have not, by themselves, been able to provide convincing arguments to support their hypotheses.[13-16]

Although there are many acknowledged methodologic problems in the studies examining skill mix in the provision of nursing care, use of a high proportion of professional staff in clinical situations has several commonly accepted advantages:

Greater patient satisfaction: The presence of highly professional staff is strongly believed to lead to greater patient satisfaction[17] and improved coordination and quality of care.[18-20]

Reduced costs: Several studies suggest that the use of nursing assistants may actually increase overall nursing costs and thus provide support for reliance on a more professional nursing staff. The reason costs are increased is that these less skilled performers require far more supervision and instruction in the use of proper procedures than do more professional nurses. This point is confirmed by studies showing that the average nursing assistant is occupied in care-related tasks only 65% to 73% of the time he or she is scheduled to work, whereas RNs are occupied, on average, 82% to 98% of their scheduled performance time.[21,22]

Findings such as these suggest that the provision of nursing services in hospitals is often too varied and unpredictable to allow them to take full advantage of the economies that might theoretically be achieved by assigning nursing tasks to the least skilled individuals capable of performing them. In addition, substantial evidence exists that a high ratio of professional to nonprofessional personnel may, at a minimum, be no more expensive than a lower ratio and in fact frequently may prove to be far less costly in terms of salary expenses and turnover rates. Methodologic uncertainties in some of the available literature make it essential that investigations in this area continue.[9,10,12-15,23-25]

CONTROLLING THE USE OF SUPPLY AND EQUIPMENT RESOURCES

Input costs can also be greatly affected by ensuring that the nurse manager prudently controls the use of available supplies and equipment. One effective management method is to compare the cost and features of a variety of equivalent supplies and equipment and then select those products that deliver the desired quality at the lowest cost. One of the best ways to implement this procedure is to have either the individual nurse manager or the institution's purchasing department use a competitive bidding process in which potential vendors submit proposals so that products can be obtained at the lowest cost.

Once the purchase is made, ensuring that supplies and equipment are used wisely can further control their costs. One of the best methods of accomplishing this is to have the individual nurse manager implement systems that closely monitor the use of supplies. A carefully developed monitoring system will serve both to reduce waste and to prevent theft. Improving the awareness of cost and increasing each nurse's sensitivity to it are also methods of reducing cost. In one reported case, a nurse manager was able to produce significant savings in her unit simply by placing price tags on all chargeable supplies. Hospital nurses who participated in this study discovered that they could substitute less expensive items, and even avoid the use of some items, with no reduction in the quality of service.[26]

Changing the Care Process

Nurse managers who want to exercise their individual creativity will find that looking for ways to improve productivity by making changes in the care process offers them a significant opportunity to do so. A comprehensive 1976 review of the literature on nursing productivity called the care process the "technology of nursing."[3] According to the definition used in that study, technology consists of "all methodologies employed in converting inputs into outputs." If this concept is still accurate, then "technology" includes all of the physical and managerial structure of nursing services, leadership and supervision, patient care delivery systems, staffing and scheduling practices, care planning, documentation procedures, and the performance of nursing activities. At the very least, such a viewpoint clearly suggests many opportunities to experiment with methods for improving the quantity and quality of nursing care provided. It would be impractical for this text to provide illustrations of all the ways the process of care could be changed. The following are some representative examples:

Adjustment of work schedules: One of the most frequently used methods for enhancing the care process is modifying nurses' work schedules. For example, it is possible to restructure work weeks by implementing different shift schedules for the available nurses. The use of four 10-hour shifts, three 12-hour shifts, or even special weekend schedules have been reported to have a significant impact on staffing efficiency while also meeting the individual nurse's need for increased leisure time.[27-30]

Job sharing or job pairing: These are programs in which two individuals divide one full-time position. This form of modification has increased flexibility for the individual nurse and also provided the hospital with the ability to schedule the right nurse into the right position at the proper time.

Reduction in rituals: It has been suggested that nursing might become more productive if nurses were to forgo some of the traditional "rituals" of nursing care. These rituals include such routine activities as changing linens and giving daily baths when not necessarily indicated. Rituals are things that are often done out of habit, and the best interests of the patient are not always in mind when they are being performed. When these rituals are

reviewed for possible elimination, however, there will be some that appear to be unnecessary at first glance but may be required to reduce the institution's liability. Therefore, a careful needs evaluation must be performed before an organization modifies these rituals to enable a nursing unit to free up time for more important work.

Changes in the direct care process: Making some fundamental changes in the direct care process may result in improvements to the quantity and quality of the patient care delivered. For example, new approaches to common clinical challenges such as incontinence and situational confusion are showing significant promise and may prove useful.

Alternative delivery methods: Organizations can also investigate alternative delivery methods for nursing care such as primary nursing or a **modular delivery system**. These alternative methods have the potential to increase productivity when used in the proper circumstances.

New or improved products and equipment: When organizations upgrade the equipment and care products they use to deliver patient care, there is typically a marked improvement in individual and group productivity rates in the nursing unit.

DOCUMENTING CHANGES

Regardless of what changes are made in the care process, it is absolutely imperative that each change and its possible consequences be effectively and efficiently measured, analyzed, and evaluated. Without careful documentation, it may prove extremely difficult to convince decision-makers that the innovations being introduced are safe, effective, and efficient and have a positive impact on the quality and quantity of patient care. Consider the following example involving a clinic specializing in midwife services:

Several years ago the staff of a clinic providing midwife services decided they would be more efficient if they replaced their existing individual approach to early prenatal teaching and orientation with a group approach. After the group approach was used several times, it became apparent that the patients, who were largely from several minority groups and many of whom had only a limited command of English and little formal education, were too diverse to make group teaching a viable alternative. Group sessions were often interrupted, and individual patients were frequently forced to wait while the instructor attended to

---

Modular delivery system is a combination of primary and team nursing in which teams of primary and associate nurses care for specific groups of patients.

language or other unique needs of other participants. Although original estimates were for a 1-hour class, classes actually stretched to several hours. Attendance dropped, and concerns grew within the community regarding the women's ability to care for themselves properly during the early stages of their pregnancies.

The clinic's staff finally decided that an evaluation of the patient teaching program was in order. When the cost of staff time, which included the time staff members were unoccupied during the class, was added to the cost of maintaining the unused clinic rooms and this total was compared with the attendance rate and knowledge outcomes, it became clear that the group approach was both inappropriate and expensive for this set of patients. The clinic reverted to the one-on-one teaching strategy.

The nurse manager should collect cost and outcome data as part of all clinical studies to evaluate the effects of changes in process. In reality, collecting this type of data requires far less work than one might expect on first examining this seemingly formidable task. The task is made easier through the use of cost-accounting methods that are easily understood and relatively easy to apply. Assistance with the financial aspects of a study can usually be obtained through the organization's financial department. It is a rare financial officer who is not eager to assist nurse managers in performing cost analyses that might result in substantial savings. Although there is no doubt that an effectively run outcome evaluation can be challenging, it is also true that when these evaluations are used for managerial purposes, they are rarely required to meet all the rigorous criteria that are applied to research studies.

CALCULATING COST

Cost can be calculated using one of the following two approaches:

1. *Estimates of direct cost:* In many instances it may only be necessary to estimate the direct costs incurred by the change (i.e., costs associated with a change in the brand of product used or with the introduction of a new record-keeping system).
2. *Estimates of total cost:* In certain cases, especially when the relevant unit of analysis is an episode of care or a patient stay, the nurse manager must estimate the total cost of nursing care. Taking the "total cost" approach may also force the nurse manager to include such things as the effects on patients of the change in practices. Fortunately, data available from the PCS can be used to compute the nursing care costs for individual patients and groups of patients.

Box 5-4 shows an example of cost estimation. The process is accomplished using the following five steps:

1. *Classification of all patients:* Using a normally accepted classification method, all patients are classified. It is critical to the accuracy of the estimation that the classification for each patient be recorded using an easily retrievable method such as the patient record form or a computer file.
2. *Determination of the cost of direct nursing care:* After the patient has been discharged, the nurse manager simply totals the number of hours of care the patient received as derived from the PCS and multiplies that figure by the hourly nursing care salary cost (total salary costs/total number of paid nursing hours). This provides the total cost of nursing provided to the patient.
3. *Addition of indirect costs:* The next step is to add all indirect nursing costs to the direct costs. Indirect nursing costs include the unit's share of the expenses of nursing administration and staff development, cost of operating the physical plant, and similar non–patient-specific expenses. These costs are generally prorated on a per-patient-day cost basis (total indirect costs/number of patient-days).
4. *Calculation of average cost per patient:* To obtain the average cost for all patients being studied, the cost of care for all patients is added together and the total is divided by the number of patients in the sample.
5. *Comparison of average costs:* The average cost before introduction of the innovation can then be compared with the average cost after its introduction to identify cost savings.

MEASURING OUTCOME

Measuring the outcome-related effects of a change in practice can prove somewhat more difficult than measuring the cost of the change. In those few cases where similar changes in the care process may have been evaluated in a research study reported in literature, nursing units may be able to duplicate the outcome measures used in the original study. In most instances, however, nurse managers must design their own methods of evaluating outcomes. The first step in this process is to identify what outcome should be measured. This is done by answering the following three important questions:

1. What is the innovation intended to do?
2. What are the potential consequences?
3. How much can the institution afford to measure?

This process can be viewed in a more practical light by considering the following example:

If a nursing manager were evaluating a new method of treatment designed to assist in the care provided to incontinent patients, the intended outcomes might be (1) to reduce the number of times patients are

BOX 5-4

Example of Cost Estimation

CALCULATE TOTAL COST OWED BY EACH PATIENT

Patient A

1. Apply workload measurement (patient classification) system:

Day 1	3 hours
Day 2	2.8 hours
Day 3	2.5 hours
Day 4	2.5 hours
Day 5	+2.3 hours

2. Compute total hours of care for entire length of stay — 13.1 hours
3. Compute cost of nursing care for individual patients (at $35/hour)* — ×$35 / $458.50
4. Add indirect nursing costs at $67.20/ patient-day ($67.20 × 5 = $336.00) — +$336.00

Total cost owed by Patient A $794.50 (1)

Patient B

1. Apply workload measurement (patient classification) system:

Day 1	5 hours
Day 2	5 hours
Day 3	4.8 hours
Day 4	4.6 hours
Day 5	+4.6 hours

2. Compute total hours of care for entire length of stay — 24 hours
3. Compute cost of nursing care for individual patients (at $35/hour)* — ×$35 / $840.00
4. Add indirect nursing costs at $67.20/ patient-day ($67.20 × 5 = $336.00) — +$336.00

Total cost owed by Patient B $1176.00 (2)

Patient C

1. Apply workload measurement (patient classification) system:

Day 1	4 hours
Day 2	4 hours
Day 3	4 hours
Day 4	3 hours
Day 5	+3 hours

2. Compute total hours of care for entire length of stay — 18 hours
3. Compute cost of nursing care for individual patients (at $35/hour)* — ×$35 / $630.00
4. Add indirect nursing costs at $67.20/ patient-day ($67.20 × 5 = $336.00) — +$336.00

Total cost owed by Patient C $966.00 (3)

Patient D

1. Apply workload measurement (patient classification) system:

Day 1	5 hours
Day 2	4.9 hours
Day 3	4.9 hours
Day 4	+4.6 hours

2. Compute total hours of care for entire length of stay — 19.4 hours
3. Compute cost of nursing care for individual patients (at $35/hour)* — ×$35 / $679.00
4. Add indirect nursing costs at $67.20/ patient-day ($67.20 × 4 = $268.80) — +$268.80

Total cost owed by Patient D $947.80 (4)

Patient E

1. Apply workload measurement (patient classification) system:

Day 1	3 hours
Day 2	3 hours
Day 3	2 hours
Day 4	+2.3 hours

2. Compute total hours of care for entire length of stay — 10.3 hours
3. Compute cost of nursing care for individual patients (at $35/hour)* — ×$35 / $360.50
4. Add indirect nursing costs at $67.20/ patient-day ($67.20 × 4 = $268.80) — +268.80

Total cost owed by Patient E $629.30 (5)

Patient F

1. Apply workload measurement (patient classification) system:

Day 1	2.8 hours
Day 2	2.8 hours
Day 3	+2 hours

2. Compute total hours of care for entire length of stay — 7.6 hours
3. Compute cost of nursing care for individual patients (at $35/hour)* — ×$35 / $266.00
4. Add indirect nursing costs at $67.20/ patient-day ($67.20 × 3 = $201.60) — +201.60

Total cost owed by Patient F $467.60 (6)

CALCULATE AVERAGE COST PER PATIENT

1. Calculate total cost (TC) for all relevant patients:
   (1) + (2) + (3) + (4) + (5) + (6) = TC

   $794.50
   $1176.00
   $966.00
   $947.80
   $629.80
   +$467.70
   $4981.20

2. Calculate average cost: TC ÷ Number of patients = Average cost
   $4981.20 ÷ 6 = $830.20

*The hourly rate shown is for example only. This rate is an arbitrary figure used to reflect an hourly rate for nursing, plus an additional percentage to account for the benefits paid to nurses. The purpose of this table is to show how cost computations are performed, not to indicate any specific rate that should be reflective of actual nursing costs.

incontinent, and (2) to reduce the skin breakdown that can be caused by frequent incontinence. Outcome measures might then include such things as (a) the number of incontinence episodes per day and (b) the degree of skin excoriation. Unfavorable consequences might include such things as (a) unsightly garments or (b) decreased patient autonomy. Procedures for evaluating patients' emotional responses could be used to assess such potential results. Each of the proposed outcomes could be measured during the patient's hospitalization period and at a relatively modest cost.

The nursing staff may also want to know the long-term outcome of the new care strategy. If so, the study will require additional effort. For example, the study will have to locate the patients after their discharge from the hospital and perform outcome measurement at some specified time. It should be cautioned that continuing the experiment beyond the patients' discharge could become a potentially expensive procedure. However, there are several ways to conduct this type of evaluation that involve little direct cost to the unit, such as the following:

- Enlist a nurse researcher interested in the problem.
- Apply for an external grant that will fund the unit so it can perform its own evaluation.
- Obtain information about patient outcomes from colleagues working in other settings. Sending evaluation forms or conducting telephone interviews with nurses working in home care or in long-term care settings can provide this type of outcome data.

USING COST AND OUTCOME DATA

Once cost and outcome data have been gathered, the nursing manager must be able to relate one to the other to determine if the innovation was beneficial. One method for doing this is to use the decision model proposed by Dr. David Fishman, which applies cost-effectiveness analysis to the evaluation of study data in a service setting.[31]

As shown in Table 5-2, quality decision-making strategy relies on careful comparison of the cost and results of two different approaches to accomplishing a similar goal. Logic says that the option that produces an equal or superior result and does so at less or equal cost should be chosen. Similarly, any option that produces inferior results for equal or greater cost should be rejected. Ambiguity arises when a superior result costs more or when the costs and results are equal for the two options. In these circumstances, the decision about which option to choose depends on whether the goals to be achieved by the options in question are more or less valuable (important) than other organizational objectives. If the goals are determined to be more important, the option in question will get the funding; if not, the funding will be applied to the more important organizational objectives. When a result leads to an ambiguous choice situation, the staff may be inspired to identify additional options for achieving the same goals at a lower cost.

The evaluation strategy for assessing the effects of changes in the care process that has been described here is but one of several that could have been used. The choice made was an arbitrary one. Regardless of which evaluation method is selected, however, the method must be chosen before any innovation or change is made. Unless an evaluation method is planned and thoroughly understood well in advance, the nurse manager will not be able to extract the data necessary to determine whether the change initiated did or did not enhance the productivity of the nursing unit.

! CRITICAL POINT

It is imperative that the evaluation process used to determine outcomes be selected well before any innovation or change in procedure is implemented. If the nurse managers responsible for determining outcomes do not thoroughly understand which method to use, the data collected will almost certainly be inconclusive.

TABLE 5-2

Cost Effectiveness Decision Matrix

Effectiveness of New Program Relative to Old Program	Cost of New Program Relative to Old Program		
	New Less Costly	New as Costly	New More Costly
New less effective	(?)	Choose old	Choose old
New as effective	Choose new	Choose either	Choose old
New more effective	Choose new	Choose new	(?)

Strategies that can be used to increase the productivity of nursing resources in hospitals include the following, to name but a few[32,33]:

1. *Do more with more:* Reduce the number of specialized staff and return some of the activities that have been assigned to other departments back to nurses. For example, it might prove to be less expensive to move intravenous (IV) treatment back to the nursing department and away from the traditionally expensive IV teams found in many hospitals. There is no evidence that patient welfare is enhanced by the use of specialized IV teams. The drawback is that an all-RN staff or an increase in available RNs might be necessary if the nursing staff performs IV therapy.

2. *Use generic care plans that have been personalized:* If 1 to 2 nursing hours are required to develop each patient care plan and an institution uses personalized generic care plans judiciously, several nurse full-time equivalents can be saved. Caution should be used to not lower the level of patient care provided.

3. *Streamline documentation:* Develop new flow sheets to reduce the amount of time nurses spend documenting patient care. Bedside flow sheets with appropriately labeled sections may contribute to efficient use of nursing time.

4. *Use group counseling and teaching methods:* When group methods are appropriate for meeting patient and family needs, these methods are preferable. In selected circumstances, group methods may be much more effective than a traditional one-on-one approach. For example, group methods could be used to give discharge instructions to patients in the same DRG or to provide baby care instruction to new mothers.

5. *Package nursing presentations and information:* Any common presentation, such as providing orientation to the unit or preparing a family to take a patient home, could be put on video or print media. Fact sheets can be prepared prior to providing medication so that patient questions can be answered without consuming valuable nursing time.

6. *Separate nursing charges from room charges:* Most PCSs specify an average number of hours of nursing care per category. The separation of room charges from nursing charges allows nursing to become a unit cost center, so that costs for each DRG can be compared across hospitals or units. Furthermore, nursing costs per DRG could be used in incentive programs.

7. *Increase the use of ambulatory surgery facilities and day-of-surgery admissions programs:* Most institu-

tions have already implemented these strategies and aggressively pursue the practices; however, for these programs to function effectively, nursing staff must work closely with medical staff.

8. *Effectively manage materials and shared services:* Every entrepreneur or business owner, regardless of educational level, understands the critical importance of inventory control and the substitution of supplies of lower price but the same quality. Many in the nursing profession, however, have not yet learned this important lesson.

9. *Think "competitive marketing" and "consumer choice":* Traditionally, the nursing profession has not viewed its services as a consumer choice, but in fact they truly are. The conduct of the professional nurse in the institution often is the only basis a patient has for forming a perception of the institution. It is the patient's experience and perception that the patient and his or her family take into the community and share.

10. *Develop new products:* Adopting a philosophy of wellness rather than acute care can suggest all kinds of new marketable programs and services in the health promotion area that can be offered to the community the healthcare institution serves.

11. *Create a learning culture among the staff:* Economics, accountability, marketing, cost containment, change management, productivity, networking, and especially human resource management are a few of the many potential topics for a learning agenda.

12. *Maximize individual and group contributions:* Especially within the professional nursing staff, this step can be accomplished through participative management, effective staff organization, professional recognition, and shared governance programs.

13. *Consider matrix staffing:* Unit-based nurses have traditionally accepted the idea that floating within their own service may be necessary to meet nursing care requirements. In matrix staffing, however, nurses develop or are hired for competencies in at least two service areas and can float between services.

14. *Develop and use nursing productivity standards and implement control systems:* Productivity standards for each DRG are essential to the efficient use of staff, and control of overtime ensures that the unit will utilizes the standards properly.

This list provides only a sampling of the kinds of things nurse managers can do in association with administrative staff and physicians to find ways to enhance the delivery of quality patient care while staying within the confines of an institution's financial objectives.

The public that is served by the nursing profession demands and is entitled to information about the efficiency and effectiveness of the healthcare services provided to it. In responding to this demand, the nursing profession has two choices: (1) develop methods to demonstrate its own value as a healthcare discipline, or (2) wait for others to provide that evaluation. The choice is clear. The nursing profession has chosen to define the product of nursing services itself, provide scientific evidence of the links between nursing intervention and patient outcome, and then use professional and scientific knowledge about productivity to influence healthcare policy.

SUMMARY

- Productivity is an indicator that describes the relationship between inputs (the resources used to produce a product or provide a service) and outputs (the quantity of that product or service produced).
- Measurement of productivity in health care in general and in nursing in particular has been difficult for two reasons: (1) the unique nature of the service provided, and (2) the lack of consensus about how best to measure output.
- Standardizing the nature of patient-days (output) and validating the measurements derived from PCSs are just two of the simple modifications that can improve the validity of current methods for assessing productivity.
- Nursing productivity can be enhanced by making changes in the use of inputs and in the processes used to deliver care.
- Nurse managers can improve the use of inputs by matching the supply of staff with the demand for care, by carefully evaluating the consequences of staff substitutions, and by controlling the use of supplies and equipment.
- Demonstrating the relative productivity of nursing services is the responsibility of every nurse manager.

FINAL THOUGHTS

Productivity is a measure of the product or work produced for a specific amount of resources and is calculated as output divided by input. For example, productivity can be measured as required staff hours divided by provided staff hours multiplied by 100.

Improving productivity means producing more work or product with a given level of input (cost). Decreasing the number of hours worked by the staff while keeping the amount of product at the same level represents an increase in productivity.

Productivity is most often calculated with reference to a PCS using some or all of the following measures:

- Average daily census
- Number of patient-days per month
- Number of patients treated
- Number of procedures performed

Many actions can be taken to increase outputs while maintaining or decreasing inputs. Recognizing the need to improve, involving the staff, creating challenges, increasing management involvement, and initiating reward and recognition programs are but a few different ways.

THE NURSE MANAGER SPEAKS

When nurse managers are looking for ways to improve productivity in their units, one of the easiest things they can do is establish an objective process for recognizing excellence in the staff.

A well-designed system of recognition can supply each member of the staff with a feeling of accomplishment and self-esteem, both qualities that are absolutely necessary to improve production with fixed resources.

Reward and recognition programs should be designed to enrich the individual's future behavior by acknowledging past excellence—what gets rewarded gets done.

Although it is traditional for managers to look for problems and implement policy to eliminate them, the nurse manager who will lead tomorrow's successes is the one who understands that nothing motivates more than positive action.

The nurse manager's primary responsibility is to produce the maximum amount of work with the minimum amount of resource depletion and expense. That does not mean that the nursing unit must be a sweatshop. To the contrary, the unit where the atmosphere is upbeat and positive, where achievement receives recognition, and where work responsibilities are shared equitably will always be the one where productivity is highest.

REFERENCES

1. Feldstein MS: *The rising cost of hospital care,* Washington, DC, 1971, Information Resources Press.
2. Hornbrook MC: Hospital case mix: its definition, measurement, and use: part I, *Med Care Rev* 39(1):1, 1982.
3. Jelinek RC, Dennis LC: *A review and evaluation of nursing productivity,* DHEW No HRA 77-15, Bethesda, Md, 1976, Health Resources Administration.

4. Office of the Assistant Secretary of Health: *Productivity and health,* DHHS No 80-14028, Bethesda, Md, 1980, American Management Sciences (AMSI).

5. Edwardson SR: The cost-quality tradeoff in productivity management. In Shaffner FA, editor: *Patients and purse strings: patient classification and cost management,* New York, 1986, National League for Nursing.

6. Giovannetti P: *Patient classifications systems in nursing: a description and analysis,* DHEW Pub No HRA 78-22, Washington, DC, 1978, US Government Printing Office.

7. Giovannetti P: Understanding patient classification systems, *J Nurs Adm* 8(2):4, 1979.

8. Buerhaus PI, Needleman J: *Nurse staffing and patient outcomes in hospitals* (study conducted for the US Department of Health and Human Services, Health Resources Services Administration), Contract No 230-99-0021, Cambridge, Mass, 2001, Harvard School of Public Health.

9. Dahlen A: With primary nursing, we have it all together, *Am J Nurs* 78:426, 1978.

10. Marram G, Barret MW, Bevis EM: *Primary nursing—a model for individualized care,* ed 2, St Louis, 1979, Mosby.

11. Osinski EG, Powels JG: The cost of RN-staffed primary nursing, *Superv Nurse* 11(1):16, 1980.

12. Nenner VC, Curtis EM, Eckoff CM: Primary nursing, *Superv Nurse* 8(5):14, 1977.

13. Burt ML: The cost of all-RN staffing. In Alfano G: *All-RN nursing staff,* Wakefield, Mass, 1980, Nursing Resources.

14. Hinshaw AS, Scofield AS, Atwood JR: Staff, patient, and cost outcomes of all registered nursing staffing, *J Nurs Admin* 11(11-12):30, 1981.

15. Miller PW: Staffing with RNs. In Alfano G: *All-RN nursing staff,* Wakefield, Mass, 1980, Nursing Resources.

16. Czaplinski D, Diers D: The effect of nursing on length of stay and mortality, *Med Care* 36:1626, 1998.

17. Ballard K, Gray R, Knauff R: Measuring variation in nursing care per DRG, *Nurs Manage* 24(4):33, 1993.

18. Georgopoulos BS, Mann FC: *The community hospital,* New York, 1962, Macmillan.

19. Miller SJ, Bryant WD: *A division of nursing labor: experiment in staffing a municipal hospital,* Kansas City, Mo, 1965, Community Studies.

20. Blegen MA, Goode CJ, Reed L: Nurse staffing and patient outcomes, *Nurs Res* 47:43, 1998.

21. Clark EL: A model of nursing staffing for effective patient care, *J Nurs Admin* 7(2):22, 1977.

22. Christman L: A microanalysis of the nursing division of one medical center, *Nurs Digest* 6(2):83, 1977.

23. Marram G, Flynn K, Abaravich W, and others: *Cost effectiveness of primary and team nursing,* Wakefield, Mass, 1976, Contemporary Publishing.

24. Forseth J: Does RN staffing escalate medical care costs? In Alfano G: *All-RN nursing staff,* Wakefield, Mass, 1976, Contemporary Publishing.

25. Corpuz T, Anderson R: The Evanston story: primary nursing care comes alive, *Nurs Adm Q* 1(2):9, 1977.

26. McVay E: Lost supply charges: would visible price tags reduce their number?, master's thesis, Minneapolis, 1983, University of Minnesota.

27. Huey F: The demise of the traditional 5-40 workweek, *Am J Nurs* 81:1138, 1978.

28. Hutchins C, Cleveland R: For staff nurses and patients—the 7-70 plan, *Am J Nurs* 78:230, 1978.

29. Kent LA: The 4-40 workweek on trial, *Am J Nurs* 72:683, 1972.

30. Mills ME, Arnold B, Wood CM: A controlled study of the impact of 12-hour scheduling, *Nurs Res* 32:356, 1983.

31. Fishman D: *Development and testing of cost effectiveness methodology for CMHCs,* NTIS Nos PB246-676 and PB246-677, Springfield, Va, 1975, National Technical Information Service.

32. Data from Sovie MD: Managing nursing resources in a constrained environment, *Nurs Econ* 3(3):21, 1979.

33. Barnum BS, Kerfoot KM: *The nurse as executive,* Gaithersburg, Md, 1995, Aspen.

SUGGESTED READINGS

Abdellah F, Levine E: Developing the nature of patient and personal satisfaction with nursing care, *Nurs Res* 5:100, 1958.

Burton EJ, McBride WB: *Total business planning: a step-by-step guide with forms,* ed 3, New York, 1999, Wiley.

Dienemann J: *Nursing administration: strategic perspectives and applications,* Norwalk, Conn, 1990, Appleton and Lange.

Dobson P, Starkley K: *The strategic management blueprint,* Oxford, 1993, Blackwell.

Douglass LM: *The effective nurse leader and manager,* St Louis, 1988, Mosby.

Marquis BL, Huston CJ: *Leadership roles and management functions in nursing: theory and application,* Philadelphia, 1996, Lippincott.

Rowland HS, Rowland BL: *Nursing administration handbook,* Gaithersburg, Md, 1997, Aspen.

Swansburg RC: *Management and leadership for nurse managers,* Sudbury, Mass, 1996, Jones and Bartlett.

Williams MA: Subjective and objective measures of staffing adequacy, *J Nurs Adm* 9(11):21, 1979.

Yoder-Wise PS: *Leading and managing in nursing,* ed 3, St Louis, 2002, Mosby.

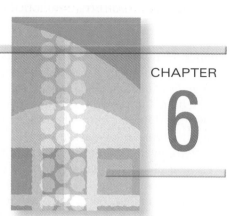

Managing Change in the Healthcare Environment

OUTLINE

LEARNING SYNOPSIS

Upon successful completion of this chapter, readers will possess a fundamental understanding of the principles for managing change in the nursing environment as well as strategies to ensure standardization of effort and practices that can make the change process easier.

OBJECTIVES

1. Describe how nurses and nurse managers can act as change agents in their environment
2. Identify ways to manage change within the systems framework
3. Identify different change theories and answer questions about the specific differences among theories
4. List the seven steps in the universal approach to planned change
5. Identify different strategies that can be used by the change agent to assist in managing change in the nursing environment
6. Identify ten skills that a nurse manager should cultivate if he or she is to be an effective change agent in a given environment
7. Describe effective methods for handling resistance to change
8. Identify ways of using internal politics to assist in the management of change

Change is not always welcome, but it is certainly inevitable. Although for many of us the thought of change produces anxiety and fear, change is absolutely essential for growth. Change involves becoming something different from what we are or doing something different from what we are used to and comfortable with, even when every aspect of the change has been well planned. Change evokes a sense of loss in many people and signals an uncomfortable alteration in what is familiar, particularly when the change is beyond our control or occurs unexpectedly. Even when change has been well planned, is eagerly anticipated, and is acknowledged to be necessary for all the right reasons, it can provoke a certain measure of grieflike reaction in some of those involved. It is very common, and perhaps even anticipated, for those who manage and initiate change to encounter resistance from those who react to it with anxiety and grief. Although change can unsettle even the strongest and most determined, however, it is the one constant in human life.

It is critical to the smooth operation of any organization that its leadership understand and anticipate a wide variety of reactions to any implemented change, and the nurse manager, in his or her role as a leader of others, is no exception. All nurse managers must possess a positive outlook and a willingness to embrace change. Although it is permissible for nurse managers to view change as a challenge, it is also obligatory that they support and encourage their colleagues to participate actively. What nurse managers must proactively guard against is becoming uncomfortable with the concept of change. To the contrary, nurse managers, as leaders in the medical community, must endeavor to embrace change and deal effectively and positively with the risk that it involves.

The healthcare system has been in a nearly constant state of change for the past four decades, and nothing that can occur in the foreseeable future will alter this fact. Change will occur in the healthcare field with or without any contribution from its nurses or their leadership. The simple truth is that, if a person is to assume the responsibilities of leadership, that individual must be willing to initiate change. If the individual does not, that makes him or her, at best, a survivor in the ocean of change that he or she will experience after stepping beyond the sheltered walls of university life. If a person is to become an effective nurse manager, that individual must become skilled in implementing the changes that he or she will initiate and that will be introduced by others. To accomplish this, the individual must learn to walk in the boardroom with the same comfort that is felt when serving patients at the bedside. To become the leader that subordinates need, the nurse manager must be able to effectively initiate and support the changes that are necessary to strengthen the practice of nursing, enhance the quality of care, and create a more capable and competent profession.

CLIMATE OF CHANGE

Absolutely no one knowledgeable in the field of health care will argue that the business is not in the midst of unprecedented change. Much of the change that has occurred and will occur is driven by economics; most has been and will continue to be generated by an ever-increasing emphasis on reducing healthcare costs. Today, the industry in under enormous pressure from the government, insurance companies, and private industry to change its historical reimbursement policies, many of which acted to create and reinforce a "blank-check" mentality. Today, there is tremendous incentive to reduce spending or absorb the difference between what providers charge and what reimbursing agents are willing to pay.

The federal regulations that established diagnosis-related groups (DRGs) created a shock wave of change that has reverberated throughout the healthcare industry. One effect has been the many changes and restrictions that have occurred in the admission practices of hospitals, one of the most expensive components of the entire system. Today, there are preset limits on what can be charged for the treatment of patients with a specific diagnosis, and even limits on how long a patient can remain hospitalized for a specific ailment. There is pressure from outside the medical industry to permit hospital admission only in the most acute cases and even then for the shortest time possible. Healthcare practitioners are being instructed to use alternative, less expensive settings whenever possible. Many of today's employee benefit programs require their members to obtain prior approval for any hospital admission and to obtain a second opinion before a recommended surgical procedure will be authorized. In some cases, employees are encouraged to use freestanding emergency centers instead of hospital emergency departments.

These are only a few of the many changes that have had a ripple effect in the healthcare industry. Today, every healthcare organization must yield to the constant demand for change if it is to survive. Most have started to accept the need for change with a positive and forward-looking attitude and are making the necessary changes even when these changes are difficult. Hospitals, for example, are reorganizing themselves into multiorganization healthcare systems. They are evolving their capabilities to include the provision of high-profit services such as those involving the use of high-tech medical equipment and basic home care. Many are specializing in providing solutions for complex and expensive-to-treat problems such as cancer and heart disease. To accomplish this, these organizations are developing special expertise in high-income treatments and are learning to handle cases thoroughly and quickly. Today more than ever, the effective management of change is requiring significant modifications in nearly every area of healthcare, but most significantly in areas such as technology, personnel, and organizational structure. In the fast-paced economic environment that is nursing today, organizational change is absolutely essential to survival, and creative change is mandatory for growth.

The climate of change has consistently produced new opportunities for the nursing staff. Those nurses who work in hospitals have found that top-level managers are now actively listening to what they have to say, and innovation is changing how everyone performs and interacts throughout the organization. Many institutions have found that they must use a participatory process, because status-quo, top-down management has proven extremely ineffective when the entire system is in transition. These demanding times continually require new ways of thinking, creative strategies, and fresh options. Today, no one can doubt that the door is finally open for those who dare to think beyond the way things have always been done.

Today, nurses who are practicing outside of the formally structured hospital are meeting the demands of a changing environment by creating new roles for themselves. The more entrepreneurial are opening businesses and are providing home healthcare services and a wide variety of preventive healthcare programs. Today, opportunities continually arise for the innovative professional nurse as third-party payers in health care seek alternatives to traditional and expensive disease-oriented institutional care. Today, regardless of whether a nurse practices independently, works in a formal organization, or forms his or her own association, one thing is constant: today's nurse must be able to understand, manage, and produce change.

NURSES AS CHANGE AGENTS

The perception of the nurse as an agent of change is not a new one. In fact, the term *change agent* has often been applied to the nursing profession and to the individual professionals who comprise it. The term also is used to identify any person or entity that brings about change. Most often, the nurse acts as an "insider," or a change agent who is a functional part of the system being altered (usually the unit he or she manages). However, the nurse can also be an "outsider" or consultant for change in other systems. The traditional training of nurses has prepared them

to function more as insiders. Nevertheless, there has never been a better time for the individual nurse—or the entire nursing profession, for that matter—to take the initiative. The traditional function of nurses, as the largest segment of the health profession, has been the day-to-day operation of the healthcare system, and this experience has provided nearly every nurse with concrete ideas about how to make the system better.

For example, although many patients are admitted to hospitals for brief periods of technologic intervention, they require around-the-clock nursing care. This means that, to a large extent, nurses control the patient's length of stay. In other words, their expertise and organizational skills can determine the overall cost and quality of the care a hospital provides.

Although it is certainly true that the provision of nursing care accounts for the largest single part of a hospital 's budget, it is also true that the quality of nursing care is a "differential advantage" for the organization. No one in the medical professional will dispute the fact that a hospital known for its excellent nursing care has a competitive edge in the marketplace. Therefore, those change-oriented nurses or change agents who can suggest changes that will help to control costs, improve quality, or offer new services are in great demand in hospitals.

Outside the hospital, nurses, acting as change agents, can effectively move the healthcare system from a medical to a nursing model. The ever-increasing demand of business to hold down the cost of health care has led to the practice of encouraging employees to follow a healthy lifestyle. This fundamental change away from treating the sick to encouraging wellness has given nurses the opportunity to create new niches in the business world. Today, nurses are developing and directing a wide variety of different prevention programs that provide "case management" for employees with many common health problems by linking them to existing services. Nurses are now creating the gap-filling services consumers require because the demand for healthcare cost reduction has forced patients to leave the hospital earlier and thus to spend much of their recovery period without the presence of competent medical professionals. In addition, the professional nurse provides the most logical solution to the problem of creating cost-effective ways to care for the elderly.

Changes such as those mentioned are continuing throughout the medical profession at a rapid pace, with and without the expert guidance of the professional nurse. This means that nurses, like organizations, cannot afford merely to survive the changes occurring around them. If nursing is to continue as a profession with expertise in addressing human responses to actual or potential health problems, then nurses must be proactive in shaping the future.[1] Nurses, especially those occupying management positions, now have a greater opportunity than ever before to change the system in which traditionally they have been allowed only to serve.

THE SYSTEMS FRAMEWORK AND CHANGE

Today, the majority of nurses still work in formal healthcare organizations. Modern organizational theory views the basic organization as a complex social system within the all-encompassing system known as society.[2] The organization is an integrated unit of mutually dependent elements that exchange information and effectiveness through semipermeable boundaries.[3] The organization also interacts with the environment that surrounds it and that it continually serves. Because of this dynamic interaction, change is inevitable. Moreover, in an organization, any change that occurs in one part of the system can produce follow-on change throughout the entire complex. Even though change is considered necessary for growth in all organizations, change must be well managed if system viability is to be preserved and performance goals are to be realized.

Successful organizations put a great deal of effort into achieving a balance with the many influences on them. This balance has been referred to as dynamic equilibrium, and it occurs when an organization responds to change by shifting to a new balance level or by modifying its goals.[3] In the day-to-day operation of an organization, every subsystem within it experiences stress, strain, and conflict. These actions or reactions are largely produced by the opposing forces that operate freely as part of the subsystem's maintenance and adaptive mechanisms. For the purposes of this chapter, *maintenance mechanisms* are defined as those things that prevent change from occurring too rapidly, whereas *adaptive mechanisms* are those that keep the subsystem evolving by allowing change to occur over a span of time. The part that these forces play in the modern healthcare organization cannot be overemphasized, because the scope and pace of all the change that occurs in an organization depends on how well these forces are managed. Although it is a fundamental responsibility of managers to reduce tension, relieve stress, and resolve conflict, these are things that must be dealt with cautiously or the overall organization may pay a large price in terms of human resources as it works to facilitate creativity, innovation, and social change.[4]

Using the systems frame of reference to understand and manage change offers a number of advantages, including the following:

It calls for integrative thinking: The individual who is managing or enacting change (change agent) must analyze the system and system-environment boundaries, mechanisms, flow of information, and energy before implementing any change. One of the fundamental elements of this process is simply recognizing that the entire system is greater than the sum of its parts. If it is carefully followed, this complex and comprehensive approach to implementing change prevents individuals from searching for casual relationships. Instead, effective managers make sure that their efforts are focused on working with the many interacting variables in the system that can be used both to facilitate and to restrict change. This effort always considers the importance of the external (environmental) factors operating on the system and carefully examines them in relation to the factors internal to the system.

It focuses attention on the hierarchical arrangement of the system: Understanding the hierarchy of the system greatly assists in achieving smooth coordination of communication and activities, and enables the change agent to understand and use the actions taking place at all levels of the system. This type of assessment normally begins with a careful examination of the overall system. What this means is that the effective management of change normally begins with those individuals in the system who are senior enough to have an overall view of the organization. This is important because external forces can have a pervasive effect on the whole establishment. Effective managers understand this fact and use it to their advantage. These professionals know, for example, that the search for organizational problems and solutions does not begin and end within the individual unit or department, or even within the organization itself. Often, it is the change that is occurring *outside* the system that holds the greatest promise and presents the greatest challenge. For example, the acute shortage of nursing personnel that has occurred in recent years has been exacerbated by factors such as the following:

State regulatory limits on hospital expense budgets, which affect professional nurses' salary increases

Reductions in federal financial support, especially those that affect educational assistance programs for professional nurses

Medicare's hospital payment procedure, which is based on medical diagnostic categories that do not take into account the intensity of nursing care required

These factors obviously represent only a bare minimum of the many outside environmental factors that influence the education and recruitment of professional nurses. In the long term, this situation affects the level of care that can be provided to the large number of general medical patients in hospitals. The potential effects of such outside influences point up the need to implement change in the overall healthcare delivery system slowly and methodically so as not to disturb the many subsystems that will be affected.

Issues such as these are serious, and they demand attention from nurse managers and force them both to adopt a broad, overall perspective and to develop strong change agent skills. Reshaping the healthcare delivery system necessitates political action, because it is largely governmental policies that determine the financing, structure, content, and process of delivering health care. If nurse managers are to have an impact in this area, they must become comfortable with and skillful in the use of the kinds of efforts necessary to influence policy beyond their units or organizations. Today, the decisions formulated in the political arena vary widely and encompass such things as what tasks nurses can legally perform, what level of nursing care third-party payers will authorize, and even such seemingly routine matters as how to dispose of syringes. Today, more than ever before, the political process is the change procedure, although there are small nuances depending on the political body (legislature, regulatory board, governmental department, etc.) that is enacting the change.

Effective, creative change is something that begins at the organizational, departmental, and unit levels, but only after careful consideration has been given to the macro perspective. Nurses, acting in their role as change agents, start the process by thinking in a broad way. As they consider the current social, political, and economic conditions, they also take the pulse of the external environment. They consider such things as competing organizations, the goals and objectives established by their institution's board of directors, and the professions that use their units' services. They must ask themselves a variety of important questions, including the following:

- What is the climate?
- What are the trends?
- What does the consumer want and need?
- What does the nursing profession propose?

As nurse managers start to connect ideas from unrelated sources, creative and innovative thinking starts to develop.[5] Creative ideas flow best from managers who think on a macro scale, brainstorm their ideas, and engage the fundamental talents of their staffs. The more flexible the nurse managers can make the vertical and horizontal organizational boundaries within their areas of influence and in their organization as a whole, the better communications will be in all directions: from the top down, from the bottom up, and in all lateral directions.

THE PROCESS OF CHANGE

Regardless of whether change is taking place on an environmental, systemwide, or unit-based level, it is a process that involves the effective use of strategy. Handling the process of change is something that can and should be learned by all nurses, especially if they desire to advance into a management position. Every nurse manager must develop a system of integrated thought which demands that problems be viewed as a whole. The ability to apply the theory of change is one of the most valuable management tools that a nurse manager can develop, inside or outside of the organizational setting. The process of change is one of simple problem resolution, much like the actual nursing process, although different experts recommend a variety of different steps or stages to follow in implementing or managing the process. However, the number and sequence of managerial steps is unimportant in managing the process of change. What is important is understanding exactly what needs to be accomplished, how to accomplish it, and why it needs to be done. If the process of change is developed and managed properly, it is both dynamic and fluid. As experience in managing change increases, the sense of this flow becomes just another tool in the nurse manager's inventory of nursing skills. In fact, those nurse managers who develop the skill of effective communication can become known as *change masters.*[5]

The problem-resolution change process described in this chapter combines elements of classic change theory, current nursing practice, and sociologic, psychologic, and organizational thought. So far, this chapter has discussed only the systems approach to implementing change, but the truly capable nurse manager, when in the process of implementing and managing change, understands that there are a great many different ways to do this effectively. The secret to success is to understand the theoretical foundations of the type of change process that is actually being implemented. To assist nurse managers and broaden their outlook on change, the key aspects of selected change theories are presented in the following sections along with a seven-step process for change implementation. Managers are strongly encouraged to consult the references that have been provided so that they can develop a fuller understanding of each of the methods. Although many readers will find similarities among these theoretical views, the unique insights provided by each can provide excellent information for implementing and managing the change process.

CHANGE THEORIES

The Force-Field Model

The book *Resolving Social Conflicts: And, Field Theory in Social Science* provides a fundamental social-psychologic view of the change process.[6] In this book, Kurt Lewin shared his vision of behavior as a dynamic balance of forces working in opposite directions within a **field**. He identified the following different elements or forces that act in the field:

Driving forces: those elements that facilitate change because they are pushing participants in a desired direction

Restraining forces: those elements that obstruct or interfere with change because they are directing the efforts of the participants along another path

According to Lewin, to effect change, one must plan effectively for change, carefully analyze the forces, and shift the balance in the direction of change through a three-step process: (1) unfreezing, (2) moving, and (3) refreezing. Change is accomplished by adding a new force, altering the direction of an existing force, or modifying the magnitude of a force. Basically, the strategies advocated for implementing change using this method are aimed at increasing driving forces, decreasing restraining forces, or both.

Lewin's force-field model and an example of how it might be applied in the nursing environment are presented in Fig. 6-1. This illustration shows graphically the opposing driving and restraining forces of change that act upon a system. These forces, which in reality are nothing more than the various parts of the system's maintenance and adaptive mechanisms, are balanced at the present, or status-quo, level. To achieve change, an imbalance between these driving and restraining forces must be created. The imbalance *unfreezes* the present patterned behavior, and the behavior *moves* to a new level at which the opposing forces are brought into a new state of equilibrium. Once participants integrate the new patterns of behavior into their personalities and relationships with others, a *refreezing* takes place. The new level of behav-

> **Field**, in this sense and as described by Lewin, can be any type or size of entity, from a unit to a department to an entire organization.

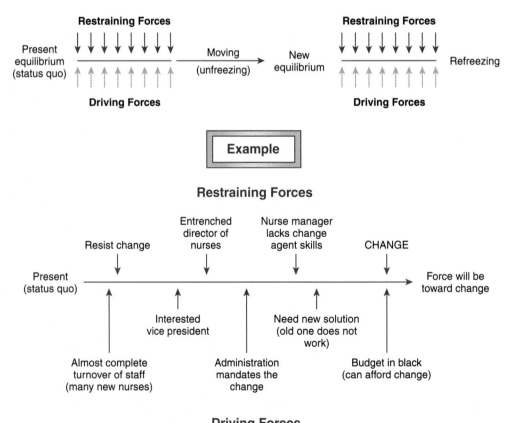

Fig. 6-1 ■ Lewin's force-field model of change.

ior then becomes institutionalized into formal and informal performance patterns.

Applying the three-step process outlined by Lewin to bring about behavioral change involves the following:

Step 1—Unfreeze: Break up the existing equilibrium. Provide motivation to the participants by preparing them in advance for the change. Carefully build trust and recognition of the need to change by encouraging active participation in the identification of the problem and in the generation of alternative solutions. This type of involvement helps to thaw attitudes.

Step 2—Move: Move the target system to a new level of equilibrium. Get participants to agree that the current behavior (status quo) is no longer beneficial. Encourage **cognitive redefinition** by helping the participants view the problem from a new perspective. Stimulate "identification" with the change process by linking participants' views to those of a respected or powerful leader who supports the change. Help them examine the environment to search for pertinent information.

Step 3—Refreeze: Cause the new system to equalize at the desired behavior level (attain balance). This is best accomplished by reinforcing the reasons that the behavior was changed in the first place and restating the benefits of the new method (how accomplishing the new behavior will benefit the individual). After the behavior has been accepted and everyone involved thoroughly understands its requirements, institutionalize it through formal and informal mechanisms (policies, communication channels, etc.).

The concepts presented by Lewin and the thinking they generated formed the foundation of the more modern views expressed by today's theorists. Clearly, what Lewin developed is a behavioral approach that many nurses find consistent with their theoretical understanding of human behavior. The simple image of people's attitudes thawing, becoming more fluid, shifting to a desired state, and then refreezing is easily understood and therefore conceptually useful. This simple symbolism helps even the most basic-level nursing staff member keep theory and reality in mind simultaneously.

Lippitt's Phases of Change

Several years after Lewin first presented his theory on the forces of change, the researcher Ronald Lippitt modified this basic theory by converting it to a seven-step process that focused more on what the change agent must do than on the evolution of change itself.[7] Lippitt emphasized the importance of active participa-

tion by key members of the target system throughout the change process but placed greatest emphasis on participation in the planning stages. Communication skills, rapport building, and problem-solving strategies form the foundation of each of the seven phases:

Phase I—Diagnose the problem: Involve key people in data collection and problem solving.

Phase II—Assess the organization: Evaluate the motivation and capacity that exist for change. Assess financial and human resources and constraints. Analyze the structure and function of the organization. Identify and prioritize the possible solutions.

Phase III—Assess self: Identify personal motivation and resources. This self-assessment is an important contribution, and one's personal commitment to change, energy level, future ambitions, and power bases must be carefully considered. Implementing a change and then giving up on it in midstream can waste valuable personal energy, expend considerable resources, and undermine the confidence of colleagues and subordinates.

Phase IV—Select progressive change components: These components include the action plan, evaluation criteria, and specific strategies that will be used during the implementation period and after the change has been completed.

Phase V—Choose a role for the change agent to play: Decide whether to act as a cheerleader, expert, consultant, or group facilitator. Whichever role is selected, all participants should be able to identify it so that expectations are made clear.

Phase VI—Maintain the change: Communication, feedback, revision, and coordination are essential components of this phase.

Phase VII—Terminate the helping relationship: Slowly withdraw from the role taken in implementing the change. The withdrawal is made gradually as the change becomes institutionalized. Those who must continually ensure that the change is maintained must be provided with the authority and accountability to do so.

Havelock's Model

In 1973, Lippitt's model was modified by another researcher, Ronald Havelock,[8] who defined a seven-step process to introduce change. This model is very similar to Lippitt's model and deviates most signifi-

> **Cognitive redefinition** is the intellectual reevaluation or change in interpretation of something. In this case, it is the redefinition of a behavior.

cantly from it in the portions that concern the planning and consolidation of change. Havelock's model identifies the following steps in accomplishing change:

1. Construction of a relationship
2. Diagnosis of the problem
3. Acquisition of resources
4. Choice of the solution
5. Gaining of acceptance
6. Stabilization
7. Self-renewal

Havelock established the change agent as an dynamic part of the implementation process and called for an assertive and participative approach in leading change.

Rogers's Diffusion of Innovation

In 1983, the researcher Everett Rogers[9] developed a broader approach to managing change than Lewin, Lippitt, or Havelock had done. He devised a five-step procedure he called the *innovation-decision process*. His new method of introducing and managing change outlined how an individual or "decision-making unit" passes through three different stages in the development of a change. He identified these stages as follows:

1. Knowledge of an innovation
2. Confirmation of the decision
3. Adoption or rejection of the new idea

Rogers' basic concept is built around what he referred to as the "reversible nature of change." This reversibility, he explained, is caused by the natural growth process of change, in which participants initially adopt a change proposal but later discontinue it. Rogers also noted that this process could take place in reverse, so that participants initially reject the change but later adopt it. His insight has provided a very useful lesson in the process of managing change, because it brings to light the fact that, if a change fails to be fully implemented the first time it is initiated or if the change agent is unsuccessful in achieving full implementation of a proposal, one should not assume that the issue is dead. Any change can be redefined and reinstituted, perhaps in a different form or context, or at a more opportune time. Moreover, and perhaps most importantly, when a change is accepted, one should never assume that this acceptance will be permanent.

Rogers outlined the following five steps in the diffusion of innovation:

1. *Knowledge:* The decision-making unit is introduced to the innovation and begins to understand it.
2. *Persuasion:* A favorable (or unfavorable) attitude toward the innovation is developed.
3. *Decision:* Activities are performed that lead to a decision to adopt or reject a presented idea, suggestion, or innovation.
4. *Implementation:* If adopted, the innovation is instituted, and through its use, reinvention or alterations may occur.
5. *Confirmation:* The individual or decision-making unit seeks reinforcement that the decision was correct. If there are conflicting messages or experiences, the original decision may be reversed.

Rogers stressed the following two important requirements for successful planned change:

1. The key people and policy makers involved in change must be interested in the innovation.
2. These key people must be committed to ensuring the successful implementation of the change.

Summary of Theoretical Perspectives Discussed

The models of change described in this text (Table 6-1) are only a very few of the many that exist. They were selected because they are classic models that

---

TABLE 6-1

Comparison of Change Models

Lewin	*Lippitt*	*Havelock*	*Rogers*
1. Unfreezing	1. Diagnosis of the problem	1. Building of a relationship	1. Knowledge
	2. Assessment of the organization	2. Diagnosis of the problem	2. Persuasion
	3. Assessment of the change agent's motivation and resources	3. Acquisition of resources	3. Decision
2. Moving	4. Selection of progressive change components	4. Choice of a solution	4. Implementation
	5. Choice of the change agent's role	5. Gaining of acceptance	
3. Refreezing	6. Maintenance of the change	6. Stabilization	5. Confirmation
	7. Termination of the helping relationship	7. Self-renewal	

show a significant degree of similarity despite their individual differences in perspective. The seven-step approach described in the following sections, which is widely used around the world and is based on the actual nursing process, is presented to help the reader abstract the common points of the classic models and to identify those that have particular significance for nurse managers in their role as change agents. Insights of current experts on innovation have been integrated into this model.

A SEVEN-STEP UNIVERSAL APPROACH TO PLANNED CHANGE

In the early 1950s, an industrywide search for a framework to use in solving problems in patient care resulted in the conceptualization of the nursing process in use today. In this conceptualization, the nursing process is recognized as encompassing the critical elements of assessment, planning, implementation, and evaluation, and these are so ingrained in the nursing profession that they have become nearly second nature to the professional nurse. In fact, today this view of the nursing process structures much of the typical nurse's thinking and forms a fundamental framework for ensuring the delivery of high-quality patient care. Essentially, the process of managing change follows a very similar path—that is, assessment, planning, implementation, and evaluation (see Table 6-1). In the discussion here, however, the process of managing change has been further subdivided into seven easily assimilated steps (Table 6-2), because many nurses are far more uncomfortable with managing change than they are with providing patient care. In developing these steps, a great deal of attention has been given to the assessment phase for the following two reasons:

1. Thorough data collection and analysis allow the process of planned change to move past the basic stage of "Wouldn't it be a good idea if we. ..."
2. Many nurses, regardless of their level of professionalism, are unfamiliar with the type of data they will need to collect and/or the methods by which to analyze them to manage and initiate change.

Two representative situations are described later that are designed to assist you in understanding and applying the steps in the change process, regardless of the type of setting or the specific problem encountered. The first situation involves a hospital staffing problem at a medium-sized medical center; the second describes a communications problem in a community health center. After reading these examples, you are encouraged to identify a situation relevant to your own practice or management role and review the change process steps with that challenge in mind.

TABLE 6-2

The Seven Steps of Planned Change: A Comparison with the Nursing Process

Nursing Process	*Change Process*
1. Assess	1. Identify the problem or opportunity
	2. Collect data
	3. Analyze data
2. Plan	4. Plan the change strategies
3. Implement	5. Implement the change
4. Evaluate	6. Evaluate effectiveness
	7. Stabilize the change

For example, if you are a nurse in private practice, you might consider the continual challenge of obtaining hospital admission privileges. Nurse managers might want to substitute the initiation of an improved patient classification system that will link patient acuity levels to staffing patterns.

Assessment

IDENTIFICATION OF THE PROBLEM OR OPPORTUNITY

Change is associated with opportunity as much as, and possibly a great deal more than, with the solution of problems. However, it is very common for nurse managers who do not practice good leadership to overlook the opportunity that is inherent in every change. These basic-management–style nurse managers spend most of their time planning to close a performance gap or remedy a discrepancy between the desired and actual state of affairs, instead of considering how they might use change to create an opportunity. Performance gaps are those gaps that occur because obstacles are confronted when trying to reach a performance goal or because a new goal has been created.

It does not really matter, however, whether the change that must be dealt with represents a problem or an opportunity. What is important in managing change is that the performance gap be clearly identified. If members of the staff perceive the challenge differently, the search for solutions will become difficult and confusing. Managers should start the process by performing a mini-SWOT (*S*trengths, *W*eaknesses, *O*pportunities, and *T*hreats) analysis, using the following questions:

- Where is the unit right now?
- What is it that is unique about us?

- What would we like our unit or business to be like?
- What can we do that is different and better than what our competitors or sister nursing units currently do?
- What is the driving motivation in our organization; that is, what is it that determines how we make our final decisions?
- What, if anything, prevents us from moving in the direction that we would like to go?
- What is the actual problem we wish to correct?
- What kind of change is required?

The last question should generate integrative thinking regarding the potential effect(s) the proposed change might have on the current system. This is extremely important, because all types of organizational change involve modifications to the system's interacting components (i.e., technology, structure, and personnel). For example, the introduction of a new technology may necessitate changes in the structure of the organization (e.g., the physical plant may require alteration and staffing levels may need to be changed if open-heart surgery is added as a new service).

The relationships among the people who work within a system change when the structure of the organization or system is modified. In addition, changes in an organization or system can create changes in personnel, as when new skills, knowledge, attitudes, and motivations are needed to accommodate a new technology. The one thing that is always true of change is that every time it involves behavioral change on the part of personnel, no matter what opportunity is presented or what problem is being resolved, management will find it challenging to complete the change as designed.

Given the current and projected transitional state of the healthcare industry, nurse managers need to define problems and opportunities with insight so they can avoid status-quo management. Developing creative insight is not a simple task and requires considerable practice.* Managing with creative insight involves looking at old challenges in a fresh and untraditional way and from a variety of different perspectives. It is highly recommended that managers do not use historical events as guides for arriving at solutions to current problems. In fact, effective managers concentrate on moving beyond the normally accepted, comfortable ways of experiencing a phenomenon or dealing with a problem to arrive at new

---

*To help you develop this skill, several exercises have been suggested to make you a more efficient change agent. See Exercises to Stimulate Creative Thinking at the end of the chapter.

insights and different possibilities.[10] Problems can result in opportunities for change that not only will solve the immediate problem but also can reshape and stimulate the system.

Situation 1: Staffing. The following narrative provides one excellent example of the use of creative insight to define a problem:

Senior management at a medium-sized medical center had recognized a staffing problem that they proposed to solve through a combination of methods, which included (a) using nurses from a temporary agency, (b) having permanently assigned staff from one floor float to another floor, and (c) requesting nurses to complete additional shifts of duty for overtime pay.

The pediatric unit supervisor saw the problem differently, however. After holding meetings with her staff, she was convinced that the problem with staffing levels was directly attributable to senior management's unwillingness to provide limited control to the staff, control that would have brought with it increased accountability and respect. The problem, in the nurse manager's opinion, was caused by senior management's failure to respond to the needs of the hospital's human resources. The nurse manager felt that her nurses, who were proficient in the care of children, resented being pulled out of pediatrics to serve the needs of a unit that did not require their specialized expertise or, worse yet, a unit that required specific expertise that they did not have. The result was that the frequent shifting of expert personnel from the pediatric unit to another unit to compensate for shortages actually led to an increase in overall absenteeism in the pediatric unit.

With the problem placed into proper focus, ideas were generated. Working with her staff and senior management, the nurse manager transformed the problem of staff shortages into an opportunity to create a children's center. The result was a decentralized unit encompassing pediatric and pediatric intensive care services. The solution required the new unit to be staffed and managed in an autonomous manner through a process of collaboration between the unit supervisor and the pediatric nurses under her jurisdiction. Nurses would not float into or out of this unit. Instead, a contingency schedule was developed that would provide staff coverage from among the assigned nurses whenever any nurse called in sick. The new schedule provided a reliable plan for the provision of qualified human resources to maintain a high level of patient care and, at the same time, to enhance professional camaraderie and accountability. Another significant benefit of the plan was that it lowered overall operational costs, especially in the area of overtime expenses. The professional relationships that developed between the assigned nurses created a situation in which they were less likely to call in sick when they knew their colleagues would be required to cover for them. In short, the depersonalization of coverage was eliminated.

Situation 2: Communication. The following example, although it has been made hypothetical to enhance learning, is based on a real-life organizational problem that occurs frequently:

> A large semirural community health agency that provides services to 22 different municipalities in a single Midwestern U.S. state consists of a main office and two branch locations, situated about 30 miles apart. The nursing staff is divided among the three offices, whereas all of the administrative staff and support therapy staff (physical therapy, social workers, etc.) are located at the home office. In addition, that location serves as the site for most of the staff meetings, the processing of referrals, and billing decisions.
>
> The agency hired a new director of professional services after the previous director retired. Upon assignment, the new director commenced an evaluation of her areas of responsibility, which led her to identify several concerns. The first and most serious was what she perceived as poor communication between the three offices and between each office and the other community agencies on which the organization relied to provide specific patient services. The new director believed that the poor communication stemmed from the physical layout of the agency (three offices) and proposed a reorganization that would consolidate the agency's three offices into a single centralized office at a completely new location. After 3 years of presenting her solution, she was unable to persuade the board of directors to adopt her suggested change. In fact, very little agreement was ever achieved, and absolutely no movement was made toward a solution.

To break the deadlock described in this example, an alternative is needed. Poor communication may be the primary issue, but because of the deadlock between the director and the board, some other solution should be considered, such as changing the pattern of communications or the technology used to communicate. For example, a simple solution might be to arrange for the administrative staff and therapists to make more frequent visits to the branch offices. A more innovative change might be to introduce teleconferencing equipment that will permit interactive electronic meetings between two or more groups of people at multiple locations. Each office will need conference rooms equipped with up-to-date communications capabilities that may include such things as speaker phones, telecommunication links, electronic mail, and interactive writing equipment or facsimile machines. These things are available at relatively low cost and can be connected by commercially available communication network services. An additional benefit of this arrangement is that other organizations with similar technology, such as regional medical centers, can be tied into any of the three agency offices for meetings, in-service education, or patient care conferences.

DATA COLLECTION

Once a problem or opportunity has been clearly defined, the professional change agent collects data from sources that are both outside (external to) and inside (internal to) the system. This is a critical step in ensuring the eventual success of the planned change. All forces that will move the change (driving) and all forces that will restrict movement (restraining) are identified so that one (driving) can be emphasized and the other (restraining) can be reduced or eliminated. To accomplish this efficiently, the political climate in the organization must be appraised and used effectively. This can be accomplished by asking the following questions:

- Who will gain from this change?
- Who will lose?
- Which of these two factions (winners and losers) has more power and why?
- Can these power bases be altered? If so, how?

Nurse managers can best assess the political climate in the organization being affected by the change by examining the reasons for the present situation. Who is in control who may be benefiting from the way things are currently structured? The levels of ego that are involved, the commitment of the involved people, their individual personalities, and people's likes and dislikes are as important to a correct assessment as are the formal organizational structures and processes. The individual encouraging the change and the individual actually managing it need to understand these matters as much as possible if they are to gauge the resistance that will be encountered.

The costs and benefits of the proposed change are obvious focal points and should never be overlooked. In addition, the amount, quality, and cost of the resources available to nurse managers as they implement and/or manage change need to be closely evaluated, especially those over which the nurse managers have control. A nurse manager who has the respect and support of an excellent nursing staff has access to a powerful resource in today's climate. Another critical source of support is the data available through current research.

Situation 1: Staffing

The pediatric unit supervisor had to collect data to support the arguments for introducing her proposal for a decentralized unit with autonomy in staffing. The following are examples of the data she gathered from external sources:

- State, regional, and local supply-and-demand statistics for general and pediatric nurses
- Statistics that reflected consumer demand for expert pediatric nursing services
- Staffing policies of competing hospitals
- Research data regarding the motivation of professional employees

Data from internal sources were obtained from the following different system levels:

Organizational level: Here the supervisor examined the hospital's philosophy, goals, and marketing plans. She sought evidence that the hospital would benefit from marketing the children's center as an organization that employed a stable staff of specialist nurses. In this case, there was no competing focus, such as might have been present if the board of directors had possessed long-range plans to market a different type of unit.

Group and individual levels: The supervisor consulted her own staff and discussed the idea with nurses from other specialized units. It is important to note here that if the staff had been organized into a bargaining unit, she would have had to investigate the bargaining unit's negotiated staffing policies and potential support for the idea.

The goal of this research was to collect data that supported the belief that the proposed change would fit into the goals, norms, and values of the organization and its members. As a nurse leader, this supervisor was also interested in demonstrating how her idea reflected the goals and values of the nursing department and the profession.

The quantitative data that were compiled helped to document the need for change. Some of these data were the historical staffing and turnover rates for this unit. These records contained information that demonstrated higher absenteeism during the periods when the relocation of nursing staff was practiced. Incident reports for unit and nonunit members documented the fact that a much higher level of care was consistently provided by seasoned specialists than by the temporary nurses. Finally, the pediatric supervisor estimated the cost savings that were possible if temporary nurses were not required.

Situation 2: Communication

In the community health agency, a cost-benefit analysis of regular teleconferencing would focus on time, communication, equipment, and quality of care. Estimates of the cost of equipping conference rooms with appropriate equipment and the cost of the training that would be necessary for personnel to use it effectively are fairly straightforward, and these costs should be outweighed by estimates of projected benefits such as the following:

- Amount of time that would be saved in travel to meetings (translates into estimated hard dollars)
- Amount of time that would be saved by teleconferenced meetings that were shorter and better managed (again translated into estimated hard dollars)
- Amount of savings expected from the reduction in transportation expenses
- Maximization of third-party reimbursement brought about by timely decision-making (key persons can be gathered quickly and conveniently) and expeditious referrals among providers (nurses, therapists, social workers, etc.)

- Improved productivity from key personnel due to the facilitation of action (i.e., participation is improved when distance is removed as a constraint to interaction and participants maintain access to important sources of information at their usual work locations)
- Improved quality of care that would be realized from productive interdisciplinary communication within the agency and between the agency and selected organizations (regional medical centers that have teleconferencing capacity)

Quantitative data might include the following:

- Deployment of staff (time spent in traveling)
- Percentage of meetings that have full versus partial participation by key persons
- Number of third-party payer rejections related to delayed or inappropriate decision-making
- Numbers of meetings that had to be repeated in each branch to communicate essential information (and associated time)

Qualitative data should also include (a) examples of miscommunication such as that related to the organization's inability to gather participants together at one time to communicate important messages, and (b) examples of instances when the quality of care was negatively influenced by delays in decision-making. Although this is by no means a comprehensive list, these examples illustrate the need for thorough and sometimes creative data collection.

DATA ANALYSIS

The importance of data analysis cannot be overemphasized, for without it, the many types of data collected—all extremely important in supporting the need for change—are useless. The individual responsible for enacting the change should focus more energy on analyzing and summarizing the data received than on collecting it. Analysis is conducted for the following purposes:

- To identify possible sources of resistance
- To recognize potential solutions and strategies
- To develop areas of consensus
- To build support for whichever option is selected

Whenever possible, efforts should extend to a complete statistical analysis of the data related to the situation and business environment. The effort will almost always prove to be worth the expense, especially when the change agent will need to persuade members of senior management who are comfortable with financial analyses, statistics, and probabilities. When developing the analysis, it is not necessary to include every piece of information that is obtained. It is far more beneficial simply to pull trends and themes from the data and thread them together to make a persuasive case. The analysis should be presented concisely and supported by the use of appropriate graphs and diagrams.

Planning of the Change Strategy

Planning the *what, who, how,* and *when* of any change is a fundamentally important step. What is the exact system that will be targeted for change? It is critical that this be identified as early as possible so that those individuals concerned with that system can be active participants in the planning stage. The more involved the affected people are at this point, the less resistance to change there will be in later, more critical stages. Lewin's "unfreezing" imagery is particularly relevant in the planning stage. Current attitudes, habits, and ways of thinking must soften so that those members who are primarily concerned with the targeted system will be ready for the new ways of thinking and performing that will be required by the change. Rigid boundaries must be broken down before the system can shift and restructure.

This is the most appropriate time to "rock the boat" or to make people uncomfortable with the current methods or systems. Initiating the acceptance of change involves giving the affected group a reason to accept the change (i.e., something that will cause them to look forward to the new system because of the improvements or benefits the change will offer relative to the existing processes or equipment). The information required will normally be found in the data collected (e.g., research findings, quantitative data, surveys of patients and/or staff, statistical information supplied by the manufacturer). The proposed change should be presented to the group in as clear, straightforward, and honest terms as possible. At no time should employees be misled with false or unclear information or half-truths. Although every attempt should be made to minimize the anxiety of the group, quality leadership dictates that everyone concerned must be given the truth first and the justification second. In short, never lie to the staff when attempting to institute change. It will always create significant problems later on.

Those managers who will be affected by the change need to plan for the resources they will require and, at the same time, establish feedback mechanisms to evaluate the progress and success of the change. The change agent should ensure that control points are established with those who will be responsible for providing the feedback. It is imperative that close liaison be maintained with these people at all times and that specific goals with time frames be established well in advance to clarify their individual roles and specify the standards of performance expected.

The initial planning stages must also identify operational indicators that will signal success or failure in terms of performance and satisfaction. When these control points are established, the time between assessments should not be too long. The more frequently the change agent is made aware of the progress being made, the easier it is to correct a mistake and the more frequently the opportunity is presented for celebrating a success. One of the best ways to keep the resistance to change at a minimum is to give the affected personnel plenty of reason to celebrate. Nothing helps attain success more than success itself. Celebrate often and take every opportunity to turn change into fun and anticipation.

Situation 1: Staffing

Potential goals (control points) and objectives (indicators) for the children's center proposal might be stated as follows:

- At start plus 6 months, the nurse manager will present a contingency schedule, prepared in collaboration with staff members, on a monthly basis.
- At start plus 8 months, the children's center will have achieved a 20% decline in absenteeism.
- By the tenth month of operation, the supervising nurse will meet with senior hospital management to report the effect of the new staffing policy on the nurses' professional identity and sense of control.
- By the end of the twelfth month of operation, the unit supervisor will submit a recommendation to continue or discontinue the new staffing policy based on such evidence as staff turnover, absenteeism, and the necessity for use of temporary agency personnel.

Situation 2: Communication

Potential goals (control points) and objectives (indicators) relevant to the community health agency situation might be as follows:

- Within 30 days, the executive director will obtain estimates from three competing telecommunications vendors and recommend one to the board of directors for trial rental of equipment.
- Within 60 days, the director of professional services will appoint a staff member to be trained in teleconferencing.
- Within 3 months from the start date, the trained staff member will begin training supervisors.
- Within 4 months from the start date, two interdisciplinary meetings will take place that involve all of the locations within the agency.
- Before the end of the tenth month, the director of professional services will report to the board of directors with tracking data regarding usage patterns, changes in staff deployment and time expenditures, and so on.
- Before the end of the first year of operation, the board of directors will decide to extend the rental of telecommunications equipment, discontinue it, or purchase the equipment.

Implementation of the Change

In this cycle, the plans are put into motion. Lewin called this the "moving" stage, and it marks the beginning of the change for most of the organization. During this period, interventions are designed to ensure that the necessary compliance occurs. The role of the change agent during this critical period is to create a supportive climate. To accomplish this, the change agent may have to act like an energizer to provide proper motivation at appropriate times, like an inquisitor to obtain and provide feedback, and like a coach and facilitator to overcome the inevitable resistance.

Managers are the key change process actors. These critical performers use implementation tactics "to install planned changes, whether they be novel or routine" (p. 16).[11] The specific activities that are undertaken to induce organizational change actually comprise the method of change—what is actually done.[12] Depending on the type of change strategy pursued, any of a variety of different approaches may be used, such as giving a presentation or forming a task force. Some of the methods used will be directed toward helping specific individuals deal with the change, whereas other methods will target entire groups.

METHODS USED TO CHANGE INDIVIDUALS

Information Giving. The most common method used to assist in changing individual perceptions, attitudes, and values is called *information giving*.[11,12] The change agent can contract with external consultants who are experts in a specific field or select resident experts from the internal organizational staff and have them prepare and disseminate the information. This form of dissemination is accomplished most often through a top-down communication flow. Providing accurate and high-quality information is essential to implementing change effectively, but it is never adequate to guarantee success unless lack of information is the only obstacle to effecting the change. Supplying information does not provide anyone with a reason to accept the proposed change, and unless individuals understand why they should change, it is almost certain that little change will actually occur. (This is the reason that the vast majority of training programs fail to achieve the degree of change they were originally designed to create.)

Training. Training is a form of assistance that usually combines information giving with practice in specific skills. As a socialization strategy, training is more a system maintenance mechanism than an adaptation mechanism because it typically shows people how they are to perform in a system, not how to change it.

Counseling or Psychotherapy. Counseling or psychotherapy can be an effective method of assisting employees, especially if they hold an influential organizational position, when they experience significant difficulty with change or are severely troubled by it. However, care should be taken when using this method, because it can be expensive and may not be accepted by the parties who need it the most. It should be reserved for individuals who are vital to the organization.

Management must remember that this is a most severe form of assistance, and extreme sensitivity should be used when considering it. Unqualified management should never attempt to provide this by themselves, and qualified management should suggest this approach to the employee only after consulting with a qualified therapist.

Assignment, Reassignment, or Termination. Assignment, reassignment, or termination can be accomplished with carefully identified individuals (normally those who are playing a key part in the resistance to the change) and exercising one of the options. Once again, extreme care should be used in these circumstances because of the backlash that can be generated, as well as the legal, moral, and ethical issues that arise. However, these are always available as an alternative in the most severe instances.

METHODS USED TO CHANGE GROUPS

Some forms of change implementation strategy are best used with groups of people rather than with individuals to obtain compliance. It is important to remember that the power of an organizational group to influence its members depends on how much authority it has to act on an issue and the significance of the issue itself. The greatest influence is achieved when group members discuss issues that they perceive as important and choose to make relevant, binding decisions based on those discussions. Research on the use of sensitivity groups has not shown them to be effective in implementing organizational change, probably because these groups are not usually composed of individuals who occupy closely related positions in the organization. A more successful strategy is the use of the *survey feedback*. In this method, groups of individuals who have closely related positions in the organization are brought together to discuss issues as an "organizational family."

There are times when the best approach is a combination of individual and group tactics. Whatever method is chosen, however, participants should feel that their input is valued, and each person should feel rewarded for his or her efforts. Some people will not be persuaded that a change is beneficial before it is actually implemented. In fact, some will experience a state known as *cognitive dissonance,* in which their established beliefs about the change become inconsistent with more recently acquired information once the change has been implemented. For these people, the behavior change actually takes place first and the individual's attitude toward it is later modified to fit the new behavior. In such a case, the change agent should be aware of participants' conflicts and reward the desired behaviors. It may take some time for attitudes to catch up.

Situation 1: Staffing

The pediatric supervisor recognized that she was initiating a unit-level change that would have systemwide implications. To ensure a smooth transition, she realized that it would be necessary to employ both individual and group methods of change. When she provided fact sheets to her own unit members, she heightened their interest. To accomplish the same thing with the supervisors of other units, she met with each one individually on an informal basis. The primary tactic used was to change existing attitudes by appealing to the professional values of both the pediatric nurses and the other supervisors. Group meetings followed the individual sessions. In these group meetings, the pediatric supervisor suggested that a trial program be conducted and solicited the participation of others in developing guidelines for contingency scheduling. After the meetings, the supervisor began to screen staff nurse applicants regarding their desire for autonomy. Finally, she persuaded the director of nursing and the nurse recruiter to visit another hospital that had already instituted a similar policy in its critical care unit so that they could be satisfied about the feasibility of the idea.

Situation 2: Communication

Individual and group methods are also excellent techniques for implementing a teleconferencing system. If the director of professional services lacks the expertise, she can hire a new manager who is more experienced in this technology to assist and ensure that proper performance is achieved. Because of the complexity of the proposed system, high-quality information and training must be provided to all managers who will be involved with the change. One of the best ways to stimulate participation by others is to create a task force and solicit input and assistance. Another method is to arrange for a seminar to be given by expert consultants and for presentations to be made by users of similar systems. This approach is often extremely beneficial, especially in swaying naysayers to support the change. In this effort, the change agent is limited by several key factors: (1) imagination, (2) allotted time frame, and (3) cost.

Evaluation

EVALUATION OF EFFECTIVENESS

It is important to ensure that the established operational indicators are monitored as planned. The change agent bears the responsibility for determining if the planned benefits are being achieved in terms of both cost and quality. After careful evaluation, the extent of success or failure is determined and an explanation is prepared for senior management. It is important to note here that the final analysis may very well reveal both unintended consequences and undesirable outcomes. What is critical is that the evaluation be performed in an objective and forthright manner. Bending the evaluation results to a particular viewpoint is not productive, beneficial, or professional.

Situation 1: Staffing

In the case of the children's center, the pediatric supervisor's evaluation might produce evidence that the new facility has helped to attract patients, retain expert staff, and reduce overall labor expenses. To provide a totally candid and unbiased presentation, however, she must also measure staff satisfaction. It is possible that the staff do not feel that covering for one another is beneficial and that these negative feelings are developing into a potential conflict. This negative point must be included if the evaluation is to be objective.

Situation 2: Communication

At the community health agency, the director would conduct an evaluation to determine if the teleconferencing process actually reduces wasted time and increases the quality of care by improving interdisciplinary communication as originally predicted. The evaluation may also uncover the fact that most of the staff are intimidated by the technology and are wasting valuable time using it. Both sides of the situation must be reflected in the evaluation so that senior management can make an objective and professional decision about whether to continue the program and purchase the technology or look for another, more practical, method of improving communication.

STABILIZATION OF THE CHANGE

When the change is extended past the pilot stage and the target system is refrozen, the change agent will terminate his or her helping relationship by delegating responsibilities to target system members. However, the change agent must continue to play the energizer role assumed earlier in order to reinforce the new behaviors through positive feedback. The sense of permanency is developed by (1) writing formal policies and (2) making sure the staff repeat the new behavior frequently and do not revert to the old familiar behavior.

CHANGE AGENT STRATEGIES

Regardless of the setting, the environment, or the actual proposed change, the seven-step change process described earlier should be followed. However, any combination of specific strategies can be used, depending on the amount of resistance that is anticipated and the degree of authority possessed by the change agent. The three classic strategies discussed in this chapter were first described in 1969 by Bennis, Benne, and Chin[13] and have been revised four times since then. They are useful and realistic strategies that can be considered when the change agent is deciding exactly what methods to use. It is critical to note that extremely few change processes will proceed exactly as these strategies envision. Therefore, any strategy recommended in this chapter should be modified to fit the individual change agent and the specific circumstances.

Power-Coercive

Power-coercive strategies are based on the exercise of power by legitimate authority or the use of extreme measures such as economic sanctions and/or political influence. Making changes through modifications in the law, modifications in business policy, and alterations in financial appropriations are examples of the use of power-coercive strategies. When these strategies are used, those in control compel and enforce change through economic, legal, political, and administrative means. So completely does such a strategy operate that many of those who are not in power are not even aware of what is happening, and if they are, there is little they can do to prevent the change from occurring. This form of change process uses the seven-step procedure detailed earlier, but there is little, if any, participation by the target system members. Resistance to the change is generally handled by invoking authority (i.e., accept the change or leave).

An excellent example of a power-coercive strategy is the federal government's enactment of the prospective payment system for reimbursement of the costs of hospitalization of Medicare patients. This system was designed to change the process of hospitalization through the effective use of economic incentives. Under this system, the hospital is not paid for a patient's care based on the number of days the patient is hospitalized. Instead, the hospital receives a predetermined fee based on the patient's DRG regardless of the length of stay. This change represented a major shift in the policy regarding admission, retention, and payment for hospitalized illness, but there was little that any hospital had to say about it because of the authoritative method that was used to enact the change.

Power-coercive strategies are useful when it is unlikely that a consensus will be reached in support of a necessary change despite efforts to stimulate participation throughout the change process. When a high level of resistance is anticipated, time is short, and the change is critical for organizational survival, this type of strategy may be necessary. An example of the application of a power-coercive strategy in a hospital administration is a case in which the vice president of

nursing exercises his or her legitimate authority to appoint a specific person to be a unit supervisor. Such a use of a power-coercive strategy is valid in some situations, such as when a unit is without a leader during a critical period (e.g., a local epidemic of measles). Although the professional autonomy of the unit's members would be better served if they were given the opportunity to interview and vote on a candidate, in the case of an epidemic, organizational and unit survival needs might take precedence, at least for as long as the epidemic lasts.

It is very important to note that the use of a power-coercive strategy often has severe consequences, and responsible management should never ignore the potential negative aftereffects of such a unilateral approach. This is especially true if the unit members have been practicing in a decentralized framework and value their accustomed autonomy. In this situation, the backlash from a unilateral decision can be devastating to the smooth operation of the unit. Resistance to the imposed change (such as an appointed leader) and decreased morale can be anticipated, and managers can build in processes to take them into account. Power-coercive strategies should not be used lightly or frequently if the nurse manager wishes to foster an environment of cooperation and a climate of acceptance of change.

Empirical-Rational

Empirical-rational change strategies differ from power-coercive strategies in that the power component is not authority but knowledge.

Empirical-rational strategies make the following two major assumptions:

1. The vast majority of people are rational and will follow their rational self-interest if that self-interest is made clear to them.
2. The individual who possesses knowledge has expert power that can be used to persuade other people to accept a rationally justified change that will be beneficial to them.

The flow of influence in this type of strategy is from those who possess the information regarding the change to those who do not have this information, or from the informed to the ignorant. New ideas are *invented* and communicated or *diffused* to all participants, as in Rogers's diffusion of innovation. This process is best used in cases in which enacting change is a simple matter of educating the people who will be affected by it and disseminating information to those who might come into contact with it. According to this strategy, once rational people are enlightened, they will either accept or reject the proposed change based on its merits and the anticipated consequences.

The problem with this type of strategy is that people often act in a manner that is anything but rational, and because people do not always respond rationally, this strategy should not be used as the only method of supporting a planned change.[14] However, empirical-rational strategies are often effective when very little resistance to the proposed change is anticipated and the overall perception of the change is that it is both rational and beneficial. Introduction of a new technology that is easy to use, that reduces the amount of time required for a nurse to perform a specific task, and that improves the quality of care is possibly a change that would be readily accepted after adequate in-service education and perhaps a trial period. Change agents can usually direct the change themselves, without a lot of staff participation in the early steps of the change process, although input from the staff is important in the evaluation and stabilization stages. The benefits the staff will gain from the change and selected research findings regarding patient outcomes can act effectively as the major driving forces. One of the best opportunities for the use of this strategy is when the introduction of a well-researched, cost-effective technology is being considered.

Normative-Reeducative

Whereas empirical-rational strategies are based on the concept that people exhibit rational behavior, normative-reeducative strategies of change are built on the assumption that people act in accordance with social norms and values. According to this concept, the mere presentation of information and rational arguments, no matter how well developed or convincing, is insufficient to change the average person's patterns of action. To introduce and manage change using a normative-reeducative strategy, the change agent must focus on the nonintellectual components of behavior as well as the intellectual components. The normative-reeducative approach holds that people's roles and relationships, perceptual orientations, attitudes, and feelings influence their willingness to accept any change presented.

In this type of strategy, the power component is neither authority nor knowledge, but skill in interpersonal relationships. The effective change agent will not use coercion or nonreciprocal influence but will rely on a campaign of collaboration. The change agent will ensure that as many members of the target system as possible are involved throughout the change process. This involvement will provide each person with the necessary level of education to implement his or her portion of the change effectively. Beyond what is learned through actual involvement,

no formal education is included in this strategy. Change or reeducation is a *normative* change as well as a cognitive and perceptual change, and participation in groups is an essential strategy for accomplishing change effectively and efficiently.[13]

Normative-reeducative strategies are well suited to the creative problem-solving environment so prevalent in nursing and healthcare today. The change agent consciously uses and emphasizes a human relations approach to the change process. As many members of the target system as possible are actually enjoined in the various steps of the change process. The value conflicts that are introduced in all parts of the system are openly and freely discussed and worked through so that the change can progress as quickly as possible.

Professional nurses, because they typically possess a comprehensive background in behavioral sciences and have better-than-average communication skills, are comfortable with this type of strategy. In most cases, the normative-reeducative approach to implementing change will be effective in reducing resistance and stimulating personal and organizational creativity. The downside to this approach is the amount of time required for group participation and conflict resolution throughout the change process. When there is adequate time or when group consensus is fundamental to the successful implementation of the change, the professional manager would do well to work within this framework.

CHANGE AGENT SKILLS

Implementing change is not easy, but developing the ability to do so is a fundamental part of every manager's job. Learning how to accomplish this primary function is made easier by the fact that most successful change agents demonstrate certain characteristics that can be cultivated and mastered with practice. These include the following:

- Ability to combine ideas from unconnected sources[5]
- Ability to energize others by keeping the interest level up and demonstrating a high personal energy level
- Skill in human relations—well-developed interpersonal communication, group management, and problem-solving skills
- Integrative thinking—the ability to retain a focus on the "big picture" while dealing with each part of the system
- Sufficient flexibility to modify ideas when modifications will improve the change, but persistent enough to resist nonproductive tampering with the planned change

- Confidence and the tendency not to be easily discouraged
- Realistic thinking
- Trustworthiness—a track record of integrity and success with other changes
- Ability to articulate a vision through insights and versatile thinking
- Ability to handle resistance

HANDLING RESISTANCE

Why do a great many people involved in the healthcare industry resist change? Those who research such subjects would say that a generalized resistance stems from fear of losing the comfort of what is familiar, no matter how inadequate it is. A great percentage of adults find comfort in clinging to the present and fear the uncertainty brought about by change. The mere idea of change can threaten those with a vested interest in maintaining the status quo, because many people view new ideas from the narrow perspective of "How will this change affect me?"

For example, the change being considered may represent a loss in social status for some people if an organization is restructured and social relationships are rearranged and altered. Decentralization may eliminate positions and decrease promotional opportunities. This represents an actual or perceived economic loss to many people and is just the type of personal loss that will bring resistance to a fever pitch. Unions may resist changes that threaten job security for some of their members, even if most of the other segments within an organization benefit—and no matter how significant those benefits might be. For some people, even the inconvenience of learning new behaviors can cause significant resistance to a proposed change.

The change agent should always attempt to anticipate, restructure, and use resistance to change, and every opportunity should be taken to aggressively look for it. Resistance to change, like change itself, is one of the few constants in life, and anyone who is a manager of change for his or her organization can make a safe bet that it will be lurking somewhere and will rear its head when and where it is least expected. A perceptive and persistent manager, however, will be able to recognize its presence by listening for statements like the following:

- "We tried that before."
- "It won't work."
- "No one else does it like that."
- "We've always done it this way."
- "We can't afford it."
- "We don't have the time."
- "It will cause too much commotion."
- "You'll never get it past the board."

- "Let's wait awhile."
- "Every new boss wants something new to do."
- "Let's start a task force to look at it. . . . Put it on the agenda."

As the individual responsible for change, the nurse manager should expect resistance and listen carefully to who is saying what, when they are saying it, and what the circumstances are that prompt them to say it. People who openly verbalize their resistance are far easier to deal with than those who hide in the closet and express their resistance only at the most inopportune moments. Managers should also look for nonverbal signs of growing resistance, which typically manifest in such things as a slowing down of performance, an increase in unsafe and poor-quality work habits, and a general lack of interest in the job and the change.

As change agents, managers should not try to eliminate resistance because it has both positive and negative effects. On the one hand, the potential for resistance forces the change agent to be clear about *why* the change is needed. The agent must know the change inside and out because it is the agent's role to defend it against challengers. The very fact that resistance to change exists demands that those trying to implement it have a sharper focus and be able to resolve problems quickly and painlessly. Resistance causes people implementing change to look for and take steps to prevent the unexpected. It forces the change agent to clarify information, work diligently to keep the interest level high, and answer effectively and honestly the key question, "Why is this change necessary?" Resistance is a stimulus as much as a force to be overcome. It may result in something as simple as motivating the target system to work with the current system more efficiently and improve on what is currently considered acceptable in an effort to avoid the change, which thus saves the organization money and time. In this case, resistance can produce a positive change in behavior.

On the other hand, resistance, if not well managed, can prove to be the death knell for the intended change, especially if it is allowed to persist beyond the planning stage and into the implementation phase. It can wear down those who support the change and redirect system energy from implementing the change to dealing with the resistance, which increases both time and expense. One critical impact of unmanaged resistance can be its detrimental effect on the morale of the organization. Left unchecked, resistance can be absolutely devastating to far more important things than the change that is being implemented.

When managing resistance, change agents must first be sure that they want to reduce it. As previously mentioned, there can be times when well-managed resistance can actually benefit the change. For example, it can be used to sharpen decisions and eventually gain consensus. If it becomes necessary to minimize resistance, however, every effort must be made first to eliminate the potential for personalizing it. Managers must remain rational, stick to the problem-solving change process, and follow these guidelines:

- Open up free communication lines with those who oppose the change. Make every attempt to use what is learned to get to the root of their reasons for opposition.
- Clarify information and provide accurate feedback.
- Be open to revisions but be clear about what must remain.
- Present the negative consequences of the resistance (threats to organizational survival, compromised patient care, etc.). Be honest and do not overdramatize.
- Emphasize the positive consequences of the change and the benefits to the individual and/or group. However, do not spend too much energy on rational analysis of why the change is good and why the arguments against it do not hold up. People's resistance frequently flows from feelings that are not rational.
- Keep as many as possible of those resisting the change actively involved and ensure that they have plenty of face-to-face contact with supporters. Encourage proponents to empathize with opponents, recognize valid objections, and relieve unnecessary fears.
- Maintain a climate of trust, support, and confidence.
- Divert attention by alerting people to other concerns. Energy can be shifted to a more important problem inside the system, so that resistance is redirected and proponents are provided with a breathing period. Alternatively, attention can be brought to an external threat to create a "bully" phenomenon. When members perceive an environmental threat that is greater than that represented by the change (such as competition or restrictive governmental policies), they tend to unify internally.
- Follow the politics of change.

THE POLITICS OF CHANGE

Energy must always be expended to effect change in a system. Power from one source or another is the main provider of that energy. Although very few nurses use coercive power, they do rely on power derived from information, expertise, and possibly position to persuade others. Whenever these classic "political" strategies are used, the change agent or change manager should exercise restraint and use the strategy effectively. The following are some suggestions that may help the change agent use the internal political structure of the organization:

- Managers should analyze the organizational chart so that they are familiar with the formal lines of authority. An additional effort should be made to identify and work with the informal authority structure that exists in every organization. This informal structure should not be overlooked as an important source of political influence.
- The key individual(s) who will be affected by the proposed change should be identified. Special attention should be paid to organizational positions of influence that are immediately above and below the point of change.
- As much information as possible should be gathered about the key people who have been identified. What are the primary things that motivate them? What causes them inconvenience, discomfort, and irritation? What interests them, gets them excited, and keeps them that way? What are the important things with which they are concerned? What is included on their important personal and organizational agendas? Who typically aligns themselves with whom on important decisions?
- The process of building a coalition of support and influence should begin *before* the change is enacted. Those key people who will most likely support the idea, those who will definitely not, and those who are most likely to be persuaded should be identified. Managers should talk *informally* with each of them to identify any possible objections they might have to the idea, and especially with those individuals with influence who might become potential opponents. One of the best ways to influence potential naysayers is by describing the benefits of the change as well as telling them what the potential costs may be. It is far better for managers to lose support because they were honest than because people found out later that they did not tell the complete truth. Identify costs and benefits in political terms. Managers also might want to ask themselves if they could modify the idea to garner more support from key personnel.

Following these suggestions will help the change agent develop the change idea in a way that will make it marketable to a wide range of different interests, or at least will help in identifying points of potential resistance. This is a broad beginning to the data collection step of the change process and will require adjustment once the idea is clarified.

The politics of change continue to be relevant through all the steps of the change process. The astute change agent is always alert to shifts in influence and struggles for power that might conflict with or support the proposed change.

One more very important thing to keep in mind when dealing with change is *never to change too much too fast*. In fact, this can be considered the cardinal rule of change management. The most effective change agents develop a sense of timing that enables them to pace the change process in tempo with the political pulse of the organization. For example, change managers may unfreeze the system during a period of coalition building and high interest, when resistance is low or at least unorganized. They may deliberately refrain from moving the project beyond the pilot stage if it looks like resistance is becoming organized or if it gains a powerful ally. In this case, the change agent employs mechanisms to reduce resistance. If resistance continues, the change manager should consider several possibilities: (a) the change is not workable and should be modified to meet the strongest objections (compromise); (b) the change is sufficiently fine-tuned but can be deferred until resistance subsides; (c) the change must proceed now and resistance must be overcome. If the last situation pertains, energy must be focused on reducing the resistance. This means that supporters will have to be mobilized and constant, consistent pressure will have to be applied to keep the change moving forward.

How effectively a change agent uses the politics of the organization to support implementation of the change often depends on whether the change agent is considered a political insider or not. Someone who is part of the system being changed knows that system, has a stake in the outcome, and is familiar with the people, language, and politics involved. However, being an insider can restrict the agent's ability to move freely throughout the system because the agent may be locked into certain roles, authority structures, and expectations. In addition, an insider's perspective may be somewhat limited. An outsider offers a fresh perspective and is independent of most of the internal politics but is unfamiliar with the system and with people's values and personal agendas. An agent in either political position can effectively accomplish change, but each must assess and use the politics of change differently.

EXERCISES TO STIMULATE CREATIVE THINKING

The ability to develop a vision is not some mystical or mysterious talent. It can be learned through the application of hard work and research. The "discipline of innovation"[15] involves a deliberate, conscious search for innovative opportunities. Any nurse, and certainly any nurse manager, not only can become an

effective change agent but also should put effort toward becoming knowledgeable in this area. By profession, nurses are highly educated, highly trained, and intellectually astute. There is no logical reason that every one of them cannot become an effective innovator. If they are to do so, however, they cannot cling to the status quo but must nurture within themselves a willingness to assume risk. The demanding environment in which nurses work is no longer the rigid place it used to be. Today, it is not enough to rely solely on logic and pragmatic, careful, small steps to find the solutions to the complex problems being faced. Nurses cannot continue to do more with less, and do it well. They must be able to do it *differently*.

The following five exercises are offered to assist individuals in developing insight and should be learned and used effectively by every nurse:

1. Keep a ledger and write down one new idea a day for a month. It can pertain to work, research, professional activities, family, or leisure, but each day's entry must be new. Consider some action on each idea (e.g., discuss it with colleagues, experiment with it, or implement it).

2. Break out of the mold. Do something unexpected, even if it pushes the envelope a bit. Learn to tolerate ambiguity.

3. Try to build the ability to look at things differently. Read a book about creativity or attend a creativity seminar. Read Steele and Maraviglia's, *Creativity in Nursing*,[16] for example. There is no need to stick to nursing references; in fact, it is not recommended. Instead, read the light-hearted *A Whack on the Side of the Head* by von Oech.[17]

4. Engage in extreme thinking. Build time for unfettered thinking into your meetings (supervisors' meetings, for example)—at least for part of the meeting, and several times each month.

5. Try to make things complex and ambiguous. Every day for a month, choose one problem or situation and look for multiple meanings and extreme possibilities. Break it apart and put it back together in a different way. Check out all the angles.

Practicing divergent thinking prepares one to use the process almost automatically in day-to-day situations, such as solving a difficult problem.

SUMMARY

■ Regardless of whether nurse managers practice in a hospital, health maintenance organization, industry, or community health setting, their function is to cause different subsystems of an organization to work effectively and diligently toward meeting the organizational objectives established by senior management. In this role, they must be able to deal effectively with the potential impacts of change because change is an inherent part of an open system.

- The systems and personnel of an organization will always experience conflict and stress as the organization strives to adapt and grow in an evolving environment.
- Regardless of whether nurses are managing or initiating change, they must possess the knowledge and skills to guide the change process effectively in a systems framework.
- Nurse managers must analyze the many interrelating factors that influence the system's response to change if they are to be able to manage the change conceived at any point in the organization, even if they do not actually become involved until the late planning and implementation stages.
- The change agent must understand how to move a change plan forward, how to use and reduce resistance, and how to evaluate outcomes before stabilizing the change.
- A seven-step process for implementing change, as described in the text, has been developed from the work of several researchers.
- Nurses will continue to confront change. They can choose to survive it or manage it. The challenge is to expand their influence by initiating change at all levels of the healthcare system.
- Nurses, and especially nurse managers, must think creatively and act accordingly.
- Many strategies are available for implementing change.

FINAL THOUGHTS

As the individual responsible for leading change in the nursing unit, the nurse manager identifies the problem, assesses the unit's motivations and capacities for change, determines alternatives, explores the ramifications of these alternatives, assesses the availability of resources, determines the availability of assistance, establishes and maintains effective cross-unit relationships, recognizes that change takes place in phases, and guides individual employees through the change process.

Basically, all of these responsibilities are the sole domain of nurse managers. Nurse managers are the ones who will facilitate any planned change by serving as a catalyst, solution provider, process helper, and resource identifier. They will clarify, share, and engage commitment throughout the unit. They will clarify by listening carefully, focusing their energy, and restating

communication. They will share with others by explaining the purpose of the change, overseeing the change, linking the change to employee concerns, and specifying how the concerns will be addressed. They will engage commitment by soliciting understanding, support, and ideas, and creating agreement on action steps.

THE NURSE MANAGER SPEAKS

The nurse manager is responsible for administering change in his or her unit. There is no doubt that it is the nurse manager who will ultimately lead the unit through the transition from old to new.

Implementing and managing change, however, is never an easy task. Many people—and frequently even highly educated individuals—are reluctant to change what has worked for them in the past. In fact, change is disturbing to a very large percentage of the working population, and many will resist any attempt to alter the status quo. Some fervently believe that, given the proper chance, the old system will always prove good enough.

Anyone who has worked for more than a day in any healthcare institution during the last two decades knows that the only constant in health care is change. It is everywhere, from the treatments available to patients to the manner in which their progress is charted. Change is here, and it is here to stay.

What advice can be given about the management of change? The best is still the simplest: *get used to it*. If you are going to be an effective nurse manager, you must not only accept change, you must champion it.

REFERENCES

1. American Nurses Association: *Nursing: a social policy statement*, Kansas City, Mo, 1980, The Association.
2. Kast FE, Rosenzweig JE: *Organization and management: a systems approach*, ed 4, New York, 1985, McGraw-Hill.
3. Chin R: The utility of systems models and developmental models for practitioners. In Bennis W, Benne K, Chin R, editors: *The planning of change*, ed 4, New York, 1985, Holt, Rinehart and Winston.
4. Yoder-Wise P: *Leading and managing in nursing*, ed 3, St Louis, 2002, Mosby.
5. Kanter RM: *The change masters: innovation for productivity in the American corporation*, ed 3, New York, 1993, Simon and Schuster.
6. Lewin K: *Resolving social conflicts: and, field theory in social science*, Washington, DC, 1997, American Psychological Association.
7. Lippitt R, Watson J, Westley B: *The dynamics of planned change*, New York, 1958, Harcourt, Brace.
8. Havelock R: *The change agent's guide to innovation in education*, Englewood Cliffs, NJ, 1973, Educational Technology Publications.

9. Rogers E: *Diffusion of innovations,* ed 5, New York, 1996, Free Press.
10. Hickman C, Silva M: *Creating excellence: managing corporate culture, strategy and change in the new era,* New York, 1984, New American Library.
11. Nutt P: Tactics of implementation, *Acad Manage J* 29(2):16, 1986.
12. Katz D, Kahn R: *The social psychology of organizations,* ed 2, New York, 1989, Wiley.
13. Bennis W, Benne K, Chin R, editors: *The planning of change,* ed 4, New York, 1989, Holt, Rinehart and Winston.
14. Haffer A: Facilitating change: choosing the appropriate strategy, *J Nurs Adm* 16(4):9, 1986.
15. Drucker P: The discipline of innovation, *Harv Bus Rev* 63(3):7, 1985.
16. Steele S, Maraviglia F: *Creativity in nursing,* ed 2, New York, 1997, McGraw-Hill.
17. von Oech R: *A whack on the side of the head,* ed 5, New York, 2001, Warner Books.

SUGGESTED READINGS

Galpin TJ: *The human side of change,* San Francisco, 1999, Jossey-Bass.
Kanter RM: *When giants learn to dance,* New York, 1989, Simon and Schuster.
Lancaster J, Lancaster W: *The nurse as change agent,* St Louis, 1982, Mosby.
Nadler DA, Nadler MB: *Champions of change,* San Francisco, 1998, Jossey-Bass.
Rocchiccioli JT: *Clinical leadership in nursing,* Philadelphia, 1998, Saunders.
Schermerhorn JR Jr: *Management for productivity,* ed 2, New York, 1998, Wiley.
Smith DK: *Taking charge of change: ten principles for managing people and performance,* Reading, Mass, 1996, Addison-Wesley.
Sullivan EJ, Decker PJ: *Effective leadership and management in nursing,* ed 6, Upper Saddle River, NJ, 2005, Pearson/Prentice Hall.

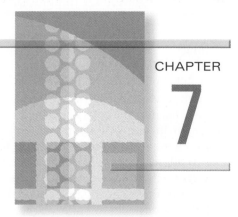

Ethics in Healthcare Management

OUTLINE

LEARNING SYNOPSIS

Upon successful completion of this chapter, readers will possess a fundamental understanding of the importance of ethics in managing health care and in building trust and the perception of quality care in patients and their families.

OBJECTIVES

1. Describe why ethics is such an integral part of the nursing profession
2. Identify two fundamental ethical approaches used in nursing
3. Describe selected principles that apply to the practice of biomedical ethics
4. Identify the elements of the ethical model MORAL and the purposes for which it is used
5. Identify special ethics-related issues faced by the nurse manager

The nursing profession is a moral enterprise whose mission is the provision of high-quality care to others. In spite of this lofty concept, however, the history of the profession is one of nearly continual confrontation with ethical dilemmas. Traditionally, issues such as confidentiality and informed consent have focused the nurse's attention on the safeguarding of patients' rights. These issues remain relevant to the profession today, and dealing with them now requires even more

motivation on the part of individual nurses and nurse managers, because the complexity of care and treatment makes interpretation of these issues even more difficult and important.

Today's medical professionals, because of innovations in healthcare technology, have the tools to keep patients alive almost indefinitely. These advances have created new definitions of life and death, and today the profession faces decisions fraught with ethical dilemmas. Treatment provides both cure and comfort, but at the same time often costs a great deal physically, financially, and emotionally. Patients and their families require assistance in making the difficult decisions that will balance the costs and benefits of the available treatment in terms of their own beliefs and values. Today, all members of the nursing profession must be able to address both intrapersonal and interpersonal conflicts in their daily practice. Nurse managers face these same dilemmas and many more in the discharge of their responsibilities. For example, it is nurse managers alone who must address the ethical implications of their management decisions. Today, more than ever before in the history of nursing, the ability to deal with ethical issues effectively is at the heart of the practice of nursing.

ETHICS: AN INTEGRAL PART OF NURSING MANAGEMENT

How nurse managers operate in their management role is influenced by their individual beliefs and values, and the experiences that form each as individuals and leaders. Personal values as well as the values of the nursing profession define their responsibilities to the patients and communities they serve. The *Code of Ethics for Nurses* of the American Nurses Association (ANA) (Fig. 7-1), the associated interpretive statements, and the ANA's social policy statement* provide each nurse with guidance for making ethical decisions that reflect the standards of the nursing profession. The Patients' Bill of Rights clarifies the rights of patients in institutional settings and implies an obligation on the part of the nursing profession to assist patients in securing those rights.

A quick review of these documents makes it clear that every nurse manager has an obligation to do the following:

- Not discriminate
- Support continuity of care
- Provide safe and respectful care
- Ensure privacy and confidentiality
- Support the policies of the hospital
- Act in accord with his or her own values
- Collaborate with other health professionals
- Support the welfare of the nursing profession
- Safeguard the public from unethical or illegal practice
- Promote efforts to meet the health needs of the public
- Maintain conditions of employment conducive to high-quality care

---

*These documents are available from the ANA, 8515 Georgia Avenue, Suite 400, Silver Spring, MD 20910; 1-800-274-4ANA; http://www.ana.org.

- Ensure that the patient has enough information for informed consent
- Follow physician orders that are in compliance with acceptable standards of care

As this listing is reviewed, what becomes obvious is that, in the process of meeting one of the stated obligations, it may become difficult for a nurse to meet another. Consider the case of a patient with acquired immunodeficiency syndrome (AIDS) who requests that the nurse not inform the spouse of the diagnosis. This creates a conflict between the nurse's duty to safeguard the patient's right to privacy and the obligation to protect the public health.

Another example of a dilemma that can be faced by nurses is the conflict that occurs when a decision has been made to conduct a labor strike. The ANA *Code of Ethics for Nurses*, Provision 6, declares: "The nurse participates in establishing, maintaining, and improving health care environments and conditions of employment conducive to the provision of quality health care and consistent with the values of the profession through individual and collective action."

There is little doubt that conflicting obligations place significant stress on nurses, and unless nurses receive help in addressing them, they can become a source of nurse burnout.[1] Ethical dilemmas, by definition, seldom have right or wrong answers; however, nurse managers can learn to deal with them effectively by preparing themselves and their staff to participate in the decision-making process. Knowledge of the theories and principles of biomedical ethics and a model for decision-making can assist in analyzing issues and provide a basic ability to articulate ethical positions.

ETHICAL APPROACHES

Compared with nursing itself, the field of biomedical ethics is fairly new. This field has become increasingly important, however, as healthcare decisions have moved into the public arena. The ongoing debate over abortion, questions relating to the cessation of life support (such as the ventilatory support that was provided to Karen Ann Quinlan), and legislation regarding brain death are examples of important issues in health care that have generated high levels of public interest in the ethical decision-making process in the medical profession. Today, it is not uncommon for philosophers, theologians, and even social scientists to contribute to the analysis of these important ethical issues.

Theories and principles invoked to address biomedical problems traditionally have been drawn from the discipline of moral philosophy. Biomedical ethics applies these philosophical concepts to specific challenges encountered in the delivery of health care. Deontology and teleology are two theoretical

---

Code of Ethics

Developed by the American Nurses Association

The *Code of Ethics* is based on a belief about the nature of individuals, nursing, health, and society. Recipients and providers of nursing services are viewed as individuals and groups who possess basic rights and responsibilities, and whose values and circumstances command respect at all times. Nursing encompasses the promotion and restoration of health, the prevention of illness, and the alleviation of suffering. The statements of the *Code* and their interpretation provide guidance for conduct and relationships in carrying out nursing responsibilities consistent with the ethical obligations of the profession and quality in nursing care.

1. The nurse respects the dignity and worth of all individuals.

2. The nurse's commitment is to the patient and all of the potential forms this may take.

3. The nurse is an advocate for the patient regarding his or her rights, health, and safety.

4. The nurse is accountable for all nursing actions including those that may be delegated to others.

5. The nurse owes the same duty to himself or herself as to others in regards to self-worth, professional and personal growth, integrity, competence, and safety.

6. The nurse fosters a healthy work site and one that is conducive to a healthy work environment and respects the rights for those who seek individual and collective action.

7. The nurse plays a role in the advance of the profession through education, knowledge creation, and practice.

8. The nurse works with others to improve the health of individuals, families, communities, and nations.

9. The profession of nursing is represented by a variety of associations that promote nursing practice, its values, its integrity, and its social policy.

Fig. 7-1 ■ The American Nurses Association's *Code of Ethics*. (Summarized from American Nurses Association, The Center for Ethics and Human Rights: *Code of ethics for nurses,* Silver Spring, Md, 2001, The Association. Full text available at http://www.nursingworld.org/ethics/ecode.htm.

approaches that are used today to address a wide range of issues in biomedical ethics.

Deontology focuses on the duties and obligations of the medical field. This philosophy holds that the features of actions themselves determine whether they are right or wrong. It assumes that these duties and obligations are universal principles or rules that are inherently good or right, independent of their consequences. Examples of these duties are "Tell the truth," "Do not kill," and "Keep promises."

Teleology, also called *utilitarianism,* gauges the rightness of actions by their ends or consequences.

Deontology is derived from the Greek word *deon,* which means "duty." It is a theoretical approach to biomedical ethics that focuses on the duties and obligations in the medical field. This philosophy holds that the features of actions themselves determine whether they are right or wrong.

Teleology is derived from the Greek word *telos,* which means "end." Also called *utilitarianism,* this theory gauges the rightness of actions by their ends or consequences. The basic principle governing this practice is that of utility, which asserts that the goal of morality is to produce the maximum benefit and minimum impairment for the greatest numbers.

The basic principle governing this practice is that of utility, which asserts that the goal of morality is to produce the maximum benefit and minimum impairment for the greatest numbers. Right conduct and duty are defined in terms of what is good or that which produces good.[2] The position taken in terms of individual, family, or society when considering the good or harm that might be achieved will influence the decisions that are made.

Application of these theoretical concepts to the actual practice of the individual professions has yielded a variety of different codes of ethics and philosophical approaches for the nursing profession. The philosophical premise chosen as a basis for the code of ethics for a specific profession defines the obligations and duties of that profession. One example is the concept of human advocacy put forward in 1979 by Leah Curtin[3] as a philosophical foundation for the practice of nursing. According to Curtin, because the purpose of nursing is to enhance the welfare of other human beings, the goal of the profession is a moral, not a scientific, one: "The good that the profession seeks centers around the relationships nurses develop with other human beings. The wise and human application of a nurse's knowledge and skill is the moral art of nursing" (p. 11). This ideal of advocacy is based on the common humanity, common needs, and common rights of nurses and patients. To operate as advocates, nurses needs to understand both the clinical and moral dimensions of the issues faced by both patients and nurses. Diseases, for example, have a physiologic impact on individuals but can obviously damage humanity as well. The ability of professional nurses to be independent, to act freely, and to exercise their right to make choices is influenced both by the medical problems faced by the patient and by the bureaucratic institutions with which the nurse and patient must interact when the patient is ill.

Nurses in their role as advocates have a responsibility to provide appropriate information on a timely basis that both will help patients make decisions within their value systems and will assist them in finding meaning and purpose in the issues they must confront.

These philosophical positions provide different frameworks for addressing ethical dilemmas, such as (a) defining which right or obligation applies, or (b) identifying the harm or good that will be produced by the action. The principles described in the next section help conceptualize these issues and make them understandable.

PRINCIPLES OF BIOMEDICAL ETHICS

The principles of biomedical ethics provide concepts and language that can be used to identify and reflect on issues and also to articulate the ethical positions one might take. A concept is "an abstraction or generalization that helps attach meaning to a phenomenon that is observed in the clinical setting" (p. 52).[4] A concept, in short, helps nurses recognize what is occurring. If a nurse says that a patient "is in shock," a fairly representative picture will appear in the minds of other equally qualified professionals. In the same way, if a nurse identifies an issue as one of "patient autonomy," an entire range of questions will arise. Respect for individuals underlies the basic nursing principles of autonomy, nonmaleficence, beneficence, and justice.

The Principle of Autonomy

Autonomy is derived from the Greek words *autos* (self) and *nomos* (rule) and is defined as self-rule or self-governance. Personal autonomy is further defined as "being one's own person, without the imposition of constraints either by another's action, or by psychologic or physical limitations" (p. 74).[2] The principle of autonomy requires that nurses respect the individuals within their care as autonomous agents who have a right to control their own lives. To enable a patient to do this, the nurse must remember that making one's own decision requires accurate information. Therefore, the requirement that a patient give informed consent is based on the principle of autonomy. Nurses often encounter situations in which a person either has not received information or has not attended to or remembered it. This means that nurses will frequently be required to provide information to patients, seek information for them, or inform them that they have a right both to receive information and/or to refuse treatment. Differences of opinion between patients and families or among caregivers are often revealed when questions such as the following are asked: "Should we tell him he has cancer?" "Does she know that the treatment will be painful and expensive, and may very well be futile?"

In the spirit of respect for autonomy, professional nurse managers must help people participate in decisions that affect them to the extent to which they are able. To be self-governing, one must be competent to act on one's own behalf. Competency assessment, therefore, is a critical prerequisite in determining who makes decisions. In cases of incompetence or in an emergency, healthcare professionals may act in what they consider to be the best interests of the patient.

To the greatest extent possible, nurses should reflect the patient's values when making these decisions. Competent patients have the right to decide their individual futures, even if the outcome of refusing treatment may be death. For example, a devout

Jehovah's Witness will refuse a blood transfusion, because in this group's belief system undergoing this procedure risks the eternal soul and thus presents a far greater threat than death.

It is difficult to allow someone to make a decision that is likely to be harmful from a medical point of view. Because of the risk of paternalism, however, to override an individual's decision, the medical professional must have *strong* evidence that the person is indeed incapable of rendering a competent decision. *Paternalism* is a word that the nursing profession uses to describe taking actions in the "best interests" of those who are being given medical care. Healthcare professionals have long acted in accordance with this precept out of goodwill, but the human rights movement of the last two decades has brought with it a major focus on individual rights and a conflict with paternalism. Today, patient autonomy is given increasing weight in the decisions made by medical professionals.

The patient's rights to privacy and confidentiality also have their roots in the principle of autonomy. The advent of AIDS has created some new questions regarding how confidentiality and privacy are to be maintained, such as "How can I protect the health of other hospital staff without disclosing the patient's diagnosis?" and "Who has the right to information in the medical record?" In such cases, the patient's right to autonomy and confidentiality must be weighed against the responsibility to preserve the health and well-being of others. The right to autonomy, while it is certainly a fundamental right of all patients, is not absolute.

The Principle of Nonmaleficence

Nonmaleficence is the principle that requires members of the medical profession to "do no harm." Adhering to this principle is often considered one of the most stringent responsibilities of every professional involved in medicine. The nursing profession's contract with society requires that each nurse provide safe care to every patient with whom he or she comes into contact. To act in accordance with the principle of nonmaleficence, members of the profession must continually conduct themselves in a thoughtful and competent manner. "Due care" requires that every nurse possess the knowledge and skill necessary to perform the tasks he or she undertakes, and the ANA *Code of Ethics for Nurses* states that the nurse is accountable for all nursing actions, including those that may be delegated to others. This means that the responsibility for maintaining professional knowledge and skills is placed directly on the individual nurse. Also, it means that if a nurse knows that he or she does not have the competency to perform a certain act, then the nurse should not attempt it.

The concept of harm includes the infliction of emotional trauma and financial expense as well as the more commonly considered outcomes of pain, death, and disability. Although this principle seems to be a fundamental one, dilemmas occur when individuals' perceptions and definitions of harm differ. Death may be perceived by the staff as the worst result of a particular action, but the patient may not agree, or vice versa. In the case of chemotherapy administration or transplantation, it would seem obvious that pain and illness are harms that one may choose to sustain in order to prevent the even greater injury of profound illness or death, but this may not be so for every patient.

The Principle of Beneficence

Beneficence, or the principle of doing good, is often placed on the same plane as the principle of nonmaleficence. However, it is less passive and requires taking action that contributes to the welfare of others as well as preventing and removing the potential for harm. Mercy, kindness, and charity are concepts related to the principle of beneficence.

Provision 1 of the ANA *Code of Ethics for Nurses* declares, "The nurse in all professional relationships, practices with compassion and the respect for the inherent dignity, worth, and uniqueness of every individual, unrestricted by considerations of social or economic status, personal attributes, or the nature of the health problems." This means that *not* providing a service that is available is a breach of professional obligation and a violation of the principle of beneficence.

The situation that occurs when the nurse's personal belief that a particular treatment is wrong confronts his or her professional obligation to provide it has been discussed for years. The outcome of these discussions most often is that the nurse may transfer to another unit where the conflicting practice is not routinely encountered. Abortion is an excellent example of a treatment that may provoke this type of conflict. In the short term, however, if a nurse is assigned to a specific patient, the nurse may not abandon the patient simply because the nurse's personal belief conflicts with the patient's right to a specific treatment. This situation exemplifies the nurse's higher obligation to do no harm, or the principle of nonmaleficence. Beneficence and nonmaleficence

---

Nonmaleficence is the ethical principle that one should do no harm and is based on the Latin phrase *Primum non nocere*, "First, do no harm."

Beneficence is the act of doing good. Mercy, kindness, and charity are concepts related to the principle of beneficence.

represent extreme ends of the treatment scale, and the distinction between the two lies in the amount of action required. The nursing profession has a special contract to provide care for the sick, and active involvement in providing or arranging for appropriate care is an act of beneficence.

The Principle of Justice

Justice, at least in concept, is frequently equated with fairness or, more precisely, with the practice of giving each individual person his or her right or due. To receive a license to practice nursing is a form of justice because each nurse who receives one has earned the right to possess it through hard work, study, and personal effort.

Distributive justice, or the just allocation of burdens and benefits within society, is a recurring theme in health care today as advances in technology and calls for increased cost control create challenges for many traditional policy decisions. For example, discussions regarding resource allocation have increased in recent years with the recognition by the healthcare profession that available resources are not without limits. At the level of the individual patient, establishing the criteria for receiving an organ for transplantation is an example of a situation in which justice must be considered. On a macroeconomic level, issues of justice are frequently addressed through questions such as, "Is there a right to health care?" and "What does a right to health care mean?" In the recent past, the realities of the medical profession have dictated that uninsured and underinsured patients be added to the ranks of those disenfranchised individuals who cannot always obtain health care. Justice, however, has caused policy makers to discuss a possible safety net to provide catastrophic health insurance to assist those individuals whose resources have run out.

It is a function of nurse managers to participate in the decision-making process that determines what institutional programs will be developed or discontinued. This participation includes active involvement in both budget development and strategic planning. Because nurse managers wear the two hats of institutional administrator and nursing professional, they must consider when making decisions their obligation to provide quality care to the patient as well as the need for the institution to operate in a cost-effective manner so that it can continue its mission—something that can give rise to a significant dilemma.

Nurse managers address questions of justice as they consider such fundamental requirements as the proper staff mix, the percentage of available staff that will be assigned to each shift, and the establishment of daily performance assignments. Nurse managers' judgment reflects the needs of the patients, the skills of the available nursing staff, and the knowledge of how the best care can be provided. The ANA *Code of Ethics for Nurses* states, "The nurse's commitment is to the patient and all of the potential forms this may take." For most nurse managers, the dilemma of best interests would come into play if they were required to treat two equally ill patients—one of them a "bag lady" and the other a hospital director—and had to decide which of the patients would be assigned the best-qualified staff.

There is little doubt that beliefs, values, and self-interest play a role in many decisions—regardless of the professional ability of the individual making the decision. Therefore, to prevent discrimination and unfairness, at least to the greatest extent possible, nurse managers need to have an awareness of their personal values and biases. Nurse managers are humans as well as professionals, and their profession requires them to make value judgments on a frequent basis. If these nurse managers are aware of their personal values and biases, they will make their decisions more consciously, although, even then, they may not do so perfectly. Because the nursing profession seldom offers clear "right" answers but rather options to be considered, a model for decision-making can help nurse managers analyze the ethical issues that confront them.

A MODEL FOR ADDRESSING ETHICAL ISSUES

Most ethical decision models are structured around the basic nursing process and incorporate the principles of biomedical ethics discussed in the last section. One such model for decision-making was developed and refined by Crisham based on research involving hundreds of staff nurses in acute care settings.[5] Crisham's model is a tool that can be used to clarify the issues when nurses face conflicting obligations. It outlines a process for identifying and articulating a position so the nurse can participate in the decision-making process (Box 7-1).

BOX 7-1

The MORAL Model for Ethical Decision-Making

Crisham's model involves five steps represented by the mnemonic MORAL:
  M: Massage the dilemma
  O: Outline the options
  R: Review the criteria and resolve
  A: Affirm the position and act
  L: Look back

Data from Crisham P: MORAL: how can I do what is right?, *Nurs Manage* 16(3):42A, 1985.

The following case helps illustrate the steps in the model.

CASE STUDY

▓ MRS. ADACHI

The nurse manager of an intensive care unit is confronted with an ethical dilemma when the staff nurses caring for Mrs. Adachi say that she is communicating verbally and nonverbally (by resisting treatments) a wish that she be allowed to die. As Mrs. Adachi's condition grows worse, the nursing staff anticipate a cardiac arrest, and they believe it would be abusive to the patient to engage in normal resuscitation efforts. Because there is no "do not resuscitate" order in the medical record, the nurses are obligated by hospital policy to initiate resuscitation efforts until such an order can be obtained.

When Mrs. Adachi's sons are approached with this information, they express the belief that a discussion of death would take away Mrs. Adachi's hope and thus might actually hasten her death. They want all possible efforts taken to sustain her life. As discussions are occurring between the nursing and the medical staff, Mrs. Adachi's condition worsens. She slips into a coma and is unable to communicate.

How does the nurse manager address this dilemma?

■ Massage the Dilemma

The first step, as in most other such processes, is to identify the problem; that is, to be aware that an ethical dilemma actually exists. Nurses, like all other professionals, are less likely to feel discomfort when they are able to identify the specific conflict. *Massaging the dilemma,* or collecting data, helps to identify what specific dilemma is being faced and who is, or should be, involved in the process of decision-making. Collecting all the relevant data available is the most crucial component in ethical decision-making.

It is important to remember that the different parties involved in a specific situation may have conflicting wishes and values. Conflicts can arise between patient, family, nurse, and doctor, or even between a nurse's personal values and the prescribed treatment. A dilemma occurs when a party believes that valid reasons exist to take two opposing actions. Phrased another way, reasons exist *to do* and *not to do* the same thing; for example, to respect the patient's wishes and not to violate institutional policy. In this case, the nurse manager's conflicting obligations are the following:

- To do no harm (not abuse)
- To provide the best possible treatment
- To support the patient's autonomy and act according to her wishes
- To support the family in a time of crisis
- To follow orders and hospital policy (resuscitate because there was no order to the contrary)
- To assist staff by acting professionally
- To make an ethical decision

In collecting data for decision-making, some issues for consideration are the following:

- What is the prognosis at this point?
- Who has the information regarding the prognosis?
- Who can make the decision?
- Was Mrs. Adachi competent when she indicated her wish to die?
- What are the relationships among family members?
- Can the sons represent Mrs. Adachi's best interests?
- How capable are the sons of making the decision? Are they in denial regarding their mother's prognosis?
- Can hospital policy be of assistance in this instance?
- What is the primary obligation of a nurse manager?

As nurse managers attempt to unravel the confusion that often surrounds dilemmas, it is helpful to consider exactly what options they have available and what tools they have at their disposal. Ultimately, nurses cannot write "do not resuscitate" orders, but they can, and frequently do, interact with others (family, physicians, chaplains) in the decision-making process. In this instance, the staff nurses have concerns about the family system, the survivors, and the dying patient and her autonomy. In this dilemma, the nurse manager's goal becomes one of assisting the decision-makers and the family to share their information and their values in the pursuit of a consensus.

■ Outline Options

The process of outlining the options should be accomplished with full staff involvement to help the staff clarify the options available and the consequences of their potential actions. The following options may be identified:

- Do nothing
- Discuss the medical diagnosis, prognosis, and medical plan with the primary physician
- Discuss with family members their perceptions of the diagnosis and prognosis, their values and beliefs, and what their mother would have wanted; this may include asking questions such as, "How is quality of life defined for Mrs. Adachi—is it awareness, productivity, spending time with grandchildren, etc.?"
- Discuss the nurses' values and clarify their reasons for not wanting to resuscitate; clarify whose best interests the staff is representing
- Schedule a care conference with the family, nurses, physicians, and whomever else may be helpful (e.g., minister, chaplain, social worker)

■ Review Criteria and Resolve

To determine exactly what the appropriate actions are, one must weigh the options generated against the principles or primary values of those involved.

Crisham provided a decision matrix such as that is shown in Table 7-1. This matrix includes principles and practical factors that should be considered in the decision-making process. The alternatives or options listed in the preceding section are put on this graph and weighed against the criteria the nurse manager may include (staff autonomy, nonmaleficence, etc.). Practical considerations such as legal impact, effectiveness, and likelihood of success can also be included in the grid.

Adding a plus or minus to each cell or applying numerical weightings can give the nurse a visual indication of the positive and negative aspects of various options. Many ethical decisions are approached by effectively weighing choices, because there is seldom one right or wrong answer when dealing with an ethical dilemma. Listening and attempting to understand the values of the parties involved is essential to collaborative decision-making.

Individuals often assess the effects of positive and negative factors differently and weigh their choices in dissimilar ways. Therefore, the tool presented here, when used with members of the staff, can help in understanding the different frames of reference of those involved.

■ Affirm Position and Act

Once a decision has been made as to what the next appropriate action will be, a strategy must be developed to ensure that this action is, in fact, accomplished. The history of biomedical ethics indicates that knowing the correct action does not have a great deal of influence on whether healthcare workers act in accordance with what they believe to be correct. To increase the likelihood of appropriate action, one should look at the organizational forces that assist or impede an action plan.

The following questions should be considered in planning for action to resolve the dilemma in Mrs. Adachi's case:

- Are the nurses able to risk stating their opinions and rationales?
- What are the consequences of following and not following institutional policy?
- Will the attending physician be willing to attend a care conference?
- Can the nursing staff deal effectively with all of the outcomes that could potentially result from a care conference?
- Does the nursing staff need additional resources to assist with the process?

Planning the specifics of the care conference is part of the nurse manager's facilitating role in ethical decision-making. Nurse managers can help their staff determine what are the appropriate time and place and who should attend so that they can participate in the decision-making process and feel supported while doing so. Participation in the care conference may also help the staff develop new skills that can be used to deal effectively with future dilemmas as they occur.

■ Look Back

To resolve Mrs. Adachi's case, the staff conduct a care conference. During the consultation, it becomes clear that the family is acting on information obtained weeks earlier and is assuming that, if treatment is successful, Mrs. Adachi will have 2 years or more of "normal" life. However, the nurses and doctors are now observing Mrs. Adachi deteriorate at a far more rapid pace and are seeing her become infected and septic. Both the nurses and physician now believe that the most that can be done medically is to prolong a painful and brutal process of dying. When family members hear the new prognostic information, they readily see that extraordinary efforts to maintain their mother's life will cause more harm than good and agree that, if Mrs. Adachi goes into cardiac arrest, she should not be resuscitated. She dies a few days later.

In this instance, the resolution is successful in that it prevents harm to Mrs. Adachi and promotes goodwill and respect among all involved. In cases in which disagreements persist, however, the nurse manager may need to go back through the process to redefine the problem, to generate options, and/or to identify consequences with all of the decision-makers. The nurse manager also may involve different specialized resource personnel to assist in the problem-solving process.

As nurse managers address different dilemmas in their management practices, the same grid format shown in Table 7-1 that lists options, values, and practical considerations can be used as a basis for reflection. Nurse managers can also add, substitute, or delete some of the categories to provide the greatest flexibility in the use of the matrix. Additional values that can be considered for use include such things as fairness, honesty, empathy, and concern for others above self. These can be listed along with the ethical principles that are being applied in the given case or they can replace them on the decision matrix, depending on what specific values are applicable to the situation.

The field of business ethics addresses issues such as corporate responsibility, conflict of interest, and honesty in dealing with consumers. Nurse managers frequently consider relationships with their staff and colleagues, their responsibility to their patients and to the organization, cost effectiveness, and sometimes community relations in their management decisions

TABLE 7-1

Decision Matrix

Options	Patient Autonomy	Beneficence	Nonmaleficence	Staff Autonomy	Interdisciplinary Relationships	Family Comfort	Compliance with Policy	Reduction of Legal Risk	Time	Clarity of Issue
Do nothing	–	–	–	–	NA	+	+	+	+	–
Discuss with physician	+	+	+	–	–	?	+	–	–	±
Discuss with family	+	+	+	±	NA	+	NA	+	–	±
Discuss with nurses	+	+	+	+	–	±	NA	+	–	±
Schedule a care conference	+	+	+	+	+	±?	+	+	+	+

NA, Not applicable.

and their supervisory relationships. Articulating the issues clearly, defining the goal one wishes to achieve, and analyzing its impact are means that can be used to increase the consciousness with which decisions are made. These steps can also enhance a manager's ability to articulate the rationale for the directions he or she intends to pursue.

SPECIAL ISSUES FOR THE NURSE MANAGER

Provision of Safe Care

The most fundamental ethical obligation nurse managers have is to ensure that safe care is provided. With the increasing complexity of care and technology, the nursing staff must possess advanced assessment skills and an up-to-date knowledge of the latest treatments and procedures available to their patients. The individual skills discussed in earlier chapters are extremely important for nurse managers to master so that they can address patient care at least from the perspective of the minimum requirement of nonmaleficence. In addition to practicing these simple management skills, nurse managers also have the responsibility of developing the patient's ability to care for himself of herself by providing basic education and the information essential for autonomous decision-making.

Confrontation of Unsafe Practices

Nurse managers also have the responsibility to deal effectively with personnel engaging in unsafe practices and with impaired practitioners in accordance with the "due care" standard, regardless of whether the poorly performing individuals are nurses or other healthcare professionals. Nurse managers need to know and thoroughly understand the institution's procedures for addressing issues of safety and professional conduct and know how to apply these principles in a variety of situations. In addition to possessing all these skills, nurse managers must also maintain a high degree of respect for others, which is an underlying principle of biomedical ethics. To conduct themselves *humanely and gently* while providing accurate data requires nurse managers to employ their best communication and leadership skills even when confronting the most painful of issues.

Support of Patient and Staff Autonomy

To address ethical issues effectively, nurse managers must also know and understand their own personal values and goals. Having this knowledge makes it easier to express personal beliefs and positions when taking an ethical stance. In addition, this knowledge increases nurse managers' objective ability to assist a patient or staff member in making decisions that are based on his or her personal value systems. Nurse managers must work hard to avoid paternalism. Language used to identify a "noncompliant" patient often suggests that the patient's value system is different from the nurse's own. For example, a patient's definition of quality of life may differ greatly from that of the nurse. To act as an advocate, the nurse must understand the patient's values and, through them, support the patient's decisions. "So often by trying to do what we think is right by our value system, we trespass upon the authenticity of the person" (p. 11).[3] It is absolutely essential that nurse managers hear and understand the values and goals of the patient and the staff to avoid infringing on their individuality.

Ethics Education and Resource Management

Ethical issues arise commonly in healthcare institutions—so frequently, in fact, that many facilities have created special resources to manage them. These special resources are most often designed to provide education, consultation, and support to both patients and staff members. Such organizations also ensure that individuals such as line supervisors, clinical specialists, and/or ethics consultants are available to provide assistance. Many institutions now have standing ethics committees, which are responsible for developing policies that protect patients' rights and for providing education and consultation in difficult cases. These committees generally have members from a wide variety of disciplines. This interdisciplinary character allows them to supply objective insight as well as an overview of the process to ensure that due care is used in the decision-making process.

Programs that ensure continual staff education and open discussion of ethical issues when a crisis is not looming are effective tools in preparing the staff to address ethical dilemmas when they do arise. Formal classes given as a part of a comprehensive in-service educational program provide a framework for open discussion of ethical dilemmas. In addition, when ethical concerns are discussed openly during staff meetings, teamwork is developed that will help in identifying issues and patterns of issues that occur frequently.

Another effective method of approaching ethical issues is to incorporate "ethics rounds." These are interdisciplinary rounds conducted by members of the nursing staff and individuals in other disciplines who frequently interact with patients and personnel within a unit. This process provides a forum in which principles can be presented and discussed openly and in which specific cases can be reviewed and debated. While participating, members of the staff can develop a common language as well as an awareness of one another's values. This shared foundation of knowledge becomes well known and is clearly understood when a difficult issue arises. A significant benefit of ethics rounds is that, as staff members gain skills and awareness, ethical issues are often identified at an earlier stage, which averts many crises. The goal of ethics education should always be to develop staff skills that can be used to deal effectively with the issues that arise frequently in professional practice.

When nurse managers create educational opportunities, they should indicate that sensitive issues are open to discussion and thus identify these issues as important parts of nursing practice. By listening, participating in problem solving, and soliciting additional resources in a nonthreatening manner, nurse managers make it possible for the staff to risk raising sensitive issues.

Nurse managers who know their own values, who respect their staff members, and who expect high-quality care are the managers who create an environment in which ethical issues can be addressed easily and resolved quickly. The time and skill required to resolve conflict and encourage creative problem solving are scarce resources in the nursing department. The capable nurse manager, therefore, is the institution's best asset for developing a professional, ethical nursing practice.

SUMMARY

- Beliefs, values, and experiences influence one's ethical decision-making ability.
- The nursing profession has delineated its code of ethics in the ANA *Code of Ethics for Nurses*. The *Code*, along with the accompanying interpretive statements (available from the ANA), guides nurses' ethical decision-making.
- Ethical principles include autonomy, nonmaleficence, beneficence, and justice.
- Use of a model for addressing ethical issues assists the nurse in the decision-making process.
- The nurse manager has a number of ethical responsibilities, including the obligations to provide safe care, thwart unsafe practices, support patient and staff autonomy, manage resources, and provide ethics training to subordinate staff.
- The staff's ability to deal with ethical issues is directly related to the nurse manager's skill in conflict management, willingness to allow risk taking, and support of staff acting in a professional manner.

- Nurse managers communicate interest in ethical issues by assisting staff in generating alternatives and developing strategies for action.

FINAL THOUGHTS

Ethics is a moral philosophy, an art of judging the relationship between the means one uses and the ends one achieves, and controlling the means so that they will serve the desired ends.

Ethics is not an easy thing to possess. It means that the individual and the organization embrace conflict, choice, and conscience in the way they do business and the relationships they establish with others. Conflict occurs in how choices are made and how these choices are influenced by the values that are held. Choice involves a decision to serve what is held to be right, just, and correct, or what is expedient, acceptable, and subjective. Ethical choices consider wants, needs, and rights, but in such a way that there is no infringement upon another person's wants, needs, and rights.

Ethics is about providing people—all people, both seniors and subordinates—with value. Value is something the receiver would freely choose, something the receiver consciously prizes.

A moral dilemma can occur when a decision that is made has advantages for one but equally unsatisfactory alternatives or impacts for another.

Nurse managers must practice ethics in the day-to-day discharge of their responsibilities.

THE NURSE MANAGER SPEAKS

Moral outrage and distress occur when conflicting systems of ethics are allowed to coexist in the same work environment. This situation creates confusion for the worker because it leaves the question of what is right and good open to perspective.

Nurse managers must practice ethics in the performance of their jobs, and this system of ethics must be fair and just for every person the nurse manager influences. This is especially true when decisions are made. The professional nurse manager makes decisions using the ethical principles of beneficence, nonmaleficence, justice, and autonomy.

Ethical situations are not objective realities. They are always influenced by the attitudes and values of the individual viewing the situation. Because ethical situations are social, conflicts will occur that reflect the different points of view held by the individuals involved in the situation.

This type of conflict occurs frequently in the nursing unit. It can be heard in the comment, "Why do I have to fight so hard for what is right and good?" Conflicts stemming from different moral points of view or moral perspectives have often led to high levels of moral distress in the nursing profession.

Because different perspectives define right and good in different ways, nurse managers must become morally reflective about their own definitions of right and good and must be aware of the definitions held by others. It is never enough to analyze a situation and find the "right" answer; nurse managers must be sensitive to others and their views of what is right and good.

REFERENCES

1. Cameron M: The moral and ethical component in nurse burn-out, *J Nurs Manag* 17(4):42B, 1986.
2. Beauchamp T, Childress JF: *Principles of biomedical ethics,* New York, 1983, Oxford University Press.
3. Curtin LL: The nurse as advocate: a philosophical foundation for nursing, *Adv Nurs Sci* 1(3):11, 1979.
4. Jillings CR: Concepts relevant for critical care nursing: the knowledge-practice connection, *Crit Care Nurs* 5(2):52, 1985.
5. Crisham P: MORAL: how can I do what is right?, *Nurs Manage* 16(3):42A, 1985.

SUGGESTED READINGS

Curtin LL, Flaherty MJ: *Nursing ethics: theory and practice,* Bowie, Md, 1999, Robert J. Bradie.

Davis AJ, Aroskar MA: *Ethical dilemmas and nursing practice,* New York, 1997, Appleton and Lange.

Jones R, Beck S: *Decision making in nursing,* Belmont, Calif, 1996, Delmar.

Laborde GZ: *Influencing with integrity,* Palo Alto, Calif, 1983, Syntony.

Marquis BL, Huston CJ: *Management decision making for nurses,* ed 2, Philadelphia, 1994, Lippincott.

Marriner Tomey A: *Guide to nursing management and leadership,* ed 7, St Louis, 2004, Mosby.

McGuffin J: *The nurse's guide to successful management,* St Louis, 1999, Mosby.

Vroom VH, Yetton PW: *The new leadership,* Pittsburgh, 1973, University of Pittsburgh Press.

Yoder-Wise PS: *Leading and managing in nursing,* ed 3, St Louis, 2003, Mosby.

Communication for Front-Line Managers

OUTLINE

LEARNING SYNOPSIS

Upon successful completion of this chapter, readers will possess a fundamental understanding of how communication affects the nursing environment and how nurse managers can use good communication skills to enhance the performance of the nursing unit.

OBJECTIVES

1. Identify and define major communication concepts
2. Describe the six steps in an effective communication process
3. Describe the basic communication process and explain why it is complex
4. Identify five fundamental characteristics of effective communication
5. Describe different methods of communication
6. Describe the various communication systems
7. Identify the different communication modes
8. Explain the importance of listening to effective communication

9. Describe what is meant by assertive communication and explain how nurse managers can use it
10. Identify the potential effects of distorted communication and discuss what can be done to reduce its impact
11. Identify seven principles of effective communication
12. Explain how effective communication applies to nurse managers

The ability to communicate effectively is extremely important to nurse managers because most of their management duties depend on their capacity to express themselves clearly. Cultivating the ability to communicate effectively is indispensable for nurse managers, who must interact with a wide variety of individuals both inside and outside the healthcare facility, including patients, family members, subordinate personnel, administrative personnel, medical staff, vendors, and other support workers. Good nurse managers must be able to listen attentively and accurately to others and express themselves effectively, both in speech and in writing. As a matter of fact, most healthcare organizations owe the effectiveness of their public relations efforts to the skill of individual nurse managers in communicating a positive image of the organization.

By definition, managers perform their work by directing the efforts of others, and their ability to do so efficiently depends largely on their capability to make themselves and their desires clearly understood. Nurse managers are no different from their counterparts in other types of business; they perform the traditional management functions of planning, directing, and organizing the daily work in their areas of responsibility. To accomplish their duties, they make informed and well thought-out decisions and carry out the standard management functions of providing leadership, supervision, and motivational support. In addition, nurse managers perform the human resource management functions of hiring, training, performing appraisals, coaching, administering discipline, and developing positive labor relations. The ability to accomplish any of these demanding functions successfully hinges on the quality and effectiveness of their communication.

The difficulty with communication is that few people are born with the ability to do it well. However, communicating effectively is a necessary skill that any reasonably intelligent individual can master. Developing this skill is not difficult and can even be compared with learning a technical skill such as aseptic technique. Once a nurse understands the principles of this technique, he or she can learn any procedure that requires it. If the nurse does not learn the principles of sterility, however, the nurse may perform procedures in an unsafe manner and risk harm to a patient. The same thing is true of communication. Once a nurse understands its principles, he or she can begin to interact effectively with just about anyone. Good communication is as essential to a nurse manager's effectiveness as a scalpel is to a surgeon. It is with the instrument of communication that nurse managers learn to plan, organize, and direct the efforts of others.

The healthcare environment contains unique challenges that sometimes limit nurse managers' ability to develop good communication skills. These include the following:

Organizational structure: The typical organizational structure of a healthcare facility is significantly different from that in other types of working environments because multiple lines of authority operate simultaneously (e.g., medical staff, administration, and nursing). Even individuals who are not employees of the hospital (e.g., physicians) wield considerable influence in the day-to-day operations of the medical unit.

Composition of staffing: The nursing profession has a great deal of influence in the healthcare facility, but traditionally it has been hampered by the fact that it has been primarily a woman's profession and has experienced bias as a result. This has presented a significant challenge, and although things have begun to change in recent years, these changes still are occurring only in the most enlightened societies. Even today, throughout much of the world, nursing is considered a woman's profession, and this causes problems for nurse managers operating in these societies. The problems generally stem from the fact that the traditional female role in society, especially when it is applied to the profession of nursing, is still largely one of subservience and of service to others. The nursing profession's orientation toward service and the attitude in the typical healthcare institution that the nurse is present only to serve the needs of others does not create an environment that is conducive to the sharing of authority.

Effective management is a process of controlling the environment and positively influencing the individuals who function in it to achieve specific results. In the medical unit, the nurse manager is the one who is responsible for this process and who exercises this control; however, many of these nursing professionals have never learned to pursue their management goals through the effective use of communication. Instead, most managers concentrate their communication efforts on developing effective patient and peer expression and give little thought to using communication as the effective management tool it is.

Good communication is a two-dimensional skill that consists of the abilities to converse effectively and to listen effectively. Good verbal (oral) and written skills enable nurse managers to articulate their ideas in a manner that others can easily understand. Careful listening allows nurse managers to learn and under-

stand others' ideas accurately, which enables them to intervene appropriately in interactions with those whom they encounter or must influence.

THE PROCESS OF COMMUNICATION

All management functions involve the ability to communicate effectively. The process of effective communication involves the following six basic actions:

1. Ideation
2. Encoding
3. Transmission
4. Receiving
5. Decoding
6. Response

Definitions of these and other communication concepts are presented in Table 8-1. The process of communication operates as shown in the following diagram:

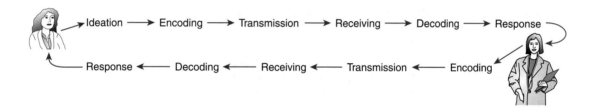

Ideation → Encoding → Transmission → Receiving → Decoding → Response

Response ← Decoding ← Receiving ← Transmission ← Encoding

TABLE 8-1

Communication: Major Concepts and Definitions

Word/Phrase	Definition
Aggressive	Strong or emphatic in effect or intent; dynamic, brazen, energetic
Assertive	Disposed to or characterized by confidence or boldness; confident in stating one's opinion or need
Communication	A process by which information is exchanged by individuals through common symbols, signs, or behavior; talk, gestures, writing, etc.
Decoding	Converting into intelligible form; recognizing and interpreting; putting meaning into symbols
Encoding	Converting from one system of communication to another; putting meaning into symbols
Feedback	The transmission of evaluative or corrective information to the original or controlling source about an action, event, or process; the information so transmitted
Fogging	Making obscure or confusing
Formal	Following or in accordance with established form, custom, or rule; for example, formal communication
Grapevine	An informal person-to-person means of circulating information or gossip; a secret source of information; an informal communications system
Ideation	The forming of ideas; the decision to share an idea
Informal	Marked by the absence of formality or ceremony; characteristic of the ordinary, casual, or familiar; not according to prescribed ways

Continued

TABLE 8-1

Communication: Major Concepts and Definitions—cont'd

Word/Phrase	Definition
Life position	Assumptions made by oneself concerning relationships with others
Negative assertion	Acceptance of negative aspects about oneself; the act of stating or declaring negatively in a forceful manner
Negative inquiry	The act of asking for more information about oneself, often in a negative context or manner
Nonverbal	Other than verbal, not spoken; referring to communicative means such as body language, voice tone, facial expression, gestures, posture, or pauses in delivery
Passive	Lacking in energy or will; inactive; acted on; tending not to take an active or dominant part
Receiving	Coming into possession of; assimilating through the mind or senses; seeing or hearing a transmitted message
Repetitive	Involving or characterized by the act or instance of repeating or being repeated; sometimes the slang expression "broken record" is used to describe something repeated on numerous occasions or the person who repeats it
Response	Something constituting a reply or reaction; feedback
Transmission	The act, process, or instance of sending an impulse across a space
Vernacular	Using a language or dialect native to a region or country rather than a literary, cultured, or foreign language

To fully understand communication and how it works, let's consider its six fundamental elements in more detail (Fig. 8-1):

1. *Ideation:* the formation of ideas and the decision to share an idea. This step begins when the originator of the content decides to share the message with another individual, believes that there is a reason to communicate, or develops an idea or concept that can be expressed. The reason the originator decides to share the information is important to the communication delivered, because it shapes the tone of the delivery. The purpose of the communication varies depending on the needs of the originator; for example, it may be to command, to entertain, to inform, to instruct, to inquire, or to persuade. Whatever the specific purpose, the originator of the communication needs to have a goal and to think clearly before communicating, or the message may become unintelligible and insignificant.

2. *Encoding:* This step involves putting meaning into a symbolic form (e.g., verbalization, composition, or nonverbal behavior). The originator's personal, cultural, and professional biases can affect the encoding process because they can change the message in ways that affect how the listener perceives it. The originator must use all of the clearly understood symbols and forms of

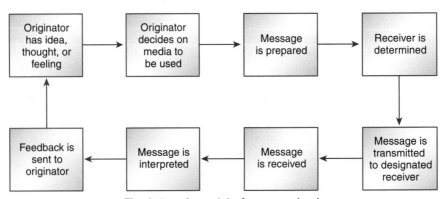

Fig. 8-1 ■ A model of communication.

communication available to move the required information to the receiver.

3. *Transmission:* This step is the actual delivery of the message, and it must be accomplished in such a way that it avoids interference. Among the causes of such interference are the unintelligibility of speech, the incomprehensibility of words, failure to match the vernacular of the receiver, the use of protracted and complicated sentences, distortion from receiving devices, noise, and even the illegibility of handwriting.

4. *Receiving:* The receiver's senses of seeing and hearing are brought to bear as the expressed message is received. This process is complicated by the fact that most people tend to have selective attention; that is, they screen out the portions of messages that do not interest them and attend to the portions containing things that they wish to hear. This selective process can easily work to create distorted and incomplete perception of the message that was actually transmitted. It is very common, for example, for a receiver to tune out a message mentally because the content of the message is believed to be known. One can also easily understand how a message can become garbled when one considers that the average person speaks at approximately 120 words per minute whereas the adult mind thinks at approximately 2000 words per minute. Because of the imbalance between speech and thought, the receiver's mind is so busy formulating a response to the message that he or she often does not hear the actual words spoken. The mind can block effective reception of a message simply by being preoccupied with other thoughts, which renders it incapable of listening effectively. Poor listening habits are one of the major challenges to overcome in developing good communication skills.

5. *Decoding:* Once the receiver takes possession of the message, the mental process of defining the words and interpreting the gestures used to convey the message begins. Less time is available for the decoding process with verbal messages than with written messages, and therefore verbal messages are less reliable. Individuals require time to determine the explicit meaning and implications of a message based on what the words and gestures signify to them. The shorter the time allowed, the greater the chance that the original message will be garbled by the decoding process. Each word, symbol, or gesture used by the originator of the message is subject to interpretation by the receiver based on personal, cultural, or professional biases and may not have exactly the same meaning to the receiver as it did to the originator. Good communication depends on the ability of the receiver to understand what has been transmitted, and often the vernacular of the receiver is far different from the vernacular of the individual sending the message.

6. *Response:* Sometimes referred to as *feedback,* this is the last step in the communication process. It is how the receiver of the message ensures the originator that the message sent was received and indicates how it was understood. Providing feedback facilitates the processes of enhancing value, clarifying, and confirming the original message. If the meaning attributed to the message and the value the receiver places on these three items matches what originator sent, then the message is considered understood. If there is no balance, then the message has not been clearly understood and must be recommunicated.

COMMUNICATION AS A PROCESS

Good communication is far more complex than simply sending a message in a straight line between the originator and the receiver, as is often thought. Communication is a *process* that involves give and take between the participants. This process entails both verbal and nonverbal transmissions that are sent back and forth by the originator and the receiver and to which both react. For example, employees may be totally silent while their nurse manager explains a new unit procedure, but their body language, facial expressions, and eye contact (or lack thereof) may indicate to the casual observer what they are really feeling. The employees hear the message, perceive and interpret it, and then send feedback to the manager that relates their feelings, emotional receptiveness, and attitude toward what has been received. Once the nurse manager receives the feedback, he or she then has information that indicates what the receivers heard and how they responded to the message. By correctly interpreting feedback, nurse managers can decide whether to continue or terminate the communication and, if it is to be continued, how to proceed. The following dialogue between a nurse and her manager provides a good illustration of a nonverbal response:

Nurse: Joanne, can I talk with you?
Manager: (Moves her head up and down and frowns.)
Nurse: You look busy. I need a few minutes, but I can wait until later.
Manager: Okay.

Even though the manager acknowledged the nurse (she indicated that she was willing to give her the time she requested and said nothing negative when she heard the staff nurse's request), she provided a nonverbal message that strongly indicated that she didn't really want to be bothered. The nurse clearly "heard" the nurse manager's negative nonverbal message and responded to it directly by switching her request to a later time period.

Many factors contribute to the ability to communicate effectively. The circumstances leading up to the communication, the environment, the relationship between the originator and the receiver, their relative positions of authority, timing, and external forces all affect the outcome of the communication. Is the setting a nonthreatening environment for both parties? A communication between a nurse manager and employee can take on significantly different aura depending on the environment in which it occurs. Is it in a break room over coffee, or in the nurse manager's office across the desk? The circumstances can place the participants on different levels. In the coffee room the two participants are colleagues, but in the nurse manager's office they are clearly boss and employee. As conditions change, so does the recipient's ability to hear and interpret what is being said. For example, is the manager talking to strangers, patients, or employees? Where, when, and how communication occurs influence the outcome as much as the spoken words.

BASIC COMMUNICATION SKILLS

An effective communicator can ensure understanding by assuming value, clarifying, and confirming the content of the communication. Identifying the merits of the communication, building on the ideas expressed, and balancing the merits of the original message with the concerns of the recipient can enhance the value of the communication. Capable managers support their employees by expressing appreciation and being specific in their communications.[1]

Assuming Value

Assuming value is nothing more than expressing an attitude about the person delivering the communication. It says that the sender is worth listening to and that the receiver is opening (or should open) the lines of communication so that he or she can clearly comprehend what the originator is thinking and feeling.

Assuming value helps the receiver of the communication understand what the speaker is saying and why it is worth listening to. Projecting the attitude that what one is communicating has value generally ensures that the other person will listen in return.

Clarifying

Clarifying is the process used when one of the parties to the communication is not sure of what the other party is saying. Simply asking a specific question such as, "What do you mean when you say ... ?" can help the receiver obtain additional information regarding the real meaning of the content. A statement such as, "I don't understand what you mean" can also be used to obtain more information to clarify previous communications. Another effective method is the use of an open-ended expression of interest such as, "And then?"

Regardless of the method used to gain the additional information, the individual must ask questions regarding any communication until he or she completely understands what has been said—not what he or she thinks *might* have been said.

Confirming

Confirming is the process used when the individual thinks that understanding has been achieved but feels that this needs to be verified. The goal is to ensure that what the receiver of the communication heard was exactly what the originator intended—that is, to verify accuracy.

Confirmation is best accomplished through a process of feeding back information about the receiver's understanding to the originator of the communication. If the receiver has heard correctly, the sender will acknowledge that the receiver has understood the real meaning; if the receiver has not heard accurately, then the originator has the opportunity to correct the receiver's interpretation of the communication.

Enhancing Value

Enhancing value is not the same as offering criticism. The process of enhancing value is used to identify the merits of the communication and build on and balance those merits—not to reject another's ideas or concepts. Criticism tells someone else what we don't like or don't appreciate about their idea, what is wrong with it, and why we feel the concept won't work. Criticism is a negative response and leads to demoralization, defensiveness, and the suppression of creativity and innovation. As supervisors of others, nurse managers will always be more effective if they refrain from criticizing and rely more on the process of enhancing value.

To enhance value, the receiver of the communication identifies the good points in what has been said and then asks himself or herself mentally how the idea or action can be improved upon without mentioning concerns and reservations. If the receiver feels that this can be done, he or she can build on the original communication by noting the merits of the idea and offering enhancements (value). Merit is anything the receiver liked about what the speaker said or did, or what the receiver would like the other person to keep doing despite the need for change. Merit may be found in part of an idea, a good intention, an important issue that has been addressed, or part of an action. If the receiver can find no merit in the communication, he or she can still ensure understanding by asking the speaker about the value of his or her idea or action. Most people have good intentions and are more than willing to share them if the receiver simply lets them know that he or she understands what they have said and is willing to hear more.

Value can often be enhanced simply by mentioning the merits of the communication and gently offering additional methods to consider or paths that might be followed in pursuit of the goal. If a merit the receiver has identified can be used as an example of what he or she wants, the change the receiver is suggesting will be viewed as an alternative and not as a rejection. This approach can also serve to reinforce the original idea holder's commitment to his or her expressed action or idea. The receiver's suggestion can take the form of a recommendation for a minor change or a refinement. The receiver simply specifies the merit and verifies with the other person that the latter thinks the suggested action is acceptable.

Balancing

If the person delivering the original communication asks for an evaluation or needs to know what might be wrong so that he or she can make necessary changes, there is a need to *balance*. The sender specifies the merits, asks for suggestions or reactions, and follows up. Suggestions are invited after the sender has clearly identified the merits in the original communication and expressed his or her concerns. This will help get the other person involved in finding a solution, obtain commitment for the original ideas, and receive the other person's ideas instead of receiving only simple confirmation of what has been said.

It is not considered the mark of a good manager to invite ideas and suggestions unless the manager intends to consider each one received. After the manager has invited suggestions and received them, the manager must provide a positive and reasonable reaction, confirm and clarify what he or she believes to have been said, provide another response, and ask for the other person's continued feedback.

Supporting

The act of supporting promotes a spirit of cooperation because it provides timely feedback about the positive aspects of another's ideas or efforts and acknowledges the value the receiver of the communication has placed on the other person's contribution. Most people need recognition for their efforts and accomplishments, and there is a direct correlation between the support a person gives others and the cooperation he or she receives in return. The ability of a person to provide quality feedback so that others clearly know what to expect from that person will save time and effort in accomplishing the goals that person has been assigned. Good managers are not reluctant to support others. They realize that support is not likely to be misconstrued as weakness or insecurity. A capable manager sees the connection between giving and receiving and is quick to communicate support when someone else shows the first signs of improvement or starts to fulfill requirements that have not previously been met. The best managers demonstrate their support for others by expressing appreciation for the work they accomplish or the help they provide. Nurse managers do not have to acknowledge everything, nor is this even recommended. If they do, people will begin to believe that the managers simply like everything or are lying. This will have the effect of diminishing any praise that is actually earned. When managers take the time to mention how other people's accomplishments are important and what others have done for the unit, they are earning the goodwill and succor necessary to support themselves when times are tough. People have a tendency to trust those with whom they feel most comfortable, and one way to make others feel comfortable is to provide praise when it is deserved. Well-deserved praise gives other people a sense of self-worth, makes them feel important, and increases their desire to continue contributing.

SOME CHARACTERISTICS OF COMMUNICATION

Author Dee Ann Gillies[2] identified the following basic characteristics of communication in her research:

The differential effectiveness of media: The usefulness of different media varies with the educational level of those exposed to them. People with less education tend to rely more on aural and pictorial media, whereas the more highly educated seem to prefer various printed offerings. This is a generalization and may not hold true with everyone.

The effect of self-esteem: People who have lower levels of self-esteem are more easily swayed by persuasive communication than those with higher levels of self-esteem.

The effect of being comfortable: The average person is far more likely to hear information that agrees with his or her individual views and is more likely to listen to messages that concern familiar topics.

Manipulation and trust: The more the audience trusts a speaker, regardless of the subject, the less likely members are to perceive that person as manipulative.

Majority opinion: An opinion held by the majority is far more effective in changing the attitude of an individual than is one voiced by an expert.

THE "FIVE S" APPROACH TO COMMUNICATION

One of the most effective methods for developing oral and written communication was devised by researchers David Whetten and Kim Cameron in 1998.[3] They called their method the *Five S* approach, and it included the following five components:

1. *Strategy:* Strategy develops the purpose for the audience and the occasion. This component involves identifying the general and specific aims of the communication, understanding the needs and attitudes of the audience, and designing a specific message that satisfies those needs. What this means is that the communication should be centered on the audience. If the environment is formal, then the communication should emulate it and be formal itself. Slang should not be used in a formal situation, although it may be permissible in a less formal environment. It is recommended that both sides of an issue be presented if the audience receiving the communication is either uncommitted or hostile.

2. *Structure:* This step translates the structure into a specific form. It begins with an outline or forecast of the main ideas to be presented. The point here is to capture audience members' attention and give them a reason to continue to listen or read. Basically, structure is an outline of the message to be delivered that allows the audience to follow the presentation easily. Simple to complex, old to new, and familiar to unfamiliar are fundamental methods of structuring a presentation. In this outline, only a few basic points should be made, and transitions should be supplied between each point. It is also recommended that the presentation end on a positive note that either calls for some form of action or creates a good feeling in the audience.

3. *Support:* Examples and graphics are used to support or reinforce the ideas presented. The effective use of audio and/or visual aids helps create credibility for what is being communicated. It is recommended that a variety of different aids be used and that each be kept simple. Each aid should be developed as a method of improving comprehension and retention.

4. *Style:* This is the method used to express the ideas. It is often as important as the ideas being expressed. If the presentation is oral, one method speakers might consider is making a few written notes to guide themselves and then practicing the presentation with their visual aids so that they become familiar with it. This will help them gain proficiency in engaging the audience through eye contact, gestures, and the effective use of physical space.

   The use of style in written communication involves both mechanical and factual precision. Tone is developed through an effective choice of words and should be adjusted to fit the formality of the situation. It is also important that the proper format be used when constructing such things as a business letter, memorandum, proposal, or research paper.

5. *Supplement:* This step is the process of providing informed responses to challenges and questions related to the presentation. The author should be prepared to answer questions and challenges to any position taken, using a specific format. It is recommended that novices use the following format:

   - The objection is restated.
   - The author's position is restated.
   - Support is offered for the author's position.
   - The impact of supporting the author's position is addressed.

COMMUNICATION SYSTEMS

Studies involving group communication have identified a variety of frequently used methods of exchanging ideas. Specific forms of group communication are shown in the following sections.

Forms of Intergroup Communication

THE CHAIN

The chain is the simplest of all forms of communication and is both a fast and an accurate method of solving simple problems (Fig. 8-2). A middle person in a chain often emerges as the leader. The chain has several drawbacks, including the following two:

1. It often generates low morale.
2. It is inflexible if used for problem solving.

THE Y AND THE WHEEL

In the Y and the wheel forms of communication, the leader emerges at the apex or center of the communication (i.e., the fork of the Y and the hub of the wheel; Figs. 8-3 and 8-4). These methods provide both fast and accurate problem solving. The people at the center of the communication are generally satisfied with the quality of the information, whereas those at the outer peripheries are generally less satisfied than they would be even if a less efficient system were used.

THE CIRCLE

The circle form of communication is both slow and inaccurate; but even more critical, the structure does not influence the emergence of a leader (Fig. 8-5). Because the process does not allow everyone to communicate with everyone else, there is little coordination of effort. On the positive side, morale is generally high in groups that use this form of communication and it provides considerable flexibility when it is used in problem-solving efforts.

THE ALL-CHANNEL SYSTEM

When the environment allows it, most groups evolve a combination of the forms of communication described previously. This combination method is commonly referred to as the *all-channel system* (Fig. 8-6). This method provides the group with the flexibility to handle complex problems by engaging in open communication among all points within the group and then shifting back to the less complicated wheel structure when dealing with simpler matters. The all-channel format allows a large amount of information to be processed as task uncertainty and the complexity of issues increase.

One important point concerning the various forms of communication described here is that there is no correct or more proper method of communication. The best form is the one that accomplishes the communication with the highest degree of accuracy and the least amount of effort, and creates the highest level of satisfaction among the members of the group.

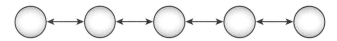

Fig. 8-2 ■ Chain communication.

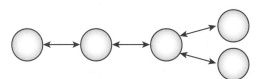

Fig. 8-3 ■ Y communication.

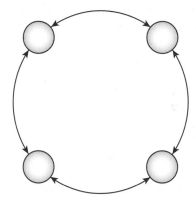

Fig. 8-5 ■ Circle communication.

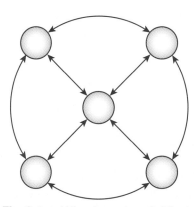

Fig. 8-4 ■ Wheel communication.

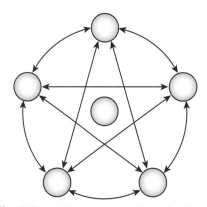

Fig. 8-6 ■ All-channel communication.

Lines of Communication

TOP-DOWN COMMUNICATION

The traditional lines of communication within an organization originate at the senior management levels and travel down through the various levels of subordinate management until they reach the actual performers (Fig. 8-7).

In almost all circumstances, top-down communication is directive and is used to help coordinate the activities that occur at different levels in the organizational hierarchy. It instructs the members of the organization in what to do and provides the information necessary for all members of the staff to relate and coordinate their efforts to meet the goals of the organization. Top-down communication employs both verbal and written forms of transmission and is used to coordinate indoctrination, education, and other informational activities that influence the attitudes and behaviors of the staff.

Common forms of top-down communication are employee handbooks, operation manuals, job description sheets, performance appraisals, employee counseling forms, letters, memorandums, messages, posters, bulletin boards, information brochures, company newspapers, the grapevine, and union transmittals.

Top-down communication produces greater dissatisfaction among the staff than does upward communication, regardless of the subject or quality of the message. Therefore, although this is an essential communication avenue in the organization, it should be used carefully and with great awareness of its potential negative connotations.

BOTTOM-UP COMMUNICATION

More enlightened management techniques encourage the establishment of a working environment that promotes delegation of authority and more personal involvement in the decision-making process by junior members of management and the staff. This evolution of the traditional authority structure has created a need to establish bottom-up lines of communication (Fig. 8-8).

Bottom-up communication provides a means of motivating and satisfying personnel by encouraging employee input. Once this input is received, the manager summarizes the information and forwards it upward to the next level for use in the decision-making process. That next management level summarizes any action it has taken using the information and forwards it to the next senior level of authority. Each level of management tends to bias the information to place it in the best light for the more senior level's review, so that the original information is filtered on its way up the chain. By the time it reaches the most senior level of management, it usually has been highly refined and purged of all elements that might reflect poorly on the intermediate levels of management.

In spite of this filtering process, this is an important type of communication to develop in an organization, because many times the staff is in a much better position to assess individual situations accurately than is management. It is not inconceivable for a nurse working on the front line to have a better solution to a problem than the nurse manager, who still will understand the situation better than will the director of nursing. Consequently, establishing bottom-up communication is a critical part of leading the modern healthcare organization and its decision-making process.

To engage productively in this type of communication, the staff must feel free to communicate both solicited and unsolicited information to their senior managers. Management must encourage employees to do so and assure them that they need not fear repercussions, or else management will lack the critically important information that allows the best possible decisions. Also, if management stifles this type of communication, staff members are likely to become

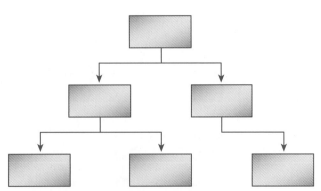

Fig. 8-7 ■ Top-down communication.

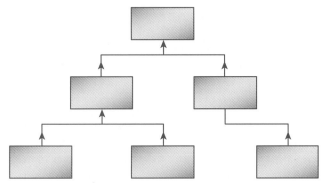

Fig. 8-8 ■ Bottom-up communication.

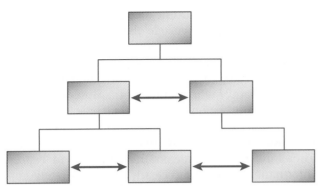

Fig. 8-9 ■ Lateral communication.

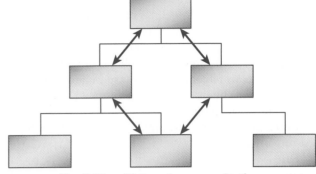

Fig. 8-10 ■ Diagonal communication.

frustrated and nonresponsive when their input is requested.

Common means of providing bottom-up communication are face-to-face discussions, interviews, open door policies, staff meetings, task forces, written reports, performance appraisals, grievance programs, exit interviews, opinion surveys, suggestion programs, counseling, ombudsmen programs, the grapevine, the inevitable informer system, and participative, consultative, and democratic management practices.

LATERAL COMMUNICATION

Lateral or horizontal communication is dialogue that occurs between departments or personnel at the same level of the organizational hierarchy (Fig. 8-9). This form is used most frequently to coordinate activities in the organization.

The need for lateral communication increases as the interdependence of the various elements in the organization increases. A classic example is the need for communication across shifts within a nursing unit. A specific job might be started on one shift and finished on the next; therefore, it is imperative that the nurses on these two shifts communicate effectively or the smooth operation of the unit and/or patient care might suffer.

This form of communication is also frequently used to transmit technical information between units or individual personnel and from time to time may concern subjective and even emotional aspects of the job. Committees, conferences, and meetings are often used to facilitate horizontal communication.

DIAGONAL COMMUNICATION

Diagonal communication occurs between individuals or departments that are not on the same level of the hierarchy and not necessarily in the same direct reporting line of authority (Fig. 8-10). This form of communication is most often informal and is used between staff groups and line functions and in organizations that carry out projects. Diagonal communication is a form of multifaceted communication and is the type of communication desired in the modern organization because it creates a constant flow of information in all directions. It helps keep personnel in different areas aware of occurrences around them and mindful of information that, although perhaps not of direct concern, may be important in eliminating repetitive actions.

THE GRAPEVINE (INFORMAL COMMUNICATION NETWORK)

The informal communication networks that coexist with the formal channels in an organization are most often referred to as the *grapevine*. This is probably the most widely used form of communication in any organization, and the news it carries travels extremely fast and is widely accepted at all points in the organization. Speed does not always mean accuracy, however, and the grapevine is rife with error, innuendo, and complete falsehoods. Nevertheless, it can be an effective form of communication to spread the word within an organization. Highly competent managers will use the grapevine to disseminate information they want to be heard by all but do not want attributed directly to themselves. They can count on the tremendous speed of the grapevine, which is due to its use of clusters or chained pathways (i.e., the involvement of groups of three or four individuals at a time in spreading the word), instead of the one-on-one transfer of the more formal passage of information. The grapevine is even faster when the information it carries is recent or anticipated or affects the staff directly (e.g., pay increases, changes in policy, gossip).

Information carried over the grapevine has a tendency to become distorted for any number of reasons, but the single most important one is that the information carried is often fragmented, and the participants have a tendency to supply the missing pieces. In addition, many participants use the spreading of information as a means of promoting their own agendas or establishing their individual importance. Others compensate for feelings of insecurity by embellishing the information they pass along. The reason for such exaggeration is simple: there is no accountability for what is transmitted or for deliberately misinforming another. Managers can gain a tremendous amount of information by listening to the grapevine, and they can do much to remedy the distortions in its communications by using this informal channel to pass along correct information.

One way to understand how difficult it is for accurate communication to be disseminated through the grapevine is to try the following simple exercise:

1. Put 10 to 20 people in a circle.
2. Have one person tell (or read) a story to a second person in a whisper.
3. Have the second person whisper the story to the next person and so on around the circle.
4. Have the last person repeat the story out loud; it is likely to be entirely different from the original.

Informal communication is sometime referred to as "the way things really get done." It moves vertically, horizontally, and diagonally. Research into communication channels in organizations notes that the grapevine serves several important purposes for people[4]:

- It satisfies a basic need for social interaction.
- It fulfills an individual need for recognition.
- It can serve as a method of communicating or acquiring information that might not be available through any other channel.

In its most prodigious use, the grapevine provides a widely accessible means for employees to find out about events before they are announced officially. For example, a nurse who has been waiting for an opening in the labor and delivery unit may hear, via the grapevine, that a nurse on that unit is leaving and therefore may approach the maternity floor supervisor to make her desires known, perhaps even before the maternity supervisor knows the other staff nurse is departing.

The truly effective nurse manager is always aware that the grapevine is operating whenever he or she talks with anyone.

COMMUNICATION MODES

Written Communication

Most people think of communication as verbal interaction. However, written communication is also widely used to interact with others, and a combination of both of these communication modes is used by nurse managers in carrying out their day-to-day management tasks. In fact, for managers, good writing skills may be among the most important skills needed to communicate effectively.

Nurse managers must be able to receive verbal and written information, decode that information, select which portions of it to pass on to appropriate people, and present these portions in an effective manner, either in writing or through verbal expression, to the person or people who require them. Most often, nurse managers are responsible for developing the written correspondence that is required by their staff members and that is used to operate the nursing unit. Therefore, nurse managers must be able to express information in writing clearly and accurately and assist each member of their staffs in doing likewise. For example, when a nurse completes an incident report, the nurse manager is the individual who must determine the accuracy and completeness of the report. The nurse manager accomplishes this by communicating effectively with the nurse to ensure that the incident is reported with sufficient detail and clarity so that it can be easily and clearly understood by others, some of whom will communicate in a totally different vernacular or simply not have the background to understand even elementary medical prose. Another example is a case in which the nurse manager must communicate a patient's prognosis to the patient's employer, who is an engineer and not a physician; the employer must be given understandable information so that he or she can make an informed decision as to whether to allow the patient to return to work.

Although it is permissible for nurse managers to use informal modes of written communication, most written communication at the management level is done in a formal style. Some of the formal written communication tasks of managers include the following:

- Preparation of employee records and materials, job descriptions, performance appraisals, or characterizing notes
- Documentation of activity and justification reports
- Documentation of committee activities, including agenda development and recording of minutes
- Development of critical incident comments (anecdotal notes)

THE MEMORANDUM (MEMO)

Memorandums (memos) are one way that nurse managers communicate with others. Nearly every manager will create a memorandum at one time or another. Two things must be remembered when using this form of communication:

- A written memorandum is always a formal communication because it is a written representation of the author to others and to the organization. Its clarity, style, tone, and content will always be judged accordingly. Do not underestimate its potential impact.

- Many organizations do not like memorandums or the people who use them. Too many people have employed this form of documentation as a means of covering up personal or questionable activities, and today the entire process is held in disdain by much of the management community.

The following are some basic guidelines to observe when drafting a memorandum:

- Analyze the situation before writing the memorandum by determining the subject, the purpose, the exact form that will be used, the intended audience, and the tone.
- Consider carefully the needs of the audience and the impact of different choices in the tone of the memorandum.
- Use this analysis to decide what particular writing skills will be used, what the exact phrasing will be, what thoughts or ideas to present, what kinds of material to include or exclude, and how the content should be organized.
- Use objective, not subjective, words and make them appropriate to the audience. Refrain from the use of jargon, especially if the communication is targeted to nonmedical personnel or individuals outside the author's specific area of responsibility. Never include vulgarity or hostile or demeaning comments, no matter how slight.
- Use sentence structure and tone to convey meaning, as follows:

  For a policy statement, say directly what is expected without being overbearing (e.g., "Lunch hour should be scheduled after 11:00 AM for the day shift").

  Don't lead a person to covet what you want (e.g., "Does anyone object to going to lunch before 11:00 AM?").

  Don't be overbearing (e.g., "No one will take lunch before 11:00 AM.").

- Use your title when referring to yourself (e.g., "Susan Hawkins, RN") and include your position (e.g., "Nursing Manager") if writing to someone outside the unit; refer to the recipients by their titles (e.g., "Ms. Jones") or as "nursing staff."
- Arrange material logically by presenting the topic, the purpose, the things that need to be done, the rationale, and the time frame.
- Include enough detail to inform but not so much that you confuse, bore, or overwhelm.

JOB DESCRIPTIONS AND PERFORMANCE APPRAISALS

Most managers dislike the task of writing job descriptions and employee performance appraisals because of their difficulty, yet both of these are vital to maintaining high productivity in a nursing unit. Accurate and current job descriptions enable an institution to instill purpose into each job in the organization and ensure efficient use of the human resources available. Job descriptions specifically identify appropriate tasks to be performed by personnel with specific job titles that are compatible with the needs of the institution. When they are properly prepared, job descriptions take much of the work out of the performance appraisal process by allowing performance appraisals to be prepared in a more objective manner and without many of the subjective personality-related elements that have traditionally been their hallmark. Reducing the influence of personality factors allows the appraisal process to focus objectively on the tasks performed and the quality of the performance.

ANECDOTAL NOTES

Nurse managers use anecdotal notes, or "noncritical incident reports," as they are commonly known, in assessing and documenting staff performance. These notes provide an effective method of documenting events, because they are written without the detail required in a formal reporting procedure. When they are properly prepared, these notes reduce both the incidence of selective remembrance and the influence of personal bias in the appraisal process. The nurse manager must use accurate, clear language to report specific behavior, however, in order to reduce the chance for ambiguity or inability to determine meaning several months after the incident.

THE JUSTIFICATION REPORT

Nurse managers must communicate effectively to others using written reports to carry out such tasks as identifying current unit conditions and forecasting future unit needs. To accomplish these tasks, managers must compile written justification reports that list specific resources and provide data to support a given request. For instance, they may identify a need in their unit for additional resources such as technical equipment, supplies, additional staff, or larger space and then develop a justification report requesting these resources. Included in the report will be the background of the situation, the rationale (to explain the need), and specific details of how the resources will be used. In addition, they must cite the benefits the needed resources will bring to the institution and, quite possibly, describe what the situation will be if the requested materials are not provided. The value of the written proposal is that it provides a record senior management can refer to in the future and use in the preparation of policies, budgets, and assessments of staffing requirements.

THE PROPOSAL

Nurse managers may also be involved in the development of a formal proposal to gain authorization for purchase of a major piece of technology, a policy change, or deviation from a prescribed course of action. These proposals are very similar to justification reports except that the changes they concern are generally larger. Proposals may involve one, several, or even all of the areas in an institution and may have far-reaching and complex consequences, both internally and externally. Fundamental information required before a proposal can be developed includes determining whether it is solicited or unsolicited, identifying the developers, and assessing the level of influence the developers have in effecting change within the institution. It is a good idea to have first-line managers participate as part of a committee when preparing proposals.

THE PRODUCTIVITY REPORT

Nurse managers are responsible for writing or presenting activity or productivity reports for their units. One example of this type of report is a monthly report of the activities carried out within the nursing unit that accounts for the productive use of both human and material resources. To develop this report, the nurse manager must collect and quantify available information on the use of staff time, salaries, equipment, and supplies, and then present it in a logical and easily understood manner. How the report is written may have a large bearing on what future assets are available to the unit and how the unit is perceived within the organization. For example, quantity is not always an indication of quality. The fact that a report is lengthy does not mean that it will be considered a high-quality document. Nurse managers must be able to see through the mire of information they have available to them and use only what best reflects the unit's performance when they draft their reports. For instance, a nurse might chart a note that says, "A.M. care given." From this, the nurse manager must determine whether the care was given (almost a certainty), whether the nurse failed to document the type of care given, or whether the observations and patient responses are unknown.

Verbal and Nonverbal Communication

Probably the most frequently used form of communication is that which is transmitted orally. Verbal communication is considered by most experts to be made up of two basic parts: (1) the things that are *spoken*, and (2) the things that are *inferred* (i.e., unspoken).

Spoken communication, often referred to as *verbal communication*, refers to the words an individual uses to transfer his or her thoughts to another. In nursing management, verbal communication is primarily used to give and receive information, report results, give directions, provide feedback, and maintain continuity in the day-to-day tasks of managing a unit. However, it also has the secondary purpose of assisting in the creation of a cooperative and professional environment and providing fundamental reward and recognition.

Nonverbal communication is the form of communication that is seen rather than heard. It can transmit information about the message and the relationship of the communicators without the support of speech. Nonverbal communication involves the following five basic elements:

1. *Kinetics:* the body movements and gestures that accompany speech
2. *Spatial relationships:* the physical space between the individuals involved in the communication
3. *Paralanguage:* the nonlanguage characteristics of speech, including pitch, tone, timing, pace, and voice
4. *Cultural attributes:* the special considerations that are part of the environment in which the participants operate and from which they originate; for example, the Japanese communicate respect with a bow instead of a verbal expression
5. *Appearance:* elements such as clothing, grooming, and hairstyle

The nonverbal message is far more effective when there is a direct relationship between what is actually said and the nonverbal message being sent, and it can be far more powerful than the spoken word. As a matter of fact, given a choice, the listener will almost always believe what is expressed nonverbally rather than what is expressed by the speaker's words. For example, if an individual asks a supervisor, "Am I doing a good job?" and the reply is, "Yes," but the supervisor's facial expression and an indifferent nod and shrug communicate "No," then "No" is what the individual will come away believing. If, however, the supervisor establishes eye contact and emphasizes the answer, "Yes," with a positive up and down movement of the head, the supervisor's positive response is far more likely to be believed. In the latter instance, the nonverbal message is similar to the verbal message and therefore tends to reinforce what is heard. In the first example, however, the negative affect of the supervisor tends to leave the words open to interpretation and does not reassure the listener or reinforce the message. Lack of correspondence between what is verbalized and what is expressed visually is one of the most significant roadblocks to effective communication because it distorts the message.

Distorted communication occurs when the receiver misunderstands the message that the sender believes was transmitted. When distortion occurs, the receiver will respond according to his or her interpretation of what has been said, and the original sender will almost certainly receive distorted feedback. Consequently, the ability to prepare and present ideas, feelings, and thoughts so that they will be heard in the way the speaker intends is critical to the nurse manager. When the level of distortion in interpersonal transactions is reduced, the result is improved opportunity to develop conditions conducive to problem solving and negotiation.

Nurse managers, in their capacity as leaders of their units, must frequently clarify communication received from other managers; for instance, they may need to explain a new hospital policy. This task is accomplished by nurse managers as they receive, decode, clarify, and then transmit the incoming message using a style and choice of words that their audience will understand. In other words, nurse managers often act as conduits and filters for communication between other elements in the organization and their staffs. The ability to help different groups to appreciate, understand, and work with each other is one of the most important assets nurse managers can develop. To accomplish this task effectively, they must develop the skills to express themselves sensibly using written, verbal, and nonverbal forms of communication.

The cultural experiences and background of the participants involved in any communication control to a large extent their ability to express and comprehend. Nonverbal factors such as body movement, gestures, tone, and the response to spatial orientation are culturally defined, and participants can be expected to best comprehend words that are within their own cultural context. A great deal of miscommunication results from participants' lack of understanding of each other's cultural expectations.

Nurse managers must also consider how presentation affects the nonverbal aspects of communication. Nonverbal cues such as posture, dress (e.g., wearing a nursing cap, having a stethoscope in one's pocket), mannerisms, and gestures all contribute to the way others "hear" what is said. Although most people believe that they pay close attention to the words that are spoken, the truth is that context and nonverbal elements set the stage, and words have impact only as they relate to this setting. When there is a lack of correspondence between the verbal and nonverbal messages sent, the listener will tend to believe the nonverbal. Therefore, effective nurse managers pay close attention to the nonverbal behaviors of those with whom they communicate and consider the total picture presented by a communication whenever possible.

LISTENING

A fundamental aspect of communicating effectively is the ability to listen clearly. Although in recent years a great deal has been written about active listening skills as they pertain to therapeutic proficiency with patients, little attention has been focused on the need for nurse managers to develop these skills. Effective listening, although it certainly can be learned by anyone, is not a simple task. The difficulty lies in receiving messages in the manner the sender intended when sending them. Listening requires that each receiver decode the message in his or her own frame of reference, and that is where the challenge comes in. Because each individual involved in a conversation is unique, it is nearly impossible for the listener to interpret the message in exactly the same way as did the originator of the communication. Each person's ability to communicate and interpret communications, both verbal and nonverbal, is affected by that person's experience, environment, biases, attitudes, perceptions, and preconceptions regarding the other person.

In addition to the myriad challenges confronted by most people in listening effectively, nurse managers have still other barriers to overcome. Two of the most significant are (1) the complexity of their responsibilities, and (2) the diverse relationships that exist between themselves, staff, and colleagues. Nurse managers also face another significant challenge, one they share with managers in every type of business, and that is the environment in which managers operate. This environment, with all of the associated stimuli, can quickly overload managers, whose attention is continually being demanded by any number of people at any given moment and who must operate on several different levels and respond to several situations simultaneously. These continual distractions often create a situation in which others believe that managers are not really listening and responding to them. This tendency makes it especially important for nurse managers to develop active listening skills.

The development of active listening skills begins with the basic requirement that a nurse manager pay more attention to the other person's message than to forming a response. When listening, the nurse manager must pay attention to the words, expressions, gestures, and context of the message and verify his or her understanding of the message with the speaker. Consider the following example:

Ms. Jones, the unit's nurse manager, has received complaints about a staff nurse, Mary Smith. She approaches Mary, and the following interaction ensues:
Ms. Jones: Mary, could I talk with you for a moment?
Mary: Sure.

Both go to Ms. Jones's office, and Ms. Jones gestures to Mary to be seated in a chair next to the desk. Ms. Jones takes a chair next to Mary.

Mary: Is there something wrong?

Ms. Jones: Yes, Mary. I've received several complaints about your behavior toward the nursing assistants. They say you have been excessively critical of their patient care.

 Mary scowls and looks away. She doesn't say anything. Ms. Jones allows a few minutes of silence before continuing.

Ms. Jones: You look upset *(reflecting Mary's expression and lack of response).*

Mary: (She nods affirmatively.)

Ms. Jones: Do you want to talk about it?

Mary: There's nothing anyone can do. It's settled.

Ms. Jones: Settled? *(encouraging Mary to explain further).*

Mary: Yes. You see, my husband's being transferred to California. *(She starts to sob.)*

Ms. Jones: How do you feel about that? *(eliciting the cause of Mary's distress and trying to confirm it).*

Mary: I love my job here. Now I'll have to start all over with a new hospital, new people, new friends!

Ms. Jones: Oh, Mary, I'll hate to lose you, but I know some hospital is going to get a very good nurse. *(She pauses to let Mary realize she is appreciated.)* Mary.

Mary: Yes?

Ms. Jones: Maybe you thought it would be easier to leave if you put some distance between yourself and the staff by being more critical.

Mary: Maybe. I didn't mean to be so cross with everyone.

Ms. Jones: Let me help you with your resume and begin your letter of reference *(showing Mary that her actions will follow her words).*

This example demonstrates the use of good listening skills. In it, the nurse manager employed basic listening principles, including the following:

- Talking in a location that offers a minimum of distractions or interruptions
- Sitting or standing so that both participants can look directly at each other
- Listening to what is being said but also paying close attention to the nonverbal cues that are being sent
- Asking questions to develop points in greater detail
- Being empathetic—trying to put oneself in the other's place (empathy should not be confused with sympathy; the latter rarely has a place in manager and employee conversations)
- Obtaining feedback regarding one's impression(s) of the other's thoughts or feelings
- Acknowledging positive contributions of the other
- Responding to the other's message and meaning
- Being patient

Positive results were reported in a study in which nursing service administrators were asked to employ active listening techniques in their meetings with hospital employees. The nurse managers who were evaluated stated that they felt they had improved feelings of understanding, and these same feelings were echoed by members of the staff when they were questioned about their supervisors' active listening practice.[5]

ASSERTIVE COMMUNICATION

Assertiveness is a term used to describe behaviors that an individual can employ to stand up for what he or she believes in without encroaching on the rights or beliefs of others. The nursing profession has seen a marked increase in the awareness of self-confident behavior as assertiveness training has become more and more popular, and as women have become more aware of their rights and have recognized that a person can be assertive without being aggressive or obnoxious. Traditionally, the nursing field has been one of subservience; therefore, it is especially appropriate for nurses and nurse managers to learn to assert themselves properly. Especially for the nurse manager, the healthcare field is an environment in which assertive behavior must be practiced carefully, particularly in relation to hospital administrators and physicians, who are frequently very influential individuals and who often desire that traditional roles be honored.

Author Melodie Chenevert[6] identified what she called the "ten basic rights for women in the health professions." Although Chenevert's focus was predominantly on the female's role, the basic rights she outlined are equally important for all members of any profession:

1. To be treated with respect
2. To have a reasonable workload
3. To receive an equitable wage
4. To determine one's own priorities
5. To ask for what one wants
6. To refuse without making excuses or feeling guilty
7. To make mistakes and be responsible and accountable for them
8. To give and receive information on a professional level
9. To act in the best interests of the patient
10. To be human

Chenevert noted that, although nurses have these basic inalienable rights, each individual is responsible for acquiring these rights for himself or herself; no one else is responsible for "giving" these rights to anyone.

Assertive behavior is situation specific and can be differentiated from nonassertive and aggressive behavior in which participants respond in a certain manner regardless of the situation. What this means is that an assertive individual tempers responses and communication based on the specific circumstances. Methods and mannerisms that work in one situation may be totally inappropriate in another.

The use of assertive techniques in communication can benefit nurse managers, their staffs, patients, and the institutions they work for, because the clear, accurate, and honest expression of ideas and feelings encourages others to respond in kind. Consider the following example:

> Ms. Jones, a nurse manager, enters Mr. Wilson's room to find him scowling. He promptly states, "That stupid nurse forgot my medicine *again!*" Ms. Jones is offered the opportunity to respond in any number of ways, including the following:
> "There now, don't worry. I'm sure it will be all right."
> "Oh, really! Well, I'll take care of her!"
> "Tell me what you missed and I'll check on it."
> "Mr. Wilson, we really don't have stupid nurses. Making an error is something that can be corrected, and I'll help you."
> If the first response is selected, Ms. Jones will impugn the patient's rights with a verbal pat on the head. This is a nonassertive response that causes her to accept responsibility for her nurse's actions without even determining the facts. If she chooses the second response, Ms. Jones is making an assumption that the staff nurse is at fault and vocalizing the concept of retribution, which can create unrealistic expectations in the mind of the patient. The third response indicates that Ms. Jones has heard the patient and is willing to take action in his behalf, but without assuming any responsibility herself and without finding fault with others. Finally, the fourth response takes the positive action of establishing ground rules with the patient and, at the same time, providing him with the assurance that his complaint will not go unanswered.

Many people who practice assertive communication actually have reported a decrease in physical symptoms such as headaches and abdominal distress. Because stress is known to contribute to a number of psychosomatic illnesses, it seems reasonable to assume that an honest expression of feelings can reduce a great deal of internal stress.

Another benefit that has been observed in individuals who use assertive techniques is that many become more likely to respond to a stimulus at the appropriate time. Nonassertive behavior often includes an attempt by the individual to avoid problems by remaining silent, even if the person is very angry. On the opposite end of the spectrum are aggressive individuals, who typically respond to the emotional aspects of a situation and end up alienating themselves from others. One of the most positive characteristics of assertive people is that they generally respond to a specific situation in the appropriate manner and at the appropriate time. Participants in a conversation may not agree with each other's particular responses, but they take the responsibility to clarify what they don't necessarily like about the other's position and accept the other's right to differ.

Open, direct, and timely interactions between management and employees encourages problem identification and facilitates a much more positive form of problem solving and decision-making. Assertive communication techniques are valuable tools for the nurse manager to use in carrying out these tasks. Being assertive in any situation calls for observing the following rules designed to guide behavior[7]:

- Avoid apologizing too much
- Avoid defensive and hostile reactions such as aggression, temper tantrums, backbiting, revenge, slander, sarcasm, and threats
- Use body language (e.g., eye contact, body posture, gestures, facial expression) that is appropriate to and matches the verbal message being sent
- Be willing to accept manipulative criticism while maintaining responsibility for a decision rendered
- Calmly repeat a (negative) reply without justifying it
- Be honest about feelings, needs, and ideas; try to use "I" statements such as "I think ... ," "I believe ...," etc.
- Accept and/or acknowledge personal faults calmly and without apologizing for them

DISTORTED COMMUNICATION

There is ample opportunity for distortion in the complicated process of sending, receiving, and responding to messages, as demonstrated by the following written correspondence between a plumber and an official of the National Bureau of Standards (p. 19)[8]:

> Bureau of Standards
> Washington, D.C.
>
> Gentlemen:
> I have been in the plumbing business for over 11 years and have found that hydrochloric acid works real fine for cleaning drains. Could you tell me if it's harmless?
>
> Sincerely,
> Tom Brown, Plumber

> Mr. Tom Brown, Plumber
> Yourtown, U.S.A.
>
> Dear Mr. Brown:
> The efficacy of hydrochloric acid is indisputable, but the chlorine residue is incompatible with metallic permanence!

Sincerely,
Bureau of Standards

Bureau of Standards
Washington, D.C.

Gentlemen:
I have your letter of last week and am mighty glad you agree with me on the use of hydrochloric acid.

Sincerely,
Tom Brown, Plumber

Mr. Tom Brown, Plumber
Yourtown, U.S.A.

Dear Mr. Brown:
We wish to inform you we have your letter of last week and advise that we cannot assume responsibility for the production of toxic and noxious residues with hydrochloric acid and further suggest you use an alternate procedure.

Sincerely,
Bureau of Standards

Bureau of Standards
Washington, D.C.

Gentlemen:
I have your most recent letter and am happy to find you still agree with me.

Sincerely,
Tom Brown, Plumber

Mr. Tom Brown, Plumber
Yourtown, U.S.A.

Dear Mr. Brown:
Don't use hydrochloric acid! It eats the hell out of pipes!

Sincerely,
Bureau of Standards

Communication is difficult enough when a conversation involves just two people; distortion increases proportionally as the number of individuals involved in the communication increases. The problem of distortion often begins with the source of the communication. The sender may write or speak without first thinking things through or may use inadequate, illogical, or even judgmental words. The originator's delivery may be too fast or too slow, or the receiver may be busy and/or distracted. The sender may use terms that are unfamiliar to the receiver or spend so much time on detail that the receiver becomes bored with the communication and misses the main points. Consider the following example of a sender's use of inadequate words at an inappropriate time.

Vice president of nursing (speaking to a nurse manager): Ms. Green, your unit's absenteeism is too high.

Ms. Green can interpret this message in one of several ways:
1. Members of her staff are missing work more often than those on other units.
2. The supervisor thinks the absences are not really illness related.
3. Ms. Green is not carrying out her responsibilities properly and is creating an environment that promotes absenteeism.

Ms. Green, acting like most people when faced with an unclear message, responds by becoming defensive and thinks to herself, "I'd like to see her manage these people and take care of all our sick patients," or, "It isn't my fault people get sick."

If the vice president makes her comment as she is passing through Ms. Green's unit on a busy day and does not sit down to discuss exactly what she means about the possible underlying problems, bigger problems will ensue. If the vice president wants the problem corrected, it is up to her to clarify her communication by taking the time to develop a plan of cooperation with Ms. Green that outlines how they can work together to solve the problem. If this is not done, the challenge will remain, and Ms. Green may come to see her senior as an adversary. The action taken by the vice president, and the reaction of Ms. Green, will set the tone for the next interaction between these two individuals.

A sender may even distort a message based on his or her relationship with the receiver. When communicating with a supervisor, for instance, a staff member may be prone to report in a way that minimizes weaknesses and emphasizes strengths and accomplishments. With the previous interaction setting the stage for assumed judgment, Ms. Green may be reluctant to report future staff problems, especially if they could possibly reflect negatively on her performance.

As stated earlier, the context of the interaction strongly determines its meaning and outcome. *Where, why,* and *how* an interaction occurs is as influential to the result as *what* was actually said. By carefully managing these fundamental elements of communication, especially if the subject reflects negatively in any way on the receiver, the sender can significantly control the potential for distortion.

Receivers have less control over the situation because they are the recipients of previously developed messages and are merely responding to them. Therefore, receivers are presented with significantly more opportunity to distort messages. In fact, their attitudes toward senders and their experience with previous messages from specific senders can distort messages almost before they are even sent. Receivers' experience with senders and others can strongly influence their objectivity. For example, if a receiver has had negative experiences with the sender of a specific communication and, from those experiences, has grown to distrust the sender, then the receiver may question everything that the sender says. On the other hand, if the sender is an individual who is highly regarded, the receiver may be overly accepting of anything that is said and thereby risk an error because of an unwarranted belief in the reliability of the message.

The suggestion has been made that commonality of experience influences the effectiveness of communication and that the greater the number of common experiences, the greater the likelihood that the sender and receiver will connect effectively with one another.[9] For example, if a nurse manager has a lifestyle that is similar to the lifestyles maintained by the staff, the staff will probably interpret his or her words and actions in the manner in which they were intended. In turn, the nurse manager will normally present his or her ideas in a way that the staff can easily assimilate.

Organizational structure also can have significant influence on the effectiveness of communication. For instance, status, position, and role expectations are environmental aspects of communication transactions. Most nurses can remember the awe they felt for registered nurses in their all-white uniforms and caps, with stethoscopes around their necks, when they were just beginning students. It didn't take long, however, before the students learned to imitate the nurses' behavior by carrying a stethoscope just so, using the "right" type of pen, and walking and talking like a professional. As graduation drew close, the difference in uniform was often the only distinguishable thing separating the students and registered nurses, so accomplished had the students become at "being a nurse." By that time, the students had also moved from the role of subordinate to that of colleague. The interactions between the two groups changed as well, as they shared experiences and became problem solvers together. In the beginning, the students assumed that the registered nurses "knew everything" and that they, as students, had little to offer; but as time progressed, they developed a more realistic view. Just as the basic roles changed, consider how the communication between the two groups of individuals might have evolved.

Not only do the obvious status and role differences have an effect, but the responsibilities of communication participants also encroach on their interactions. On most weekday mornings, the nurse manager of a busy surgical unit has a hectic schedule, with several patients awaiting surgery, preoperative medications to be administered, families and patients to be reassured, and postoperative cases from the previous day to be monitored. It is not the proper time for the vice president to initiate a talk about staff nurses' absenteeism. The senior manager should consider the nurse manager's responsibilities and subordinate status. The nurse manager may think that any request made by his or her senior is more important than intended and neglect patient care to attend to the ill-timed inquiries.

People translate or convert messages into their own language, a vernacular that is the product of their previous experiences and acquired knowledge. The limiting nature of experiential learning, however, creates the possibility of incomplete interpretation or erroneous translation of a message's real meaning. It therefore benefits both sender and receiver to pay close attention to each other's discussion, responses, meanings, and interpretation. In addition, it is vital that each person involved in a discussion both request and provide clarification and feedback frequently.

PRINCIPLES OF EFFECTIVE COMMUNICATION

To develop and increase communication skills, nurse managers must understand the principles of effective communication. Many intrusive influences have been discussed in this chapter, but their effects can be minimized if nurse managers are aware of and abide by the following seven basic management principles:

1. *Providing information is not communication:* For discourse to be communication, participants must interact. Communication requires that both receivers and senders provide input in the form of dialogue and feedback to one another. Although many of the responsibilities of management involve giving directions and sharing information, managers must be careful to remember that receivers' responses are necessary for communication to have taken place.

2. *The sender is responsible for clarity:* Frustration with others' actions is part and parcel of a manager's job, and nursing management is no exception. However, this frustration can be greatly reduced if nurse managers take the time to ensure that their messages to their staffs are clear. Managers must remember that the responsibility for communicating ideas clearly is theirs and not their staffs'. The situation is the same as with ads in the advertising business. If a new ad fails to increase sales, the reason is assumed to lie with the advertising agency and not with the customer. In communication, the responsibility for clarity always belongs to the sender.

3. *Simple and precise language should be used:* In both written and spoken communication, using words precisely and stating the message in the simplest terms possible greatly improves the chances that the transmitted communication will be understood by listeners. This means that managers should speak in such a way that their listeners will be capable of understanding and

willing to listen to the message. It is the sender's responsibility to determine which words will be comprehensible to the listener. A wise old sage once said, "An intelligent person is one who speaks in the vernacular of the audience," or, to put it more simply, "in words the audience will understand."

4. *Feedback should be encouraged:* The best way to be sure one's message has been accurately interpreted is to obtain feedback from those who receive it. Insufficient feedback is a common cause of future misunderstanding. In fact, it has been referred to as a method of modifying future actions by using experience gained from past performance.[10] Feedback will help clarify the points in the communication that are unacceptable or objectionable to the receiver.

Just receiving feedback is not enough, however. Managers must also learn how to evaluate it; that is, to place it into the proper perspective so that any disturbing aspect can be dealt with in a positive and constructive manner. To respond effectively, managers must learn to be skillful in encouraging feedback and in observing and evaluating verbal and nonverbal responses to their communications.

5. *The sender must have credibility.* The personal and professional credibility of the information giver is often more important in establishing the desired outcome than the content of the communication.[11] Trustworthiness, reliability, and competence are characteristics of a credible professional and have a tremendous impact on the communicator's ability to generate understanding in an audience. The ability to communicate effectively is much like trust—it doesn't just happen but must be nurtured carefully and guarded like a precious commodity. Managers should always "say what they mean and mean what they say." Finally, managers should never knowingly mislead anyone, because such an action will always undermine respect and professionalism, as well as all of the aspects of management associated with them, such as effective communication.

6. *The contributions of others should be acknowledged:* In years past, nurse managers may sometimes have been reluctant to acknowledge the contributions of others because of how others might have responded, especially if the work performed was viewed as competitive with the nurse managers'. In today's employment atmosphere of cooperation, however, recognition of individual contributions is viewed as complementary

and motivating. The active and positive acknowledgment of another's contribution, especially if the person is a subordinate, is encouraged at all points in the management chain.

Although acknowledging staff members' contributions is easier when their opinions match those of the manager, it is just as important, if not more so, to acknowledge the work of those with opposing opinions. The suggestion has been made that sharing opposing opinions can provide satisfaction for the participants if each explicitly acknowledges the other and if the entire truth is told by each.[12]

7. *Direct channels of communication are best:* Whenever possible, nurse managers should communicate directly with the individuals for whom their messages are intended, simply because the more people that filter the message, the greater the opportunity for distortion. In addition, face-to-face communication is preferable to written or phone communication, especially if the news being conveyed is negative or could be interpreted as being so. In a direct dialogue, each participant receives immediate feedback, both verbal and nonverbal, which reduces the chances for misunderstanding. This face-to-face exchange and evaluation enable both participants to engage in a facilitative dialogue that will conclude the discussion positively. Body language and facial expressions can also be read in a face-to-face discussion, and their impact can have a significant bearing on the outcome.

Adherence to all the aforementioned principles can be expected to save nurse managers time and improve their ability to perform in their units. In contrast, distorted communication and misunderstanding almost always result in unproductive use of time, poor patient care, and frustration for everyone concerned. There is real truth in the maxim that settling problems after they have occurred takes more time than preventing them through the use of clear and appropriate communication.

APPLICATIONS FOR THE NURSE MANAGER

The positive effects that clear, concise, and effective communication can have on the performance of nurse managers and entire nursing units are too numerous to mention. The following sections present some guidelines for implementing the principles of effective communication to achieve such positive effects in several broad areas that are very relevant to nurse managers.

Communication with Subordinates

Depending on the policies of the specific healthcare institution, nurse managers' responsibilities may include selecting, interviewing, counseling, and disciplining employees; handling their complaints; and settling conflicts. The principles of effective communication are especially pertinent in this manager-employee relationship, because in almost all cases communication is the adhesive that builds and maintains an effective work group.

The communication channels used by nurse managers may be downward, upward, or diagonal as shown in Figs. 8-7 through 8-11. Top-down communication is usually directive and generally includes specific instructions for subordinates. This is an effective method to coordinate activities among personnel and to make efficient use of staff time and abilities.

To give directions and achieve the desired results, however, nurse managers need to develop a message strategy. Suggestions discussed in the following sections should help to increase the chance of effective responses from receivers.

KNOWING THE CONTEXT OF THE INSTRUCTIONS

As front-line supervisors, nurse managers should be certain that they know exactly what they want done, who will accomplish the task, how much time is available, and, in some cases, what steps should be followed to perform the task. They should have the information the staff will need to carry out the instructions clear in their minds before discussing the effort with their employees. In addition, they should have a clear vision of what the outcome of the task will be if the instructions are carried out and how that outcome will be evaluated. Only after they have the answers to these questions are nurse managers ready to give proper instructions.

WARNING!

When communicating with subordinates, nurse managers should avoid giving instructions to the point of micromanaging the effort. Employees need to receive clear and well-structured instruction, but they do not need their managers to hover over them providing minute details to guide their performance. Good managers provide easily understood, broad descriptions and allow their subordinates to grow through the process of self-directed performance.

OBTAINING POSITIVE ATTENTION

Managers should make an earnest effort to eliminate the conditions that interfere with effective listening on the part of staff members. One of the most effective means of doing this is simply to inform the audience that the instructions are about to be given. A simple statement that precedes the actual presentation will garner the positive attention needed. When managers provide instructions, they should be careful to highlight the background and justification for the task to be performed and the importance they are placing on the instructions being given.

GIVING CLEAR, CONCISE INSTRUCTIONS

Managers should talk in an even tone of voice and avoid becoming defensive or offensive. Managers' instructions should include all of the information necessary to complete the task but should not be so precise that they remove the necessity for subordinates to think for themselves. One of the best ways to provide instructions is to recommend a procedure. Remember that part of the nurse manager's job is to develop capability in subordinates. If managers are too detailed, they run the risk of forcing their employees to be mechanical and nonthinking in their performance and highly resentful of what will be perceived as a micromanagement style.

OBTAINING FEEDBACK

Managers must ensure that the various members of the audience (the receivers) understand the instructions being given. Managers should openly solicit feedback and verify understanding. The best way to do this without offending is to simply ask questions. Managers should not be condescending and should not talk down to employees when obtaining verification. They should avoid the use of phrases like, "All

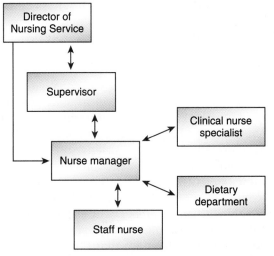

Fig. 8-11 ■ Communication channels in nursing.

right, everyone understands what we are going to do, right?" Such questions are rhetorical, and everyone knows it. Instead, managers should ask open-ended questions that require more than a yes or no response.

PROVIDING FOLLOW-UP COMMUNICATION

Just because instructions are understood does not mean performance is guaranteed. It is absolutely essential that managers follow up aggressively to determine the outcome of their instructions. When doing so, they must continually reinforce their original instructions by providing positive feedback to the performers.

At the risk of being redundant, it is important to restate that *providing direction does not constitute communication*. For communication to occur, the person providing the instructions must receive feedback from those who receive them.

Nurse managers have the responsibility to provide a quality environment for individual employees to work in and a quality environment for the provision of patient care in the unit. Achieving a good balance between these two responsibilities is critical. One of the best methods of doing so is to ensure that individual staff assignments are distributed equitably. If nurse managers allows their assignments to be influenced by the individual desires of their subordinates, the quality of patient care delivered can suffer because of the imbalance in performance responsibilities. To ensure that this responsibility is discharged professionally and without bias, nurse managers can use the communication principles that have been discussed. If they take the time to acknowledge the special needs of individual employees, especially if those needs conflict with the needs of the unit, and speak directly with those concerned, stating clearly and accurately the rationale for their decisions, there will be far less resentment over the assignments made. It is not essential that the staff agree with the manager's decisions, but it is important that their needs be respected. This can be accomplished by outlining the reasons that decisions have been made. Fairness and respect, coupled with well-orchestrated instruction, will go a long way toward developing a positive and enthusiastic attitude among staff.

Communication with Senior Managers

Nurse managers' interactions with senior members of management are very similar to their interactions with subordinates except that the roles are reversed. Junior managers must recognize that their senior managers have different types of responsibilities from theirs. Senior managers' responsibilities generally cover much broader areas, such as all of the nursing service or the entire institution. In this situation, junior managers need to remember that they are communicating with people who, very much like their own subordinates, typically are thinking on a different communication level than their own. However, most of the principles outlined earlier for communicating with subordinates remain appropriate for bottom-up communication with seniors.

Junior managers must communicate their needs clearly, explain the rationale for requests, suggest possible benefits for the larger unit, and use appropriate communication channels. In addition, they must be prepared to listen objectively to the responses provided by their supervisors and be willing to consider the potential conflicts between their needs and those of other areas. This is, of course, the description of an ideal communication between a junior manager and a senior manager, in which both participants practice good communication skills. This may not always be the case. There are as many poor communicators among senior management as there are in the rank and file, and, on a percentage basis, perhaps even more. Being a member of senior management does not mean being good at communication. In fact, junior managers can serve as role models to both subordinates and seniors by consistently demonstrating good communication skills.

Communication with Medical Staff

Communication with the medical staff can be difficult for nurse managers because of the traditional nature of the physician-nurse relationship:

- The medical staff, although not generally employees of the institution, wield enormous influence in the typical healthcare organization.
- The historical relationship of physicians and nurses has been that of senior and subordinate.
- A gender disparity often exists between physicians and nurses.

Added to these significant challenges is the fact that the medical staff itself is extremely diverse. A typical healthcare facility's medical staff consists of physician employees, residents, interns, private practice physicians, and consulting practitioners, with some of the more specialized physicians, such as pathologists, radiologists, and anesthesiologists, working on a contractual basis. Obviously, the principles of effective communication are extremely important when interacting with any member of the medical staff.

When communicating with people with influence, it is important to remember that the best results are achieved when an environment of mutual respect is established. Although nurse managers may not always have control over this situation, as professionals they should always extend respect. Showing respect is not and should not be considered a submissive act. Rather, it is simply a means of developing rapport and cohesive performance within the unit.

Communication with Other Healthcare Personnel

In addition to having responsibility for patient care in their units, nurse managers also have the difficult task of coordinating activities in their units with the activities of many other personnel at various levels of authority and with various types of training and responsibilities. The coordination responsibilities of the nurse manager can best be understood by considering the care provided to patients. Although the care of a given patient is the responsibility of a specific unit, the patient may also receive care from personnel assigned to other units in the hospital. For instance, a patient may receive nursing care from a nursing assistant and registered nurse assigned to the primary unit but also may receive regular care from nonunit personnel such as respiratory therapists, physical therapists, and the dietary staff.

Nurse managers must engage in good interdepartmental relations and use communication skills effectively when working with personnel and managers from other departments. In this situation the communication moves in a horizontal or diagonal direction depending on whether the nurse manager is communicating with other managers or directly with their staffs. The horizontal communication between managers usually follows formal channels, whereas the diagonal communication between managers and subordinates is generally informal.

Communication in Groups

The development of groups is a normal part of human activity. People join groups for a variety of reasons, including the following:

- As a means of fulfilling affiliative needs (e.g., security, belonging, companionship)
- As a source of information and reward, and as a means for accomplishing a goal

When people are involved in a group, they behave in ways that are systematically different from the ways individuals typically behave when they are not part of a group. Nurse managers can do a great deal to facilitate the benefits of group membership. For example, when they are planning work schedules and making performance assignments, they can increase the interdependence of group members. They can foster the sharing of common interests and exert con-

siderable control over rewards for the attainment of performance goals. Nurse managers can do a great deal to foster effective individual and group performance by exercising constructive influence on this performance through the careful demonstration of leadership. Indeed, this is one of their primary roles in the healthcare environment.

Nurse managers also act to guide the group in the best direction possible to achieve unit, department, and organizational goals. They bring staff members' attention to the goals, clarify issues in terms of how they relate to the unit's goals, and evaluate the group's progress toward the goals on a frequent basis.

All of this occurs in a context that is usually referred to as *group dynamics.* Behavioral scientists have known for a long time that group interactions and group output are different from those of a set of individuals working alone. For one thing, people are excited and energized by the presence of others. Frequently, this increased enthusiasm is transformed into enhanced motivation, especially when the individual's contribution to the group is clear and measured. In addition, groups tend to take more risks than do individuals; for example, work groups are more likely to go on record as supporting unusual or unpopular positions than are individuals. Group leaders tend to be less conservative than individual decision-makers and frequently display more courage and support for unusual or creative solutions to problems.

Although it might be the intention of the group to establish equality among members, in fact some people have more influence on group processes and group decisions than do others. Orwell said it best when he wrote, "some are more equal than others."[13] Groups generally influence the nature and process of communication and generate competition and political activity on a much larger scale than might be expected through individual behavior. In short, groups are greater than the sum of their parts, and they can bring out the best and the worst in individuals.

Groups are clearly different from individuals, and influencing group processes toward the attainment of organizational objectives is the direct responsibility of nurse managers. This is best accomplished by establishing a professional group environment in which group members feel free to talk about what concerns them, critique, offer suggestions, and experiment with new behaviors without the threat of retaliation.

SUMMARY

- Good communication skills are essential tools for nurse managers to use in managing their units.
- Communicating effectively is a skill that can be learned by anyone.

- Communication is an interactive process that occurs between a sender and a receiver. The form may be spoken (verbal), nonverbal, or written.
- Lines of communication operate as both direct (formal) and indirect (informal) channels in an organization.
- Nurses have become increasingly aware of the need to express their ideas, opinions, and desires without violating others' rights. Assertive communication training provides the necessary skills.
- Distorted communication occurs because the communication process is complicated and is affected by extraneous variables. Understanding the source of these influences can help reduce distortion in messages sent and received.
- Principles of effective communication include accepting responsibility for sending a clear message, using precise language, and encouraging feedback.
- Communication between the nurse manager and subordinates, senior managers, and physicians revolves around their mutual tasks.
- Nurse managers convey the institution's image of competency and professionalism to the public.

FINAL THOUGHTS

Nurse managers can ensure understanding if they make certain that their own communications contain value and are clear and concise, and if they take time to confirm the content of the messages they receive.

Assuming value is an attitude within the listener that says, "This person is worth listening to." This simple thought process opens the lines of communication and allows the receiver to understand what the speaker is saying and feeling as he or she speaks. Another benefit of this attitude is that it can influence other parties to the discussion by instilling a willingness to listen to what is being said.

Clarifying is the process used by nurse managers when they play the role of listener in the conversation. When they are not sure exactly what the speaker is saying, they clarify the conversation by asking simple questions to solicit more information, such as, "What is meant by … ?" or "Exactly what do you mean when you say … ?" Alternatively, by asking the open-ended question, "And then what?" nurse managers can easily obtain more details to help clarify the information previously shared.

Confirming is the process used when the listener believes he or she has understood what has been spoken and seeks verification from the other person that what was heard is what was actually said. This can be done by paraphrasing the previous conversation, as in, "What you said was … ." It is not good enough simply to say, "I understand what you said," because this really means only that the listener *thinks* he or she understands. Restating what has actually been said, at least in part, is a much more accurate way of confirming the true content of the conversation.

Enhancing value is far different from criticism because it identifies the merits of the conversation, builds on its content, and balances what has been said instead of rejecting it. Instead of telling a speaker that his or her ideas are not appreciated, pointing out what is wrong with what was said, or indicating that the idea suggested will not work (i.e., delivering criticism), wise nurse managers focus on adding value to the conversation by building on its merits. To accomplish this, they simply select any part of what has been said that they like or approve of and ask for clarification. If they have difficulty identifying anything in the conversation that they like, they ask the speaker to place value on his or her idea. After they have heard the speaker's opinion of its value, they can easily add information that highlights its merits and expresses sensitivity. They can also suggest slight refinements or changes that offer other approaches to reaching the same goal.

The goal of communication is to create common ground, cooperation, and understanding. These things are not achievable unless nurse managers focus on finding value in other people, their ideas, and their conversation.

THE NURSE MANAGER SPEAKS

Not all of the people with whom a nurse manager will communicate or attempt to communicate will be nice, professional, or even reasonable. Many will range from difficult to extremely forbidding. Such hostile-aggressive people frequently seem to be in an attack mode when addressed and often turn on the speaker in an abrupt, abusive, and intimidating manner. The intent is to push the speaker into acquiescence even if it is against his or her better judgment.

Difficult people often seem to feel that they know what others should do—or at least they give this impression. At the very least, they have a need to prove themselves right. They almost always lack trust and seldom seem to care about other people.

As a nurse manager, you must be able to stand up to such a hostile, aggressive onslaught or risk being run over and losing the respect normally received from others. You must do this without losing control or allowing the confrontation to escalate into an argument or fight.

Standing up for what you believe in the face of strong opposition or threat often begins by letting the oppressive individual run himself of herself out of emotion and then carefully interrupting to exercise the right to stand up for your convictions. This may not always be easy because verbal assaults are hard to bear, and, quite frankly, it may be difficult to find an opportunity to speak between the other person's sentences. Once you try to speak up, it is also quite common for the strong personality to interrupt your first attempt. If this occurs, simply inform the other person, "You interrupted me" — preferably with a smile.

You must get the oppressive individual's attention to engage in real problem solving. The most efficient way to do this is simply to speak the person's name or to stand up. When you gain the person's attention, state your ideas in a forceful but sensitive manner that does not belittle the other.

When dealing with confrontation, stand up for what you believe, but do not to give in to the desire to retaliate. Stay in control and remain professional.

COMMUNICATION AND CAREER

Management is, at best, an extremely complicated, multifaceted function that demands extensive knowledge and skill. Nevertheless, one thing must be very clear to anyone who wants to become a nurse manager: managing others in today's healthcare institution is a *communication process*. The inability to communicate automatically leads to the inability to direct the efforts of others, no matter how much one knows about leadership, organizational theory, or nurse management. Thankfully, good communication is a skill and can be learned by almost anyone. All nurse managers must learn to communicate effectively and must be able to do so with widely diverse groups of people. The requirements for effective communication are continually broadening; for example, only recently were financial and consumer relations responsibilities added to the job of nurse manager, and with them came the requirement for an entirely different type of communication skill. No one really knows what tomorrow will bring, but if nurse managers make it their business to continue their growth through learning and can communicate effectively what they have learned, they will enjoy success.

REFERENCES

1. Xerox Corporation: *Advanced effective learning*, Stamford, Conn, 1981, The Corporation.
2. Gillies DA: *Nursing management: a systems approach*, ed 2, Philadelphia, 1989, Saunders.
3. Whetten DA, Cameron KS: *Developing management skills*, ed 6, Upper Saddle River, NJ, 2004, Prentice Hall.
4. Reese BL, Brandt R: *Effective human relations: personal and organizational applications*, ed 8, Boston, 2001, Houghton-Mifflin.
5. Smith MJ: *When I say no, I feel guilty*, New York, 1978, Bantam Books.
6. Chenevert M: *Special techniques in assertiveness training for women in the health professions*, ed 4, St Louis, 1994, Mosby.
7. Smith MJ: *When I say no, I feel guilty*, New York, 1996, Bantam Books.
8. Scannell E, Donaldson L, Scannell ES: *Human response development: the new trainer's guide*, ed 3, New York, 2000, Perseus Books.
9. Douglas LM: *The effective nurse: leader and manager*, ed 5, St Louis, 1996, Mosby.
10. Wang RY, Hawkins JW: Interpersonal feedback for nursing supervisors, *Superv Nurs* 11:40, 1980.
11. Costley DL: Basis for effective communication, *Superv Nurse* 21:105, 1973.
12. Fulton K: Acknowledgment supports effective communication, *Superv Nurse* 8(March):62, 1981.
13. Orwell G: *Animal farm*, 50th anniversary edition, New York, 1996, Signet Books (originally published in 1928).

SUGGESTED READINGS

Barr L, Barr N: *The leadership equation*, Austin, Tex, 1989, Ekin Press.
Berne E: *Games people play: the basic handbook of transactional analysis*, New York, 2005, Ballantine Books.
Bramson RM: *Coping with difficult people in business and life*, New York, 1999, Doubleday.
Brown SJ: Communication strategies used by an expert nurse, *Clin Nurs Res* 3(1):43, 1994.
Davidhizar R, Dowd SB: The dynamics of rumors in the clinical setting, *Nurs Stand* 11(13-15):40, 1996.
Davis LL, Cox RP: Looking through the constructivist lens: the art of creating nursing work groups, *J Prof Nurs* 10(1):38, 1994.
Dowd SB, Davidhizar R, Dowd LP: Rumor and gossip: a guide for the health care supervisor, *Health Care Superv* 16(1):65, 1997.
Fiesta J: Communication: are you listening?, *Nurs Manage* 25(9):15, 1994.
Gilovich T: *How we know what isn't so: the fallibility of human reasoning in everyday life*, New York, 1993, Free Press.
Hanna B: Improving communication ... "over the sink," *Nurs Manage* 25(7):88, 1994.
Hein EC: *Contemporary leadership behavior*, ed 5, Philadelphia, 1998, Lippincott.
Heineken J: Patient silence is not necessarily client satisfaction: communication problems in home care nursing, *Home Healthc Nurse* 16(2):115, 1998.
James M, Jongeward D: *Born to win*, New York, 1996, Perseus Press.
McMahon B: The functions of space, *J Adv Nurs* 19(2):362, 1994.
Peterson LW, Halsey J, Albrecht TL, and others: Communicating with staff nurses: support or hostility?, *Nurs Manage* 26(6):36, 1995.
Tannen D: *You just don't understand: women and men in conversation*, New York, 2001, Harper Trade.
Williams D, Brown DL: Automation at the point of care, *Nurs Manage* 25(7):32, 1994.
Wywialowski EF: *Managing client care*, ed 3, St Louis, 2004, Mosby.

Leadership in Healthcare Supervision

OUTLINE

LEARNING SYNOPSIS

Upon successful completion of this chapter, readers will possess a fundamental understanding of the theories of leadership and their applications in the healthcare institution and the typical nursing unit.

OBJECTIVES

1. Describe ways of defining leadership in the nursing unit
2. Identify different ways in which the personality, behavior, and style of the leader affect the unit
3. Describe different theories of leadership
4. Explain the social learning approach to implementing leadership in the nursing unit
5. Identify factors that influence the demonstration of leadership within the group

When an individual advances to the level of nurse manager, the assignment brings with it the mixed blessings of new opportunities, freedoms, privileges, responsibilities, and pressures. Although most individuals who are not and have never been in a position of authority view management as a repository of prestige, power, and privilege, the truth is that a management position carries far more responsibility, hard work, and pressure than privilege, rights, and freedoms. The following are some of the multitude of responsibilities that nurse managers inherit with their position:

- Administering the health care and needs of a variety of patients; in most cases, these patients will be the more serious cases and those with special needs—certainly those at high risk
- Guiding the performance and conduct of subordinate personnel
- Developing, implementing, and controlling a budget
- Acting as a liaison between senior management and front-line employees
- Managing a specific portion of the overall communication and control process for the organization
- Directing the day-to-day operations of the unit for which he or she is responsible

A management position, regardless of the level, demands that the holder possess a variety of capabilities, not the least of which is the ability to demonstrate effective leadership. So critical is this requirement to the successful operation of a nursing unit that properly defining what leadership is may be as important as learning how it is exercised. Clarification of this concept is vital to the discussion in this chapter, and so is a clear understanding of the meaning of leadership to every person who would accede to a position of responsibility. Therefore, let's start discussion at that point.

WHAT EXACTLY *IS* LEADERSHIP?

One can best define exactly what leadership is by understanding what it is not. Leadership, as it must be demonstrated by managers—or by anyone else in a position of responsibility who has control over the performance and lives of others—is *not* an act of management. In fact, leadership and management are many times diametrically opposed to one another. The following are the definitions of both words used by the major business organizations in America:

Management: the act of bringing about, accomplishing, taking charge of or responsibility for, or conducting operations for others

Leadership: The ability to influence or guide the direction, action, and opinion of others

Leadership is *not*, as many of the old school management personnel would have you believe, the exercise of power and influence through interpersonal interaction to ensure the execution of assigned tasks. This is the classic definition of management. Leadership goes beyond the simple use of power and influence to affect the functioning of others.

Leadership is a set of qualities that causes others to follow. This definition makes it clear that leadership cannot exist without the presence of someone who is willing to be led. Getting another person to follow one's lead takes far more than promotion to a position of responsibility. Leadership is an emotional, interpersonal relationship in which the leader demonstrates specific courses of action and strategies that have the collective effect of influencing followers toward the accomplishment of specific goals. The act of leadership influences others to go beyond what they believe themselves capable of and thereby ensures that, through collective effort, the group will reach goals and objectives previously thought unattainable. Leaders build this synergy in the following ways:

- By inspiring trust
- By acting consistently
- By motivating through words and deeds

Reduced to its fundamental aspect, leadership is the willingness to accept responsibility and accountability and the ability to effectively and consistently demonstrate the following three vital skills:

1. *Obtain the collaboration of others:* A leader must be able to get others to accept his or her vision of the future and the correct way to achieve it.
2. *Listen effectively:* An individual who would lead others must have information, and to obtain it and qualify it, he or she must be able to hear what is being said as well as what is not being said.
3. *Place the needs of others above one's own:* The leader must be willing to sacrifice for the greater goal.

Management, in contrast, refers to the formulation and coherence of resources through processes, such as planning, organizing, directing, and controlling, in an effort to accomplish specific objectives. Thus, when a person who occupies a position of authority is exercising management skills, he or she is primarily concerned with planning for, scheduling, and overseeing the use of resources through the accomplishment of predetermined tasks. A desired characteristic of a manager is the ability to create an environment in which required objectives can be achieved without the creation of dissension or animosity.

The act of supervising, or supervision in general, is also frequently confused with leadership. *Supervision*, for the purposes of this textbook, is defined as coordinating and administering the basic performance activities of the organization in accordance with approved plans and procedures. It involves overseeing the work activities of others and is directly concerned with leader-subordinate interaction.

It is not only possible but also highly desirable for all managers and supervisors within an organization to be effective leaders. However, this is not the case in the vast majority of businesses, including those in the healthcare industry. In fact, there are many people occupying both managerial and supervisory positions in every organization who have little or no real leadership ability and very few if any management skills. The reality is that management skills and leadership ability are not inherent in any position of authority. Leadership and management result when the individual performs a series of routine tasks that anyone can learn and accomplish effectively. There is nothing mystical about either process. One thing is critical in the development of these abilities, however: every person occupying a position of authority needs to realize that he or she must expend effort to become an effective manager and leader. The qualities and capabilities necessary are never inherited with the promotion.

BLENDING THE QUALITIES

Although leadership and management have been discussed in detail, there is really only one point to be made here, and this point is that a distinct difference exists between the *act* of management and *art* of leadership. Understanding the difference between these two is critical to any individual in charge of any part of a healthcare organization today, no matter the size of his or her area of responsibility. Each is absolutely essential to the successful operation of a healthcare unit, and neither is more important than the other. To understand why both management and leadership must be undertaken enthusiastically by anyone wishing to lead a successful unit in a healthcare facility, the following well-known but much more practical definitions of both terms are offered:

Management focuses on doing things right.

Leadership focuses on doing the right thing.

When the concepts are expressed in this manner, it is easy to see why neither can stand alone in today's healthcare industry. Even to approach success in a managerial role, one must combine the proper proportions of each in every action. Doing things right has little value if one is not doing the right thing, and doing the right thing is useless if one is not doing it properly. Every person fulfilling any role, on any level, in any healthcare facility is responsible for combining these qualities in the proper proportion to positively influence the employee and the patient. This is how *moments of truth** are won.

Every person in every organization who desires success must continually apply his or her unique combination of leadership and management skills in a way that increases the ability to generate positive influence. This is accomplished through a program of constant and consistent self-analysis. Only when people form and maintain a clear mental picture of themselves as they would have others perceive them can they truly manage their impact and influence on others. Leaders must constantly look into themselves for what they expect to see in others, so that they can provide a positive example of what it is they wish emulated.

Leader is the noun in the sentence of life; *manage* is the verb. One shows action and the other defines who the person is. The two must be combined effectively to create a meaningful perception for one's employees and patients.

DEFINING LEADERSHIP IN THE MEDICAL UNIT

As stated previously, leadership is the effective use of one's ability to influence another's willingness to follow. Although it may be true that everyone has a different potential for leadership, the individual skills required to cultivate it have been identified and can be learned by anyone who is willing.

In the healthcare industry, leadership has traditionally been considered a relationship between people, a process of influencing the activities of an organized group toward goal setting and goal achievement.[1] Historically, nurse managers have been the individuals assigned responsibility for directing the activities within the unit, which include (but obviously are not limited to) the following:

- Making patient care assignments
- Scheduling
- Planning inservice education

Moments of truth is a phrase first brought to importance in the book *Leaders* by Warren Bennis and Burt Nanus (New York, 1983, Dell). The phrase was used by Jan Carlzon, president and chief executive officer of Scandinavian Airlines (SAS), when he was engineering the modern business miracle of turning SAS from a near-bankrupt airline into one of the world's most profitable travel-based conglomerates. The phrase describes the opportunity that is presented each time an employee meets, talks to, comes face-to-face with, or influences a customer. It is said that a moment of truth is won when the customer comes away feeling positive about the entire organization through that single contact. Carlzon believed that SAS had a minimum of 50,000 moments of truth daily.

How effectively nurse managers accomplish these tasks depends a great deal on their leadership style and skill.

The effective demonstration of leadership, as was stated earlier, requires more than a person who wishes to lead. It also requires the presence of people who are willing to follow, and an appropriate relationship between these two elements. As was stressed before, appointment to a position that requires the ability to exercise leadership does not guarantee that the person so appointed is capable of effectively leading anyone. Neither does it ensure that the group will accept the individual occupying the position or that the person can elicit a willingness to follow. A leader must be able to *inspire* others to achievement. This skill should not be confused with *making* people want to accomplish something—it is not the same. One is leadership and the other is manipulation.

If one accepts the fact that leadership is the interpersonal process of influencing the activities of an individual or a group toward achievement of a goal in a given situation,[2] then it is clear that leadership does not involve domination. Leadership is the careful elicitation of work done through the actions of other people. To give one recognizable example, effective leadership occurs when a nurse manager identifies a personality conflict between two staff nurses and uses his or her ability to work through the difference to achieve agreement on a patient assignment calendar.

Leadership can be either formal and informal, regardless of the hierarchical position or status of the nursing staff involved. Leadership is viewed as *informal* when a team member who does not occupy a position of authority within the unit demonstrates it. In a group of peers, when one nurse exerts influence over another in accomplishing the work of the unit, that nurse is usually thought of as the leader. Informal leadership can be complementary or contradictory to the goals of the unit or the institution. Leadership is considered to be *formal* when it is demonstrated by the person responsible for the unit, regardless of how subtlely it may be exercised.

BASES OF POWER

As noted earlier, leadership, or the willingness to accept responsibility or exercise influence, involves an individual's attempt to achieve a goal by carefully directing the behavior of others. It usually means bringing some kind of influence to bear on the followers in an effort to persuade them to act in accordance with the leader's vision and goals. An individual who is exercising leadership possesses a certain degree of authority over the group that is limited by the following:

The leader's ability to obtain cooperation: Leadership is a process of offering something for something.

Implicitly, what a leader does is to trade a goal or vision focused on the future for struggle and hard work in the present. The goal must be real and attainable, and it must fit the needs of the people being led.

The leader's ability to listen effectively: Leaders must make listening a critical skill. To direct the efforts of others, the leader must be able to assess the mood of the group. If the leader cannot listen, he or she will not be able to hear the advance warnings of problems occurring at all levels.

The leader's ability to put the needs of others before his or her own: Regardless of whether a leader is facilitating or is developing a plan that will take the group to where it wants to go, to be effective the leader must be altruistic and continually place the needs of the group above his or her own. The leader who focuses on the trappings and perks of the management position rarely enjoys a long tenure in that position.

To a certain degree, followers may be motivated by an individual exercising authority because (1) the followers believe that the individual exerting control will use rewards or punishments to support his or her request for assistance; (2) the group members either greatly fear or highly value the outcomes that may result; and (3) the group members have few, if any, alternatives—that is, little way to change or decrease the pressure that the person in authority can exert. Authority exercised in such circumstances is not leadership, however. To the contrary, it is, at best, a manifestation of an inept use of power.

Realism dictates that the exercise of power be thoroughly discussed if one is to have an appreciation for the qualities of leadership. Nurse managers must know about some of the resources they can bring to bear in a leadership situation. Studies of the manipulation of authority or power have led to the identification of the following six primary sources of power[3,4]:

1. *Reward power:* This type of power is based on the incentives the leader can provide to group members in exchange for their performance and on the value group members place on those incentives. For example, nurse managers may have considerable influence in determining what compensation a nurse receives or how vacation time is structured for a specific staff nurse. Reward power, in these circumstances, is based largely on a leader's formal management responsibilities.

2. *Punishment:* Sometimes referred to as *coercive power,* this influence is based on the negative motivational actions that an individual occupying a position of authority has at his or her disposal and can invoke to control an individual group member or the group as a whole. For

example, nurse managers have the authority to assign a staff nurse more than a reasonable share of unsavory tasks within the unit, issue a verbal or written reprimand, recommend a temporary salary reduction or loss of another form of compensation, or, in the most severe circumstances, recommend termination.

! CRITICAL POINT

In almost every healthcare or medical service provider facility, discipline or punishment is a closely monitored process. It is not realistic to believe that nurse managers can mete out unwarranted discipline except possibly for assignment to unsavory tasks without facing, at the minimum, reversal of the measure or, at the maximum, some sort of disciplinary action, up to and including termination, taken against them by the organization. Even the assignment to unpleasant duties, if it is later determined to be unreasonable, unfair, or a result of prejudicial retaliation, will be dealt with swiftly by the organization. Although these unprofessional acts still continue to occur, today's business environment and the risk of court action faced by the organization creates an atmosphere in which these acts, if discovered, are only very rarely condoned or ignored.

3. *Informational power:* This form of influence is based on the principle that those who are in the know have an advantage over those who are not. The degree to which access to information is controlled determines the amount of power that can potentially be wielded. Nurse managers may possess this type of influence. For example, a person who occupies a managerial position is frequently made privy to information that is not shared with nonmanagerial staff. Much of this information is sensitive, and managers are frequently directed not to make it available to members of the staff. Therefore, it is realistic to assume that nurse managers do have information at their disposal that staff nurses do not. This unbalanced possession of information does not become a problem unless nurse managers fail to share information that is supposed to be passed along to the staff and the absence of this information makes it more difficult for staff members to perform their responsibilities or in some way impairs the performance of the team or the organization.

4. *Legitimate power:* This influence is almost inherent in a position of authority. It is derived from the perception of subordinate personnel that a person who holds a position of authority has a legitimate right to make a request of a subordinate and a right to receive a reasonable and positive response. Even the most junior of personnel on their first day on the job understand that members of management have authority delegated to them so that they can perform their jobs. The amount of legitimate power the manager is perceived to have depends, at least initially, on the position of the manager in the management hierarchy.

5. *Expert power:* This form of influence is rooted in the fact that management personnel are usually more experienced and/or knowledgeable than front-line staff in specific areas and, in some cases, in general. This may be because the senior person has a higher level of education, a particular knowledge, and/or a skill that is not possessed by the staff. Typically nurse managers are appointed based on extensive technical experience, demonstrated technical ability, or completion of advanced education, and generally these factors qualify them as the individuals to whom others should look for instruction on what to do in a given situation. For example, staff nurses frequently consult nurse managers for advice in difficult or unique situations, for guidance when they are unsure of particular procedures, and even for assistance in operating special equipment.

6. *Referent power:* This form of influence is often the most powerful that a leader has available and is rarely possessed by a hard or severe manager. This is a type of power given by a single individual to a specific person who may or may not occupy a position of authority. In fact, such influence quite commonly is held by a member of the staff who is especially competent. This referent power is based on the deference and regard that one individual feels for another. This type of influence is demonstrated when a staff nurse seeks out the nurse manager to discuss a personal problem that is occurring away from the work environment. Referent power is developed less through the position the individual holds than through the personal qualities that the person exhibits.

As can be seen, power or influence can stem from a variety of different sources and can arise for quite a few different reasons. How much power is actually available to a specific nurse manager is almost always directly proportional to the actions taken by that nurse manager and to his or her approachability and professionalism. In addition, only very rarely is influence derived from a single source. The following two points regarding power and influence are important to remember:

1. Power (influence) is fleeting. It can be lost far more easily than it was gained. This is especially true of referent power but is applicable to any type.

2. The most effective form of power is that exercised with restraint and compassion, and through responsible action focused on what is best for the team or organization. How power is exercised should depend on the situation at hand and the goals and objectives of the team or organization. It must be exercised dispassionately, with care taken that prejudice and other such influences do not affect the people involved.

One can never stress enough that the exercise of power is something that requires patience, concern, professionalism, and care. Although there are some very general principles regarding the use of power, it is an extremely subjective process in most cases, and how the individual exercises power is almost always critical to the success of both the individual who wields it and the organization that grants it. The exercise of power is a responsibility, not a privilege. It must be done carefully with the intent of enhancing the individual, the unit, and the organization. If power is used to advance one's personal agenda—and it often is—the person foolish enough to do so will ultimately pay a significant price. It is absolutely certain, especially in today's environment, that personnel who exercise authority or power over others will be held accountable for their actions.

Truly professional managers know that subordinates are far more likely to comply when legitimate, expert, and referent power are exercised than when reward or coercive power is used. In fact, considerable agreement is found between the type of power managers prefer to use and the type subordinates prefer to have used in a specific situation. Nevertheless, professional nurse managers must be aware that some important differences exist between how power is wielded and how it is perceived, both at the level of the individual manager and at the level of the organization as a whole. Some managers adopt an autocratic style in exercising their authority, whereas others rely on a more participatory style. Regardless of the style used, however, all managers must realize that the exercise of power does not become an act of leadership unless it is intended to benefit the individual staff member, the team, or the organization, and this benefit is put ahead of any gain that might be realized by the individual who exercises the authority. Truly effective leaders tend to rely more on expertise and referent power or social pressure to accomplish their goals, and this is sometimes difficult if the overall organization tends to emphasize autocratic control in its management systems.

The responsibility for the use of influence is held by the individual exercising it. In every instance, that person will be the one held accountable.

THE EFFECTS OF PERSONALITY, BEHAVIOR, AND STYLE

For many years, researchers have searched, without much success, for a relationship between the demonstration of effective leadership and specific personality traits or personal attributes. Every time investigators have identified certain characteristics in successful leaders, they have found examples of leadership failure on the part of individuals possessing these same qualifications. Nevertheless, research has continually demonstrated that the specific situation in which leadership is demonstrated can be a major factor in determining the extent to which the characteristics of the leader influence leadership effectiveness.

From the late 1950s to the early 1980s, researchers studying leadership at several highly esteemed universities began to focus on what it is that leaders do in addition to what personal characteristics they possess. Following are the results of research at three universities:

1. *Harvard University:* Study of leadership at this renowned center identified factors such as "activity," "task ability," and "likability" as contributors to the behavior identified as leadership.[5]

2. *Ohio State University:* In field research, Buckeye investigators asked nonmanagerial workers to describe the behaviors or traits they felt were exhibited by people they worked with and identified as leaders.[5] Their responses could be grouped into the following two broad categories:
   Consideration: This refers to the actions (behavior) of the individual holding the leadership position that convey mutual trust, respect, friendship, warmth, and rapport with a member or members of the team. Consideration establishes an environment in which the employee learns to expect that the person occupying the leadership position will hear a complaint or react to dissent in an open and professional manner and does not normally fear reprisal.
   Initiation of structure: This refers to the behavior demonstrated when the person in a leadership position determines and fixes the limits of the work that is expected to be accomplished and establishes well-defined, predictable work patterns, communication channels, and methods of performance. For example, nurse managers might provide their subordinates with explicit job descriptions that cover each subordinate's area of responsibility, a copy of the organization's personnel policies, and specific procedures for requesting special consideration (time off on a holiday).

3. *University of Michigan:* Researchers here also conducted their research in the field but asked the leaders themselves to describe what they did.[5]

This effort identified two major dimensions of leadership behavior: job centered and employee centered.

The results of these independent research projects show a remarkable consistency. In each study, the following two areas were identified as major contributors to leadership behavior:

1. *Interpersonal relationships:* consideration, likability, and employee-centered behavior
2. *Concern for the task:* ability, initiation of structure, job-centered behavior

Although the consistent findings of these early research efforts are encouraging, the exact relationship between the behaviors demonstrated by leaders and their effectiveness in leading continues to be an enigma. Follow-up studies have shown that specific task-oriented behaviors and interpersonal behaviors, or any given combination of them, do not necessarily produce effective leadership. In addition, studies have failed to demonstrate a correlation between interpersonally oriented or task-oriented leadership styles, or any combination thereof, and consistently higher achievement and competency. Instead, it has become quite evident that it is the situation in which leadership is demonstrated that has the most profound influence in determining the relationship between leadership behavior and the performance of those led.

Although this early research did not produce the correlation that was hoped for, it provided a significant advance in understanding leadership effectiveness. If nothing else, these studies gave birth to research into the effects of different leadership styles or clusters of leadership behaviors. There is high expectation that this research will result in the identification of particular patterns and/or styles of leadership that can be employed in specific situations.

Leadership styles, at least in the research venue, are typically identified as *sets or clusters of behaviors.*[6] In the real world of nurse managers, a leadership style is the manner in which individuals use their interpersonal behaviors to influence the accomplishment of goals in the unit for which they are responsible.

Every individual's behavior is heavily influenced by the experiences and environments of his or her formative years and the collective effect of his or her past; thus, each individual's leadership style is unique. Because extensive research found it impossible to identify specific characteristics or individual traits that are present in all successful leaders, the focus of study shifted to determining how successful leadership is accomplished and identifying exactly how people in leadership positions have achieved success in delegating tasks and communicating with their followers. The most exciting finding of these studies is that, unlike personal traits, the behaviors that result in effective leadership can be learned.

The fact that the character, disposition, and collective experience of leaders helps to create their specific leadership styles does not mean that their styles cannot be enhanced, modified, or changed. In fact, one startling characteristic of nearly all individuals recognized to be excellent leaders is that they rarely use the identical style in varying situations. Styles of leadership run the gamut from very authoritarian to very permissive, and almost all of them are subject to change as the situation changes. For example, a nurse leader may use one style when responding to an emergency situation such as a patient's cardiac arrest (authoritarian), another to encourage creative problem solving in planning the care for a patient with multiple problems (democratic), and even a third when attempting to generate ideas for the implementation of a new procedure within the unit (permissive). The style of an effective leader is the one that best complements the organizational environment, the tasks to be accomplished, and the personal characteristics of the people involved.

Authoritarian

Sometimes referred to as *autocratic,* the authoritarian style is primarily characterized by the issuance of directives, and because of its single-minded orientation, many people do not consider this type of direction to be leadership. One specific feature of this style is that the people employing it tend make decisions alone and unassisted. Although this behavior might well be more expedient and may even achieve the desired result, this type of leadership style is rarely able to garner the same degree of support from the group as might be realized by a more collaborative effort. Autocrats are concerned primarily with accomplishing the task at hand—or at least far more so than with demonstrating any real concern for the people who perform the tasks that result from their directives. These classic "directors" consider their decisions to be fundamentally correct simply because they are the ones who bear the burden of responsibility and have been granted authority. These managers typically expect their subordinates to respect them because of their position and obey their directions without question. Such individuals may go through the motions of listening to suggestions but rarely are substantially influenced by them; in fact, many will seek retribution from a subordinate bold enough to suggest that the manager's ideas are not perfect. These individuals do little to encourage personal initiative, creativity, or even cooperation within their areas of responsibility.

People who use an autocratic style frequently exercise their authority (power) through manipulation and coercion. Typically, these individuals have personalities that are rigid, persistent, self-confident, and controlling. They like to be the center of attention and rarely share credit with others. The classic autocrat views subordinates as naturally indolent, without aspiration, irresponsible (or at least not desiring of responsibility), and in need of someone to direct their efforts. The classic autocrat is assumed to be self-centered, indifferent to organizational needs, resistant to change, not very bright, and lacking creative potential.[7] People of this type in positions of authority have little trust or confidence in those who are compelled to work for them and vice-versa. (Can you see why such people are not typically considered leaders?)

In spite of the many negative aspects of this leadership style and the fact that it is not even considered leadership in most typical situations, nurse managers must understand that autocratic direction is necessary in periods of crisis when there is no time for group decision. It is a form of leadership that all managers will, at one time or another, demonstrate. In a hospital, this type of directive behavior is needed when a patient's life is threatened and there is no time to convene a meeting to determine a course of action; a cardiac arrest is a prime example. In a dramatic situation such as this, being confident, directive, and controlling is entirely appropriate leadership behavior.

Another situation in which this type of behavior might be acceptable is a case in which the nurse manager is the only one who has the essential information or skills to accomplish a specific task or treatment. In this situation, however, the directive, controlling behavior should be demonstrated in a teaching mode and not solely as a performance style. The idea may be to get the task done correctly, but effective leaders understand that their primary job is to nurture performance in others. Therefore, when they must demonstrate this behavior they do so with the intention of instruction, not domination. In these specific situations, inexperienced staff members will expect to be told what to do and may not expect to provide input on how something might be done. For example, in a disaster the best course would be to inform a recently graduated nurse of correct procedures through direct, uncomplicated instructions issued with the expectation of blind obedience.

Democratic

When the democratic or participative style of leadership is demonstrated, the manager is generally concerned with the welfare of the followers (people oriented). People exercising this style focus much of their energy on interpersonal relations, teamwork, and the creation of a work environment that is conducive to the enhancement of the working group. In this environment, cooperation and teamwork are emphasized and the leader is viewed as a facilitator

responsible for guiding the team's efforts and promoting harmonious teamwork. Much effort is expended to develop a sense of worth in the team members by encouraging them to make independent contributions—even in sensitive and difficult situations. Communication is an important part of this environment and is kept open and bidirectional. Not only is there a spirit of collaboration and joint effort between the followers and the leader, but both sides work actively to promote closer relations. As a result, the individual members of the team enjoy much more freedom and satisfaction and are far more willing to take personal risks by being creative and by offering suggestions for improvement.

The following is an example of democratic leadership in the nursing unit: A patient who is recovering from a recent myocardial infarction is repeatedly found walking in his room even though he is supposed to be on complete bed rest. The nurse manager, exercising a democratic leadership style, makes arrangements for members of the team to attend a case management conference at which they can collectively explore methods of encouraging the patient to remain in bed and promote recovery.

The democratic leader's primary goal is to gently facilitate the group's advancement in the right direction. The basic assumption of managers who employ this style is that, if followers are treated as important contributors, they are likely to respond in a professional manner. Democratic leaders make an effort to create situations that will enhance a follower's feeling of self-worth and importance.

Of course, there are situations in which the leader, regardless of his or her desire to do so, simply cannot be completely democratic. In these situations, the true democratic leader will make the decisions necessary to meet the challenge at hand but in doing so will encourage as much participation as possible so that staff members will continue to identify with the democratically oriented work environment.

It has been proven over and over again that active participation promotes the acceptance of goals and elicits the staff's cooperation in carrying out the activities decided upon. It also provides the opportunity for individuals to grow because it compels them to change or improve their performance and helps them understand that even mistakes are opportunities if they are used as learning tools.

Early studies of this style of leadership found that it did not consistently lead to high productivity but that it had significant positive impact on employee job satisfaction.[8] Later studies, however, have shown that, although this form of leadership may take longer to produce results, the benefits derived and the levels of performance achieved are far greater than those realized in an autocratic environment.[9]

Permissive or Laissez-Faire

The permissive or laissez-faire style is another method of exercising authority that is not considered leadership by much of the research and business communities. The individual tasked with providing direction (nurse manager) who uses this form of influence rarely has established goals or policies and consciously refrains from directing the efforts of the staff. The general climate is one of permissiveness with no central direction or control. The leader wants everyone to feel good, fosters freedom for everyone, and avoids responsibility by relinquishing power to the staff.

The degree of effectiveness of this style depends on the quality of the individuals who comprise the group. One of the most common failings of this type of leadership is that it almost always requires the leader to be physically present for the group to function effectively. The basic belief held by the permissive leader regarding staff members is that they are industrious, creative, dependable, adaptable, energetic, intelligent, and willing to accept the goals and objectives they are given. On the surface, this type of leadership may seem able to accomplish little, but when it is used to direct the efforts of highly professional and motivated groups, it is actually one of the most effective styles. However, it is rarely used by nurse managers directing the efforts of a unit in a highly structured healthcare delivery system. Because of the diversity of people and backgrounds found among staff in a healthcare facility, the situation rarely is conducive to loose control, and most of these facilities are organized to provide a much stronger exercise of authority.

Bureaucratic

Another style of leadership frequently found in clinical settings is the bureaucratic style. Leaders who use this form of control appear, at least on the surface, to be much like individuals employing an autocratic style. Most people who adopt a bureaucratic style are relatively insecure in their positions and are unsure about their ability to lead others. Such individuals feel safe and comfortable following the organization's established policies, often word for word. They exercise their influence over their teams by referring to established rules and are rarely flexible in their operations. In the units they direct, exercising personal or group initiative is generally discouraged, and the environment is usually cold and clinical. These managers rarely allow variations from standard policy, and when they do, they expend a good deal of personal effort to ensure that the rules are followed. Individuals using this style feel comfortable in their official capacity, have difficulty relating to staff members except in an impersonal or official manner, and rarely make a decision unless the risk inherent in it can be mitigated by adhering to organizational standards and guidelines.

Mollifying (Appeasing)

About halfway between the bureaucrat and the autocrat sit those managers who exercise their influence using the mollifying approach to leadership. These managers are raging storms of turmoil—they are worried that staff members have too much autonomy and, often at the same instant, are concerned about satisfying them as a first priority. Nurse managers of this type usually have good rapport with the staff and communicate with staff members on a variety of professional and personal levels. They typically listen well and actively solicit input from the staff regarding the operation of the unit. They are almost always ineffective, however, especially in the long term, because although they provide the staff with the opportunity to participate and appear, at least on the surface, to be team oriented, they rarely follow through on the information they learn while listening. Instead of using the ideas they elicit, they do what they had planned to do before they had any discussions with the staff. The problem with this approach is that the staff, especially the educated and professional members, will pick up on this inconsistency; at the very least they will stop providing input, and at the worst they will stop supporting the nurse manager.

Parental

Managers who adopt a parental style are "too good" to the members of their staffs and rarely, if ever, exercise discipline within the unit. Instead, they foster dependence in the staff and reward those members who seek their guidance and advice. Communication within the unit is mostly downward and rarely is upward dissent encouraged. Managers of this type are often insincere and condescending in manner and inconsistent in performance. They typically maintain a loose form of control within the unit until a challenge or difficulty occurs. When challenged, they tend to tighten control and become highly directive. The parental manager is rarely effective, and this style is not recommended for day-to-day operations; however, that does not mean it does not have its place. There are times, and individuals, that require this form of supervision, and if it is used sparingly and carefully, it can be a positive managerial tool.

Multicratic

The multicratic style of leadership incorporates the best elements of three styles discussed earlier—autocratic, democratic, and laissez-faire—and typically produces the best results in a professional unit. Individuals using a multicratic style of leadership integrate flexibility into their management technique and, at the same time, have a genuine concern for the members of the staff. Their focus is on attaining the goals of the unit and providing competent management.

• • • •

Simply knowing what the different styles of leadership are does not prepare nurse managers to assume leadership roles or help them determine which style will be the most effective under specific conditions. In fact, none of the styles discussed earlier considers the unique circumstances and effects of a specific leadership situation. The inability of leadership research to effectively address these shortcomings led to the development of several contingency theories of leadership. These theories attempt to incorporate a variety of leadership traits, behaviors, and situational characteristics into a single conceptual framework that can explain the circumstances under which effective leadership occurs. This framework is designed to help individuals holding positions that require leadership to understand what might constitute effective leadership and to predict what type or types of leadership behaviors will be the most effective under specific circumstances.

THEORIES OF LEADERSHIP

The Contingency Model

Researcher F. E. Fiedler studied leadership style, and his book *Theory of Leadership Effectiveness* was first published in 1967.[10] According to the model of leadership presented by Fiedler (known as effectiveness contingency), the style of leadership used must be harmonized with the conditions of the situation in order for an individual to provide effective leadership. Fiedler very carefully defined *effectiveness* as *the performance of the group itself*, not as the performance of the leader as indicated by some arbitrary rating. He identified two fundamental styles of leadership, which he referred to as (a) relationship oriented, and (b) task oriented.

Fiedler determined basic leadership style using a questionnaire he called the *Least-Preferred Co-worker* scale. Using this tool, leaders evaluated their least favorite co-worker(s) along seventeen scales secured at either end by contrasting adjectives (e.g., capable–incapable, efficient–inefficient, friendly–rejecting). If leaders described their least-preferred co-workers in positive terms, then they were categorized as having essentially a relationship-oriented motivational style. If leaders described their least-preferred associates in relatively negative terms, then they were said to be basically task oriented.

Fiedler defined leadership as a *process of influence* and categorized the leadership situation in terms of the ease with which the individual exercising leadership can influence the members of the group. According to Fiedler, this leadership dimension, which he termed *situation favorability*, is determined by the following three elements:

1. *Leader-member relations:* the degree to which the leader enjoys the loyalty and support of his or her subordinates
2. *Task structure:* the degree to which the task or result of effort is described or to which there are standard operating procedures that guarantee successful completion of the task; that is, how easy it is for the leader to determine how well the work originally assigned was accomplished
3. *Position power:* the degree to which the leader is able to control the rewards and punishments associated with the performance achieved (essentially a matter of legitimate power)

When leader–staff member relations are relatively good, when the task is relatively structured, and when leaders have a high level of position power, it is relatively easy for them to influence the group toward the accomplishment of organizational objectives. Fiedler believed that the leader-member relations component is the most critical, followed by task structure; formal position power is the least important determinant of situation favorability.

Fig. 9-1 shows the leadership styles Fiedler believed were best for specific combinations of the situational characteristics listed earlier. According to his model, leaders are most effective when their leadership style matches the situation in which leadership is being exercised. Fiedler recommended that leaders make a conscious effort to develop situations and environments for which their predominant leadership style is most appropriate. When a mismatch does occur, he recommended that the leader attempt to change the characteristics of the situation or change his or her specific leadership style to accommodate the requirements of the new situation.

The Path-Goal Theory

The path-goal theory was developed by R. J. House and T. R. Mitchell and was described in their 1974

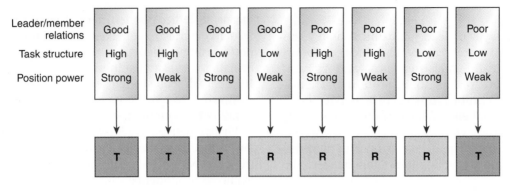

Leader/member relations	Good	Good	Good	Good	Poor	Poor	Poor	Poor
Task structure	High	High	Low	Low	High	High	Low	Low
Position power	Strong	Weak	Strong	Weak	Strong	Weak	Strong	Weak
	T	T	T	R	R	R	R	T

T = Task-oriented style   **R** = Relationship-oriented style

Fig. 9-1 ■ Optimal leadership styles for specific combinations of situational characteristics according to the contingency theory of leadership.

article, "Path-Goal Theory of Leadership."[11] This theory views leadership effectiveness in terms of human motivation and task performance. More specifically, the theory focuses on the fact that a primary responsibility of a leader is to motivate the individual members within a group to work toward the attainment of organizational objectives. Path-goal theory proposes that this motivational function is accomplished best when the leader focuses his or her energy on performing actions that will remove obstacles from the path of goal attainment and on ensuring that all of the personal rewards provided to members of the group are contingent on attainment of the desired goals. In this theory, the leader's function is one of coaching, facilitating, guiding, and providing performance incentives that ensure a high level of performance. The theory also suggests that the behavior of the leader directly affects the amount of job satisfaction obtained by individual group members, at least to the extent that the leader is responsible for making rewards available, and that the leader's conduct itself is a source of satisfaction for team members.

The requirement that a leader provide motivational opportunities to the members of the team grows out of the expectancy theory of work motivation that is discussed in Chapter 25. According to expectancy theory, team members work for rewards that they find attractive and that are likely to be awarded for desired performance. In other words, every individual works for what is in his or her own best interests. Expectancy theory also suggests that staff members must firmly believe that their efforts will lead to high performance before they will become highly motivated. Thus, the leader's purpose is to clarify the nature of the task to be accomplished (the performance objective), facilitate the employee's attainment of that objective by providing the proper resources and training at the appropriate intervals, and ensure the coordination and cooperation of all other parties whose actions are required for task completion.

According to path-goal theory, to fulfill his or her role, the leader must adopt one of the following four basic forms of leadership behavior:

1. *Supportive leadership:* The leader considers the needs of subordinates in the decision process, displays concern for employee well-being, and creates an open, professional environment within the unit.
2. *Directive leadership:* The leader informs subordinates of exactly what they are expected to do, provides specific guidelines for the performance, ensures that applicable rules and procedures are followed, and schedules and coordinates the task.
3. *Achievement-oriented leadership:* The leader establishes attainable and challenging goals, continually pursues performance improvements, stresses high-quality performance, and demonstrates a belief in the subordinate's ability to perform to high standards.
4. *Participative leadership:* The leader seeks consultation from team members and considers their opinions and suggestions before making decisions.

Staff members will interpret and respond in different ways to the form of leadership behavior depending on situational factors such as the following:

■ Characteristics of the individual team members
■ Type and difficulty of the task
■ Setting in which the task is to be accomplished

Specifically, team members' needs for achievement, affiliation, and autonomy; their ability to perform the task (e.g., job skills, knowledge, experience); and their personality traits (e.g., self-esteem) form part of the environment within which the behavior of the leader produces specific effects. This environment includes the characteristics of the task and the setting in which it is to be accomplished. The setting includes things such as the extent to which the job is automated and the degree of formalization required by the organization (e.g., written job descriptions, regulations, procedures, and performance standards). In simpler terms, the effect of leadership behavior on the satisfaction and effort of subordinates is directly related to the situation in which the leadership behavior occurs.

SUPPORTIVE LEADERSHIP

Supportive leadership behavior is typically more effective when team members perceive their jobs as tedious, undesirable, stressful, or in any way unpleasant. As the leader attempts to make the job more tolerable, he or she can directly affect the level of employee satisfaction and possibly even increase the desirability of the work. Once the work begins to be perceived as interesting and enjoyable, however, the maintenance of supportive behavior may not continue to increase the level of job satisfaction or motivation and may not even be able to sustain it at a given level. Also, when a team member has a relatively high level of self-esteem or little fear of failure, supportive leadership may have little or no effect on the person's motivation.

DIRECTIVE LEADERSHIP

Directive leadership behavior reduces uncertainty regarding the role of the staff in a specific set of circumstances provided staff do not have previous experience with that particular situation. When they do have such experience, engaging in directive behavior will lead to an increase in dissatisfaction. When staff are inexperienced, however, the use of directive leadership can eliminate many of the questions that might otherwise remain unanswered and thus increase the level of satisfaction. For example, when the nurse manager takes the time to explain the relationship between performance and rewards to a group of new nurses, performance levels and job satisfaction should increase. If the nurse manager repeats the same presentation to a group of experienced nurses, however, performance and overall satisfaction in the group may decrease.

In addition, nurse managers who practice directive leadership can affect the desirability of outcomes among staff members by manipulating the magnitude of rewards and punishments and linking them directly to task success. The measure of success here, however, will be directly proportional to the degree of control the nurse manager has over specific rewards and punishments. The characteristics of the given situation also have a strong influence on whether or not directive leadership increases staff motivation and satisfaction.

ACHIEVEMENT-ORIENTED LEADERSHIP

The behaviors that comprise achievement-oriented leadership increase staff members' confidence in their ability to achieve challenging goals. The higher a goal is set, as long as it is perceived as realistic and attainable, the higher the level of performance will be, even if the goal is not always attained. What this means is that the simple act of setting a goal is both an expression of confidence in subordinates' ability and a viable method of increasing employee motivation. This is especially evident when the task is non-repetitive and even somewhat ambiguous (i.e., relatively unstructured).

PARTICIPATIVE LEADERSHIP

Participative leadership behavior is generally most effective when employees' tasks are unstructured. Working toward attainment of the task and participating in the decision-making process, especially when it concerns setting goals and developing plans and strategies to attain those goals, provides staff nurses with an opportunity to learn something about an unfamiliar requirement. Such participation directly affects employees' understanding of what has to be done and how they must go about accomplishing it, and this enhances individuals' confidence levels.

Typically, staff members who have records of high achievement and who enjoy a good deal of autonomy respond more favorably to participative leadership than do staff members who have less desire for achievement and autonomy and prefer structured tasks in which they have little responsibility for decision-making. In fact, the latter type of individual may find participation intimidating and disagreeable, will respond with lower levels of individual job satisfaction, and may become a source of problems for the nurse manager.

● ● ●

In summary, the effect of specific leadership behaviors on levels of employee satisfaction and motivation is directly related to the situation in which these behaviors are used (particularly the degree of task structure) and the unique characteristics of employee in the unit.

The need to focus on nurse managers' behaviors to improve staff performance was supported by research conducted by R. L. Jenkins and R. L. Henderson in the early 1980s.[12] Their research centered on how staff nurses, who perform the bulk of patient care, perceived the behaviors of charge nurses. They concluded that, when a nurse manager's behavior showed respect for the staff's needs for belonging, love, social activity, self-respect, status within the organization, recognition, dignity, and appreciation, high levels of individual motivation and a high quality of patient care were achieved.

How useful is the path-goal theory of leadership? The question is difficult to answer with any degree of certainty, because the majority of studies testing this theory have had conceptual or methodologic flaws. In addition, the theory itself is quite complex, and the definitions provided for the four categories of leadership behavior are very broad and otherwise less than perfect. The structure of any given assignment depends not only on the task itself but on the manner in which it is introduced to the employee and the degree of preparation needed for task accomplishment, which adds to the complexity of the problem.

Many nursing tasks are highly structured; however, many aspects of nursing (e.g., patient relations, orientation of new staff members, some special projects) are relatively free of structure. Therefore, it is virtually impossible to prescribe a specific leadership behavior that will be more successful than others for a given combination of task and employee. In short, there is no substitute for the exercise of common sense and the judicious application of basic motivation and leadership principles on the part of the nurse manager. Leadership is difficult to accomplish because it is hard to identify clearly. The best advice is to follow the three principles emphasized previously.

1. Elicit cooperation; don't demand it.
2. Listen effectively to what is being said and what is not being said.
3. Place the needs of others before your own; make sure you never do something or expect something from a staff member out of a quest for personal gain.

The Normative Model of Decision Participation

Researchers V. H. Vroom and P. W. Yetton provided a workable model for determining the optimal amount of participation in decision-making for different situations.[13] In essence, the model these researchers developed helps the individual manager "decide how to make a decision." The model examines the following two characteristics of the decision process that determine the effectiveness of the decision:

1. The character or quality of the decision and its rationale
2. The potential for acceptance by the individual members of a team and the willingness of a subordinate to commit his or her energy to execute the decision effectively

In their research, Vroom and Yetton found the following to be true:

1. Managers can and do make decisions with varying degrees of participation by subordinates.
2. The amount of participation that occurs depends on whether or not staff members' acceptance of the decision will be required to implement it effectively and whether or not the manager had all of the information necessary to make a quality decision at the time it was rendered.

Fig. 9-2 presents a matrix based on these ideas that the nurse manager can use in deciding whether to allow staff to participate in the decision-making process and what degree of participation might be appropriate.

Participation in the decision-making process is not an all-or-none proposition; participation can be implemented to varying degrees and by managers who employ many different leadership styles. For instance, nurse managers may take any of the following approaches:

Delegate: Give the decision authority to those at a staff meeting and agree to live with their decision.

Join: Grant the decision authority to those at a staff meeting and participate actively in the meeting as an "equal" member.

Consult: Meet with members of the staff on an individual basis or in a group, make the decision, and then inform the staff.

Sell: Make the decision without involving the staff and then "sell" it to the group.

Tell: Make the decision and then inform the group as a matter of fact.

It is easy to see how the effectiveness of each of these approaches may differ depending on the type of decision being made. Fig. 9-3 is a decision tree designed to assist nurse managers in deciding when to use each approach in making leadership decisions.

Combination of Situational Characteristics

	Yes	No
Yes	Use some participation	Participation absolutely required
No	Need no participation	Use some participation

(vertical axis label: Staff Member's Acceptance Needed to Effectively Implement)

Fig. 9-2 ■ Decision matrix for determining the degree of staff participation in decision-making.

Nurse managers must ask themselves the following three basic questions when deciding whether or not to involve their staffs in the decision-making process:

1. Is all of the information required make the correct decision present?
2. Is acceptance of the decision by the staff necessary to ensure effective implementation?
3. If the choice is made to delegate the decision, is there sufficient reason to believe that the staff will render a decision that can be lived with?

Fig. 9-3 also indicates how time affects the selection of an approach. Rather obviously, the approaches that involve less staff participation require less of the manager's time per decision.

The following is an example of how Fig. 9-3 can be applied:

Ms. Nelson is the nurse manager of the neurologic intensive care center and is interested in changing her unit from the team nursing system to the primary care system. She has garnered the support of the administration and now must consider her staff's reactions. Fig. 9-3 can be used to help her work through the following three questions:

1. Do I posses the information necessary to make the decision?
   Ms. Jones decides that the answer to this is no; she still needs to know what staffing patterns will be required and how that will affect personnel costs.
2. Is acceptance by the team necessary to ensure effective implementation?
   In this case, the answer is obviously yes.
3. If the decision is delegated, will the team make one that can be lived with?
   Regardless of whether Ms. Jones decides that the answer to this question is yes or no, she remains ultimately responsible for the outcome of such a major change. However, if she feels that the team cannot render a decision the unit can live with, she may be compelled to make the final decision on her own or at least after consulting with key members of the staff.

According to Fig. 9-3, the leadership style to use in this case is either sell or consult. Ms. Jones can mount a campaign to convince her staff that primary nursing will have many benefits and gain their acceptance (i.e., sell) or she can continue to gather information on staffing, costs, and other possible consequences to the unit and the hospital and engage in discussions with

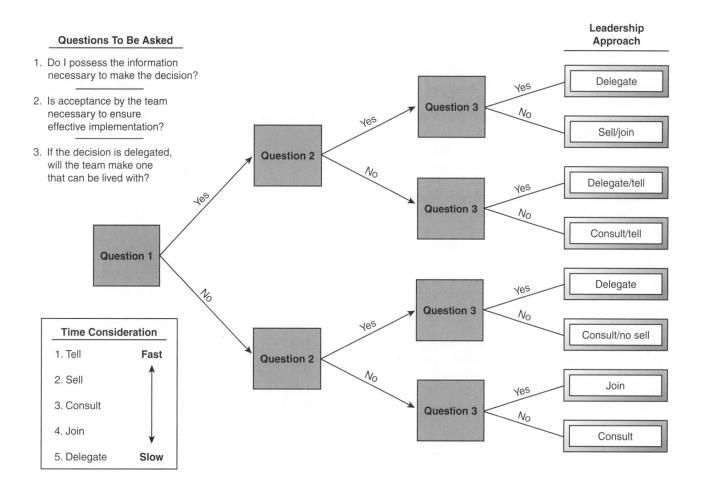

Fig. 9-3 ■ Decision tree for selecting an appropriate leadership approach.

the staff regarding the pros and cons of implementing primary nursing, ask for their recommendations, and then make the decision (i.e., consult).

A SOCIAL LEARNING APPROACH TO LEADERSHIP

Social learning theory recognizes the fact that, although formal education is certainly an effective way human beings learn what to do in various situations, most of what people learn throughout life does not come from formal classroom training or even on-the-job coaching. In fact, the average 2- or 3-year-old child, who has never attended a day of formal training, has leaned an incredible number of different behaviors, largely without the benefit of formal parental assistance. Rather, the child has learned these behaviors by observing different models (e.g., parents, siblings, television personalities) and then rehearsing the behaviors either covertly or overtly until they can be performed well. The age-old expression, "Out of the mouth of babes..." recognizes the fact that children practice their developing behaviors without having yet fully learned why these actions are done or when to do them. The point is that social learning begins at a very early age (even before birth, many professionals believe) and continues throughout life. Although various behaviors are learned, however, most of them cannot be performed effectively unless they are reinforced through practice.

For example, participating in a course on how to become an effective nurse manager or, more specifically, studying this chapter on leadership skills, will not make anyone an effective nurse manager or a leader. Students may well have the knowledge of what to do and the intelligence to be able to do it, but unless their educational experience is reinforced by practice and practical experience, their actual performance capability will be minimal. Being well educated does not necessarily make a person capable. Much can be learned about being a nurse manager, both what to do and what not to do, by observing nurse managers in other units, but even that will not prepare a person sufficiently to become one. In short, although this textbook will provide you with considerable information about being a nurse manager, none of it will truly be yours until you actually combine it with practical experience. Only the combination of education (stimulus) and performance (practical application) can change behavior (how something is done).

How can nurse managers use what social learning theory has to offer them in developing their ability to manage and supervise nursing units with professional and nonprofessional staff? Consider this: Nurse managers are very visible and serve as very important role models for the staff members whom they lead. If they feel it is important for the staff to be able to accomplish a particular task, then they should use their expertise by acting as practical and knowledgeable models; that is, they should demonstrate a procedure's relevant behaviors by showing the right way to do the task. As they progress through the procedure, they should point out the challenges and demonstrate the practical experience they have gained. Once they have demonstrated the correct procedure several times, they should ask each of their staff nurses to perform the task. As each nurse moves through the procedure, he or she should provide encouraging and appropriate feedback and guidance, keeping it as positive as possible, even if a mistake is made. The more nurse managers can involve other nurses in the actual training, especially in the feedback and social support necessary to assist the learning process, the more effective training becomes.

What about those situations that cannot really be classified as training? How do nurse managers deal with them? What about the nontechnical behaviors that are critical to successful nursing performance? What about teaching the staff the importance of arriving for work on time, or even a few minutes early, to allow time for reports to be compiled without inconveniencing the departing shift? What about the professional responsibility of maintaining a spirit of cooperation, sensitivity, and tact when dealing with other members of the team, different units, doctors, and patients? Remember that nurse managers are role models and that the behavior they exhibit always serves as a guide for the behavior of others. By being conscious of what it is that they actually do and how and when they do it, they can become more proficient at diagnosing the successes and failures of staff members.

When a member of a unit does not fulfill his or her responsibilities according to the manager's expectations or organizational standards, the manager should take the time to ask himself or herself whether he or she has engaged in the appropriate behaviors, as expected of a role model. If the manager is sure that this has been done, then the manager should simply draw attention to the appropriate behavior and gently but firmly remind the errant subordinate of what is expected. Part of correcting a situation is making sure that a subordinate never departs a counseling session without the nurse manager's taking the time to reinforce the positive things that the staff member is doing; this will help soften the corrective actions and can be instrumental in returning the employee to the work environment with a positive outlook. A good nurse manager never underestimates the power of balancing reprimands with appropriate praise when he or she deals with staff members.

If, on the other hand, a nurse manager's analysis indicates that his or her behavior as a role model has been less than expected, even deficient, it might be practical to acknowledge the deficiency to subordinates and explain the importance of behaving in the appropriate manner and his or her intention to do so in the future. This requires courage and timing. Having the courage to face one's deficiencies is tough enough, but when they must be acknowledged in front of others the task is even more difficult. Timing is important. It is never really appropriate to call a meeting to confess shortcomings. Instead, things like this should be done when a learning event can be created. For example, when a staff nurse fails to demonstrate a desired behavior, it might be time to share with him or her the fact that others have problems with the same behavior and offer a plan for improving performance. If a change in behavior can be accomplished, the new approach will be noticed by the staff and, in most instances, emulated.

PYGMALION EFFECT

The *Pygmalion effect* was named as a tribute to George Bernard Shaw's play of the same name, which was popularized in the Broadway musical *My Fair Lady*.[14] The term refers to what is known as a *self-fulfilling prophecy,* in which an individual or a situation becomes what one expects it will be. In *My Fair Lady,* the professor envisioned the poor, illiterate flower girl as an enlightened duchess, which, in typical Broadway style, she eventually became. The magic of Hollywood aside, this phenomenon has been demonstrated in real life to be both subtle and profound.

For example, a sample of elementary schoolchildren was tested at the beginning of the school year and the children were paired on the basis of measured intelligence quotients (IQs).[14] Within each pair with similar IQs, one child was randomly assigned to a "high expectation" group and the other was assigned to a "low expectation" group. The fact that the students in each pair possessed identical IQs was not shared. In fact, their classroom teachers were told only of the high or low performance expectations for each student in the coming year. The teachers were instructed to make every attempt to treat each child as an individual, and each gave the students the attention and training required for development based on their expectations about each child's potential for improvement.

At the end of the school year, each child's IQ was again determined. The IQs of the children who were fortunate enough to be in the high expectation group had increased significantly above those of the children who were in the low expectation group. How and in what subtle ways the teachers' expectations were reflected in intelligence scores at the end of the school year is unknown, but the fact is that teachers' expectations produced differences in the children's test-taking behavior.

It is fairly easy to understand how a self-fulfilling prophecy can affect human beings, who have a high capacity for perceiving and interpreting the responses of others around them. The power of this effect, however, was even more apparent in a study in which graduate students conducted research using laboratory rats.[14] The students were told that the rats had been bred either for faster learning (smart) or slower learning (dull). In reality, however, the rats were litter mates, born of the same mother and reared in exactly the same environment. The only difference lay in what the graduate students were told about the expectations for each group.

The students trained their rats to learn a succession of left and right turns to traverse a standard laboratory maze. The "dull" rats were given the same number of opportunities to learn the maze as the "smart" group. The results showed that the rats in the "smart" group learned the correct sequence of turns significantly faster than did those in the "dull" group.

How the graduate students conveyed their expectations to the rats in each group in unknown. Obviously, the behavior of the researchers was very subtle and could not have involved formal language as cues or hints regarding their expectations. Nevertheless, the behavior of the two groups of rats was distinctly different, which illustrates the very potent effect of expectations.

The Pygmalion effect is closely related to social learning, in which behaviors are observed and learned vicariously. Study of the phenomenon has repeatedly demonstrated that not only modeled behaviors but attitudes are learned. Applying the findings described to the healthcare environment, one might conclude, "If these attitudes can easily be learned by an animal as simple-minded as a rat, then how easy must it be for intelligent, well-educated professionals such as staff nurses to perceive and respond to them?"

How might a nurse manager's expectations be reflected in the motivation and performance of staff nurses? For one thing, there is little chance that staff nurses will perform well if they perceive or believe that the nurse manager thinks they are incapable of accomplishing an assigned task. In the nursing unit, as everywhere else in life, it is extremely difficult for most people to hide their true feelings and expectations, and thus it is equally easy for others to see these beliefs and expectations. If a nurse manager does not think a staff nurse can accomplish an assigned task, then there is every reason to believe that the nurse will know. This makes assigning the task to that particular individual irresponsible, because the task will almost always prove to be too difficult. The key to successfully managing others is to maintain *realistic expectations* about another's individual ability; that is, to expect a performance that is challenging but that is also attainable for that specific individual. In dealing with staff members as a nurse manager, one must always project a positive attitude. All thoughts and actions must convincingly convey to a staff member the attitude, "I *expect* you to be what you *can* be."

Shaping of behavior, which is discussed at length in Chapter 25, is the selective reinforcement of behaviors that are successively closer approximations to the desired behavior. A key factor in this process, just as in the Pygmalion effect, is to have realistic expectations regarding the degree of approximate behavior to be achieved while maintaining a conscious effort to nurture the actual behavior desired. In short, it is not good management, and it is bad leadership, to accept "close" as good enough; only "acceptable" or better should be considered good enough. The nurse manager also must never forget that what is good enough today may not even be close to what will be good enough 2 weeks from now, or what might be good enough under different circumstances or when dealing with another patient. This is true because every realistic expectation can realistically change. Also, professional nurse managers understand that if an expectation is truly realistic, then it is never unattainable. To be realistic, an expectation must be sufficiently difficult to challenge the performer and must be supported by coaching and positive expressions of confidence in the subordinate's ability to achieve success.

How does the true professional nurse manager accomplish this? Personal example is certainly one way. Also, competent nurse managers know that achievement-oriented leadership behavior stresses the attainment of challenging goals and that directive and/or participative leadership behaviors require that the nurse manager not only clarify what the staff nurse is to do but also ensure that he or she understands how to do it. Modeling is an excellent way to facilitate this kind of learning, as has been stated earlier. Finally, supportive leadership behavior can be used to express pleasure with the subordinate's success and, at the same time, reinforce the subordinate's willingness to accomplish the task again.

In the final analysis, the successes achieved by subordinates will be their nurse managers' successes as well. If nurse managers take pride in their staffs and do everything within their power to bring about success, then they will indeed be effective leaders. Keep in mind that one's true beliefs and attitudes do not have to be expressed to have impact, because they can be heard loud and clear through one's subtle and even unintended behaviors. If leaders form realistic expectations and provide genuine assistance to develop their employees' performance, the chance that their units—and themselves, for that matter—will be enhanced is vastly improved.

DEMONSTRATING LEADERSHIP IN THE GROUP

Nursing in a hospital environment, in its simplest form, is a continual problem-solving and interactive group task. Because members of the nursing staff work in close proximity and frequently depend upon one another to accomplish their work, the quality of the environment in which group interaction occurs is extremely important. An example of an excellent performance atmosphere is one in which all staff members feel free discuss those things that concern them, to critique and offer suggestions, and to experiment with new behaviors without threat of reprisal. This type of environment can be sustained only when the work group is open, supportive, and relatively free of interpersonal conflicts and political infighting. Maintaining such an atmosphere is a difficult task and a major responsibility for all nurse managers.

To develop a clear understanding of this leadership task, one must first consider exactly what is meant by the term *group,* how and why groups are formed, and what factors influence their effectiveness.

What Is a Group?

A group might be defined in a number of different ways. For example, consider the following descriptions offered by R. M. Steers in his book *Introduction to Organizational Behavior*[15]:

Perception: If two or more individuals see themselves as a group, then a group exists.

Structure: If two or more individuals interact in a manner that allows them to cooperate in the performance of a task, have a set of formal or informal role relationships, and have norms that govern their behavior, then a group exists.

Motivation: If there is a gathering of people whose presence is rewarding to each individual, then a group exists.

Interpersonal interaction: If several individuals communicate and interact with one another regularly over time, then a group exists.

These concepts can be integrated into the following definition:

A group is two or more individuals who, over time, share a set of norms, have specific role relationships, and interact with each other to pursue common goals.

Group Formation

The two primary types of group are the following:

1. *Informal:* groups that evolve naturally as a result of individuals' self-interest and are not part of any organizational design or appointed structure; an example is a group of people who regularly who eat lunch together
2. *Formal:* work units developed by the organization, regardless of whether they are temporary or permanent, such as sections, departments, and committees

It is not uncommon for informal groups to form and work both in support of and in conflict with formally established groups. In fact, most individuals are simultaneously members of many formal and informal groups both in and out of the organization that employs them.

People join groups for many reasons, including the following:

Security: People form groups to obtain protection from threats and other forms of protective support.

Proximity: People often come together because they are located close to one another.

Goal advancement: People form groups to pursue goals that cannot or should not be achieved alone (the idea of strength in numbers).

Economics: People join together to pursue economic self-interest (e.g., collective bargaining organizations).

Social benefits: People form groups because they want a sense of belonging, because they want to be needed, or because they want to lead or be a part of something they feel is important.

Self-esteem: People often join prestigious groups to increase their sense of personal worth.

Finally, as groups arise, they typically progress through the following steps:

Formation: Participants come together.

Development: Participants establish leaders and roles.

Creation: Participants adopt goals and rules for acceptable behavior.

Performance: Participants agree on basic purposes and activities and perform some sort of work.

Group Effectiveness

Many factors determine a group's effectiveness after it emerges or is formed by an organization.

TASK

The task provided to or created by a group can influence the group's effectiveness because it affects the motivation of individual members and because the nature of the task imposes certain requirements or processes. For example, if the task to be performed is tedious, inefficiently designed, or undesirable, or does not satisfy members' needs (such as the needs for independence, feedback, or significance), each group member's effort will decrease to the degree that he or she is influenced by it.

Typically, the more people who are involved in an *additive* task (one in which group performance is the sum of individual performances), the greater the resources that can be devoted to achieving it. With a *disjunctive* task (one in which the group succeeds if only one member succeeds), the addition of more people increases the likelihood that someone in the group will be able to solve the problem. With a *divisible* task (a task with a division of labor), the presence of more people increases the likelihood of and opportunity for specialization. When a group is given a *conjunctive* task, however (the group succeeds only if all members succeed), the presence of additional people increases the likelihood that the success of the group will be limited by a single member. Thus, it is easy to see how group productivity often depends on the size of the group and the task it was formed to accomplish.

When the group is given a divisible task, the level of interdependence in the group is important. For the purposes of this discussion, three kinds of interdependence are identified, as follows:

1. *Pooled:* Individual members of the team contribute, but none is dependent on any other member. A good example is a committee.
2. *Sequential:* Each member of the group must coordinate his or her activities with the members to each side, above, and/or below him or her. This form of activity is classically demonstrated in a production assembly line.
3. *Reciprocal:* Each member must coordinate his or her individual activities with every other individual in the group. Any sports team provides an example.

GROUP SIZE

Although in most cases increasing the number of people in a group will increase productivity, on least in some occasions a phenomenon called *social loafing* can occur. Social loafing is seen when the size of a group increases and each individual member is required to contribute less of his or her potential. In addition, an excessively large group size is often associated with low satisfaction, higher absenteeism, and greater turnover.

GROUP COMPOSITION

Group performance normally is directly proportional to the sum of the capabilities and contributions of the members. However, coordination of effort, proper utilization of abilities, appropriate task strategies, and harmony in the group also play a significant part in determining what a group can actually produce. For example, homogeneous groups (groups with members of similar backgrounds and/or interests) tend to function more far more harmoniously than do heterogeneous groups, which are often plagued by internal conflict.

Homogeneity is not always a characteristic to strive for when constructing a group, however, because it also carries significant risks, such as a tendency for the individual members to fall into what has come to be known as *groupthink*—a failure to explore alternative approaches or ways of thinking because the majority of the group thinks in a certain manner. Another disadvantage is the fact that homogeneous groups tend to show large redundancies in specific strengths and weaknesses. Because the members of the group come from similar backgrounds and share other characteristics, they also tend to do things similarly. This is an especially difficult situation when the group has been formed to deal with change.

GROUP COMMUNICATION

Who actually interacts with whom is an essential consideration when forming a group. Closed groups (i.e., those in which members rarely interact with individuals from outside of the group) typically are not as creative as open groups. It is also important to ensure that the interactive patterns formed in a group relate to the task before it. One of the best ways to accomplish this is to maintain open communication in the group, because this tends to enhance performance, especially when complex or uncertain tasks are involved.

Research has revealed the following important considerations relating to communications among group members[1,16]:

Leadership is derived from central positioning: Group leadership is most likely to arise from among those individuals who have key roles in the communication network developed within the group. Those in central positions frequently have more information available to them and, as a consequence, are perceived to be more capable.

A correlation exists between position and participation: An individual's feeling of participation is directly related to his or her position in the communication network of the group. If an individual feels left out of the loop, the willingness to participate quickly wanes.

Positioning affects outcome: Groups within over-centralized communication networks are generally far more effective in implementing tasks than they are in developing new strategies. These centralized groups have a tendency to maintain the established direction and are usually not comfortable developing their own sense of purpose.

Too many cooks spoil the soup: Information is lost or distorted if it must travel through too many people.

REWARD STRUCTURE

American organizations are prone to reward individuals rather than groups, but competitive or individualistic reward systems can be destructive in groups in which members must cooperate to achieve success. The group as a whole must rewarded for the efforts of the group, or the group will deteriorate as a result of internal struggles over the correlation between reward and level of effort.

GROUP COHESIVENESS

The ability of group members to combine their efforts toward a common goal is directly proportional to the extent to which members of the group are motivated to remain in the group. Members of highly cohesive groups tend to put more effort into group activities, are more satisfied, are absent less, and are more influenced by group goals. Group cohesiveness can be increased by several means, including the following:

- Making admission to the group difficult
- Ensuring that rewards are presented to the group as a unit
- Increasing the status of the group
- Encouraging member participation in goal identification
- Increasing the frequency of interactions
- Developing trust among the members of the group

Traditionally, healthcare organizations have used many of these means to increase organizational cohesiveness, especially in the groups formed by professional care givers.

Group Norms

Norms are those expectations developed and shared by the members of a group that define the proper conduct and attitude for the group. Norms play an important part in the overall success of a group because they provide a means for an individual member to predict the behavior of other members in specific circumstances. In addition, norms serve as standards for determining expectations and for judging the individual behaviors of group members. Those members who deviate from established group norms are likely to find overt and covert pressure brought to bear to ensure conformity. The key for nurse managers in developing group norms is to match them to the level of work effort required of the members. If the established norms conform to organizational goals, the group will be perceived as being effective.

Groups are viewed as most effective when the following apply:

- The members want to belong to the group.
- Group size, heterogeneity, and structure match the task to be accomplished.
- Norms and goals of the group support established unit and organizational goals.
- Individual members trust one another.
- Group members are motivated to communicate openly and cooperate with one another.
- The group is rewarded for goal attainment.
- Social loafing is discouraged and, if discovered, effectively reduced.

Groups have traditionally been successful in solving many problems that were considered insurmountable by even the most highly qualified individuals because they bring diverse expertise to bear and are far more likely to take risks and be creative in devising solutions and outcomes than are individuals. The formation of a group is not always the road to success, however, because many engage in groupthink or diffuse responsibility (i.e., groups tend to be less responsible than individuals). Groups do not offer a universal solution to all problems, but they can be used effectively and dynamically to solve the problems encountered in many situations. To ensure the effectiveness of a group, nurse managers must have some understanding of group dynamics.

Intergroup Conflict

It is a rare group that does not have to interact with other groups or other parts of the organization. Because this is so, the development of effective intergroup relations is an important element in the success of organizations. An organization must promote good coordination among its groups in order to be productive, yet it is very common for different groups to develop rivalries and open animosity. The primary reason is that one group is commonly pitted against another (i.e., the groups must compete for rewards, status, resources, and privileges).[17] The following behavior is frequently observed in groups in competition:

Within the competing groups
- Group cohesion increases.
- Members become more task oriented.
- Authority becomes more centralized.
- Activities become more organized.

Between competing groups
- Other groups are viewed as adversaries.
- The strengths of one's own group tend to be overestimated and the strengths of opposing groups tend to be underestimated.
- Communication between competing groups decreases.
- When one group is forced into interaction with a competing group, only those things that reinforce the original predisposition toward the other group are heard.

According to E. H. Schein,[17] there are two approaches to managing intergroup conflict: (a) deal with the competition as soon as possible after it occurs, and (b) take constructive action that prevents its occurrence in the first place.

Strategies for minimizing ongoing competition between groups include the following:

- Identify a common adversary that all groups can focus on.
- Appeal to a goal that can be supported by all groups.
- Bring representatives of the competing groups into direct contact with one another on a repetitive basis and ensure that they understand that individual success is contingent on organizational success.
- Train members of the competing groups to understand the negative potential of conflict with the intent of minimizing it.

Actions to be taken to prevent intergroup conflict include the following:

- Base rewards for the groups on their contributions to the organization and its overall success.
- Make part of the reward system available only to those groups that cooperate with other groups.
- Ensure frequent interaction between members of various groups.
- Make plans to reduce isolation and withdrawal of groups from other groups.
- Rotate members between groups.
- Avoid situations of lose-lose or win-lose competition between groups.
- Emphasize the sharing of resources among groups.

Conferences and Committees

Almost all nurse managers actively participate in both formal and informal groups. Formal groups include such entities as conferences and committees, whereas informal groups are those that occur whenever people gather for some period of interaction. Conferences are usually one-time affairs, held for a limited time and a specific purpose, such as to deal with a certain patient's problem, whereas committees may have an ongoing assigned task. All of these groups can be classified in relation to their purpose, membership, and leadership. Table 9-1 lists various types of conferences and their purposes. The purpose usually determines the members and the leader. For example, a nurse manager might call a report conference to request an update from staff members regarding the effectiveness of a new staffing procedure.

Committees are almost always semipermanent groups that enjoy institutional or organizational approval. They are usually formed to coordinate the efforts toward a specific goal, most have some mechanism for selecting members, and virtually all of them have the authority to make recommendations or decisions. Committees are usually formed when the input of a variety of people is necessary for information gathering and decision-making, and when having representation from several units in the organization might be beneficial to implementing the decisions that are made. Assignment of a given task to one or two individuals rather than to a committee may be preferable, however, if the task is complex and requires a high degree of coordination. According to Vroom and Yetton,[13] whose work was discussed previously in this chapter, the decision to use groups is based on the quality of the required decision, the need for acceptance of the decision by subordinates, and the time available to make the decision. The advantages of assigning tasks to groups and to individuals are shown in Table 9-2. The structure of the organization, the nature of the task, and the preferences of the manager and other administrators influence the choice to assign certain tasks or decisions to committees or to individuals.

Prudent nursing managers carefully weigh the disadvantages of using a committee against its advantages. Assigning a task to a committee is generally far more expensive for both the unit and the organization when one factors in the hourly pay of the members, preparation time, secretarial help for taking minutes, and other administrative tasks such as making calls or writing memos reminding members of the time and place of meetings. These disadvantages must be weighed against the benefits of group input and participative decision-making as well as other advantages before a committee is organized for problem solving.

A number of group characteristics influence the nature and effectiveness of communication in small groups. First, the past experiences of the members; their current relationships, both individually and as a group; and the expectations and preconceptions they have of each other influence the communication patterns they use. The structure of the group also imposes certain patterns of interaction. If a committee member's supervisor is chairperson of the committee, for instance, that individual will almost always interact with the chairman in the same pattern used by the two in their superior-subordinate relationship. Time and place are also determinants of communication. When and where meetings are scheduled may facilitate or hinder participation by specific members. A final consideration is the expertise of each member in relation to the assigned task. All of these factors

---

TABLE 9-1

Types of Nursing Conferences and Their Purposes

Type of Conference	Purpose
Direction giving	Provide job assignments
	Provide patient care information
	Outline specific areas of responsibility
Patient centered	Analyze a specific patient's problem
	Discuss alternative solutions
	Develop a plan to implement solutions
Content	Learn new information related to the nursing profession
Report	Inform leader about member activities
General problem	Discuss problems such as communication difficulties that might exist among group members

---

TABLE 9-2

Advantages of Task Assignment to Groups versus Individuals

Assignment to Group	Assignment to Individual
Effective use of resources and opinions	Reduction of pressure toward conformity
Rapid response to errors	Encouragement of individual initiative and performance
Increase in member motivation	Centralization of responsibility and motivation
Increase in acceptance of group decisions	Faster problem solving and decision-making

must be considered and weighed against what might be gained before organizing a committee.

It is also important to understand that each member of the group may behave in a different manner toward the group. For example, each member of a group may be positive, negative, or neutral in his or her attitude toward the group's goals. Members may contribute very little or they may use the group only to fulfill personal needs. Some members may assume most of the responsibility for the group's actions, thereby "helping" less participative individuals to be noncontributing members. Ensuring that all group participants do the following can facilitate the group's activities:

- Come to the meetings prepared with the necessary information.
- Make it a policy to listen to other members with an open mind.
- Request clarification of information if something is not understood.
- Stimulate action by asking other members for their ideas and opinions.
- Make sure that all remarks are focused on the topic—avoid personal comments, especially if they malign other members or other groups.
- Recognize opposing points of view and avoid ridiculing or belittling them.
- Encourage all other members actively to contribute information, ideas, and opinions.
- Be willing to openly disagree and make sure that when disagreement occurs a rationale for the disagreement is given.
- When appropriate, volunteer to help with the implementation of decisions and encourage other members to do so.

The behaviors demonstrated by the group's leader can facilitate group communication and movement toward acceptable decisions. Facilitative leaders do the following:

- Establish an atmosphere that promotes participation and cohesiveness.
- Encourage active participation by all members.
- Keep the group focused on the task assigned.
- Do not allow one person to dominate the group.
- Focus the discussions on one topic at a time.
- Allow persons with dissenting opinions to explain their points of view.
- Summarize discussion and ask the group to arrive at a decision.
- Determine a plan of action for implementing any decision reached.
- Request arrangements for follow-up and ask for volunteers to handle it.

As in one-on-one interactions, nurse managers can use their participation in a group, as either leaders or members, to effectively perform all of the tasks of management, including motivation, training, and conflict resolution. However, nurse managers' skills may be severely challenged in group interactions. Managers must make sure that they attend to individual interactions in the group as well as stay focused on the group process.

GROUP MEETINGS

In their 1980 book *Management Strategies for Women*,[18] A. M. Thompson and M. D. Wood described a meeting as a "play calling for a script, preparation of the actors, and a competent director to insure a successful performance" (p. 37). They summarized the contributions of the various components as follows:

The director: Also known as the *chairperson*, this is the individual who is responsible for planning the meeting, preparing the agenda, directing the meeting, and following up any plans that have been made.

The script: Also referred to as *the agenda*, this premeeting document is critical in determining the effectiveness of the group's activities. Thompson and Wood provided the following guidelines for agenda preparation:

- If it can go in a memo, it should not be put on the agenda.
- The chairperson should have a clear purpose behind every meeting he or she holds and behind every item on the agenda.
- Every item on the agenda should require some kind of action by the group.

The chairperson should have an idea of the outcomes he or she expects to achieve in the meeting in terms of group discussion, plan of action, formation of smaller subgroups for specific purposes, or policy decisions to be reached. In addition, the chairperson should plan the agenda so that the meeting will move along and keep the participants involved. Careful planning, such as determining the order of priority of agenda items and their potential impact on the group, is essential to an effective meeting. Thompson and Wood also suggested sending out the agenda and all necessary materials a week prior to the meeting so that all participants can be prepared.

The performers: Otherwise known as the *group members*, these people are not part of an audience that has come to be entertained; they are the participants and should be expected to contribute. Their responsibilities are to come prepared, to respond to others' ideas and comments, and to make contributions in a clear, concise, logical manner.

The stage: Also known as the *meeting room*, this is where the meeting is to be held and where people sit. These seemingly unimportant aspects of a meeting appear at first glance to have no influence on what happens in the meeting and the outcomes it produces, but in fact they have a significant part to play. If, for example, conflict between participants is possible, and especially if one participant is a great deal more powerful than others, then the site chosen for the meeting should be in neutral territory.

The head of the table is the most powerful position and usually should be occupied by the chairperson. Those who sit on the sidelines may see themselves as being less important to the group's activities or may become adversaries. The seat at the foot of the table is a common spot for a potential adversary.

SUMMARY

- One of the responsibilities of a nurse manager is leadership—the use of specific behaviors and strategies to influence individuals and groups toward goal attainment in specific situations.
- Leadership differs from management, which is a broader concept encompassing planning, organizing, directing (supervising), and controlling. Leadership behavior can be learned.
- Leadership is the exercise of power. Power can come from several sources: control over rewards and punishments, control of information, authority given by the healthcare facility, expertise, and personal qualities that elicit respect and deference on the part of others.
- The search for leadership characteristics has focused on personality traits, leader behaviors, and leadership styles. None of these approaches has adequately defined successful leadership.
- Leadership styles include authoritarian, democratic, permissive, bureaucratic, mollifying, autocratic, parental, and multicratic.
- Fiedler took the study of leadership beyond the identification of styles and behaviors with his development of contingency theory. He maintained that successful leadership is an interaction of leadership style and situation.
- House and Mitchell developed the path-goal theory of leadership, which asserts that a leader is effective to the extent that he or she helps subordinates identify goals and paths to those goals.
- Vroom and Yetton provided a model of participative leadership that is prescriptive—it tells the nurse manager which style of leadership to use in different situations.
- Nurse managers must pay attention to the examples they provide to staff and their expectations of staff members. Both will influence staff behavior.
- Hospital nursing is a team effort. Nurse managers must develop an understanding of group communication and interpersonal relations and use that understanding to create a supportive climate that fosters group cohesiveness.
- Nurse managers interact in many group settings, including conferences and committees. Knowledge of group theory and group dynamics is critical.

FINAL THOUGHTS

Nurse managers, as the leaders of nursing units, must be more than simply the ones in charge. They must be able to reach out and draw forth the performance capabilities of every member of the unit through a combination of charisma, character, example, honesty, and objectivity.

Leadership is having the courage to stand in front of others and say, "I am responsible." In fact, leadership begins with the willingness to embrace responsibility. It is not enough simply to accept what is given; if a nurse manager is to be recognized as a leader, he or she must be willing to step forward and say, "I want to do that!"

With the acceptance of responsibility also comes accountability. Accountability means that the nurse manager is continually saying to others, "If things go wrong, I'm ultimately the reason why." If nurse managers cannot accept the responsibility for failure, they will never actually become leaders. If they look outward for an excuse instead of inward for a reason, they will have a very hard time earning the respect of others; and without that respect, they will find it extremely difficult to elicit cooperation—no matter what their title.

Leaders have the ability to inspire people to go beyond what they think they are capable of doing and thus make it possible for the group to achieve goals that were previously thought to be unattainable.

Leadership is about working with people and developing performance through the example of excellence. Leadership is not management, and the two are not always compatible. Leadership is not command. Command is the authority to lead. It is inherent in a position and focuses on the management of tasks, not the leadership of people. Command is the act of keeping the organization moving in the direction it is already headed, rather than finding out if another direction is needed.

Good leaders are generally likable individuals. They know how to get along with people—not just the people who follow them or admire them, but even those who have every reason to despise them. They do not rise to the bait of a fight with an enemy but search for common ground on which to build a compromise that can be viewed as a win-win solution by both camps. Leaders will never push an opponent until they are forced to respond.

The job of leaders is to offer opponents an opportunity to retreat at the place where their positions are least reasonable. Leaders never sacrifice the goals of the group in order to make a point.

THE NURSE MANAGER SPEAKS

Leadership is a temporary event in the life of the nurse manager. It starts at the beginning of every contact with another individual and ends with the other individual's perception of the manager's performance quality. In this regard, leadership can be aptly described by these words from *The Rubáiyát* of Omar Khayyám: "The moving finger writes; and having writ, moves on."

Leadership occurs because a need, a goal, and a person willing to accept responsibility intersect, and it often depends on the leader's being in the right place at the right time. Followers realize the temporary nature of leadership and will allow a chosen leader only so many opportunities to lead before they look elsewhere. Leadership is transient for the following two very good reasons:

1. *The situation that requires leadership may come to an end.* Leading is about helping others reach goals, and when those goals have been attained, there is no further need for it.
2. *Times and circumstances change.* Today's respected leader may be out of touch with the realities of tomorrow. Tomorrow's struggle may, in fact, be diametrically opposed to everything a leader stood for today.

It is foolish to believe that the staff will follow you just because you have been given the title of nurse manager. This is a mistake that has led to catastrophic results for many a manager. The right to lead is earned and reearned; it is never automatically given, nor is it part of any job description. When you hold the position of nurse manager, you can demand obedience, but the performance that results from such a demand will never reach the level attained when support is freely given. People perform best for those who value that performance the most. If you want results, provide inspiration, and the motivation will come from within the individual.

Leadership is the dynamic aspect of being in charge; management is nothing more than ensuring movement in the direction established by another.

REFERENCES

1. Stogdill RM: *Individual behavior and group achievement,* New York, 1959, Oxford University Press.
2. Moloney MM: *Leadership in nursing: theories, strategies, and action,* St Louis, 1979, Mosby.
3. French JRP, Raven B: The basis for social power. In French JRP, Raven B, editors: *Group dynamics,* ed 3, Evanston, Ill, 1996, Row, Peterson
4. Mitchell TR: *People in organizations,* ed 3, New York, 1998, McGraw-Hill.
5. Conger JA, Kanungo RN: *Charismatic leadership in organizations,* Thousand Oaks, Calif, 1998, Sage Publications.
6. Levenstein A: Do you want to be a leader?, *Nurs Manage* 16(3):74, 1985.
7. McGregor D: *The human side of enterprise,* annotated edition, New York, 2005, McGraw-Hill.
8. Schweiger DM: Participation in decision making. In Staw V, Kramer RM, editors: *Research in organizational behavior,* ed 2, Greenwich, Conn, 2003, JAI Press.
9. Loeb M, Kindel S: *Leadership for dummies,* Los Angeles, 1999, IDG Books.
10. Fiedler FE: *A theory of leadership effectiveness,* ed 3, New York, 1991, McGraw-Hill.
11. House RJ, Mitchell TR: Path-goal theory of leadership, *J Contemp Bus* 3(81):72, 1974.
12. Jenkins RL, Henderson RL: Motivating the staff: what nurses expect from their supervisors, *Nurs Manage* 15(2):13, 1984.
13. Vroom VH, Yetton PW: *Leadership in decision making,* ed 2, Pittsburgh, 1990, University of Pittsburgh Press.
14. Patton BR, Giffin K: *Interpersonal communication in action,* ed 2, New York, 1981, Harper and Row.
15. Steers RM: *Introduction to organizational behavior,* New York, 1991, HarperCollins.
16. Filley AC: *A note on current organization theory: a summary and analysis of Stogdill's theory of individual behavior and group achievement (Wisconsin project reports),* Madison, Wis, 1965, Bureau of Business Research and Service, School of Commerce, University of Wisconsin.
17. Schein EH: *Organizational psychology,* ed 3, Englewood Cliffs, NJ, 1979, Prentice-Hall.
18. Thompson AM, Wood MD: *Management strategies for women,* New York, 1980, Simon and Schuster.

SUGGESTED READINGS

Henderson RL: Path-goal theory of leadership, *J Contemp Bus* 3(81):11, 1974.
Hoffman G, Graivier P: *Speak the language of success,* ed 2, New York, 1997, Putnam.
LaMonica E: *Nursing leadership and management: an experimental approach,* Monterey, Calif, 1983, Wadsworth.
Marriner Tomey A: *Guide to nursing leadership and management,* ed 7, St Louis, 2004, Mosby.
McGee RF: Leadership styles, *Nurs Success Today* 1(2):26, 1984.
Melohn T: *The new partnership,* New York, 1996, Wiley.
Roberts W: *Leadership secrets of Attila the Hun,* New York, 1987, Warner.
Swansburg RC: *Management and leadership for nurse managers,* Sudbury, Mass, 1996, Jones and Bartlett.
Swansburg RC: *Introductory management and leadership for nurses,* Sudbury, Mass, 1999, Jones and Bartlett.

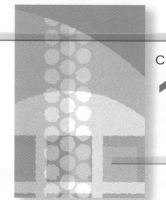

Time Management for Healthcare Managers

LEARNING SYNOPSIS

Upon successful completion of this chapter, readers will possess a fundamental understanding of how effective time management and delegation can enhance their own performance capabilities as well as those of the nursing unit staff.

OBJECTIVES

1. Describe methods for organizing personal performance
2. Identify potential and classic time wasters that affect the nurse manager and methods for controlling them
3. Explain scheduling and describe methods for accomplishing this vital task
4. Identify methods for handling paperwork in the nursing unit
5. Describe procedures and principles to follow in delegating work to the nursing staff and methods for following up and controlling their efforts

Most managers never seem to have enough time to get things done at the office. They work hard and put in long hours but often feel that they are not making headway. So they come in early, stay late, and work weekends, and when they finally get home, they are so worn out that they have no time or energy left for themselves or their families. The tried and true time management techniques that worked so well for them when they were employees simply don't work now. The world around the manager is so different, so unique, compared to that experienced when the manager was working as a member of the staff that those old methods are not enough.

Adding to the dilemma is the fact that the business world itself continues to evolve. For example, there used to be a time management principle which declared that a person should handle a piece of paper just once; if the individual could do that, it was said, he or she could certainly become more efficient. Today, we still have paper, and probably more of it than we used to have, but we also have electronic mail, voice mail, and a wide variety of wireless communications systems. We also have the Internet and an almost unlimited number of online services available to assist us. It often seems only a few moments ago that the world was revolutionized by the opportunity to send a letter via an overnight delivery service and have it reach its destination by early the next morning. Today, we just electronic mail or fax the letter directly from the computer on our desk to the computer in our customer's office and it takes but seconds to make the trip.

Not so long ago, the typical healthcare organization employed hundreds of secretaries and kept each of them busy typing memos, letters, and reports, and creating presentations. Back then, managers worried if their secretaries' typing speed fell below 60 words per minute. Today, most of those secretaries are gone, and in their places are incredibly fast personal computers that perform trillions of operations per second and give managers the capability to personally compose their own letters, memos, and presentations. Today we even have spell and grammar checkers to correct our mistakes automatically.

Thus, today's managers must do more than just get organized. They must do a better job of staying on top of unfinished work, tasks, and projects. Simply improving the systems used to follow up can do this. By using an efficient follow-up system, the modern manager can convert time that was previously spent in meetings and dictation into time that can be used to run the unit more efficiently, effectively, and productively. Jeffrey Mayer, in his book *Time Management for Dummies*,[1] called the process of converting wasted time into productive time "addition by subtraction." He

said that if people can eliminate the time they waste in nonproductive endeavors, more time will be available to spend on personal and professional things that are far more important. When time is managed effectively, managers might just be able to get their work done, leave the hospital at a reasonable hour, and find some time to spend in the pursuit of career advancement or leisure activities with family and friends.

Mayer was right on track. Work is not necessarily the same thing as performance. It doesn't become so until the person doing it stops measuring its effectiveness by volume and starts measuring it by impact. It is the quality of the work performed that is important, not the quantity. Most people, if asked what they do with their 8-, or 10-, or 12-hour days, would be hard-pressed to provide a good answer.

In the competitive world of the healthcare organization, working additional hours doesn't guarantee that the unit will prosper. Today, being successful is measured in productivity, efficiency, and profitability, not in total hours worked. As a matter of fact, the higher the number of hours worked in a day, the lower the productivity and efficiency of the individual as an hourly average. It could be argued that the key to success, then, is not longer hours but more productive and efficient ones. As a manager, one should be aware that it takes more than hours to become effective. The healthcare industry is filled to overflowing with people who put in long hours, but careful analysis of most of their work shows that they are not necessarily high-quality performers. In fact, continually recording extra-long working hours often is a smoke screen used by the truly mediocre performer. A prudent manager will examine the productivity of staff members putting in long hours before lauding them for their dedication, especially if they are being paid by the hour. One of the authors (J. A. Hawkins, president of JHawk & Associates, a Honolulu-based educational consultation corporation) has an interesting story about a long-hours worker[2]:

When I first started my business, I had an employee who seemed to always be at the office. I would come to the office before 7:00 AM, and she would be there, hard at work. When I would leave, often after 8:00 PM, she would still be there, calling out for me not to set the alarms.

Being a big believer in rewards for quality individuals, I researched this woman's performance and found her to be my very most productive employee. The amount of work that she was able to produce was nearly double what we received from her peers. So we promoted her along the internal advancement route until she was ready to become an officer of the company. After that promotion, she was made a salary-exempt employee, and no longer received pay for the overtime hours she worked.

What a change! The person who had met me each morning at 7:00 AM for over 2 years, with a smile and a desk full of work, was gone. In her place stood an individual who now dragged herself through the door at 8:00 AM. My late nights were now spent alone as my one-time, long-hours hustler now hit the bricks at 4:30 PM on the dot.

When I talked to her about the change, she told me, "Oh, I don't get paid for those hours now, so why should I work them?" (p 6-37)[2]

Many people simply don't know the difference between working hard and working well—between being busy and being productive. A point is reached in every person's work cycle at which the returns start to diminish. Once the person is past that point, the work produced per hour steadily decreases, and, even more alarming, the quality of the work is significantly reduced. Errors increase and sloppiness abounds. In today's hectic world of downsizing and ever-increasing workload, nurse managers must carefully gauge themselves and their staffs, so that all can effectively balance their work with their personal lives.

The term *time management* is actually a misnomer, because it is physically impossible for anyone to manage time. There are always going to be 60 seconds in a minute, 60 minutes in an hour, 24 hours in a day, and so on. That cannot be changed. What can be managed is how one uses the time that is available. To say that it is important to do this wisely is, without a doubt, one of the most inane statements ever uttered, because everyone knows that each of us is given just so much time to use. However, there are few people for whom the effective management of time is more important than for a manager.

The nurse manager, like all other managers, must use time wisely. The manager's workday may be broken into a variety of segments, the most common of which is the work shift, which is usually an 8-hour period that begins and ends with reports and is filled with an almost limitless variety of activities and events. Activities performed on a single shift include scheduling staff, conducting daily rounds, counseling patients' families, reading and responding to mail, training new staff members, writing incident reports, counseling subordinate employees, attending meetings, and a myriad of other activities of greater and lesser importance. In addition, the unexpected emergencies and crises that occur on some days must be absorbed into the manager's schedule, and the 8-hour shift often becomes a 10- to 12-hour workday.

Most nurse managers don't make the mistake of thinking of the work shift, or even the work week, strictly in terms of the activities and events that occur and onto which they must impose some sense of organization. They realize that very few shifts, and certainly extremely few longer work periods, will ever be normal. To compensate for the hectic environment in which they work and to meet the requirements under which they labor, effective nurse managers plan and schedule their work time to ensure that their most important work is completed and that sufficient time is available to deal with the inevitable emergencies and crises. Effective use of available time (time management) can ensure that these professionals achieve clearly measurable outcomes and still meet the challenges of the nursing unit. One of the most important reasons that success is achieved in nursing units is that professional nurse managers make sure their focus is on the outcomes that can be achieved in the allotted time and not on individual activities and events.

As everyone knows, time is nurse managers' most critical resource and the one of which they typically have the least. Behind all the concern for the effective use of this precious asset is the fact that if an hour or even a minute of the work shift is wasted, it is lost forever. Although managers can certainly increase the number of hours they put into the workday to complete some important tasks, time itself is not really affected. Working longer to complete required tasks is not time management, it is simply using more time.

The work carried out in nursing units is demanding, and nurse managers may become so overloaded with responsibilities that they have more to do than can possibly fit into the time available to them. This is so typical in healthcare organizations that it is considered by many to be normal. In fact, many nurse managers feel that there is never enough time to get involved in all the activities, situations, and events in which they would like to participate. Professional nurse managers know that they do not have the time to do everything they want to do but realize that there is always enough time to do the most important things. To ensure that time is available to complete these important tasks, nurse managers begin their planning and scheduling of the work shift by establishing priorities.

ORGANIZING PERSONAL PERFORMANCE

For the purposes of this chapter, *personal organization* is defined as what occurs when managers have developed clear priorities that are based on well-defined, measurable, and achievable objectives. In organizing themselves, nurse managers remember that they do not work alone but are one part of a professional team. Therefore, their priorities and objectives are always in harmony with those of the organization, are often coordinated with those of many other professionals, and are accord with the objectives of the unit's patients and their families. In fact, much of the time available to nurse managers is spent resolving conflicts among the needs of these competing groups.

Setting Priorities

Most nurse managers want to do more—or at least have more to do—than is actually possible given their time. In addition, those who influence the position of nurse manager may place more demands on the person filling it than can possibly be satisfied, regardless of how competent the nurse manager is. Therefore, one of the most important functions of the nurse manager's job is to determine exactly which of the demands placed on the nurse manager should be considered to have highest priority. This is fundamental to performing well because it ensures that the most important things being asked of the nurse manager are the ones that are accomplished first. The function of establishing priorities and its importance to the performance of the nurse manager can be better understood when the word *priority* is well defined. Most dictionaries provide two separate definitions, as follows:

1. That which is most important or most valuable
2. That which come first

Priorities cannot realistically be established unless both meanings are considered. To do this when there are several functions, activities, or events competing for time, it is helpful for managers to ask themselves the following simple questions:

1. *What is the level of importance of each request?* When one is comparing the relative importance of the items on a list, the process can be more complicated than one might anticipate. Consider the level of importance (critical need) of the following: (a) compiling the unit's input to the annual division report, (b) completing a subordinate's performance report, (c) investigating and satisfying a patient's complaint, and (d) attending a routine staff meeting.

2. *What is the comparative urgency of each request?* At first glance, attending a routine staff meeting might seem to be the least important of the tasks listed earlier; however, if there could be dissension among the staff at the meeting if the nurse manager does not attend, then perhaps it might be a higher priority. Investigating and resolving a patient's complaint (usually a very serious concern) might be given a lower priority than normally if the patient is a chronic complainer and previous investigations have turned up no reason for concern.

Considering both of these aspects of what constitutes priority is critical, because the process will help nurse managers decide which of their many tasks will be the first to receive attention.

Fig. 10-1 is designed to assist the nurse manager in establishing priorities within his or her job requirements. This easy-to-use matrix has two dimensions: (1) urgency, and (2) importance. Evaluating prospective tasks along these two dimensions can be of great assistance to the nurse manager in preparing for the demands of the performance day.

Fig. 10-1 not only can help managers establish priorities for the current workday but also can assist them in analyzing how decisions on work priorities are currently being made and in determining the relative priorities of future activities so that these activities can be scheduled appropriately. The process begins by listing each work requirement and asking the question, "Is it important?" If the answer is yes, then the task fits into the left-hand column of the matrix; if the answer is no, then the task should be placed in the right-hand column. Next, how pressing the task is (i.e., whether it should be placed into the

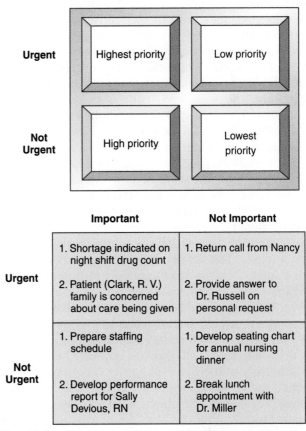

Fig. 10-1 ■ Decision-making matrix demonstrating the relationship between importance and urgency.

first or second row) is determined by asking, "Is it an urgent matter?" If the activity or event is both important and urgent, then it should be put into the box labeled "high priority." If the task is not important and not urgent, then it should be put into the "lowest priority" box. Managers should be very careful to classify nothing as "highest priority" unless it is truly an emergency, a crisis, or an action that must be taken to prevent a crisis. The basic rule is that a task that falls into this category must be done, and it must be done now. Any activity or event that is categorized as "lowest priority," on the other hand, probably should not be done during the workday, because it may be a waste of precious work time. These things are neither important nor urgent.

The "priority" box is where managers put those tasks or requests that may be important but have not yet become urgent (i.e., they do not require immediate attention). By now, it should be easy to see what is taking shape with regard to priorities. If the items placed in the "priority" category are not completed in a timely fashion, they will get pushed against their deadlines.

The closer the time gets to the deadline, the more urgent those items become, until eventually each turns into a crisis or emergency. For instance, if a nurse manager does not take the time to complete a staff member's performance review, writing the review will become a crisis when the deadline is reached and the review still has not been finished.

Activities and events that may be urgent but are not important are the ones that must be monitored carefully. The tasks and requests that are typically categorized as "low priority" are often difficult and compelling. They have a tendency to draw managers toward them and can create an internal desire to deal with them. If managers are judicious when they place the items into this level of priority, however, then these tasks remain not important, just urgent, and nurse managers must remember to allocate their time appropriately.

It is recommended that the priority matrix be used on a regular basis to determine current priorities and to evaluate the manager's conduct during the previous day. Before yesterday's activities and events are removed from their boxes and relocated within the matrix or deleted due to completion, they can be evaluated to determine their importance and urgency. Nurse managers will want to know whether they wasted any of their time or, at the very minimum, to what degree they used it effectively. Fig. 10-1 can also provide insight about what can be expected tomorrow. Writing the next day's activities into the appropriate boxes within the matrix can help managers focus on exactly where they should be spending their time. Finally, the matrix does more than help managers analyze the past and predict the future; it can help direct today's activities. What is it that the manager is doing right now? Is it important? Is it urgent? Establishing effective priorities is seldom an easy task, but the fact is that everyone who juggles multiple tasks almost always establishes priorities. The truly professional manager sets these priorities through a conscious effort, and the marginal manager through an unconscious one, but both managers, good and bad, make prioritizing part of their performance. All managers who occupy positions as responsible as that of nurse manager must make their decisions conscientiously.

Using Objectives to Manage Time Effectively

Personal organization is the key to using time effectively. Well-organized nurse managers place their primary emphasis on planning and scheduling the activities that fulfill their fundamental responsibilities and result in the achievement of the unit's objectives. In fact, nurse managers' personal objectives are derived from their basic responsibilities and the established objectives of the unit. Therefore, defining personal objectives and then managing the unit to accomplish them is a fundamental key to achieving success in the unit.

Knowledgeable and experienced nurse managers often subdivide their objectives and share the responsibility for attaining them with their subordinate staff such as an assistant nurse manager, unit clerks, and staff nurses. This process, normally referred to as delegation, allows the efforts contributed by subordinates to meld with those of the nurse manager to achieve the unit's objectives. This process of sharing is the normal action of a responsible and professional nurse manager. In fact, a key characteristic of a truly proficient manager is the willingness to achieve unit objectives by working through others.

Nurse managers, like most other managers, are evaluated in terms of how well and how efficiently their units accomplish specific objectives. Organizations know this, and that is one of the reasons such great effort is expended in creating realistic and achievable goals. Unless a well-thought-out and well-planned system of measurable, realistic, and achievable objectives is assigned to the performance units, the organization will not be able to determine achievement and evaluate performance. This same process is followed at the unit level, where nurse managers distribute their overall performance objectives down to the actual performers within the unit. They can then evaluate all of their subordinates in the same way that they themselves are reviewed (i.e., on how well their subordinates have accomplishment the subobjectives they have been assigned and how well they have fulfilled their role responsibilities).

To help get and keep themselves organized, truly professional nurse managers continually address the following five key issues:

1. What are the specific objectives that must be achieved?
2. What are the specific activities that must be done to achieve these objectives?
3. How much time will be required to successfully complete each activity?
4. Which activities can be planned and scheduled simultaneously and which must be dealt with sequentially?
5. Which activities can be delegated to staff?

One of the most important and most often neglected aspects of establishing and working toward objectives is simply recognizing that not all of the objectives that must be accomplished are equally important. Some are routine, some are important, and a few—in most cases very few—are urgent, as are the activities required to achieve them.

If the activities that must be performed to meet an objective are to be achieved in a timely manner, they must be planned and scheduled according to priority, and one of the most crucial aspects of doing this is estimating how much time each one will take. Once the time required is determined, any activity can be planned and scheduled so that sufficient time is allocated to ensure satisfactory completion. For nurse managers, this process is critical to managing time efficiently, because unless they have an effective plan in place, they can very easily become involved in activity traps (i.e., activities that cannot be tracked back to the requirements of an objective). These nonessential activities or traps are rarely planned for or scheduled, and they are almost always major causes of the wasted time in a nurse manager's schedule. Examples of such activity traps are shown in the "lowest priority" box in the bottom part of Fig. 10-1.

In all cases, determining the relative importance and urgency of the nurse manager's objectives and role responsibilities enables the nurse manager to clearly define priorities and work on the highest priority items first.

Plans and schedules should be developed with one important caveat in mind: they will rarely turn out exactly as they were conceived or written. This truism follows from the simple fact that it is nearly impossible to develop a perfect plan and a perfect schedule, and even if one could, unexpected events and problems will occur during the performance period to unsettle them. Another truism is that scheduling time for the performance of a specific activity is rarely an exact science, especially in a field as dynamic as the one in which the nurse manager operates. Some activities will take longer than the time allotted to them, regardless of the amount of effort that went into planning and allocating time for them or the level of professionalism of those who perform them. Why? Because things happen that were never and could never be anticipated (e.g., emergencies occur).

The purpose of an effective plan and schedule, then, is not to maintain exactness but to provide the user with a base from which to operate. When unscheduled events, emergencies, or nonessential activities draw nurse managers away from their planned approach to performance, the plan and schedule provide a track to follow that will return the unit to normalcy and keep nurse managers moving toward the intended path. This process of moving toward a goal only to be sidetracked by an unforeseen event and then returning to the original path occurs often in the nursing unit. To compensate for such a diversion, nurse managers should continually review the priorities that were originally established for the day and reschedule those tasks that require it. If this practice is followed, the nurse manager can ensure that the remainder of the work shift will be devoted to accomplishing those tasks and objectives that have the greatest importance and urgency.

TIME WASTERS

Time, it has been said, is wasted by the professional (i.e., the nurse manager) when it is spent on anything that really did not have to be done. This definition of time wasting can be expanded by noting that time is also wasted when more time than necessary is spent doing something, no matter how important that something is. What are the time wasters? Surprisingly, the biggest offenders are simple interruptions and casual distractions. Almost none of these nuisance matters deserve the attention of the nurse manager, and when they do, they do not merit the level of attention they are often given.

Interruptions

For the purposes of this chapter, an interruption is something that occurs any time the nurse manager is stopped in the middle of one activity to give attention to another. Although interruptions are generally considered an ineffective use of time, not all of them are negative. For example, an interruption can be positive when an emergency or crisis occurs during daily rounds. This emergency or crisis may be far more important and urgent than completing rounds at that time, so that responding to the interruption is a productive use of the nurse manager's time.

Typically, nurse managers experience many, many interruptions during the course of a normal work shift, and many of these unplanned events have a negative impact on their overall performance. An example of a negative time waster is interruption by a staff member who drops in or telephones when the nurse manager is in the middle of writing a report. The key to managing interruptions is first to make an effort to determine what kinds of interruptions are actually experienced so that action can be taken to eliminate as many of the negative ones as possible.

It is highly recommended that nurse managers keep a *time control log* (Fig. 10-2) that will track these events for several days. The log should record the following:

- The person who caused the interruption
- The nature of the interruption
- The time of day during which the interruption occurred
- The length of time the interruption lasted
- The topics discussed and their level of importance
- Any time-saving actions that might be taken

The data gathered by the time control log can be analyzed carefully to identify patterns. These patterns can suggest ways to reduce the frequency and duration of the small interruptions that consume so much of the typical day. For example, the nurse manager might notice that certain staff members are the most

Time Control Log

Employee's name: _____ Date: _____ Department: _____

Who	T/V	I/T	Time	How Long?	Topics Discussed	IMP	Time-Saving Actions

Who = Who discussion was with; **T** = Telephone; **V** = Visit; **I** = I Initiated T or V; **T** = They initiated T or V; **Time** = Time of interruption; **How Long?** = Length of interruption; **Topics Discussed** = List items discussed vertically; **IMP** = Level of importance: **A** = High; **B** = Moderate; **C** = Low; **U** = Unimportant; **Time-Saving Actions** = What can be done to save time.

NOTE: More than one line may be required to chronolog a single call or visit.

Fig. 10-2 ■ Sample time control log for time management.

frequent interrupters, and recognition of this pattern can aid management efforts by indicating that these individuals have excess time.

Analysis of the topics discussed may also reveal to the nurse manager some definite patterns. For example, a large portion of the in-office conversations might involve current events, family activities, or personal matters and not work-related topics. Other interruptions, and the topics discussed in them, might relate to important hospital policies or nursing concerns that need resolution or clarification.

The nurse manager might also find that many of the interruptions occur during a certain part of the shift or on specific days of the week. The pattern of interruptions may also show that there are specific time periods during which staff members and co-workers are more likely to waste the nurse manager's time. Fig. 10-3 illustrates a record of the interruptions experienced by a nurse manager on a typical shift. The goal of using an interruption sheet such as shown in Fig. 10-3 is to develop information that might lead to time-saving actions.

Identification of patterns should help the nurse manager take corrective action. The nurse manager must realize that he or she is an essential part of whatever patterns are found and that one can be a part of the problem and not realize it. The nurse manager is either causing these patterns to develop or allowing others to create them; therefore, it is the nurse manager's responsibility to control how time is used.

Behavioral patterns identify what are commonly known as *habits*. In many cases, these actions are so automatic that people are actually unaware of their use and their effects. In addition, these patterns of interruption may result from vicarious learning or direct positive reinforcement (i.e., people learn how to act by observing the behavior around them or by being rewarded, or seeing others rewarded, for certain behavior). What this means to nurse managers is

Time Control Log

Employee's name: _____   Date: _____   Department: _____

Who	T/V	I/T	Time	How Long?	Topics Discussed	IMP	Time-Saving Actions
John Clerk	V	T	9:20 AM	4 min	Printer ink	B	Told Clerk to order ink
Dr. Milson	V	T	9:41 AM	11 min	Req Extd Trmt time	A	Stand up during conversation to reduce socializing
					New car, children	U	
Joan, LPN	V	T	10:15 AM	15 min	Boyfriend problem	U	Do not ask about BF
Patient's family	V	T	10:42 AM	15 min	PR with patient's wife	A	
Sharon, RN	T	I	10:51 AM	2 min	Remind lunch appt	U	
Alice, RN	V	T	11:21 AM	6 min	Discussed patient	A	Checkout procedure
Dr. Bingham	T	T	11:34 AM	17 min	Patient's treatment	A	
Ruth, RN	T	I	12:21 PM	3 min	Lost otoscope	U	
Marcia, RN	V	T	12:51 PM	6 min	Requested time off	C	Post timeoff procedures
Sharon & Ruth	V	T	1:00 PM	2 min	Rpt back from lunch	B	Do I encourage socializing?
Dr. Michaelson	V	T	1:15 PM	8 min	Discussed patient	A	
Bill Candel	T	T	3:40 PM	2 min	Confirmed dinner	U	Remind not to call unit
Susan, RN	V	T	4:15 PM	3 min	Kill time at end of shift	U	Discourage practice

Fig. 10-3 ■ Example of a completed time control log to help assess the use of time. For list of abbreviations, see Fig. 10-2.

that their individual behaviors may act to reinforce unnecessary interruption, which increases the probability that such interruptions will recur, or that they may actually be providing examples of (i.e., modeling) such behavior, which is then emulated by staff members. One thing is certain: if nurse managers, as leaders of their units, do not demonstrate respect for time through their actions, then neither will those with whom they interact.

Effective communication is one of the essential elements of good management. Nurse managers must understand that keeping open bidirectional communication between themselves and those with whom they maintain contact is essential. Effective communication is defined as discourse that provides the necessary information to perform correctly. Both too much communication and too little can have a devastating effect on the success of a unit. A classic example of the overcommunication that can occur in a nursing unit is the often misunderstood and frequently abused organizational concept called the *open door policy*. In many organizations, this approach to leadership has come to mean that any person can walk in on or telephone any other person at any time and take as long as he or she chooses to communicate a point. This type of interaction should be referred to as an "open communication policy," because it is not truly an open door policy. An open door policy simply means that when an individual has something important to discuss, time will be made available to discuss it. It does not necessarily mean that the time will be made available at any desired point or at that individual's convenience, and most certainly not on the spur of the moment.

Telephone Calls

Telephone calls are, beyond a doubt, the most seriously abused source of interruption within the nursing unit. Proper use of a time control log can provide the nurse manager with considerable insight into the nature of incoming telephone calls. In today's fast-paced environment, it is nearly impossible for nurse managers to function effectively without a telephone; unfortunately, however, a large percentage of people do not function effectively when they use one. A ringing telephone is highly imperious; it draws people's attention and makes most people feel that they absolutely must do something about it immediately. In fact, studies have shown that very few will allow a telephone to ring unanswered. Because of the duties they are assigned, in any given shift nurse managers will receive many telephone calls, and a good percentage of them will cause a waste of valu-

able time. Almost all inbound telephone calls can be controlled, and if nurse managers do not make a positive attempt to impose such control, then the calling parties will be the ones who exercise it. The following sections provide tips on how to handle telephone calls effectively.

MINIMIZE SMALL TALK AND SOCIALIZING

Many telephone conversations start with polite social-speak such as, "Hello, how are you?" The caller may take more time than is available, or than the receiver of the call would like to make available, to answer this single question. Instead, nurse managers can try something slightly different, such as, "Hello, how can I help you?" This is a more business-like approach and will get nurse managers past the social niceties that often waste valuable time. Nurse managers must always try to be warm, friendly, and courteous in their conversations, but that does not mean that they must allow others to waste their time with inappropriate or extensive small talk.

PLAN CALLS

Professional nurse managers make conscientious attempts to plan their telephone calls so that they do not waste anyone's time, including that of the person called. Using a computer note pad or simply keeping a small pad or piece of note paper by the telephone will allow nurse managers to jot down discussion topics before they make a call. When their discussion has covered all these topics, they end their conversations professionally and hang up. Rigorous attention to planning a telephone call will lead to less time spent in calling back to inform the other party of an important point that was neglected or to discuss a forgotten question.

SET A TIME

Quite often, the duties of nurse managers keep them away from their offices for extended periods. This creates a backlog of calls that must be returned as well as several that must be initiated. It is best to set aside a specific part of the day—perhaps just before the shift ends or immediately after the shift begins—to handle routine phone calls.

AVOID CALLING FOR INFORMATION

When a telephone call is made, it should not interrupt what is being done at the moment. For example, if the nurse manager is in a meeting and a specific question must be answered before the project can be continued, then the phone call is important enough to make; if not, the nurse manager should phone for the information at a later time. Only rarely will the lack of information on a specific point impede the advancement of a project during a meeting, and unless it does, it is professional and proper to wait until after the meeting has been completed.

USE A TIMER

Although using a timer to monitor calls may at first seem like a bizarre idea, most people don't realize how long they spend on the telephone. The starting time should be written on a note pad when a call is first received and the stop time entered when the call is done. Most people will be surprised to discover that the vast majority of telephone calls actually last much longer than they think. A time control log makes recording the length of telephone conversations easy and provides a convenient method for tracking the length of all telephone conversations. Timing calls will help make the nurse manager more time conscious.

STATE AND ASK FOR PREFERRED CALL TIMES

If a party the nurse manager calls is not available and a request is left for that person to return the call, the manager should designate two different time periods during which he or she will be available to receive the return call. For example, "I will be in the office from 11:00 to 12:00 this morning and from 3:30 to 4:00 this afternoon." This approach will help the intended conversation partner manage his or her time and will eliminate that common annoyance referred to as "telephone tag." The telephone merry-go-round is one of the single biggest time wasters in the nursing unit.

Intercoms, Pagers, and Cellular Telephones

For many years, the intercom paging system was the critical communication tool in the hospital. Not only was this system ineffective, but it was downright disturbing to many. Technologic advances have since replaced most of these annoying intercom calls with the beep-beep-beep of electronic paging equipment and the soft ring of cellular telephones. These extremely effective devices are essential to manage emergency and crisis situations in which immediate relay of messages is critical. Unfortunately, pagers and cellular telephones frequently disturb activities that should not be interrupted. The key to effective use of these devices is to make good decisions about whether an individual should be called. In a hospital there are few unimportant activities; therefore, before paging or dialing a cellular phone number, the caller should consider that the person he or she wishes to talk with is currently engaged in an important activity. The zeal to contact someone should be tempered by the realization that high-priority activities should not be interrupted by low-priority messages.

Conversely, there are times when the users of pagers and cellular telephones should determine for themselves that they should not be interrupted unless there is an emergency or crisis. Turning a pager off might not be appropriate, but placing it in "vibrate" mode will create far less disturbance than the annoying beep-beep-beep for which pagers are notorious. Cellular telephone calls can be forwarded to an answering service or voice mailbox to avoid interruption at an inappropriate time. Then, as soon as the user is free, he or she can check for messages. These devices will continue to be important to the nurse manager, but professionalism dictates that they not be misused or abused.

Drop-In Visitors

The role of the nurse manager makes it certain that he or she will have many visitors. Although being a professional requires that the nurse manager treat all visitors as important, what many wish to visit about may not be. Even the topics that are important may not be urgent enough to warrant spending time on them. Although the nurse manager may need to spend time with a visitor, the visit may not be important enough to dictate that the time be spent immediately. The following sections present several important principles for handling visitors and visiting others.

MEET VISITORS OUTSIDE THE OFFICE

Whenever possible, visitors should be met in a reception area or in the hallway. This practice keeps the visitor out of the nurse manager's office and allows the manager to decide when or if the person should be invited into the office.

KEEP VISITS SHORT

Standing up when a drop-in visitor appears will help keep the visit short. It has been proven time and time again that conversations are likely to be shorter when participants are standing than when they are sitting. If the visitor wants to discuss an important and urgent topic, the nurse manager can always invite the person to sit down. Besides providing this additional control, standing up is also considered more professional and courteous than remaining seated. When it seems appropriate to end the conversation, taking a short step and gesturing toward the door or, if seated, simply standing up communicates the point to the visitor.

GIVE A FEW MINUTES, BUT STAY IN CONTROL

When the nurse manager is interrupted unexpectedly and he or she has a few minutes available, the manager can ask the visitor the nature of his or her business and let the person know how much time can be provided. When that time is up, it is the nurse manager who should decide whether the discussion continues, the conversation is terminated, or the visitor is asked to return at a more appropriate time. If the nurse manager wishes to remain in control, then he or she must assert this control appropriately. If the manager feels that the conversation is important enough to continue, the visitor is told that the allotted time is up but that the topic is too important to stop the discussion and it can continue. If the discussion is less important and urgent than other pressing matters, the conversation is ended politely but firmly and an appointment is set up to continue the discussion at a more convenient time.

ENCOURAGE APPOINTMENTS

Routine matters should be dealt with during routine appointments or at least at planned intervals. Emergencies and crises are not routine and should not be treated as such. The nurse manager will have many conversations a day with co-workers, staff, and superiors. If regularly scheduled meetings are established with those who need to see the nurse manager, these individuals will save routine matters for discussion at these appointments. Drop-in visits are most likely to occur when others are not certain when they will be able to see the nurse manager. Their philosophy becomes "catch them when you can." A well-organized nurse manager lets others know in advance "when you can."

KEEP STAFF INFORMED

Nurse managers can minimize unexpected visits if they keep staff members informed. The recommendation is to use a method of providing information that fits with managers' schedules, such as a program of "management by wandering around" (MBWA)* or discussion at morning staff meetings or at other such appropriate times. Because most memos are not taken seriously, no one should write a lot of them unless a response copy or space for responding is included and the staff are made aware that they will be monitored for compliance. Also, many senior managers and professional staff view a memo-writing supervisor as someone intent on covering his or her tracks. Sadly, there have been too many people who have hidden behind memos to avoid responsibility in the past, and today's more demanding, energetic workforce expects something better.

ARRANGE THE FURNITURE

Nurse managers who arrange their offices so that the view from the desk allows immediate eye contact with passers-by or drop-in visitors are asking to have their day continually interrupted. Instead, the desk should be turned 90 or even 180 degrees from the door so that troublesome eye contact can be minimized. If the office has several comfortable visitors' chairs, they too can be an invitation to the casual visitor. If a manager must have chairs in the office, it is recommended that they be less comfortable and more functional. In fact, the act of moving a chair into the position needed to provide seating for an important visitor can be used as a professional gesture, whereas keeping chairs stored out of the way makes it plain that an invitation must be extended before visitors seat themselves.

GO SEE THE PERSON

One of the most effective ways to discourage unwanted visitors is also one of the simplest: get up out of the office and go see *them*. This is especially important when dealing with the exceptionally long-winded people with whom every nurse manager must cope. Many people simply have no concept of time and have never learned when to quit talking and leave. If the professional nurse manager needs to communicate with one of these long-winded people, he or she will often go to that person's office and, when through with business, immediately get up and leave. When the necessary conversation is completed, it is far easier to say, "I have to go now" than "I need you to go now."

Management by wandering around is a performance-enhancing practice first used by the Hewlett-Packard company in the 1970s and popularized by Tom Peters and Robert H. Waterman in their 1982 book *In Search of Excellence*. The process teaches supervisors to move indirectly but deliberately when going from place to place within the work environment. As managers move about, they recognize performance, make minor corrections, offer encouragement, and converse with the staff. For example, instead of *walking* to the radiology department, a nurse manager might *wander* past Nurse Jones and comment on her professional appearance, then walk past the orderly and thank him for helping move Ms. Smith to surgery, and then go into the coffee lounge to tell the nurses gathered for lunch about an upcoming program. The key is to make the wandering appear to be part of task performance and not a rough attempt to placate the staff. Nothing should be said that isn't true, and no recognition should be given unless it has been earned.

RESPECTING TIME

One of the keys to effective management of interruptions and distractions is to have a great deal of respect for time, both one's own and that of others. This attitude is contagious, and nurse managers who have it are likely to find others developing it as well. The same values and attitudes are required to respect time as to respect others. If others see the nurse manager setting an example by acting professionally, there is every reason to believe that they will act professionally as well. Nearly all people want to be associated with the best and will emulate the outstanding qualities they perceive; conversely, very few will do what they have been told by someone who routinely breaks the rules to fit his or her own purposes. Therefore, professional nurse managers are people with high regard for others' time. Professionalism dictates that the proper procedure for talking with someone is to arrange an appointment, particularly if the matter is routine. On the other hand, professionalism also dictates that emergencies and crises always be handled immediately.

SCHEDULING

After nurse managers have established their objectives and priorities, they can concentrate on scheduling their activities. Once this is accomplished, a system should be maintained to keep track of regularly scheduled meetings (e.g., staff meetings), infrequently occurring events (e.g., annual report due dates), and appointments. One example of a usable system is a calendar combined with a file. Each meeting is entered on the calendar, along with the purpose of the meeting, who will be attending, and the time and place; in the file is arranged correspondence or reports that concern each meeting. The file should be organized by date so that the information it contains is readily available at the appropriate time. The file can also be used as a preparation device by filing information in it at an earlier date to allow the nurse manager sufficient time to become acquainted with it and prepare for the meeting.

Using a calendar makes it easy to know what is coming up and helps in generating ideas for future events. For example, if a nurse manager knows that he or she will be meeting with a superior the following week to discuss the next year's unit budget, the manager can start preparing early. Many managers maintain two calendars: a larger one at work with room for details (often this is a calendar function built into their personal computers) and a smaller one to carry to meetings and take home. Always having a calendar handy (e.g., while waiting in the dentist's office) provides more opportunity to jog one's memory. Nurse managers should also investigate technologic aids to determine how they might assist in scheduling time. For example, hand-held personal data systems can be very effective in managing the schedules of busy people.

PAPERWORK

Hospitals, it has been said, float on a sea of paper. Although this statement is perhaps hyperbole, it is true that a dynamic institution cannot function effectively without good information systems. In addition to making and receiving telephone calls and participating in face-to-face conversations, nurse managers spend a good deal of time writing and reading many different forms of communication. Increasing government regulations and the ensuing desire of organizations to avoid legal action; the development of new treatments and medications; and the availability of data processing, word processing, and a myriad of electronic media are but a few of the things that continually increase the pressure on the nurse manager to cope with a mass of paperwork that seems to grow exponentially. In today's high-technology world, the amount of communication available to the average nurse manager staggers the imagination. Too much communication and the waste of time, money, and effort that is typically associated with it are becoming as much of a challenge for the nursing unit as too little communication ever was.

Computer terminals are everywhere in the hospital—at the nurse's station, on top of nearly every desk, and in the offices of the nurse manager and every other administrator. Nurse managers of today and the future must know how to interface with these new technologies and must ensure that the incredible amount of information now available doesn't handicap them or their nursing units.

Word processing, electronic mail, the Internet, and other information systems have replaced most of the traditional manual methods of managing information. Regardless of the state of the technology in the nurse manager's particular unit, the nurse manager must be able to fulfill his or her responsibility to process information. Whether the information is handwritten, typed by a high-speed printer, or flashed across a computer terminal, there are some basic principles to be followed.

Plan and Schedule Paperwork

Writing and reading reports, forms, letters, electronic mail, and every other type of memo are essential performance requirements of the nurse manager's job, and they cannot be ignored. These duties can become a major source of frustration, however, when nurse managers do not plan for and schedule them as an integral part of their daily activities. All nurse managers must learn their organizations' information systems and their peculiarities as well as their organizations' requirements and expectations immediately upon assuming the responsibilities of the position. They must analyze the paperwork requirements of their position and make significant progress on that part of the job daily. Allowing paperwork to pile up is the death knell of professionalism.

Sort Paperwork for Effective Processing

Implementing a system to sort mail can be very helpful. The system need not be elaborate; a few large folders or envelopes will work just fine. For example, one system is to put all paperwork requiring action into a file labeled "A" (for "action"). These items can then be managed effectively according to their relative importance and urgency. All paperwork that is informational and/or related to current work is placed in a file labeled "I" (for "immediate"). The "I" file should contain only those things that must be read immediately. Reading materials such as professional journals, technical reports, and other items that are good or even important to read but that do not directly relate to the work currently facing the unit are placed in a file labeled "R" (for "routine"). Any material placed into the "R" file should be considered low priority, and reading it should be something that can be postponed to a later time.

Nurse managers should not be afraid to throw things away or erase them from the memory of the electronic information system. When items no longer have value, they should not be allowed to become clutter, because they will slow down the system and can arbitrarily cause errors to occur. Every nurse manager needs a wastebasket; the manager should get a big one and fill it often.

Share Paperwork Responsibilities

Nurse managers should not be afraid to delegate some of their administrative (paper) work to others in the unit. The process of delegating can help managers build depth in the unit by allowing their subordinates to perform at higher levels. It is usually permissible to delegate both routine and nonroutine paperwork functions, but managers should make sure that they delegate a variety of work. Delegating what the nurse manager doesn't like or doesn't want to do is not really delegation; it is called dumping, and that process has little team-building value. Teaching staff members to handle paperwork effectively strengthens a unit by broadening the capabilities of the staff. In fact, a professionally designed process of delegation often results in a high level of satisfaction among staff, especially when those involved are highly educated and professional personnel.

Write Effectively

In today's high-technology world, clear, concise writing is essential for all nurse managers. Regardless of whether nurse managers are developing a letter, a report, or a simple staff memo, what they write should be comprehensible, to the point, and never verbose. The dictation machine has just about vanished from the halls of the modern healthcare institute, but if one is used, the manager doing so should remember to enunciate properly and speak clearly. Writing is a critical part of all managerial positions, and nurse managers should never forget that, when something is written down, people will judge the author by its quality. They should never allow bad grammar, poor penmanship, or spelling errors to slip by in any document they pass on to anyone.

Analyze Paperwork Frequently

Filing policies and rules should be reviewed regularly, and files should be purged at least once each year. All standard forms, reports, and memos should be reviewed annually or as often as may be required by the organization. Each piece of paper should justify its continued existence and its present format. Managers should not be afraid to recommend changes and, when possible, initiate them.

Avoid Becoming a Paper Shuffler

Many members of the management community believe that they are far too busy to handle a piece of paper more than once. Although this sentiment is admirable in concept, it has little place in practice because it is an almost impossible task. It is more appropriate to insist that each time a piece of paper is handled, some action be taken that furthers its processing. Paper shufflers—people who continuously move paper around on top of their desks—can create unreasonable delay in any project requiring action and can become an intolerable menace to the success of the unit as the paper problem escalates. A manager's desktop is a working surface; it is not a file for piles of paper.

DELEGATION

Delegation is a major tool in time management. Delegation is defined as sharing responsibility and authority with subordinates and holding them accountable for their performance. It is not the same as direction.

Delegation is a high-level skill that relies on the manager's ability to trust that subordinates possess all the skills and knowledge necessary to accomplish something. *Direction* is simply the process of telling another person what one wishes to be done. Delegation is the process of giving junior personnel a task and the resources to accomplish it and then getting out of the way while they do it.

Delegation is a two-way process (Fig. 10-4). Those at the higher levels of the administration pyramid share their responsibilities and authority downward with their subordinates, who in turn share with their subordinates. Accountability, however, always flows in the opposite direction (i.e., upward). As noted in an earlier chapter, the small sign that President Harry S. Truman kept on his desk reading "The buck stops here" exemplifies the true meaning of accountability. The person at the top of the chain of command is the individual who retains the ultimate accountability for what occurs within an organization. For nurse managers, this means that they are the ones account-

able for everything that happens in the nursing unit, regardless of whether they personally performed a given task or it was accomplished by another.

Managers are not only accountable for the failures of their subordinates but they also share in their successes. Therefore, just as nurse managers must take ultimate responsibility for all of the problems and failures of every employee in their units, they also have the right to share credit for their units' successes and achievements. Obviously, those who delegate effectively will have more opportunities to share in success and achievement than in problems and failures.

As can be seen in Fig. 10-4, nurse managers are both subordinates and seniors in the hierarchy of the typical healthcare organization. Work is delegated to nurse managers by their immediate seniors, and they, in turn, must decide which of their many job responsibilities will be shared with their subordinates. What to do and what to delegate are questions that every nurse manager faces daily.

The specific job description detailed by an organization for nurse managers will help them make many of their delegation decisions. In addition, formal job descriptions for the assistant nurse manager, registered nurses, licensed practical nurses, nurse assistants, and unit clerks help in making delegation decisions. Nurse managers must understand the full range of job responsibilities for the unit and delegate appropriately to ensure that all responsibilities are met. No one, under any circumstances, should be delegated a job he or she is not qualified to perform.

The nurse manager's job itself must be thoroughly understood. Along with planning, organizing, and controlling the work within the unit, experienced nurse managers set aside time to ensure that they accomplish all of their specific duties. It is imperative that nurse managers understand that they are responsible for managing, not performing, the details of the unit's work. They must work effectively with and through their staff members and, in doing so, provide an environment that is conducive to developing the motivation necessary for staff members to *want* to do their jobs effectively.

The foregoing does not mean that nurse managers never get involved in the work being performed by their subordinates. In smaller hospitals with limited staff, during emergencies, or when there is a staff shortage, nurse managers often find themselves performing the detailed and routine work of the unit. The more time they spend in the performance of these activities, however, the less time they will have to carry out those functions and activities specific to their job, the ones that cannot be delegated.

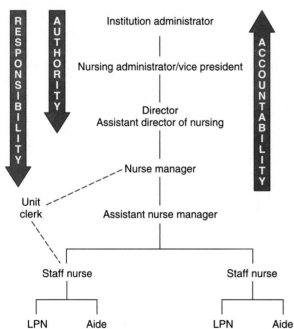

Fig. 10-4 ■ Responsibility, authority, and accountability in delegation within the hospital hierarchy. *LPN*, Licensed practical nurse.

Through good delegation, nurse managers can also develop the potential of their staffs. To ensure that the delegation process is effective, however, they must first be aware of the characteristics of their staff members. The more they know about each person's background, experiences, knowledge, and skills, the more effective their delegation efforts will be. Taking the time to develop a skills profile for each member of the staff can help managers identify individual strengths that can be relied on and areas in which well-applied delegation can be used to train staff and eliminate any known weaknesses. Nurse managers who do not develop the abilities of their staffs are those who will become increasingly involved in the daily routine and detail work of the division.

Effective delegation leads to the development of a confident and capable staff; but beyond this obvious benefit, it also reduces the risk for errors and mistakes in the unit. Working with others, no matter what their skill levels, always involves additional risks, especially for managers. These risks typically result from, or at least are increased by, mediocre communication, skill deficiencies, or the differences in values and perspectives that are always present in the working environment. Nurse managers can reduce such risks if they are aware of the competencies of their subordinates and delegate only in a responsible way.

To become effective delegators, nurse managers must understand and apply the following three fundamental concepts:

1. Responsibility
2. Authority
3. Accountability

Each of these concepts is different from the others; however, many people, especially managers, frequently confuse them. The Vroom and Yetton model discussed in Chapter 11 and the discussions in the following sections provide an easily understood method for planning and implementing delegation to enhance the performance of the nursing unit.

Authority

Most professionals view authority as the legitimate power inherent in a management position. If this concept is correct, then authority is something that is assumed with the position, not something developed within the person holding it. The position of nurse manager carries with it a certain level of authority and power.

Nurse managers can share authority with the members of their staffs, just as they share responsibility. In fact, when a subordinate is assigned the responsibility for completing a task, he or she must also be provided with sufficient authority to complete it. For example, when a nurse manager asks the assistant manager to represent the nurse manager at a decision-making meeting to discuss new procedures, the nurse manager must give the assistant sufficient authority to make decisions for the unit; not to do so would be detrimental to the performance of the assistant nurse manager and the unit as a whole. If a nurse manager feels that he or she cannot delegate the authority to perform a specific task, then the nurse manager should not delegate the responsibility for that task.

Before a nurse manager delegates to anyone the authority to perform a given task, he or she must carefully answer the following two questions:

1. What areas of authority or what resources must the person control to achieve the expected results?
2. What will be the limits or parameters for each area of authority or resource to be used?

Nurse managers who have the responsibility for maintaining adequate supplies will need the authority to authorize spending from the unit budget. Exactly how that authority is given, however, may differ from organization to organization. For example, the authority to spend money on supplies may be limited to a certain amount that cannot be exceeded; it may be granted to purchase only specific supplies, or it may be given for the purchase of supplies in general.

Another example of the delegation of authority is granting authority to a member of the unit to assign other staff members to a project. The nurse manager may place restrictions on how many personnel may be assigned, for how long they may be assigned, or which specific tasks each individual may be allowed to perform. Generally, the delegation of authority is limited to the specific project and to a time period ending with the deadline for its completion.

The power associated with the nurse manager's formal position of authority is an essential tool of management that ensures effective functioning of the unit of which the manager is in charge. However, such formal power is not without limits. Managers can deplete the formal power they inherit with the job by relying on it too much to get the job done. Managers who constantly remind their subordinates of their authority can create frustration, hostility, and even sabotage within their units. No one likes to feel that he or she is being pushed, ruled, or forced to comply. The heavy hand of the "A"-style manager almost always produces negative effects in the working environment, and yet manager after manager continues to follow this approach. The reason is most likely a lack of self-esteem or confidence on the part of the manager in his or her ability to do a proper job. Such behavior may also be associated with a manager's lack of confidence in his or her subordinates. But whatever the source, heavy-handed management is not conducive to excellence and should be used only in special circumstances (i.e., when nothing else works) or in times of emergency or crisis.

The opposite of the heavy-handed manager is the manager who does not use authority when it should be used. Being unwilling to invoke authority when necessary can be just as detrimental as using it too much. Managers must, when appropriate, take corrective action on procedural problems, discipline subordinates for excessive violation of performance standards, make decisions in a timely manner, and take control during emergencies or crises. Neglecting these vital managerial responsibilities will never make managers "good guys" in the eyes of their employees—only failures.

Authority is like dynamite. If it is used in the proper amount, at the right time, and in a professional manner, it can be one of the most effective tools available. However—and this cannot be stressed enough—it should never be misused. Proper use of authority increases the individual manager's credibility with both superiors and subordinates by ensuring their confidence and trust. When used properly, the manager's authority is actually a protection for the staff; for example, a manager should immediately take steps to discipline an employee who violates unit performance standards. By doing so, the manager reinforces the staff's belief in his or her ability and concern for their welfare. Nurse managers must remember that their credibility is based on their confidence, fairness, and consistency, and on others' perception of these qualities in them.

When a nurse manager delegates authority, the manager must ensure that he or she maintains loose control of the assignment, because, in the end, the nurse manager is always the one responsible for a successful outcome. This loose control can be maintained by following up with the subordinate frequently and checking progress or holding the subordinate accountable for the use of the resources over which he or she has been delegated authority. The nurse manager should work closely with the subordinate to whom the task has been delegated to monitor continuously whether the assigned resources are sufficient or whether additional resources are needed. Are the limits placed on the use of these resources adequate? What could be done to ensure sufficient authority for the subordinate to carry out the assigned responsibilities? All of these things can be done without causing the employee to feel as if the assign-ment is being micromanaged simply by asking open-ended questions. It is always better for a manager to ask if he or she can help in a specific area than to direct the subordinate's activities in that area.

To maintain effective control over delegated projects, nurse managers should establish feedback and information processes that will allow them to be continually aware of the progress of the work they have delegated. Before an assignment is given, they must decide exactly what feedback they will need and how they expect to receive it. Nurse managers must ensure the progress of the delegated tasks and the proper use of the delegated authority without inhibiting subordinates' growth.

The amount of control that will be used should be considered thoroughly when objectives are established and before an assignment is given. Control actions should never be forced on the performing subordinate as an afterthought. For example, a staff nurse may be given the responsibility for administering medications and with that responsibility may be provided the authority to access drugs, draw up medications, and administer them to patients. The nurse may be held accountable through several means of control, which may include restricted access to the narcotics key, end-of-shift drug counts, and review of patients' medication charts and shift reports.

Assignments

There is no possible way for nurse managers to complete all of the work for which they are responsible without engaging in effective delegation. In fact, delegation is one of the primary methods professional managers use both to develop the capabilities of their staffs and to get their own jobs done. One of the most common forms of delegation used in the unit is day-to-day patient care assignments. How well nurse managers ensure that their staffs effectively carry out these assignments determines how much time they will have available to perform the activities that they alone can do.

The responsibility for ensuring the effective of task delegation lies with the person doing the delegating. This means that nurse managers must be cognizant of the duties necessary to complete a specific task before they delegate it. If they themselves do not know the specific results they want achieved by the subordinate's activities, then the subordinate certainly cannot be expected to know them. It is not only unprofessional but also foolhardy to expect a subordinate to commit to an assignment that he or she does not thoroughly understand. Nurse managers must think about the assignment, analyze it thoroughly, and be able to describe it in specific, measurable terms before delegating it to a subordinate. The junior member of the unit cannot be expected to produce satisfactory results unless the nurse manager has done his or her job well.

Explaining the intricacies of an assignment is not as easy as managers might think. Even having the subordinate restate the assignment after it has been presented is no guarantee that it was understood; it could simply mean that the junior remembered the assignment long enough to repeat it. When a nurse manager is delegating an assignment for the first time or when it is anything other than a routine assignment, the nurse manager should confirm understanding. This is done by asking open-ended questions that require more than a simple yes or no response. These probing questions and the discussion they will create will minimize potential misunderstandings and provide both parties to the assignment with a larger measure of confidence.

Delegation through task assignment creates a team relationship between the nurse manager and the subordinate. The level of professionalism that each of them demonstrates in holding up his or her end of the delegated assignment will determine whether they experience a winning or losing outcome. Do not doubt that every nurse manager's success is achieved through the demonstrated abilities of his or her subordinates. Teamwork, in the nursing unit and in life, results when a coach and a player work together to achieve a common goal. In nursing management, the nurse manager is the coach and the staff are the players. Although there have been many effective player-coaches, no player-coach has ever been considered truly exceptional, and no team led by a player-coach has ever achieved greatness.

Planning assignments together as nurse manager and staff and then working as a team to carry out those assignments effectively is the foundation of teamwork in the unit. Certainly the conscientious nurse manager will follow up to ensure that assignments are performed successfully and that the effort expended is in line with unit and organizational standards. The greatest benefit of delegation, however, is the teamwork and esprit de corps that it develops within the unit. Effective delegation through task assignment should be a team event, even if the nurse manager's leadership, motivation, communication, and analytical skills are required to develop these assignments. Helping subordinates grow and expand professionally is far more than part of the nurse manager's professional responsibilities; it can be an extremely gratifying experience.

The following sections provide advice on how to achieve effective delegation.

PLAN BEFORE DELEGATING

Thinking about how to effectively use the time available before attempting to use it will save a great deal of it. Truly professional nurse managers take the time to write out assignments and carefully analyze them before meeting with the staff to arrange a plan of delegation. Fig. 10-5 provides a tool that can be used to accomplish this. The following thought should be kept in mind when any effort is planned: the more complex the assignment, the greater the need to plan it. Although even the simplest of assignments requires some degree of thought and analysis to reduce the possibility of errors and omissions, the need for this planning becomes pronounced for complex assignments. Another important point to consider when planning is that there are no easy assignments. Each job that is delegated should be thought out and discussed, because even simple assignments can become as critical as the most complex ones. Good managers never assign any task without thoroughly thinking it through.

DEFINE THE RESPONSIBILITY TO BE ASSIGNED IN TERMS OF SPECIFIC RESULTS TO BE ACHIEVED

During the planning process, nurse managers should write down the specific results they expect to be achieved. Then they should ask themselves the following three questions:
1. Do these results make sense?
2. Are they measurable, realistic, and achievable?
3. Will the subordinate understand what is to be accomplished?

It is also a good idea for nurse managers to write down questions to ask the subordinate to determine his or her understanding of the assignment and to think about questions the subordinate might ask in return so that they can be prepared with competent answers.

The more complex and critical the task and the less skilled and experienced the subordinate, the greater the need to structure the assignment. Professional nurse managers rarely state their assignments without considering the skill level and experience of the staff member who will be charged with the duty. Risk of failure in a delegated assignment is mitigated by discussing how complex the task is, when completion is expected, where the work can be done, and specifically who may do what. However, delegation involves letting the staff determine many of these factors. If supervisors micromanage the delegated assignment, they may as well do it themselves. Nurse managers must decide the trade-offs between the burden of personal involvement and the risk involved in delegating a critical assignment.

Delegation Planning and Analysis Form

Date assigned: _____   Date of expected completion: _____

Anticipated follow-up dates: (1) _____ (2) _____ (3) _____ (4) _____

Level of importance: 1   2   3   4   5

Description of responsibility (in terms of expected results)

_____

_____

_____

_____

_____

Authority limits/criteria   Accountability

1. _____   What? _____

2. _____   _____

3. _____   When? _____

4. _____   _____

5. _____   How? _____

Fig. 10-5 ■ Form for delegation planning and analysis.

DETERMINE THE AUTHORITY TO BE DELEGATED AND THE APPROPRIATE LIMITS

Determining the authority to be delegated means considering what resources must be made available to the subordinate in order for the subordinate to complete the assignment and what limitations should be placed on these resources. If the subordinate is granted too little authority, it might be difficult or even impossible for the person to accomplish what is expected. If the limits of authority are not carefully spelled out, their absence may be interpreted as a granting of unlimited authority, which may prompt the subordinate to take actions or make commitments that may be unacceptable. Limits also help identify the specific points at which the nurse manager expects to be asked for assistance. Handled properly, limits do not appear to subordinates as restrictions but instead provide a comfort zone within which they can function independently and feel comfortable.

DO NOT COMPLETE THE ASSIGNMENT FOR THE SUBORDINATE

Often nurse managers' concern regarding staff members' lack of progress on an assignment leads them to take over, rather than guide the team toward completion. This is a real problem, especially for the dynamic performer turned manager. Because many nurse managers have advanced to the position they currently hold because they were top performers, they may be reluctant to let go of doing things themselves and trust others to do a good job. Professional managers don't expect a delegated task to be done as they would do it; they expect it to be done to meet the established standards and satisfy the requirements. Nurse managers should keep in mind that doing something for someone is often a precursor to having that someone not want to do the next thing that needs to be done.

HOLD THE SUBORDINATE ACCOUNTABLE AND MONITOR TASK PROGRESS

Nurse managers must decide what information or feedback they will need from the team to stay in touch with the delegated project. Being in touch doesn't mean being in control of the performance, but nurse managers must never fully relinquish their hold. Nurse managers bear ultimate responsibility and have the right to be made aware of the progress of an assignment. If they do not remain aware, they will frequently end up not meeting the goals that their seniors have established for them and their units. Delegation does not mean that managers do not have to pay attention. How they stay in touch is important: they should stand back, ask questions, and expect to be kept informed.

Before providing the assignment, the nurse manager should work with the team to decide whether written reports are necessary or brief oral reports are sufficient. If written reports are required, the manager should let the staff know how they should be constructed and whether support items such as tables, charts, or other graphics are necessary. The nurse manager should be specific about reporting times and deadlines and above all make sure that staff comply with these schedules. One effective method of doing this is to establish critical events or milestones and request to be notified when these events or milestones are reached. Nurse managers must decide how closely the assignment will be supervised. However, controls should never be so tight that they limit subordinates' opportunity to grow and expand their capabilities.

Instructions for the delegated assignment must provide subordinates with enough information to prepare them to succeed, including both what should be done and what should be avoided. Although it is true that staff should be given the opportunity to make mistakes within defined limits, it is also important that those limits be fixed so that any damage done is within the nurse manager's capability to repair. Managers can avoid costly mistakes and nuisance errors by preparing their staffs as fully as possible before turning over assignments to them.

When giving instructions or setting deadlines, managers should avoid generic phrases and statements that are too vague. Nonspecific statements such as "do what's necessary to get the job done" and "let me know if you have any problems" should never be used. Another idiom to avoid is the phrase "as soon as possible." Instead, set a specific deadline and make sure the staff understand that this date is firm unless other arrangements are made well in advance.* If a subordinate is told, "Do whatever is necessary," she or he just might do so! It is not possible to anticipate or discuss with a subordinate every problem that might arise; it is usually not worth the time or effort, and no one has perfect knowledge anyway. However, nurse managers should think about what problems may occur and discuss with their subordinates how they might be resolved.

---

*"Well in advance" in this discussion means in sufficient time to allow the manager to properly schedule any change necessary and to accommodate the need to provide for makeup periods.

SELECT THE SUBORDINATE FOR THE ASSIGNMENT CAREFULLY

Selection of the individual to whom a specific assignment will be delegated should not be taken lightly, and the choice should never be made out of friendship or a desire to please or impress. The person selected is the manager's direct representative for the task to be completed. It is the manager's reputation, the manager's career, and the manager's success that are at risk; therefore, the manager should make the decision as to who gets the job based on the education and/or skill required and the experience, demonstrated capability, and work habits of the subordinates available. The following are other important factors to consider:

- The level of results desired
- The amount of authority to be delegated
- The closeness with which the nurse manager wishes to supervise the performance of the assignment
- The unit subordinates' skill profiles

Although delegating an assignment to the most experienced, best-qualified person on the staff should always be considered, nurse managers must also remember that even the newest staff members must be delegated tasks, especially those that can test and enhance their knowledge and skills. These delegated assignments will allow nurse managers to evaluate the true capabilities of every member of their staffs.

Because most truly effective staff training and development occurs through experience, it is imperative that nurse managers routinely provide all of the members of their staffs with the opportunity to grow professionally. They can do this by making sure that they delegate to subordinates assignments that will expand their experience and skills. Personal growth and achievement can occur within definable and controllable limits without excessive restrictions.

MAKE THE ASSIGNMENT EFFECTIVELY

Nurse managers make a myriad of simple yet important assignments every day. If they give even brief consideration to the six points discussed earlier, they will reduce potential ambiguities and confusion, and the assignments that are made will be carried out more effectively. However, highly complex and important assignments should be thought through carefully, because they have inherent difficulties that can be mitigated only by attentive preparation.

When nurse managers have prepared themselves sufficiently, meeting with a subordinate and making the assignment can be an enjoyable and gratifying experience for both parties. The following nine steps are highly recommended in the delegation of assignments:

1. Set aside sufficient time to make the assignment professionally.
2. Make an appointment with the subordinate and take the necessary steps to minimize interruptions or distractions during the allotted time.
3. Give the subordinate an overview of the assignment and explain why he or she was chosen to do it.
4. Thoroughly explain and discuss the results expected.
5. Describe the authority the subordinate will have and the limits within which the subordinate will work.
6. Emphasize the control arrangements necessary for a successful assignment.
7. Listen carefully to the subordinate's questions; providing the right answers before the assignment begins can eliminate ambiguities and confusion and can also strengthen the subordinate's confidence in dealing with highly complex or critical assignments.
8. Don't demean the subordinate or be critical of the questions asked.
9. Be supportive.

Insufficient Delegation

The leading cause of insufficient delegation (under-delegation) is the attitude many nurse managers have about someone else doing part of their work. Some of these attitudes are developed out of legitimate concerns, such as the risk involved in delegation, time constraints, doubts about subordinates' capabilities, and a strong need to prove oneself. Others, like the desire to maintain control, fear, and distrust, are not legitimate reasons. The researcher G. W. Poteet, in a 1980s study,[3] identified some obstacles to delegation, which are listed in Box 10-1.

A manager who has any doubts about whether or not he or she is an effective delegator can ask himself or herself the following five questions:
1. Do I work long overtime hours?
2. Am I unable to get to important projects?
3. Am I doing the staff nurses' jobs?
4. When I come back from a day off, do I find my desk stacked with work?
5. Have no innovative plans been developed recently?

If the answer to most of these questions is yes, then the manager needs to explore ways to delegate more effectively.

Delegation is a major skill that all nurse managers need to cultivate. It is nurse managers' responsibility to develop the capabilities of their staffs, and failure to delegate is tantamount to failure in the performance

---

BOX 10-1

Obstacles to Delegation

Job confusion
Fears about personal job security
Fear of losing control
Poor time management
Crisis management orientation
Fear of managerial incompetence
Failure to set goals and timetables
Competition for managerial positions
Ignorance about the delegation process
Desire to control upward communication
Lack of confidence in subordinates' abilities
Anxiety over the prospect of losing technical competence
Lack of commitment to the employee development process
Incomplete transition from staff nurse to nurse manager

Data from Poteet GW: Delegation strategies: a must for the nurse executive, *J Nurs Adm* 14(9):18, 1984.

---

of this duty. In addition to the negative impact on staff development, other significant effects such as low employee morale, increased turnover, and excessive sick time can result from a lack of delegation within the unit. If nurse managers constantly solve the problems that subordinates should be taking care of, they will not have the time to do those things that require more knowledge, skill, and authority—in short, to manage. In addition, nurse managers who deprive their staffs of opportunities to grow as professionals and as persons contribute only a fraction of what truly professional managers need to offer.

What Should Not Be Delegated

Although nurse managers cannot do everything that needs to be done, there are many functions and activities that simply cannot be delegated. Examples include the following:

Rounds: Some nurse managers conduct daily rounds—a responsibility that should not be delegated to the assistant nurse manager or a staff nurse.

Performance reviews: It is the manager's job to write performance reviews. Delegation of this fundamental responsibility may put the nurse manager in violation of employment laws or, at a minimum, organizational procedure.

Drug control: In some situations the nurse manager may be personally required to give out or even administer certain drugs.

Goals and objectives: The nurse manager may be required to write the annual objectives for the unit.

Reports: The collection of information for and the submission of drug usage reports or incident reports should not be delegated.

In addition, the following are three important areas for which responsibility should never be delegated:

Discipline: The nurse manager should not delegate responsibility for disciplining a member of the unit or a subordinate. Few things can destroy the staff's confidence more quickly than the inability of the nurse manager to discipline effectively. This responsibility should never be delegated upward to a superior or to the personnel department, although either or both might be involved in the disciplinary procedure. Staff members must view the nurse manager as the key person responsible for maintaining control of the unit.

Morale problems: The nurse manager should not delegate responsibility for handling morale problems in the unit. Obviously, advice may be sought from superiors and other professionals, but it is primarily up to the nurse manager to create a satisfactory work environment and good working relationships among all employees in the unit. Being an effective delegator is an essential element in maintaining a highly disciplined staff with high morale.

Legal responsibilities: The nurse manager should not delegate anything for which he or she has legal accountability. Terminating an employee and handling a patient complaint that could potentially result in litigation are examples of management tasks that should never be delegated.

SUMMARY

- Nurse managers must use time wisely to accomplish everything that is expected of them; this takes planning. Without effective time management, only more time will help.
- Time management begins with the establishment of priorities. Role duties and objectives can be used as guides in priority setting.
- Establishing priorities includes deciding what not to do as well as what to do. Writing out the next day's activities in a prioritized list is important, but one should remember that even well-written plans rarely work out as envisioned; open time should be scheduled to allow for emergencies.
- Nurse managers experience many interruptions during the work shift. Keeping a time control log can help identify patterns of interruption so that ways to reduce unnecessary interruptions can be planned.

- Telephone calls are a major source of interruption; they can be controlled by minimizing small talk, planning calls, using a timer, and stating preferred call times.
- Drop-in visitors are also a source of interruption. Nurse managers should meet visitors outside the office, keep visits short, encourage appointments, keep staff informed, and arrange furniture to discourage unscheduled visits.
- Nurse managers who respect their own time are likely to find others respecting it also.
- Written communication can also cause interruptions. Planning and scheduling paperwork, sorting, delegating, writing effectively, and using an effective filing system can minimize these often untimely interruptions.
- Delegation is a major tool in time management. Nurse managers must understand their own role and their staff members' abilities to delegate effectively. When authority is delegated, nurse managers must set the limits of responsibility. Assignments must be given clearly and precisely.
- Several steps can be taken to ensure effective delegation: plan before delegating, define responsibility in terms of results, define authority limits, don't complete subordinates' assignments, hold subordinates accountable, and select subordinates who are capable of performing the assigned task.
- Three things should never be delegated: disciplining immediate subordinates, handling morale problems within the unit, and performing activities for which the manager has legal accountability.

FINAL THOUGHTS

Most nurse managers never have enough time in their schedules to get done everything that is required in a normal shift. In fact, almost all nurse managers find themselves working harder and working longer but still don't feel that they are making any headway in reducing the mountain of administrative duties and clinical practice activities that must be accomplished. The normal pattern is that nurse managers come in early, work late, and work weekends, and are so worn out when they finally get home at the end of a long day that they don't have any time or energy left for themselves. Previous methods of time management don't seem to work anymore, and this is largely because the world in which the nurse manager works today is nothing like the world that existed a decade ago.

Nurse managers used to be taught that the work would get done if they simply handled a piece of paper just once. But today, they have paper plus electronic mail, voice mail, and wireless communication systems. On their desktops are superfast computers that are networked to others throughout the hospital and perhaps to hundreds more. They are in contact with people they have never met via the Internet and online services like AOL, MSN, and SBC.

Two decades ago, nurse managers were thrilled that they could send a letter via Federal Express and get it to someone across the country by 10:00 AM the next morning. Today, they simply fax it from their desktop computer to the recipient's computer and it arrives in seconds.

Nurse managers used to have secretaries or unit clerks who assisted with letters, memos, and reports. Today, these personnel have been replaced by blazingly fast personal computers that nurse managers must use to write those same letters, memos, and reports.

Today's nurse managers don't handle paper anymore, they handle information; and the time frames within which they must process their work continue to shrink.

To succeed in the new millennium, nurse managers must do more than just get themselves organized. They must do a better job of staying on top of their unfinished work, tasks, and projects, and the only way to do that is to improve their follow-up system. They must use an efficient tracking system that will help convert the normally wasted time found in every workday into time that can be used more efficiently, effectively, and profitably.

This conversion of wasted time into productive time can be called *addition by subtraction*, and if it is accomplished efficiently, the nurse manager will have the time to get the work done, leave the hospital at a decent hour, and enjoy life, friends, and family.

THE NURSE MANAGER SPEAKS

Did anyone ever tell you that it is the quality, not the quantity, of work you do that is important? Sure, you've heard that a thousand times, but no one ever stops giving the nurse manager more and more work—all of which is expected to be done to a high standard of quality.

With their workloads swollen by the downsizing fervor that has swept the healthcare industry, all nurse managers are working harder today than ever before. But most are not finding the time to get even important work done to the level of quality they would like.

So what do nurse managers do during their 8-, 10-, or 12-hour days? The truth is that most don't have the slightest idea. It's just one big swell of pile after pile after pile.

What one must realize is that the number of hours worked is not in any way related to the success that one achieves. Success comes from productivity, efficiency, and effectiveness—not from being busy. When productivity increases, the quality of work improves, things are done on time, and more tasks are accomplished with less effort. Nurse managers get paid for the results they achieve, not for the number of hours they work.

Many nurse managers try to impress others with the number of hours they work. To them, their 70- and 80-hour work weeks are a badge of honor. In almost every instance, however, the overtime is a smoke screen that covers up inefficiencies and poor work habits. If the quality of the work produced by these champions of overtime is analyzed, it is usually easy to see that they really are not superstars; in fact, most are just barely getting by. Most rarely get their work done on time, and the quality of what they produce is minimally acceptable. In fact, if the organization were to compare the number of hours they actually work with the output they produce, the poor rate of return achieved would be quickly identified.

Working longer hours doesn't make a nurse manager more productive. In fact, studies show that those longer hours actually lead to the production of less work per hour spent. Quality, not quantity, is what is important. Working too many hours ensures that more mistakes will be made and that stress levels will be higher. Don't let too many hours burn you out.

REFERENCES

1. Mayer JJ, *Time management for dummies,* ed 2, Foster City, Calif, 1999, IDG Books Worldwide.
2. Hawkins JA: *Moving business forward,* ed 5, Honolulu, 2005, TDC Publishing.
3. Poteet GW: Delegation strategies: a must for the nurse executive, *J Nurs Adm* 14(9):18, 1984.

SUGGESTED READINGS

Allen KR: *Time and information management that really work,* Los Angeles, 1995, Affinity.

Bennis W, Mason RO: *High-speed management,* San Francisco, 1993, Jossey-Bass.

Covey SR: *The 7 habits of highly effective people,* New York, 1989, Simon and Schuster.

Eliopoulos C: Time management: a reminder, *J Nurs Adm* 14(3):30, 1984.

Hansten RI: *Clinical delegation skills,* Gaithersburg, Md, 1996, Aspen.

Kossen S: *Supervision,* New York, 1981, Harper and Row.

Lakein A: *How to gain control of your time and your life,* New York, 1973, Signet.

McCormack MH: *What they don't teach you at the Harvard Business School,* New York, 1992, Bantam.

McGuffin J: *The nurse's guide to successful management,* St Louis, 1999, Mosby.

Meyer C: *Fast cycle time,* New York, 1993, Free Press.

Miller ML: Implementing self-scheduling, *J Nurs Adm* 14(3):33, 1984.

Solving Problems and Making Decisions

OUTLINE

LEARNING SYNOPSIS

Upon successful completion of this chapter, readers will possess a fundamental understanding of how effective problem solving and decision-making can enhance the performance of a nursing unit.

OBJECTIVES

1. Describe various methods for solving problems
2. Identify individual types of problems and the techniques that might be used to resolve them
3. List the eight steps in the problem-solving process
4. Describe methods to develop problem solving within a group
5. Identify potential obstacles to group problem solving
6. Define the terms *satisficing, optimizing*, and *maximizing*
7. Describe the part that risk, certainty, and uncertainty play in the decision-making process
8. Explain why creativity is needed in the nursing unit and what steps the nursing manager can take to promote it

In recent years, it has become very clear to hospital administrators that subordinate managers, such as those leading nursing units, must use advanced problem-solving and decision-making strategies to discharge their responsibilities successfully. In the late 1970s, researcher A. Latz investigated how nurse managers made decisions and discovered that the vast majority showed poor management skills in this area for the following reasons[1]:

They tended to rely on short-term planning: Most were reactive not proactive in discharging their duties.

They made decisions by themselves: They made decisions mostly alone, without the collaboration of other members of the management team or their unit staffs.

They decided on a course of action while under stress: Decision-making under stress was caused mostly by a lack of planning on the nurse manager's part. Most tended to wait to make a decision until there was pressure to comply or a deadline was near.

They seldom resolved potential or nonroutine problems: Their lack of planning caused them to spend so much time accomplishing routine matters that they did not have time to head off unscheduled challenges.

As a result of the poor managerial skills identified in the research, the average nursing unit studied was a reactionary environment (i.e., the focus was on responding to problems as they occurred, instead of preventing them). In addition, the stress and pressure under which most nurse managers operated contributed strongly to low levels of satisfaction among the staff, as indicated by unusually high turnover rates and unacceptably high rates of absenteeism within the units.

Nurse managers work under demanding circumstances and in an environment in which there is little room for error. Stressful circumstances require managers to make decisions based on objective evidence to reduce the chance of failure and to work diligently toward overcoming their personal prejudices and mitigating the lack of experience and knowledge in their units. Therefore, they must spend as much time thinking about potential problems as they do solving existing ones. This chapter provides a background in the problem-solving and decision-making processes that nurse managers should use daily.

Historically, throughout much of the healthcare industry the terms *problem solving* and *decision-making* have been used inconsistently and often interchangeably. Although it is true that, at first glance, the two processes appear similar and may even depend on one another in some circumstances, the terms are not synonymous. For example, solving a problem may involve making several decisions; conversely, a major decision may provide the solution for several related problems.

Many of the decisions typically made by nurse managers do not involve problem solving (e.g., decisions regarding budgets, equipment, or other similar matters that have no direct bearing on selecting a future course of action). Similarly, many of the problems that are dealt with in the nursing unit do not involve decision-making as a deliberate process. For example, problem-solving solutions that involve habitual action or result from a purely behavioral response may be forms of problem solving, but they do not require much in the way of higher mental processes (e.g., walking deliberately and slowly while traversing a wet hospital corridor or stopping a patient from pulling out his intravenous line).

Most of the time, however, decision-making is closely linked with problem solving. Situations that involve both processes are most often dynamic ones in which the nurse manager recognizes that (1) something is wrong, and (2) a reaction or solution is needed.

In short, the process of decision-making is the behavior exhibited by an individual when selecting and implementing one course of action from among alternatives that may or may not involve a problem.

PROBLEM SOLVING

Definition of the Problem

The most fundamental part of solving any problem is correctly identifying the problem itself. Once the problem has been properly identified, it is usually a routine matter for the nurse manager to determine the solutions or implement changes. For the purposes of this discussion, a problem is defined as a departure from what is considered acceptable or desirable as perceived by the individual who is responsible for dealing with the situation (i.e., the nurse manager).

The importance of correctly identifying the problem can be seen by considering the following situation that occurs frequently in the nursing unit.

The nurse manager has expressed her desire to have all patient care plans updated daily, but the majority of the nurses assigned to the unit are unable to complete this task. The nurse manager might identify the problem as the failure on the part of the staff to complete the care plans in accordance with her expressed wishes. The causes for this situation may be very diverse and might include reasons such as the following:

Fatigue: The staff may have been working long hours due to the admission of a large number of critically ill patients. Although this may not be a desirable situation, it may be understandable.

Apathy: The staff nurses may simply have failed to do the work because they feel that the requirement is unfair. This situation is neither desirable nor understandable.

A problem should be expressed as a descriptive statement outlining a state of affairs, not as a judgment or conclusion. If the nurse manager begins the statement of a problem with a judgment, the solution at which he or she arrives will almost always be equally judgmental. When the problem is identified in this way, critical descriptive elements of the deviation from the desired state are almost always overlooked. For instance, if the nurse manager in the care plan example described earlier defines the problem solely as noncompliance with her instruction and immediately proceeds to write interpretive notes before spending time discovering the facts, she could turn a minor problem into a full-blown crisis.

Therefore, the most important step in problem solving is the first one taken—that is, proper identification of the situation that appears to be a problem and its classification as a potential, actual, or critical problem, as follows[2]:

Potential problem: a situation that may not have to be dealt with immediately; it can emerge at any time and involve virtually any area

Actual problem: a situation that requires prompt action but may not be urgent

Critical problem: an urgent situation that requires immediate intervention

What solution is applied to a problem will depend on how the problem is identified. As noted earlier, properly identifying a problem begins with stating the problem in descriptive and nonjudgmental terms. This is a critical issue. If the problem is not identified well (it is prematurely or incorrectly diagnosed), the solution that is applied will be inadequate at best and may precipitate a crisis situation at worst. The successful diagnosis of a problem involves the following three basic steps:

1. *Getting all the facts:* Nurse managers should not rush to start making decisions before the whole story is known.
2. *Separating facts from interpretations:* Nurse managers should ensure that they are dealing with what really happened and not their own or someone else's interpretation of the events.
3. *Determining the scope of the problem:* Nurse managers must ascertain how big the problem is, how critical it is, and what its potential impact is.

The following example shows how these three principles can be applied:

A registered nurse (RN) on the night shift has complained that one of the junior nurses on the shift consistently fails to take the vital signs of the patients assigned to her but charts that she has done so.

Because the identified situation involves two levels of staff, the nurse manager needs to gather her facts from reliable sources at both levels. She should carefully question the RN regarding the situation and then conscientiously and nonjudgmentally talk with the junior nurse as well. She can corroborate the statements of both nurses by subtly asking the junior nurse's patients about the situation. If the nurse manager's investigation does not help her clearly separate the facts of the issue from interpretations of facts, she should seek the assistance of an unbiased third party. If the situation is not handled carefully, the nurse manager runs the risk of acting on her own interpretation of the facts as if it were reality; that is, either the junior nurse is lazy, dishonest, or both, or the RN has not relayed the facts properly.

If nurse managers prematurely interpret the facts surrounding an incident, they can alter their ability to deal with the situation in an objective manner. Instead of acting prematurely in the situation described earlier, a professional manager will look for other possible reasons or explanations for the alleged behavior that do not imply negative assumptions about the character of the junior staff nurse.

In addition, how well the scope of the problem is assessed will determine whether a lasting solution must be implemented or a temporary one will suffice. For example, is this a situational problem requiring only intervention with a simple explanation, or is it a more complex issue that involves the integrity of the staff nurse or the reporting processes used by the RN? Whatever the situation, the example clearly shows that problems must be carefully diagnosed and classified before any action is taken or any decision-making is begun. This is a critical step in positive management and should never be overlooked.

Methods for Solving Problems

There are about as many methods for solving problems as there are managers trying to solve them. The techniques include tried and proven formulas and haphazard and counterproductive procedures. Often, which methods are used is related directly to the manager's level of experience.

TRIAL AND ERROR

It is not uncommon for managers with only limited management-level experience to use a trial and error technique. In this approach, one solution after another is thrown at the problem until either it is solved, it improves, or by some miracle it goes away. With little or no experience to draw upon, many new managers are unable to judge the potential effectiveness of their intended efforts and most often have little time to conduct any significant research. A "shoot from the hip" solution is often what is put into effect, with results that are frequently dubious at best. Alternatively, solution after solution may be attempted until the problem is resolved. The following is an example:

> A rehabilitation unit shows an increasing incidence of decubitus ulcers. The unit manager first employs a trial and error problem-solving method and uses various treatments to decrease the size of the ulcers (e.g., heat lamps, Betadine and a cold hair dryer, hydrogen peroxide and Elase ointment). After considerable attempts have produced no results, the manager changes her technique and decides that standard preventive methods would provide a better solution. She implements a turning schedule for the patients and personally sees that it is enforced. As a result, the problem is decreased, and the prior low level of ulcer incidence is restored.

An approach such as trial and error can often be far more time consuming than is desirable and may even be detrimental to patient care and the operation of the unit. Although without question learning does occur, the nurse manager risks being perceived as a poor problem solver who has wasted a great deal of time and money in implementing ineffective solutions. In extreme cases, this approach can place a patient at risk and put the organization in a position of financial liability.

EXPERIMENTATION

Experimentation as a type of problem solving is much more rigorous in its application than is the trial and error approach. For example, experimentation might be implemented through the execution of pilot projects or limited trials. Depending on how it is used, experimentation can achieve a variety of different results that range from creative and effective to weak and unproductive. Experimentation, when used as a major method of problem solving, often evolves into a trial and error process. However, if all previous methods of problem solving have failed, it may be beneficial to experiment with various solutions. The following is an example:

> A nurse manager finds herself in a situation in which she is being challenged by the disagreement of a single staff nurse; the result is that the subordinate continually undermines the authority of the manager in these disputed matters. The subordinate's inappropriate comments and criticism and the disagreements they have created have carried over to the rest of the staff and are now causing trouble within the unit. The manager has attempted to counsel the staff nurse, but that action only resulted in further confrontation, and the desired results (i.e., mutual alliance, improved morale, and productivity) have not been achieved.

Although at first this situation looks clear-cut, in reality it is one in which the manager may want to experiment carefully. Rather than simply initiating action to terminate the employment of the disgruntled nurse, the manager may elect to assign her to a special project that requires a good deal of personal initiative and the assumption of specific responsibility for a defined time. Why not just fire her? The reason is really very simple; if the manager fires an employee, that is tantamount to failure. It is a manager's job to obtain cooperation and respect from the employee. Failure to do that is not resolution of a problem but more often the precursor to another. The assignment to a position requiring personal initiative might provide the stimulus that is missing from the staff nurse's routine, and if the assignment proves innovative, solves the problem, and salvages the employee, then the manager has discharged her responsibility. Moreover, the person who replaces an employee who is let go may be worse that the one who left.

Although some disagreement is inevitable and can be useful in task accomplishment, uncontrolled and unprofessional behavior of a subordinate, especially if it undermines the manager's authority, should not be tolerated. If the manager has applied solid leadership skills, offered alternative performance challenges, and provided counseling and yet the problem persists, then the dilemma becomes a human resources issue, and termination of employment might be the action of choice.

CRITIQUE

Critique is a problem-solving technique in which the manager assumes the role of listener and facilitator, providing feedback and constructive criticism to assist the staff in proper identification of problems. This technique is especially effective in situations in which the communication process has deteriorated to the point that it is difficult to identify the actual problem. Managers can engage their staffs in a series of brainstorming sessions, work closely with them, and carefully critique their findings until the problem has been correctly identified and resolved to the satisfaction of the participants; or the managers can simply listen and make the necessary changes themselves. The following is an example:

> A staff nurse has been heard complaining bitterly about the new admission assessment form developed by the nursing service department. By listening carefully to the concerns of the staff nurse, the nurse manager discovers that this particular nurse had developed and submitted a set of forms to the policy and procedure committee, but the forms had been rejected. The rejection has never been resolved, and the employee has become distraught over the handling of the issue. After the manager looks into the matter and discusses it carefully with her subordinate, she is able to establish a fair and unbiased critique of the nurse's perception

of how the situation was handled. The result is that the real problem (rejection) is identified and brought out into the open so that it can be resolved.

LAISSEZ-FAIRE

Some problems are self-limiting. In other words, if the problem is permitted to run its natural course, it will be solved by those personally involved. A laissez-faire approach has been known to achieve excellent results in many situations, especially when highly professional or well-educated employees are involved, but there is no guarantee that uniform application of such an approach will solve all of the problems that can occur in the nursing unit.

Professional managers do not ignore their supervisory responsibilities when they use this method but may often find an ideal resolution simply by allowing the participants to discover their own solutions to a problem. This form of leadership can be used, for example, when a newly graduated RN joins a unit in which most of the staff are licensed practical nurses (LPNs) with many years of experience. If the new RN becomes defensive and overly assertive in his or her role, the LPNs may grow to resent the organization's substitution of level of education for lack of experience. If the nurse manager intervenes prematurely, a problem that most often will be worked out by those involved can become an ongoing source of conflict. In fact, many different staffing problems, role conflicts, and interpersonal relationships can be resolved by the individuals involved if the nurse manager is willing to take an ancillary position temporarily and allow those involved to solve the problem. The skill here lies in knowing when to do nothing!

METAPHOR-BASED TECHNIQUES

Metaphor-based techniques are creative problem-solving methods that attempt to break conventional thinking patterns and suspend judgment in order to elicit a number of highly original ideas within a short time through a process of free association.[3] In this technique, the staff (or the nurse manager acting alone) identify certain concepts or ideas and, using them as a base, create new ideas. This is an analytic approach in which analogies (including fantasy or symbolism) are used to develop creative thinking to increase the output of individuals or groups. It employs ideas that do not necessarily fit into the traditional model in an effort to discover new alternatives to traditional responses. A conscious effort is made to look at old problems from completely different viewpoints. The following is an example:

A terminally ill patient with bone metastases has been difficult to care for because the staff has repeatedly had difficulty positioning him comfortably. Instead of looking at the situation in the traditional way, such as by suggesting the use of a tub or heated swimming pool, the nurse manager encourages her staff to employ a metaphorical approach. The staff members employ their collective imagination to see themselves in a magic bed, trying to find with their own bodies the ultimate comfortable position. There are no limits on the imagination in this process. The staff can fantasize about strings holding up their extremities or a magic carpet carrying them off that applies no pressure whatsoever to their weakened bodies. As a result, the traditional problem is viewed from very different perspectives and a wide variety of metaphorical solutions are discussed.

This method may at first seem useless because it involves simple-minded and easy-to-perform exercises that often produce limited or no results. Certainly, it is often easy (and unproductive) to think up metaphors, and actually implementing the ideas generated can require a great deal of energy and may achieve only limited results. The rewards of this approach, however, may lie less the results it produces than in the teamwork and professionalism it creates.

BRAINSTORMING

Another approach that is widely used in the modern business world is very similar to metaphor-based techniques. This method, called *brainstorming*, is designed to help people generate creative ideas. It was first discussed as a serious approach to problem resolution by A. F. Osborn in his book *Applied Imagination*.[4] In this process, a group of people collectively use their brains to "storm" a problem in commando fashion, with each participant courageously attacking the same objective. To obtain maximum creativity from a group using the brainstorming technique, the following four basic rules must be understood and observed:

1. *Critical judgment is not allowed:* Criticism of the ideas generated must be withheld until later.
2. *Freewheeling ideas are encouraged:* The wilder the idea that is expressed, the better; this is based on the belief that it is easier to reduce a wild idea to a workable solution than to come up with the solution on its own.
3. *Quantity is the goal:* It is not the quality of the ideas but the quantity of ideas, regardless of how simplistic or bizarre they may seem, that is most important. The thought is that the greater the number of ideas generated, the greater the likelihood of producing an idea that will solve the problem.
4. *Imagination and improvement are sought:* In addition to contributing their own ideas, participants are encouraged to suggest methods of turning another's ideas into better or more workable approaches and to propose ways of joining two or more ideas to create still another idea.

Although the ideas that result from these brainstorming sessions, considered individually, may seem wild and unproductive, they frequently lead to very creative solutions. Some of the criticisms of this approach are its relatively high cost, the amount of time consumed, and the superficiality of many of the solutions suggested.

DECISION TREE

In all of the methods discussed earlier, possible problem solutions are evaluated qualitatively. The decision tree provides a more quantitative approach to the analysis of solution alternatives. A decision tree, as illustrated in Fig. 11-1, is a graphic model that incorporates risks, options, outcomes, preferences, and other pertinent information to facilitate resolution of a specific problem. A decision tree can provide nurse managers with a means of visualizing decision alternatives and their possible consequences. The process begins with identification of a primary problem that has at least two possible solutions. The predicted consequences of each alternative are considered, along with the probability that each consequence will occur. The model resembles a tree as the decision points are diagrammed.

The problem being considered in Fig. 11-1 is one that has arisen in virtually every nursing unit in the healthcare industry, namely, the staff have expressed a desire to have every other weekend off. The following are the alternative decisions considered:

1. Use the float pool
2. Continue to give staff one weekend off a month
3. Employ staff from temporary agencies
4. Work short-staffed

Below each alternative, certain consequences are listed, and each is rated according to probability of occurrence. Simple but arbitrary rating systems are generally used, such as the numbers from 1 through 5, with 1 representing the lowest probability and 5 the highest.

Inspection of the decision tree shows that, if the float pool is used, there is high probability (5) that such personnel will be familiar with the hospital, moderate probability (3) that the staff will have some weekends off and be content, and low probability (2) that float personnel will be unable to meet staffing needs. If, however, the nurses continue to have only one weekend off per month, there is very high probability (5) of poor morale, decreased productivity, and increased overtime, and moderate probability (3) of increased turnover.

The outcomes diagrammed on the tree largely represent the subjective opinions of the nurse manager and are based primarily on his or her experiences

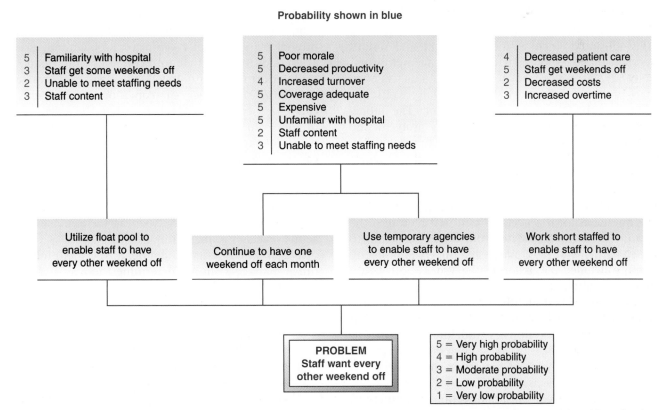

Fig. 11-1 ■ Decision tree for analyzing risks, options, outcomes, and other pertinent information considered in selecting a problem solution.

and judgment; but they may also be supported by factual data. The decision tree is not a rigorous quantitative method that will always indicate the correct decision; rather, it is a technique that produces varied data on which a reasonable decision can be based after consideration of different alternatives and their probable consequences. Although a decision tree is perhaps more reliable at producing a workable solution than a brainstorming session, it most often yields a somewhat biased solution that reflects the opinion of the manager who uses it. With this method, the quality of the results achieved depends the objectivity and skill of the manager applying it.

When managers use a device such as a decision tree, they must realize that their subsequent decisions may depend on future events and that even the original decision is subjective at best. Nevertheless, the decision tree is an effective tool for short- and medium-term planning as well as for decision-making. When used correctly, the decision tree takes into account the probability of occurrence of each consequence of each possible alternative and provides a means of placing a value on each alternative. The decision is then made by identifying the choice that most effectively minimizes loss and maximizes gain.[5] The reality in the nursing profession, however, is that most nurse managers hesitate to use devices such as the decision tree because of their complexity.

VROOM AND YETTON DECISION-MAKING MODEL

La Monica and Finch[6] applied the Vroom and Yetton[7] decision-making model to nursing management situations. Their research suggested that managers who employ this model achieve significantly more effective outcomes than managers who do not. The model allows managers to diagnose a given problem and determine the most effective approach to resolving it.

To use the Vroom and Yetton[7] model, managers answer seven questions that require a yes or no response. Each subsequent question addresses a more specific aspect of the problem being analyzed. Together, the questions form a decision tree that identifies the appropriate leadership style (from strictly autocratic to group participation) for addressing the given problem. A more detailed discussion of the Vroom and Yetton model is shown in Chapter 9. The model has, however, been modified slightly here to reflect the specific points of this dialog. In broad terms, the decision model provides the following guidelines:

- If the decision must be accepted by the group, then involvement of the group in the decision-making process is essential.
- If the quality of the final decision is important, then experts should solve the problem.

- If both quality and acceptance are required, then a combination of expert input and group participation must be used to solve the problem.

The purpose of the model is to integrate variables such as quality requirements, need for group acceptance, availability of information, and degree of problem structure in order to suggest a decision-making style that will yield a solution in the shortest time given the difficulty of the problem.

The Problem-Solving Process

The general process of problem solving can be divided into eight steps that can be applied to arrive at the best possible alternative. The realities of the nursing unit are such that nurse managers may not always be able to leave the floor and go the library to search out solutions to a problem, because far too many problems faced in this demanding environment require immediate action. Therefore, understanding basic principles, learning an organized method for problem solving, and honing one's problem-solving skills through a process of critical thinking are fundamental to making the best decisions and arriving at the best solutions. The eight basic steps in problem solving are described in the following sections.

1. DEFINE THE PROBLEM CLEARLY

The first suggestion of a problem may be the recognition of a number of seemingly small indicators that, taken individually, mean nothing but together provide evidence that a significant problem may exist. These indicators include unit conditions such as poor staff performance, antiquated care plans, and low staff morale. At first glance, the conditions might seem to call for a specific type of relief, such as the assignment of more nurses or more overtime; however, when nurse managers examine such situations with a critical eye, they may discover that they are drawing conclusions too quickly. To arrive at the best possible decisions, nurse managers may conclude that they must consider other factors that may be contributing to decreased productivity, such as increased patient acuity levels or a fluctuating census.

When attempting to define a specific problem, nurse managers should determine the area it affects and ask themselves the following questions:

1. Do I have the authority to deal with this issue by myself?
2. Do I have the knowledge and experience to provide the proper corrective action?
3. Do I have the time to see the problem through to correction?
4. Would it be proper to get someone else to do it or at least to provide assistance?

5. What are the benefits than can be expected from solving the problem?

A list of the potential benefits can provide some of the criteria needed to evaluate and compare alternative approaches to problem resolution. The list can also aid in assessing potential costs and in assigning a priority to the solution.

2. ACCUMULATE INFORMATION

Before a problem can be accurately defined, nurse managers must gather information concerning the problem. They can use this information to develop and evaluate possible solutions and to follow up on the results of the solution after it has been implemented. The information gathered will probably be a combination of hard facts and emotional opinions. It is extremely important that all information gathered be verified and not simply accepted. Only relevant, valid, accurate, and detailed information should be considered, and it should be obtained only from persons or sources with knowledge of the subject. When possible, every attempt should be made to obtain the information in writing, because this typically encourages people to report facts accurately. If a source declines a request to provide his or her statement in writing, that in itself is a good clue as to the accuracy of the comments that would have been made.

The nurse manager must decide who will be required to provide information, and it is fully within his or her right to ask that everyone involved do so. Although this approach may not always yield the highest-quality information, it may reduce misinformation and it provides everyone concerned with an opportunity to tell what he or she thinks is wrong in a given situation.

Experience by itself is a very good source of information. This experience can include the nurse manager's personal knowledge as well as the wisdom of other concerned staff members. Staff should not be discounted as a prime source of information, because most will have excellent ideas on what should be done about the problem, and many of these ideas will represent good information and valuable suggestions.

WARNING !

In the data collection process it is all too easy to acquire inaccurate or biased information. Professional managers always take the time to verify all information they receive. Not all people can remove their emotions from their professional duties, and that failing often taints the information they provide. The professional manager remains slightly skeptical of all sources of information and makes a concerted effort to omit personal conjecture or opinion from the information received.

3. VERIFY AND ANALYZE THE INFORMATION RECEIVED

Not all information received will be accurate or honest, or bear directly on the problem. This point cannot be stressed enough. Objectivity is very difficult to maintain, particularly if people have already formulated their own opinions regarding the problem or feel that they might be affected by the decision made to rectify it.

After all of the information has been gathered, it should first be sorted into some orderly arrangement, verified for accuracy, and then analyzed. The following is one method that can be used to sort acquired information:

Categorize the information in terms of its reliability: This step is not as easy as it sounds. Determining reliability requires a good deal of objectivity on the part of the person sorting the information. This process must be done without emotion, favoritism, or prejudice.

Divide the information into most important, important, and least important: Again, this process requires as much objectivity as possible.

Organize the information into a time sequence: Insofar as possible, a determination is made of what happened first, what occurred before what, and what the contributing circumstances were. This also should be an objective process; care should be taken not to allow subjectivity or personal desire to slip in.

Set up the information in terms of cause and effect: What is causing what is determined (i.e., is A causing B, or is it the opposite way around?).

Classify the information: The information is placed into broad categories, for example:
- Human factors
- Personality
- Education
- Age
- Relationships among concerned individuals
- Problems that might exist outside of the hospital
- Technical factors such as nursing skills, equipment, or the type of unit
- Time factors such as maturity, length of service, overtime, type of shift, and double shifts
- Length of time the problem has existed (i.e., How long has this been going on?)
- Other influences (organizational policy, rules and regulations, other potential contributing factors)

There is always a very good chance that the information collected will not be complete, and therefore it will be difficult to use it as the single source for determining a solution. To fill in the gaps left by missing information, managers will have to make certain assumptions. Managers must ensure that these assumptions are based on critical thinking. Managers must also recognize that whenever a problem involves people, the value systems of the people concerned will influence their analyses of the situation.

It is imperative that all information gathered be verified for accuracy and applicability. Nurse managers must understand that all of the information that surrounds a problem may not be accurate. Before using any information, nurse managers must determine its truthfulness and potential.

4. DEVELOP SEVERAL DIFFERENT SOLUTIONS

As the gathered information is analyzed, it is very possible that a number of excellent ideas regarding possible solutions to the problem will suggest themselves. When they do, they should be put in writing, and managers should start developing ideas around them. This type of problem resolution should not be restricted to a single solution, because doing so may limit thinking and lead to too much concentration on only a portion of the opportunities available. If, instead, managers focus on developing several alternative solutions, they will have the opportunity to combine the best parts of several good solutions to create a superior one. Also, alternatives are valuable in case the first one proves impossible to achieve.

When exploring alternative solutions, managers should not be critical of the way the problem had been dealt with previously. Very commonly, a problem requiring resolution has existed for a long time. One reason is that many of the staff are reluctant to bring problems to the attention of the nurse manager and instead will have applied their own quick fixes. If staff members are made to feel that management finds their attempts or those of others to be inadequate, they are less likely to embrace the solution provided by the manager.

Instead, the attempts that have been made to resolve the problem should be viewed as a record of past experience, and although they may not always supply an answer, they can aid the thinking process and help prepare for future problem solving. It is very good practice and shows professionalism for nurse managers to review the literature, attend relevant seminars, and brainstorm with others when they are attempting to solve a problem. Sometimes others will have solved similar problems, and their methods can be applied to the current problem. This collective brain trust should never be disregarded. In fact, research conducted at the Sloan School of Management at the Massachusetts Institute of Technology in the 1990s

and the first 2 years of the current millennium suggests that the brainstorming of problems is a vital part of organizational knowledge management.*

5. CONSIDER THE CONSEQUENCES OF EACH SOLUTION

A critical part of determining the best solution is considering the short- and long-term consequences of each possible alternative. One recommended method of comparing the anticipated consequences is to ask the following questions:

- How far has the situation deteriorated?
- Must drastic steps be taken or can time aid as a cure?
- Is this a new problem or has it existed for a long time?
- What will be the effect of each possible solution on the quality of patient care?
- Is there a solution that is readily applicable and that will produce quicker results?
- Have these solutions been used before? If so, what were the results?
- For each solution, are there reasons for potential worker dissatisfaction if that method is used? How high might the level of dissatisfaction be?
- For each solution, are there reasons for improved worker satisfaction if that method is used?
- What is the anticipated cost of each solution?
- How does the potential cost of each solution compare with the potential results it might achieve?

6. DECIDE WHICH SOLUTION TO USE

Different solutions require implementation at different times to achieve maximum effectiveness. For example, solutions that are intended to rectify matters of discipline or poor patient care need immediate implementation. To accommodate the need for rapid action, the nurse manager should be aware of his or her level of authority to act in the given situation and the types of penalties that can be meted out for specific infractions.

If the solution to a problem involves a change in the method of performance or new equipment, it may be met with resistance by the staff. Almost all people are disturbed by changes that reorder their habitual patterns or threaten their security or status—no matter how much they may say they are not. Change

---

*Dr. Erik Brynjolfsson, Schussel Professor of Management at the Sloan School of Management, stated in the September 9, 1996, issue of *Information Week*, "The same dollar spent on the same problem may provide an invaluable asset to the organization as a whole" (p. 26).

can be an extremely difficult process to manage and requires specialized training for all those concerned. If a recommended solution to a problem involves change, it is highly recommended that the personnel responsible for implementing the change receive the proper training prior to implementation. Many well-founded and highly anticipated plans have failed because the leader did not recognize that the change process must be set in motion before solutions can be implemented and that follow-up must be conducted during and after implementation.

Those who will be affected by the change must be fully informed of the goals and reasons for the change prior to implementation. If resistance runs high in the working environment, any change, regardless of its quality and potential, is unlikely to succeed unless an effort is made to sell the idea. This selling begins with making sure that everyone concerned with the implementation of the idea is fully committed to it. Nurse managers, in their role as change agents, should spend time with the individuals concerned, explain the reasons for the change, and elicit their responses and cooperation. Managers must be as objective as possible in this process and take the time to ensure that all of the outcomes, both positive and negative, are identified.

Exactly how change is implemented within a specific working environment can vary greatly, depending primarily on the scope of the change and the value attached to the process that will be changed. No formula can be provided that will measure the reaction to any specific change. The best possible way to deal with change is to develop strong relationships with staff before the change is attempted. The more staff members trust and respect the individual filling the position of nurse manager, the more willing they will be to accept the changes he or she requests. A manager who does not enjoy such a trusting and respectful relationship should, whenever possible, attempt the change in a limited area so that difficulties can be identified and steps taken to correct them before the change is forced on the entire unit. It is never good management to impose a sudden change on the staff. In fact, change is far easier to accomplish when the manager gets the staff involved in its creation as early as possible. Regardless of how highly educated the nurse manager may be or how well he or she may meet the demands of the profession, the implementation of change will always offer significant challenges to success because it involves an emotional acceptance and response from others. The intelligent manager anticipates resistance and involves the staff as early as possible in creating solutions.

One of the best ways to prepare for the challenges of implementing change is to understand what has been referred to as the "zone of acceptance" in executive decision-making.[8] This remarkable concept was first put forward in 1937 by C. I. Barnard, and understanding it has enabled managers to make positive decisions ever since. The essence of this idea is that most employees will cooperate only with directions or orders that fit into their zone of acceptance. Some instructions will clearly be unacceptable, some will be neutral, others barely acceptable, and some fully acceptable; however, only fully acceptable instructions lie within the zone of acceptance.

One of the classic rules of management is never to issue an edict that one knows will not be obeyed. Therefore, if managers know that they must give instruction or directions that they feel may not be obeyed, they must commit themselves to providing education and motivation if they expect the staff to comply. They must sell the change to the staff and obtain the staff's commitment to it before implementing the change. Failure to do so can cause severe damage to the credibility of nurse managers and to the welfare of their units. The following provides an example:

> A nurse manager decides that the best possible solution to the unit's short-staffing problem is to supplement the staff with personnel from temporary agencies. The manager's staff, however, has strong ideas about the use of agency nurses and the quality of these personnel and are not willing to cooperate with them to make the required transition go smoothly. If the nurse manager cannot educate the staff regarding the benefits that can be achieved by using agency nurses or motivate them to interact positively with them, the solution, no matter how good, will fail. The manager must ensure that the solution is well within the staff's zone of acceptance before implementing the procedure.

7. IMPLEMENT THE DECISION

Once a decision has been made regarding the action to be taken, implementation should follow as quickly as is prudent. If the implementation creates a series of new problems that the nurse manager had not previously considered, then these impediments must be evaluated as carefully as were the potential consequences identified for the original solution alternatives. The implementation period is a trying one, and as noted earlier the implementation process is frequently met with initial resistance; therefore, managers must be very careful not to abandon a workable solution simply because someone objects to it. In fact, it is almost certain that someone on the staff will not like the change, regardless of how good or beneficial it is. If the previous steps in the problem-solving process have been followed, then this solution has already been carefully thought out and potential problems addressed, and implementation should not be delayed. Nurse managers understand that (a) there is no such thing as a perfect solution, (b) all change is disruptive, and (c) not everyone is going to appreciate the new modification. One way to understand the importance of these points is to remember that a person who does nothing *is* taking action and is making a strong statement about the situation.

8. EVALUATE THE SOLUTION

After the solution has been implemented, the results should be reviewed. Nurse managers need to compare the actual results and benefits achieved with the objectives that were established and the outcomes that were expected when the decision was made. The fact that a change has been "implemented" does not mean that the new practice is actually being followed. People show a very real tendency to fall back into old patterns and fervently provide lip service to the change while actually engaging in the same old behavior. Because of this human failing, nurse managers must continually ask themselves the following questions:

- Are the objectives being fulfilled? If not, why not?
- If they are being fulfilled, are the results better or worse than originally expected?
- If the results are better, what reasons may have contributed to the success?
- If the results are not better, why are they not?

Conducting a continuous follow-up keeps the change on course and provide nurse managers with invaluable insights and experience that might be useful in other situations.

The outcome of every change implemented should be studied just as a coach studies replays of a game. While viewing the tape, the coach continually seeks answers to the following vital questions:

- Where were mistakes made?
- How can they be avoided in the future?
- What decisions led to successes? Why?

If nurse managers evaluate and build upon experience, they can develop valuable problem-solving skills that can be used throughout their management careers.

Group Problem Solving

In an authoritarian environment, the traditional, status-quo approach to decision-making is used. Historically, nurse managers, when confronted with problems in the nursing unit, took it upon themselves to develop solutions. Today, however, the approach to problem resolution is rapidly changing. Factors such as the increasing complexity of the problems being faced and the heightened desire among staff members to be involved in the development of solutions are creating the need for staff participation in the decision-making process and for group approaches to problem solving.

Participative problem solving is a process that joins the efforts of staff with those of management in the decision-making process. The participants may include all ancillary personnel, only nurses, or a few hand-picked employees. The proper mix is dictated by the problem being considered and the ability of the staff to provide objective input. The problem-solving process may be formal or informal, and the involvement of participants may be intellectual, emotional, and/or physical.

The principal argument in support of group involvement is that it allows a greater quantity and often a higher quality of information to be brought to bear on the selection of alternatives. Involving a variety of different members of the staff can produce information that is more complete, more accurate, and less biased than information obtained from a single individual, because it has been clarified through exposure to the group. The discussion and participation of group members during information gathering and analysis enhances their cooperation in the implementation of the problem solution. Because nurses at all levels perform their duties under significant time constraints, the data-gathering phase of this process is usually limited by the job setting.

In practice, the degree of group participation will be determined by the following factors:

- Who initiated the idea being considered
- How much subordinate support is required for implementation
- How effectively employees carry out each phase of decision-making (i.e., diagnosing the problem, identifying alternatives, evaluating consequences, and making choices)
- How much importance the nurse manager attaches to the ideas received
- How much knowledge staff members have about the matter being considered

PARTICIPATORY MANAGEMENT

Studies conducted by R. Likert in the early 1960s found that, when individuals are allowed to participate in determining a solution to a problem, they function more productively and implementation becomes easier because of the feelings of ownership generated by the process of shared problem solving.[9]

Participatory management is not without its failings. For example, it can be time consuming. However, even this drawback is mitigated by the fact that the diverse opinions and information which typically emerge as a result of the process often allow a group to make a decision faster than an individual, who must spend more time gathering information and analyzing it. Another disadvantage often cited by opponents of participatory problem solving is the potential for benign tyranny to emerge within the group; that is, members of the group who are less informed or less confident may allow stronger, more informed members to present all the solutions and make all the decisions. This can lead to the emergence of a power struggle between the nurse manager and a few assertive members of the group. However, the advantages of group participation so strongly outweigh the disadvantages that it is rapidly becoming the preferred method of problem resolution. In fact, it is almost universally the process of choice in Fortune 500 companies.

THE QUALITY CIRCLE

Another form of participative decision-making is referred to as the *quality circle*. The quality circle, or representative committee, was adapted from W. Ouchi's theory Z,[10] a management concept that first came into popularity in the United States in the early 1980s and was based on similar business practices used in Japan. Using quality circles to develop solutions to problems has since become as successful in this country as in the country where the practice originated. This method of decision-making, which can easily be adapted by the nursing profession, is based on trust between management and workers and on the involvement of workers in making the decisions that affect them. In Japan, the system emphasizes consensus-based decision-making, lifetime job security, and a strong commitment to the goals of the organization. Although the process is somewhat different in the United States, it has been very successful in promoting similar ideas. In both countries, the desired results of a vibrant quality circle process are increased job commitment, higher productivity, and lower turnover.

Z management, as it is applied through quality circles, has been used to a small degree in healthcare situations, but because it thrives best in areas in which total organizational decision and commitment are present, it has not achieved wide acclaim in the more conservative and authoritative environment of the hospital nursing unit. For example, nurse managers would not ordinarily use this technique unless their institution was promoting it. However, it is useful to understand the process so that pieces of its quality might be applied in other more readily accepted areas of decision management. The following is an example of how it might be applied in the nursing unit:

To establish its quality service process, a large Midwestern healthcare facility divided the nurses on each floor into quality circles of eight or ten individuals and appointed a facilitator for each circle. Each circle meets on a regular schedule to discuss problems encountered in the nursing environment and tries to develop solutions for each. Each circle is a thoroughly disciplined entity committed to training, development of group skills, and rigorous step-by-step improvement procedures. Whenever a policy or procedural change is suggested, there is continuous discussion within the circle until a consensus is achieved.

The facilitators from each floor circle form another circle, which interfaces with circles at higher and lower levels within the hospital authority structure, so there is reciprocal representation at all levels.

In an organization truly committed to this approach, many management decisions are actually made in the individual quality circles, and few decisions are finalized until every member has had a part in the decision and agrees with the outcome. As is obvious, this can be a laborious and time-consuming process, but once consensus is reached, implementation is instantaneous and the net effect is always increased productivity and enhanced employee satisfaction. In other forms of participatory decision-making, the simple majority makes the decision, which often leaves a dissatisfied and potentially unreasonable minority who may impede the implementation of the solution. In an organization with consensus-based decision-making, everyone feels that he or she is a vital part of the process, has a voice in the decision, and is therefore a winner. Although research on this decision-making practice has produced varied results, one study did conclude that organizations using quality circles showed improved morale, decreased alienation, and greater incentives for productivity.[11]

The System 4 theory developed by Likert[9] and his colleagues closely approximates the management-by-consensus process of Ouchi's theory Z. The research that led to the development of System 4 supports the conclusion that, the more employees are encouraged (allowed) to participate in the management process, the greater the likelihood of superior performance. However, one critical limitation to System 4—and a very important point to consider—is that, although this approach is compatible with Japanese culture, much less emphasis is placed on teamwork in the West, and in the United States independent accomplishment is the revered value. Because of this fundamental difference, group decision-making has become highly successful in Japan but has been less successful in the United States.

Another important factor, especially in the healthcare industry, is that quality circles may be more useful when their members are drawn from various interacting units or disciplines. This decision-making approach is something that warrants further research because of its potential to provide long-term rewards to the organization. This approach shows great promise for use in an industry in which innovative management has not reached the levels found in many other sectors.

WARNING !

The actual experiences of healthcare and other organizations since the appearance in 1982 of R. Moore's article[11] on the use of quality circles in a hospital setting have not shown that significant results are achieved through their use. In fact, a number of people currently believe that many rank-and-file employees view quality circles in an indifferent or even negative way. The reason lies not in the quality circle process itself but in the way the process has been applied by many organizations. In many instances, managers who wished to create a consensus environment were not willing to relinquish their right to make final decisions and thus weakened the participatory process. In addition, when a suggestion from a circle was implemented and, for whatever reason, failed to achieve the expected outcome, the circle was held accountable. The result was low participation and a loss of support among the performing ranks.

THE COMMITTEE

Another form of group participation is the use of a committee, a group of people chosen to deal with a specific problem. Formal committees are part of the organization and are normally provided with the authority to deal with specific issues. Informal committees, on the other hand, are primarily used to facilitate discussion on a particular subject and have no delegated authority. An ad hoc committee is a formal committee that is appointed for a specific purpose and a limited time. Ad hoc committee members are often given the task of collecting data, analyzing it, and making recommendations. One of the best uses of committees is for planning and formulating organizational policy. Committees offer the following two advantages:

- They represent group participation.
- Individuals with specialized knowledge of and a direct interest in a given matter can provide information that will help in the search for a suitable and timely decision.

The hope that management holds for committee work is that a resolution of differences can be achieved after these differences have been openly discussed in committee meetings. When establishing a committee, the nurse manager must determine the size, scope, and authority of the committee and must appoint a chairperson who will help the committee operate effectively.[5]

In theory, the use of committees to facilitate group discussion is good; however, the process is not without significant shortcomings, as follows:

- The committee may reach a compromise that may not satisfy any of the participants.
- The committee may be bound by organizational rules.
- The committee may look for solutions and make decisions with too narrow a focus.
- The committee may take too long to make decisions.

THE NOMINAL GROUP TECHNIQUE

Another example of group participation is the nominal group technique (NGT). Developed through the research of A. L. Delbecq, A. H. Van De Ven, and D. H. Gustafson[12] in the mid-1970s, NGT centers on the formation of a titular group, or a group that exists in name only because no social exchange is allowed between its members. NGT consists of the following:

- Each member of the group silently generates ideas and writes them down.
- Group members report their ideas in round-robin fashion, and each idea is recorded in a succinct phrase on a flip chart or other display device.
- Each recorded idea is discussed in turn by the group to provide clarification and ensure shared understanding of the idea.
- Each individual votes privately on the priority of the ideas, and the group's decision is derived mathematically through rank ordering or rating.

Although research into NGT is relatively new, NGT is expected to come into wider use, because some evidence suggests that NGT may be better than the traditional committee approach for the following reasons:

- Silent, independent generation of ideas, followed by further thought and listening during the round-robin procedure, results in ideas of higher quality.
- The structured process used forces equal participation by all members in generating ideas about the problem.
- Chances are minimized that the more vocal and persuasive members of the committee will influence the less forceful individuals. Members work and think individually and are not unduly swayed by others' ideas or presence.

Nurse managers need to assess the capabilities of their units to determine if a participatory process would enhance their decision-making efforts. One key is to assess whether staff members possess similar qualifications and work well together. If this is the case, perhaps a quality circle could be instituted with success, or at least a version of it could be created that would fit the needs of the unit. If group members are extremely diverse and individualistic, however, NGT might prove to be more beneficial. If only a few staff members have leadership potential, then a committee might achieve greater success. The decision-making method used must be matched to the characteristics of the staff.

Potential Obstacles

Of the many obstacles to effective problem solving, inexperience is probably the most often encountered. Another key factor is the nurse manager's past experience, which will often determine how much risk will be taken in a given circumstance. How much and what has been learned from the past, both positive and negative, can affect every manager's current viewpoint and can lead the manager to make subjective and narrow judgments or very judicious ones. Other obstacles that can potentially stand in the way of good problem solving are described in the following sections.

PERSONALITY

There is little doubt that a single individual can and often does affect how and why certain decisions are made. Many nurse managers are selected for the position because of their historical clinical abilities, not their managerial skills. These technically oriented managers often start out feeling insecure about their new responsibilities and resort to a wide variety of unproductive activities. Many an insecure nurse manager has made it a policy to base decisions primarily on approval seeking. This is most often manifested when a truly difficult situation arises. Rather than lose face with the staff, the insecure nurse manager will frequently base his or her decision on what will placate subordinates rather than on what might achieve the larger goals of the institution.

On the other hand, nurse managers who demonstrate an authoritative or A-type personality are prone to making unreasonable demands on the staff. For example, such a manager might grant very few requests for a weekend off and provide absolutely no compensation for extra hours worked because of his or her own "workaholic" attitude.

Similarly, lazy or indifferent nurse managers may cause a unit to flounder because any ideas or problem solutions introduced may demand action they are unwilling to take.

Personality traits are difficult to change, but awareness tests taken at management seminars or evaluations from staff may indicate to an individual manager that his or her attitudes are not conducive to productive leadership.

RIGIDITY

An inflexible management style is another obstacle to problem solving. This style may result from experience with ineffective trial and error solutions or an internal fear of risk taking, or it may be an inherent personality trait. As discussed previously, ineffective trial and error problem solving can be avoided if the nurse manager gathers sufficient information and determines a means for early correction of ineffective or wrong decisions. Also, to minimize risk in problem solving, the goal is to have a thorough knowledge and understanding of the solution alternatives and their expected results. If the tendency toward rigidity is a personality trait, however, perhaps the nurse manager who has this flaw should seek a position outside of management.

Managers who use a rigid style to solve problems easily develop tunnel vision (i.e., the tendency to look at new things in old ways and from established frames of reference). Once this tunnel vision has manifested itself, it becomes very difficult for the manager to see things from another perspective. This myopic viewpoint often turns the problem-solving process into a procedure in which one person makes all of the decisions with little information from other sources. In the current dynamic healthcare setting, rigidity in a nurse manager not only will create a significant barrier to effective problem solving but may well end in failure for the nurse manager.

PRECONCEIVED IDEAS

It is not possible to become an effective manager if one starts out with the preconceived opinion that one course of action is correct and all other possibilities are wrong. Nor does the effective manager ever assume that only his or her ideas are acceptable and all others inferior, especially those received from subordinate personnel. In short, a highly skilled manager has a personal commitment to ascertain why members of the staff might disagree and is not concerned with who might have the correct answer. When staff members perceive a challenge in a different light, the manager should investigate their reasoning thoroughly and then retain the information so that it can be used to solve future problems.

The reality, however, is that too many managers operate from a preestablished point of view. These individuals have their own thoughts about the nature of problems and the way to solve them. The difficulty with this is that individuals who believe that only their own perceptions of a challenge are accurate will be very reluctant to accept any decision reached by others and quite possibly will ignore the entire discussion process. Individuals who occupy positions of responsibility, however, have an explicit duty to be objective in their problem solving and decision-making. To do this effectively, managers must put their personal ideas aside while they gather enough information to view the situation impartially.

Satisficing, Optimizing, and Maximizing

Satisficing, at least at first glance, appears to be a misspelling. To the contrary, it is a legitimate strategy in which a manager chooses a solution that may not be perfect but either is sufficient under existing circumstances to meet minimum standards of acceptability or is the first acceptable alternative examined.[13]

An *optimizing* approach is one in which the manager first identifies all possible outcomes, then assesses the probability of achieving success with each solution, and finally takes the action judged to have the best chance of resulting in the desired outcome.[13]

A *maximizing* strategy, on the other hand, is a process in which the manager evaluates all of the possible solutions and then selects the first one that meets minimally satisfactory standards.[13]

The use of a satisficing strategy in the patient care environment can lead to a multitude of follow-on problems that are often difficult to resolve. The following provides an example:

> Because of a lack of open beds, a poststroke patient has been temporarily placed on a busy surgical floor until a bed can be found in the rehabilitation unit. The patient requires a great deal of individualized care and is unable to communicate with the staff or with his family. In addition, early contractures are noticeable. In designing the proper care plan for this patient, the nurse manager uses a satisficing solution. Her reasoning is based on her knowledge that the patient will soon be transferred to the rehabilitation unit. Because she knows that the transfer is already planned, the nurse manager decides that range-of-motion exercises, which the patient's doctor has prescribed to be performed every 4 hours, need not be done if the patient is placed in a chair every day.
>
> Satisficing behavior may also occur in another way. If the nurse manager chooses to *maximize* the solution and implements a plan requiring full care, which fulfills all of the possible goals for that patient, the staff may still *satisfice* in carrying out the treatment plan by completing only those portions of the order they feel are absolutely necessary because they know the patient will be transferred soon.

Usually it is nurse managers who lack the ability to maximize who solve problems using a satisficing criterion. Such managers tend to view their units as an uncomplicated model of the real world. They become content with this interpretation because it allows them to make decisions by following a few simple rules or by acting out of habit and does not demand their full capacity for thought. However, not only does this approach increase the likelihood of poor performance within the unit, it may also open the hospital to significant risk and even litigation. This type of manager rarely, if ever, solves problems on anything that approaches a long-term basis.

DECISION-MAKING

Managers typically make their decisions under the following three conditions, and nurse managers are no exception to this rule:

1. Risk
2. Certainty
3. Uncertainty

Risk and Certainty

Decisions that involve *risk* are more difficult to make than decisions that involve *certainty*, because under conditions of risk usually only limited information and experience are available and each alternative can have many different outcomes. It is in making such decisions that traditional methods break down and the technique of mathematical probability analysis provides its greatest contribution.

One type of probability analysis that can be applied to decisions involving risk is the analysis of *objective statistical probability*. This is a precise mathematical technique that permits the decision-maker to calculate possible outcomes and make logical deductions. This type of analysis is used when decisions are based on experience or alternatives with known outcomes. The simple act of tossing a coin into the air illustrates the concept of statistical probability. If a person tosses a coin into the air 100 times and it lands 50 times showing heads and 50 times showing tails (i.e., the coin is unbiased), then on the 101st toss the statistical probability will be 0.5 (or 50%) that the coin will land with a head (or tail) up.

Most nurse managers working in hospitals do not have as much relevant experience as does the person tossing the coin in this illustration. Furthermore, the coin tosser can be positive that there is a 50-50 chance that the 101st toss will be heads.

The circumstances of the healthcare environment make it necessary for the nurse manager to put all of his or her eggs in one basket, so to speak (i.e., the next outcome). There just isn't the time or resources to let probability work itself out. Therefore, the use of objective statistical probability analysis in this type of situation has constraints. Despite these limitations, however, statistical probability, when applied and interpreted properly, has proven effective in helping middle managers make risky decisions. For example, the director of nursing instructs all of her nurse managers to staff for minimum requirements during the Christmas and New Year's holidays. A quick review of hospital records for the holiday season for the previous 2 years can provide a fairly representative estimate of patient load and acuity levels. Using these statistical data, nurse managers can, with a fair amount of precision, staff their units to handle the expected patient load.

Decision trees and utility models are also effective quantitative methods that can be used when a risky decision is contemplated. Other types of quantitative approaches also may be considered when highly statistical methods are needed to make high-risk decisions. Among them are the following:

Computers and management information systems: These are important tools that can be used when decisions involve risk and uncertainty. Many hospitals make available to managers computer terminals that access statistical software packages. The proper use of these resources, however, requires that nurse managers become familiar with the decision-making software available and ask the following three questions: What data are important? What will be done with the data compiled? How will it fit into the decision-making process?

Minimax analysis: In this approach, nurse managers attempt to calculate the worst possible outcome for each solution alternative and then select the alternative that will be the least disastrous if everything goes wrong. The following example illustrates the use of this approach: A hospital contracts with the local university's school of nursing to allow nursing students to work on a unit that admits a large number of seriously ill patients and has a high turnover among personnel. The nurse manager of the unit, in considering how to respond to this situation, lists the worst possible outcomes for each way of handling the situation so that she can choose the alternative which offers the most acceptable results. Table 11-1 shows her minimax analysis. Careful study reveals that choices 4, 5, and 7 could possibly be negotiated and implemented to bring about a positive nursing presence in a unit already besieged by low morale and turnover. Alternative 6 may be the one choice whereby doing nothing more than making a simple assignment presents the least amount of difficulty.

TABLE 11-1

Example of a Minimax Analysis

Problem: Hospital-mandated participation by nursing students in a unit that has a large number of acutely ill patients and a high turnover rate among permanent staff

Alternatives for Nurse Manager to Consider	Worst Possible Outcomes
1. Refuse to cooperate	1. Manager dismissed from hospital
2. Request admission clerk to distribute acutely ill patients evenly to other floors	2A. Clerk refuses 2B. Clerk agrees but fails to follow through
3. Set a maximum number of students to be allowed on unit	3. School and hospital fail to comply—confrontation
4. Work closely with instructor to assign students to low-acuity cases	4. Instructor refuses to comply—confrontation
5. Insist that instructor be present for all procedures and/or treatments in which student nurses participate	5. Instructor cannot or will not comply
6. Assign every patient to two students	6. Patients irritated by increased stimulation
7. Selectively orient students and instructor prior to clinical rotation	7. Students and instructor refuse to participate

Uncertainty

Decisions involving a degree of uncertainty are generally the most complex and difficult ones to make. Extreme cases of uncertainty occur when no knowledge of the situation exists, no meaningful experience is held, or no probabilities can be assigned to outcomes. In such cases, the nurse manager has no rational basis for choosing one alternative over another, because rational choice requires an assessment of the desirability of each identified outcome. It is important to determine if the decision-making situation is really uncertain, however, or if the uncertainty perceived by the nurse manager is due to lack of adequate information or error. If the uncertainty stems from misinformation or lack of knowledge, the situation can be corrected. Once this is done, the nurse manager will be able to recognize potential new outcomes and perhaps even predict the probability of each outcome.

NEED FOR CREATIVITY

Very few will disagree that a realistic approach, the presence of a good management climate, and an environment conducive to hard thinking and evaluation are all-important to problem solving and decision-making. However, none of these things, by itself, can turn a mediocre problem-solving team into an excellent one. To do that, quality and originality of thinking—in other words, creativity—must be present. Simply defined, *creativity* is the ability to develop and implement new and better solutions to overcome the challenges of existing problems. Creativity, in fact, is the only way to keep an organization alive. Those organizations that discourage creativity and choose to operate through rigid rules and regulations, and, through these actions, stifle creativity in the workplace or in employees, are inflexible at best and are definitely on the road to oblivion.

Research conducted by G. Steiner in the early 1960s found general agreement among scholars and top managers regarding the intellectual and personality characteristics of creative individuals.[14] According to Steiner, creative people do the following:

- Generate ideas rapidly
- Are flexible and are able to discard one frame of reference for another and/or change approaches spontaneously
- Have the capability to provide original solutions to problems
- Prefer complex thought processes
- Are independent in judgment and maintain a realistic belief in themselves even under pressure
- Exhibit distinct individualistic characteristics and view themselves as being different from their peers
- View authority as conventional rather than absolute; that is, accept authority as a matter of expedience rather than as a personal allegiance or moral obligation
- Are willing to entertain and express personal whims and impulses and exhibit a more diverse fantasy life on clinical tests
- Are likely to introduce humor into situations

Because creative people are far less likely to view authority as being absolute than are their more traditional associates, they tend to make fewer black and white distinctions, have a less dramatic view of life, show more independent judgment and less conformity, are willing to give consideration to their own impulses, generally have a good sense of humor, and tend to be less rigid in their performance. However, there is convincing evidence that the creative performer is not a source of difficulty. In fact, very few present control problems in the workplace.

A great deal of research has been conducted in an effort to define the steps in the creative process, and most of the results look much like the steps in the problem-solving process presented earlier in this chapter. A more descriptive definition of the creative process is "that sequence of thinking leading to ideas which sooner or later will be regarded as novel and worthwhile. It is seldom completed in a step-by-step procedure, but is more often characterized by long delays, inactivity, and the large unpredictable leap" (p. 503).[14]

Identifying the characteristics of a creative person and the creative process are necessary before nurse managers can act to stimulate creativity. Managers have the responsibility to develop their units as environments that stimulate creativity. They typically do this by the following means:

Being creative themselves: There is no substitute for day-to-day example.

Developing carefully designed plans: This is a method of work simplification built on the premise that most people cannot increase productivity simply by working harder. Instead, increased productivity is ensured by creating an environment in which people learn to "work smarter." One of the ways of implementing this growth cycle is to introduce creativity conferences. The focus of such a conference is any problem that is creating difficulties for the unit or an individual that any member of the group chooses to bring up. The conferences are not a venue for complaint or whining about procedures, policies, or practices. Instead, problems are attacked using intellectual methods and in a creative manner. To facilitate progress at these conferences, the group usually selects one or several of the issues members submit and then gathers the relevant facts. The group then looks at the problem from as many different angles as possible, challenging every detail. Through lively discussion, the conference members develop workable solutions and either implement change or make recommendations for improvement.

Constructing creative environments: Truly expert managers work diligently to create an environment in which their staffs are not afraid to use their intellectual abilities to solve problems on their own. For instance, good managers do not rail against staff members who make mistakes while attempting something new or trying something old in a new manner. Instead, they call each mistake to the attention of the staff and use it as a learning opportunity. Certainly every effort is made to eliminate as many mistakes as possible by working carefully with the staff to build trust and confidence and by providing an example, but good managers know that mistakes are inevitable and use them to their advantage.

If staff members are reluctant to demonstrate their personal creativity, managers may want to institute programs in which they meet with their employees routinely to discuss solutions to problems. This works very well with new employees who are not encumbered with the details of accepted practices and can offer prior experiences or insights before they undergo organizational socialization and their innovative ideas are turned off. The advantages offered by new employees should be thoroughly explored, and no new idea should be discarded as being impossible to implement.

Building a philosophy of creativity: Nurse managers must adopt a philosophy that stresses creativity and must personally take steps to encourage it. If creativity is given high priority in the unit, then any reward system instituted should be geared to and commensurate with that priority. The organization can contribute by ensuring that those who regularly demonstrate creativity are promoted into positions in which they can use their creativity. For example, a creative RN who has devised innovative ways to provide nutrition to pediatric patients probably should be promoted into an area in which she can expand her original ideas, not promoted to an outpatient clinic where pediatric nutrition is not an issue. The staff nurse who has shown tremendous flexibility in working with many different types of patients should not be held back from promotion because he or she is the most productive nurse on the unit. Advancement and status should be provided within the area of creativity, and creativity should be used as an element of the promotional cycle (i.e., if a person demonstrates a willingness to take personal risk by developing and initiating new procedures, this willingness should be viewed as a positive asset).

Promoting creativity requires a certain amount of outside contacts, a willingness to accept new and different ideas, provision of proper research assistance, the willingness to provide legitimate freedoms, and even some flexible management. The development of creativity does not require permissiveness, negligence, or acceptance of any reduction in the level of performance. To the contrary, the best creative environments are those that follow the rules, have good discipline, and encourage excellence. These highly produc-

tive units encourage their members to continue their education through both formal and informal means. These units demonstrate a willingness to organize in a flexible fashion and to work hard to make the unit opportunity oriented. This means being willing to abolish needless communications, to eliminate barriers to action, and to improve the processes that identify opportunities.

Stimulating creativity: Nurse managers should try to stimulate creativity by experimenting with methods such as brainstorming. One of the best ways to do this is to make sure that the creative individual is given full credit for any success achieved as well as held accountable for any failings. If nurse managers make it important to be successful and ensure that praise and recognition are provided for the creative act, then they will stimulate creativity. People do what gets rewarded. This fact has been called the biggest secret in the business world. Consider the following two critical points[15]:

1. *Every action has consequences:* The response to an expression of creativity should be appropriate; that is, the creative person should receive recognition (consequence) for his or her effort (action).

2. *Future performance depends on the consequences of past action:* If the consequences are rewarding, it is likely that the action will be repeated. The creative nurse will feel that the recognition he or she receives is rewarding and so will be eager to create an opportunity to receive more recognition.

Keeping ideas alive: A climate must be created that ensures the survival of potentially useful ideas. It is unprofessional when someone works to develop a good idea but circumstances do not allow it to be used. New ideas are extremely perishable commodities, largely because their creators are most likely their sole supporters. It is almost an unwritten law that other people will not be supporters, because the normal reaction to something new is either to ignore it or to point out its defects. The environment in every unit in the hospital must support giving new ideas a fair and proper hearing to reduce the tendency to destroy all creative processes within the organization, the group, and the individual.

The major limitation on developing creativity stems from the initial cost. The greater the creativity sought and the greater the departure from present practice, the greater the investment will be. In the long run, however, it has been proven that creative environments produce ideas that significantly reduce costs and in fact are very cost effective in themselves. The challenge is to encourage the creative exchange of ideas so that any new gain realized acts to enhance vitality and productivity.

SUMMARY

- Understanding the problem-solving and decision-making processes is essential for nurse managers.
- The following three guidelines must be kept in mind in diagnosing problems:
  1. Obtain all the facts
  2. Separate facts from interpretations
  3. Determine the scope of the problem
- Methods of problem solving include trial and error, experimentation, critique, metaphor-based techniques, brainstorming, decision trees, and the laissez-faire approach (knowing when problems are self-solving).
- The problem-solving and decision-making processes follow principles that expand problem-solving skills and develop critical thinking. The decision-making process begins with the proper identification of the problem in terms that are as specific as possible. Decisions cannot be made unless the exact nature of the problem is understood.
- Risk and uncertainty are factors in problem solving and decision-making, but methods can be used that lead to appropriate decision-making with a maximal probability of success.
- Some of the obstacles to problem solving and decision-making are personality characteristics, rigidity, and preconceptions.
- Various types of group decision-making are helpful for nurse managers because they require interactions with others and the perceptions and ideas of other people often provide multiple alternatives that help in resolving the problem situation.
- Creative decision-making is critical, but a supportive management climate is required to turn mediocre problem solvers into individuals who develop innovative solutions.

FINAL THOUGHTS

Problem solving, the process of selecting one course of action from among all the alternatives, is a continuing responsibility of all managers. Hospitals and other healthcare organizations usually provide broad guidelines for handling routine situations, but the exceptional situations must be dealt with by the individual manager through well-developed and timely decisions.

The basic problem-solving process involves the following eight major steps:

1. Define the problem clearly
2. Accumulate information
3. Verify and analyze the information received
4. Develop several different solutions
5. Consider the consequences of each solution
6. Decide on which solution to utilize
7. Implement the decision
8. Evaluate the solution

Good problem solving is a skill that can be easily learned, and the nurse manager's mastery of this skill is absolutely critical to the success of any nursing unit.

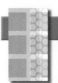

THE NURSE MANAGER SPEAKS

Making decisions is important to the discipline of nursing in dealing with problems arising from resource management and clinical practice. Nurse managers must continually determine the best course of action for managing staff members, budgets, resources, patient care, scheduling, and a myriad of other critical elements.

Decisions must be made concerning the nursing actions required to assist patients in the unit and help must be given to patients so that they make the proper decisions for their personal well-being.

Nurse managers, in all of their decision-making capacities, make a significant impact on the delivery of health care. Make your impact wisely!

REFERENCES

1. Latz A: *An investigation of the managerial techniques of nursing service directors,* St Louis, 1977, Saint Louis University.
2. Barnum BS: *Nurse as executive,* ed 4, Gaithersburg, Md, 1995, Aspen.
3. Gillies DA: *Nursing management: a systems approach,* ed 2, Philadelphia, 1989, Saunders.
4. Osborn AF: *Applied imagination: principles and procedures of creative problem-solving,* ed 3, Hadley, Mass, 1993, Creative Education Foundation.
5. Marriner Tomey A: *Guide to nursing management and leadership,* ed 7, St Louis, 2004, Mosby.
6. La Monica E, Finch FE: Managerial decision making, *J Nurs Adm* 7(5):20, 1977.
7. Vroom VH, Yetton PW: *Leadership and decision making,* Pittsburgh, 1976, University of Pittsburgh Press.
8. Barnard C: *Functions of the executive,* ed 10, Cambridge, Mass, 1988, Harvard University Press.
9. Likert R: *New patterns of management,* New York, 1961, McGraw-Hill.
10. Ouchi W: *Theory Z—how American business can meet the Japanese challenge,* Reading, Mass, 1981, Addison-Wesley.

11. Moore R: On the scene: quality circles at Barnes Hospital, *Nurs Adm Q* 6(3):20, 1982.

12. Delbecq AL, Van de Ven AH, Gustafson DH: *Group techniques for program planning,* Glenview, Ill, 1975, Scott Foresman.

13. Gillies DA: *Nursing management: a systems approach,* Philadelphia, 1982, Saunders.

14. Steiner G: *The creative organization,* Chicago, 1965, University of Chicago Press.

15. LeBouef M: *How to win customers and keep them for life,* New York, 1997, Bantam.

SUGGESTED READINGS

Beare P: Decision making in nursing practice. In Lancaster W, editor: *Concepts for advanced nursing practice: the nurse as a change agent,* St Louis, 1982, Mosby, pp 146-70.

Benner P: *From novice to expert: excellence and power in clinical nursing practice,* Menlo Park, Calif, 1984, Addison-Wesley.

Carnevali DL: The diagnostic reasoning process. In Carnevali DL, Mitchell PH, Woods NF, and others, editors: *Diagnostic reasoning in nursing,* Philadelphia, 1984, Lippincott.

Corcoran SA: Task complexity and nursing expertise as factors in decision making, *Nurs Res* 35(2):107, 1986.

Duxbury ML: Head nurse leadership style with staff nurse burnout and job satisfaction in neonatal intensive care units, *Nurs Res* 33(2):97, 1984.

Grohar-Murray ME, DoCrose HR: *Leadership and management in nursing,* Stamford, Conn, 1997, Appleton and Lange.

Huber GP: *Managerial decision making,* Glenview, Ill, 1980, Scott Foresman.

Janis IL, Mann L: *Decision making: a psychological analysis of conflict, choice, and commitment,* New York, 1977, Free Press.

Keen P, McKenny J: How managers' minds work, *Harv Bus Rev* 2(May/June):16, 1979.

Paul R: *Critical thinking,* Santa Rosa, Calif, 1993, Foundation for Critical Thinking.

Peterson ME: Motivating staff to participate in decision making, *Nurs Adm Q* 7(2):63, 1983.

Prawka J, Warner DM: A mathematical programming model for scheduling nurses in a hospital, *Manage Sci* 19(4):18, 1972.

Smith HL, Reinow FD, Reid RA: Japanese management—implications for nursing administration, *J Nurs Adm* 14(9):33, 1984.

Steele SM, Maravaglia FL: *Creativity in nursing,* Thorofare, NJ, 1981, Slack.

Leading and Coaching the Professional Team

OUTLINE

LEARNING SYNOPSIS

Upon successful completion of this chapter, readers will possess a basic understanding of how the nurse manager's coaching of the team toward success can assist the nursing unit in achieving its goals, what the nurse manager can do to position himself or herself as coach, and what the nurse manager must do to be perceived as a coach by the staff.

OBJECTIVES

1. Cite the basic rules that must be followed by the nurse manager who aspires to be a coach
2. Identify the characteristics that must be displayed by anyone wishing to coach a nursing unit
3. List 10 steps that can be used by the nurse manager to position himself or herself as a coach within the nursing unit

/CRITICAL POINT

The titles leader, coach, *and* nurse manager *and the terms* leadership *and* coaching *are used throughout this chapter to designate the individual tasked with an influential role in the guidance of others and the actions taken by such an individual to facilitate the direction of a team (nursing unit). In actuality, leadership and coaching employ many of the same actions. It can be argued that all great coaches are proficient leaders, but not all people in positions of leadership are proficient coaches; all great leaders employ effective coaching techniques, but not everyone occupying a coaching position can be correctly called a leader.*

The intent of this chapter is to describe the actions of an effective coach. Here, a coach is defined not as a person occupying a certain position but as any individual who helps others achieve excellence. The authors believe that this definition crosses all professional lines and can legitimately be applied to a person holding virtually any position.

Regardless of whether nurse managers are directing their own personal efforts, leading their units toward the accomplishment of a goal, or building winners out of their nursing staffs, the best approach is to *coach for improvement, not perfection.* The meaning of this is simple: it is better to ask for and expect small improvements on a regular basis than to demand large gains over a short (or even a long) period of time.

The human animal likes to lead a relatively simple life. Because of this tendency, focusing the unit's energy on the attainment of large gains is seldom beneficial. People need to be able to visualize their goals and are motivated to excel by the emotional rewards gained through success. Focusing on large goals limits the degree of success an individual can attain. It is far easier for the average employee to focus on a few small goals and share in their successful achievement than to strive for the attainment of a larger and more distant goal. The following saying expresses this concept clearly:

The best way to eat an elephant is one piece at a time.

When nurse managers are directing their units, or any segments of them, they must be pursuing more than the accomplishment of goals. Managers must avoid the pitfall of measuring success only by looking at numbers and counting projects. Goal attainment, although certainly critical to the nursing unit's continued success, accounts for only a small fraction of the big picture that unit managers must keep in focus. If managers have built their staffs properly and are currently operating with employee rosters that include superior people, it is reasonable for the managers to expect superior results on every project. The unit's recipe for continued growth should be *realistic, attainable goals accomplished through participative, well-coached*

action under leadership that demands superior accomplishment and provides for recognition and reward.

Most nurse managers already possess most of the qualities they will need to be effective coaches. The two most important are the following:

- The ability to judge character well
- Basic common sense

These qualities are so critical to the successful growth of a nursing unit that it is safe to assume that any person who has successfully led a busy nursing unit for any length of time possesses them. However, being an effective coach requires a blending of other skills and behaviors. This chapter discusses the qualities of leadership that apply to coaching a nursing unit effectively and reintroduces the role of health team leader as one of coach and facilitator. The intent is to help nurse managers become successful coaches in the dynamic arena of the nursing unit.

Almost all nurse managers completed the primary process of building a successful unit when they recruited, hired, and trained a team of superior performers. The next steps must be taken to protect and nurture the success of that team. Highly competent individuals don't like their leaders to exert command and expect a certain degree of freedom to use their talents, creativity, and capabilities. If the work environment does not permit or encourage these qualities, truly capable performers will move on—away from the nurse manager's team—in search of one that does.

Capable and imaginative people who encourage excellence in others build quality organizations. Those would-be leaders who exercise command to secure their dominance over others stifle the energy and motivation necessary for any group to become truly effective. In a command setting, the manager creates the vision, develops the goals and objectives, and assigns the staff their roles in the implementation process. In a team-oriented setting, however, the nurse manager works with the staff to create the vision and develop goals and objectives, and together they work to accomplish the task. Nursing units whose staffs are established as teams, *real* teams, develop a relationship of two-way trust between nurse managers and staff members. Those nurse managers who win the confidence and support of the staff members continually reinforce their value to the unit by not violating any part of their trust.

After trust is established, the achievement of real proficiency becomes possible. The actual road the nursing unit travels may be filled with detours and challenges, but these will be overcome as the nurse manager gently but firmly guides the staff in a direction consistent with the vision that has been created for the overall organization. The accomplishment of interim goals provides every member of the staff with the opportunity to celebrate achievement and gives the nurse manager the opportunity to recognize excellence and reward performance.

THE RULES OF SUCCESSFUL COACHING

One of the most basic of all the leadership requirements nurse managers must fulfill is the coaching of staff members inside the organized structure of the unit. Although many administrators and managers willingly devote time and energy to coaching, few of the people occupying management roles become really good coaches. Too many nurse managers, for example, bring along their own emotional baggage when coaching their staffs. This extra baggage causes a nurse manager acting in the role of leader-coach to become unhappy and lapse into a more command-oriented mode as he or she deals with the challenges of coaching others. The unhappy leader-coach transfers his or her emotional burden onto the shoulders of the individual staff members and they, in turn, become unhappy. The result is that the unit performs poorly, important contributions are lost, and the organization suffers.

Coaching a nursing unit and its individual members is far more demanding than commanding one. Effectively directing the individual efforts of a group of enthusiastic and dynamic performers can be very difficult. Leadership is a dynamic process that requires the person exercising it to show compassion, understanding, discipline, persistence, flexibility, and infinite patience. Coaching a unit's staff requires the leader to define success as more than simply compiling a good record. Obviously, the achievement of goals and the attainment of proficiency are significant contributors to success, but for a well-coached team, real success comes from two other factors:

1. *The players remain:* Coaches, regardless of whether they are working with Little League ballplayers or a dynamic healthcare unit, are responsible for helping the individual team members develop skills they can use throughout their lives, not just in the achievement of an immediate goal. A good coach works to instill a high level of desire in team members so that they will be willing to work hard and give of themselves enough to outlast long, demanding shifts, stress, deadlines, and pressure. The coach teaches that the inner ambition necessary for each team member to perform comes not from the possibility of becoming a star but from the knowledge that he or she has a future with a dynamic team. The drive to accomplish is fueled when the coach encourages the team members to play in the real game and

when they are never allowed to just sit on the sidelines observing those in managerial positions make all the moves. If a staff member is not motivated to stretch and achieve through a positive demonstration of capability, then he or she should be encouraged to exercise the option of taking another path—one that may lead away from the dynamic nursing unit and into a less demanding environment.

2. *Team members don't join the competition:* The average functional nursing unit accomplishes a great deal every shift. The staff make it through the emergencies and critical care procedures, they overcome impossible challenges, and they grow in capability and character as a result. The effort that it takes to become a successful and professional nursing unit is almost immeasurable. Through it all, an important constant remains: the competition is aware of the nurse manager's achievements and the opportunity inherent in knowing his or her ideas. The nurse manager's record of achievement has caused others to respect what the manager has accomplished; this respect can take the insidious form of another unit's desire to employ members of the manager's staff. Well-coached employees are invaluable assets to other organizations. Just as the nurse manager wants to hire the very best, so do his or her fellow nurse managers, and if they want the manager's staff badly enough, they can generate offers that are very hard to refuse.

The trust that is shared in well-coached teams carries a big benefit for the organization: loyalty. Individual performers who are respected, treated well, and provided with a work environment that recognizes the value of individual contribution rarely will look elsewhere for employment. So precious are the values operating in a well-coached team in the nursing profession that few are willing to give them up. People work for different things, and for most professionals, money does not top the list. A survey conducted in the 1970s showed that the things employees prized most in a professional relationship were, in order of preference, (1) recognition, (2) appreciation, (3) opportunity, (4) responsibility, and (5) money. These things remain valued today.

The best way to continue the exceptional performance of the unit is to retain its superior performers. It is these superior performers who will be first to leave if the nurse manager does not provide a nurturing environment.

Although many things go into becoming a good coach, the nine principles presented in the following sections are considered the primary rules for successful coaching.

1. Don't Assume

The story that follows, taken from the book *My Season on the Brink*,[1] illustrates one of the most fundamental lessons that can be learned by a coach in the nursing profession:

"I always start my practice by numbering the bases."

That statement came from a neighbor who had been coaching for 10 years and it had been rattling around in my head ever since I got the phone call telling me that I was going to be in charge of a team.

"What are you talking about?" I had asked him. "It's simple," said Tom, the neighbor and a father of three, who had coached everything from soccer to track as his kids grew up. "The first year I was coaching Little League, I laid out the bases. Then I had the kids line up and said, 'To warm up, let's have everyone jog around the base path.' The first four kids took off toward third. Ever since, I've numbered the bases and explained that you have to run them in order. You'd be amazed at the number of kids who go from first to third by cutting across the pitcher's mound." (p. 37)

The message: No matter where the nurse manager is coaching or at what level, the manager should never assume that team members know everything that he or she does, or that they need to. It is the leader's responsibility to explain everything.

2. Delegate

Leading and coaching a nursing unit is an incredibly difficult job, simply because there are so many things that have to be discovered, performed, and followed up. The effort will be eased if nurse managers involve the staff as their assistants. In addition to helping managers fulfill their duties, these assistants can provide managers with the following two extremely important assets:

1. *Someone to talk to:* The responsibility of leadership is demanding, and much of it must be shouldered alone. However, if nurse managers involve their staffs in their projects, they will have others with whom to discuss the challenge, people from whom to receive input and opinions, and different perspectives to draw upon.

2. *Strength in numbers:* Individual staff members may not appreciate their nurse manager's leadership style and will gravitate toward someone else. In fact, the higher the proficiency of the performer, the greater the tendency to move toward a leader who can demonstrate specific requirements better than the one for whom he or she currently works. Having several assistant coaches ensures that each member of the staff will get enough attention and eliminates the possibility of any staff member's being excluded.

Consider the following story:

When I first took over my new job as the Director of Nursing for a group of units within a large Midwestern hospital, I inherited a group of individuals who had been abused almost past the point of salvation. The previous manager had lied, manipulated, and deceived every junior manager and nearly every subordinate employee. There was no sense of "us" unless you counted the "us" (employees) as opposed to "them" (management).

However, a strong sense of bonding had occurred as a result of the previous leader's abuse. No doubt from a sense of preservation, the members of the various nursing units had formed themselves into a sort of subteam that looked to one of the more gifted nurse managers to protect them from their previous boss. This particular individual possessed remarkable influence over nearly every employee, as her efforts had saved many from termination or, at a minimum, excessive rebuke from the former manager. I knew that my success would be realized only if I could elicit the support of this remarkable leader (her name was Tracy).

I tried talking with Tracy and, at one point, even asked for her help when things looked bleak. But each time I approached her, she sidestepped, and I missed the opportunity to make my pitch. Tracy saw her duty as protecting all of the other employees from the person who occupied my job, and I felt that she was not willingly going to assist me in anything.

Leading the nursing staff was a tough job made even harder by the demanding and inadequate individual to whom I was forced to report. The burden saw me working from 6:00 AM to nearly 10:00 PM daily, and the toll that was being taken was becoming evident. One day, I called Tracy into the office and told her I needed her help completing an important task. I explained the requirements, how a successful job would benefit the entire staff, and how I was willing to let her have a free rein in how the task was accomplished as long as she would permit me to occasionally check with her on the progress being made. Reluctantly, Tracy agreed to perform the task and did a marvelous job. That first job led to many more, and soon Tracy was my number one assistant. Several months later, at an off-site, all-employee nursing meeting, I stunned everyone in the crowd by having small plastic fluted glasses passed out, and we uncorked enough champagne to fill everyone's glass for a toast.

I asked Tracy to come to the front of the room and lifted my glass and commended her, in front of every nurse in the room, on the excellence of her performance. I talked about Tracy's years of commitment and tireless efforts on behalf of the employees of our group, and unknown to anyone I had arranged a promotion for Tracy to Assistant Director of Nursing (she had been a nurse manager for nearly 10 years), and the Hospital Administrator was on hand to make it official. I told the assembled nurses how critical Tracy had been through the past difficulties, how essential her leadership had been to me since I had come on board, and how unselfishly Tracy had performed her role—never asking for herself but giving everything to help the other members of the team. I concluded by asking everyone to help me thank Tracy for her professionalism, her spirit, her loyalty, and her sense of teamwork. When I finished, there wasn't a dry eye in the house.

Within weeks, our organization started the difficult climb out of the basement that had been dug for it, and with Tracy's cooperation and assistance (now freely given), we continued to increase our productivity and enhance the quality of our patient service and new business development, and we witnessed a drastic reduction in sick time and turnover of our professional staff. We stayed in those leadership positions throughout my tenure as Director of Nursing, and it was due, in a very large part, to the commitment and dedication of a woman named Tracy.

3. Involve All the Stakeholders

Many truly successful organizations have a rule that every stakeholder* must take a turn at some activity, even if that activity is as simple as providing credible feedback or showing up at an open house. These organizations have found out that it pays to bring as many of the stakeholders as possible into the decision-making process and to listen carefully when one of these interested parties speaks.

Involving the stakeholders in the leadership and coaching process produces far more benefits than simply providing another source of information. This involvement allows an individual staff member, by taking an active role in the development of the unit, to garner support for the organization's efforts within the community and provides the nurse manager with a tangible method of coaching individual performers. The actual coaching role takes shape in how each nurse manager incorporates the information received from the stakeholders into the whole of the unit's experience. Involving the stakeholders shows the unit members the results of their efforts, lets them see the challenge of growth being faced, and showcases

---

*The term *stakeholder* is used in this discussion to mean any person who has a stake in the success of the nursing unit. The stakeholders include (but are not necessarily limited to) administrators, vendors, patients, the community at large, and other associated nursing units. A stakeholder is anyone who benefits from the manager's continued success or could potentially be harmed if the manager's unit should fail to meet its goals.

the nurse manager as a patient, understanding, and flexible leader.

Involving the stakeholders is a preemptive strike against the "unhappy performer" syndrome because it addresses the concerns of the unit through feedback received from people who have something to lose. The staff are no longer simply listening to the nurse manager, they are seeing, feeling, and being placed in direct contact with the product of their efforts. The stakeholders should be involved as early and as often as possible in the unit's growth process.

4. Look for the Positive

The following are some words of wisdom from a coach who knows:

> My general managerial instructions included such comments as, *"Come on, show some hustle,"* went over fine with the people sitting in the bleachers watching our Little League game, but others like *"John get your body in front of the ball"* as another ground ball slid by Johnny G. into left field, did not. After being glared at by Johnny G.'s parents, I resolved to only say positive things (e.g., *"Nice try Johnny, but maybe next time you could think about . . ."*) for the remainder of the season. (p. 42)[1]

Criticizing an individual in front of his or her peers is not good for the nurse manager, the unit, or the organization. If a team member has done something wrong, he or she should be pulled aside and the issue addressed privately. The nurse manager should never demonstrate dissatisfaction with an employee in front of the other members of the unit. The nurse manager should never, never, never make one member of the staff the scapegoat for any part of the unit's failure. Even in sports such as hockey and soccer in which a single member of the team has the responsibility to protect the goal, the goalie isn't totally responsible when the opposing team scores. The other team's ability to score almost always indicates a breakdown of the entire defense, which is the coach's responsibility, rather than the poor play of the goalie.

In nursing management, as in sports, when a single member of the team fails to perform on a consistent basis, one gets rid of the player, but when the entire team fails to perform, it's time to start looking for a new coach. There is real truth in the maxim that what is expected is what gets done. If the unit sees the nurse manager looking for good things and recognizing excellence only in front of others (this does not mean that the manager doesn't correct errors in private), they will be motivated to improve their performance. Everyone wants his or her 15 minutes of fame.

The nurse manager's words should be kept encouraging and positive. As the leader of the unit, the nurse manager's job is to elicit the cooperation of the team and its individual members, not to turn the team's environment into an adversarial pressure cooker.

5. Coach the Team to Win

Every goal, every objective, and every effort is independent of every other if the nurse manager chooses to perceive it as so. Therefore, the nurse manager should go into every new challenge with the desire to win, to overcome, to succeed, no matter what the unit's previous track record has been. There are slogans everywhere that proclaim the opportunity to win, but none is so easily understood as the belief in the possibility of victory voiced by the National Football League in its slogan, "On any given Sunday, any team can beat any other."

People win more consistently than they lose, and the nurse manager's unit has proven this through its ability to help the manager get the organization into the successful position it now enjoys. Even if the nursing unit suffers bitter defeat, the nurse manager needs to draw on his or her strength and provide inspiration to the staff, because next time, everything will come together and success will be achieved.

No one can win if the nurse manager doesn't coach to win. Knute Rockne would not have inspired many people if he had said, "Let's go out and *lose* one for the Gipper." The nurse manager must hold to an absolute belief in the inevitability of success.

A large part of winning is mental. If people believe that they can overcome, they almost always can. If people believe that failure is an option, however, the chances are good that they will settle for that option. It is the nurse manager's job to instill a will to win, a belief in the inevitability of success. Managers need to do more than talk about winning; they must be living embodiments of the positive attitude—the certainty of victory—the example for the team to emulate.

6. Coach Players to Take Advantage of Opportunity

It is highly unlikely that the nursing unit staff will start out as well tuned, efficient, and confident in its achievement. Few do. Units get that way through a long process of hard work coupled with the experience of success. It's like coaching a small child's T-ball team. The chances of seeing a well-executed play are almost nonexistent.

Things happen every day and on every shift, and the unit staff should be taught to take advantage of the opportunities presented by unusual situations and circumstances. If one of the staff members has a success, it should be shared with the entire unit, but everyone should be kept moving in a positive direction while this is done. Don't *stop* and celebrate; *move faster* and celebrate.

Coaching the staff to seize opportunities has the following advantages: (1) Individuals work better if they know that they can control the tempo of the job by being slightly aggressive. It makes the game of nursing fun and challenging. (2) Good performance on the part of the unit has a way of eliminating the potential for mistakes by another unit or at least helping to reduce the level of these mistakes. This can provide the staff with a reputation for effectiveness—something that can only have a positive effect on future performance. Success builds two things that are critical to future success: confidence and the willingness to take future risk.

7. Don't Play Favorites—Play Performers

Most leaders develop relationships with their individual staff members that vary depending on the contributions received. The more the staff member contributes and works, the more willing the leader is to listen to and share with that staff member.

Although it may sound commendable for nurse managers to try to spread their time evenly among their staff members, the reality of nurse managers' demanding position is that it will almost never be possible to do that. For this reason, nurse managers must commit their time to those who contribute the most. The 80-20 rule, applied to the nursing unit, states that typical nurse managers spend 80% of their time with 20% of their staffs. The problem is that in most cases nurse managers spend that 80% of their time with the wrong 20% of their staffs.

If 20% of a unit's staff (call this Group A) performs 80% of the work, it is a mathematical process to determine where the nurse manager should spend his or her time. Assume that there are 100 employees in the unit. This means that 20 of these employees (Group A) will do 80% of the work. Now suppose that the work assigned is to move 100 barrels from one side of the room to another. This means that 20 people will move 80 barrels, which is 4 barrels apiece. The other 80% of the team (Group B) will move only 20 barrels, or only $\frac{1}{4}$ of a barrel each. Let's add one more condition: let's say that the barrels have to be moved in 1 hour. Therefore, the work performed by each person in group A is 4 barrels per hour, whereas each member of Group B works at a rate of only $\frac{1}{4}$ barrel per hour, or at an efficiency 16 times lower than that of Group A's high performers. Quite a difference.

Now, assume that the nurse manager can improve the performance of each member of the team by 10%

for every hour the manager spends with that person. If the work efficiency of a member of Group A is 16 times higher than that of a member of Group B, it stands to reason that the time the manager spends with a member of Group A will be 16 times more effective than the time spent with a member of Group B.

Competent nurse managers spend most of their time coaching the better performers and let it be known why they are doing so. Coaching the staff does not mean giving everyone everything equally. People should get what they earn. Top performers should get the lion's share of everything. This does not mean that poor performers should be totally excluded, but it does mean that nurse managers must direct their efforts efficiently. The job of the nurse manager is to obtain results, so individuals occupying this position should put their time and effort where they will do the most good. (If staff members do not try to improve or do not seek help to do so, they should not be allowed to remain. If they must be kept in the organization, a place must be found for them where they can do no harm.)

! CRITICAL POINT

At first glance, the previous discussion may appear to make the leader-team concept meaningless, but it is critical for nurse managers to understand that choices must be made, and these choices must be made for the overall improvement of the unit. This textbook has consistently encouraged nurse managers to make a significant effort to bring all of the unit's members up to acceptable performance levels. However, nurse managers must understand that at some point efficient use of time must be considered. If the nurse manager has expended valuable time to assist a staff member and that member has not responded with improved performance, the nurse manager has coached for improvement and still the staff member continues to perform poorly, and the staff member's performance continues to have a negative effect on unit performance, then it may be time to consider replacing that staff member.

Nurse managers have only so much time. Spending it all with poor performers is not a good use of that time unless the time spent can somehow enhance the performance of the entire unit. The point is that nurse managers should apply their time where it will do the most good.

8. Don't Cheat

People have a tendency, no matter how slight, to bend the rules a little when the unit is falling behind and to be very literal about the rules when the staff are enjoying success.

In the organization and in the unit, the nurse manager is the one who determines whether something is right or wrong. The nurse manager should not make the mistake of awarding all the good calls to one group or to one individual. It is far better to have some calls occasionally go against the manager's own unit than for the manager to develop a reputation as an individual who takes unfair advantage or who cheats to slant benefits.

A good nurse manager has the trust of his or her staff. Cheating, no matter how innocent or well intended, is always considered a negative action. To cheat is to work against the trust the nurse manager has worked so hard to attain. Employees generally think in fixed patterns and in black and white. If they see the nurse manager cheat once, that manager is a cheater—*period*.

9. Keep Things in Perspective

One of the great joys of coaching a team is being able to teach other people. Nurse managers are expected to give of themselves for the benefit of others. The effort a nurse manager expends to help others become better at things at which they want to excel can be tremendously beneficial to the overall success of the nursing unit. There is always a chance that the nurse manager will get lucky and that a staff member will stand up in front of the assembled unit members and publicly recognize the nurse manager's contribution, but this should not be the motivation for wanting to assist others, and it is a situation that rarely occurs.

The number of people who are willing to share their individual successes with their managers is very small. The nurse manager should keep this in mind when the job starts to seem unrewarding and the manager feels unappreciated. The fact that the nurse manager is not receiving feedback on his or her successes does not mean that the manager is not having them.

The nurse manager's job as a coach is to teach the staff to love the game for the benefits the game can provide, to perform at peak capability because it feels good and adds to the enjoyment of the work. Work should be fun, and if the nurse manager, when performing as a coach, focuses on the welfare of the team and works hard to teach each staff member to enjoy their efforts, the entire business environment within the unit will be improved.

People work for their own reasons, not for management's. Therefore, the nurse manager should not establish unreasonable expectations for staff members. Instead, the manager should prepare the team to win and celebrate its victories. Unlike playing in sports, participating in a professional nursing team involves far more than simply how each person plays the game. In the nursing unit, whether one wins or loses *does* count. But winning without some measure of celebration is meaningless, and losing without learning from the process is not professional.

CHARACTERISTICS OF A GOOD COACH

Nearly every nurse manager truly desires to excel and to be successful. Many, many of those who take on the job with the highest of ideals, in possession of raw talent, with excellent academic backgrounds, and with great intentions, well-rounded experience, and tremendous personal drive never succeed. The ones who do succeed will tell anyone who will listen that they did so because they focused on helping others achieve success before they worried about their own.

Different people in different places, working under different sets of criteria, call "helping someone else" by different names. Some call the process "leadership," some call it "mentoring," others refer to it as "coaching," and still others call it "management." Regardless of what it is called, those who help others succeed and do it well have the following three basic characteristics that have been emphasized in previous chapters. These attributes perhaps occur in different degrees and are applied differently, but every successful leader, every successful mentor, coach, or manager, possesses them:

1. *The ability to elicit cooperation:* Cooperation must be obtained first from oneself and then from others.
2. *The ability to listen:* Self-awareness, self-regulation, and empathy all begin with the ability to listen, both to one's inner voice and then to the voices of others.
3. *The ability to place the needs of others over one's own:* Self-control and confidence begin with the ability to put others before oneself, the willingness to do for others and forsake oneself, and the willingness to take personal risk that will benefit another.

These qualities do not stand alone, however. They are supported by a variety of other characteristics that are called upon in varying degrees to meet the requirements of specific situations. Although many different traits are interwoven into the fabric of a good coach, this chapter confines its discussion to the 10 that appeared the most frequently in a study of America's top corporate leaders conducted by Burt Nanus and Warren Bennis as research for their book *Leaders.*[2] Bennis and Nanus identified these 10 characteristics, described in the following sections, as typical of a good coach and leader.

1. Enthusiasm

This textbook has repeatedly stated that people in leadership positions embrace responsibility as a fundamental part of that role. The word *embrace* has been chosen here because part of its definition is to "take up gladly or willingly."

People who want to be examples for others or to assist (coach) others in their performance do not simply accept responsibility as part of the job. They step forward and grab hold of it, even when the acceptance of responsibility means they will have to perform an unpleasant task. Anyone can do agreeable tasks, but only an individual of character accepts responsibility when faced with a challenge that others refuse and then performs the distasteful duty in such a way that later the others wish they had become involved.

Coaches look for opportunities to showcase the abilities and talents of others. A good coach is willing to work long, arduous hours attempting what others deem impossible and expects no extra compensation for it. Being a good coach is working with a struggling employee who is trying as hard as he or she knows how but is failing to achieve. It is showing and sharing, assisting and encouraging, in a manner that provides the recipient with dignity, self-worth, and opportunity.

Anyone can be a leader and look for ways to showcase his or her own abilities and the abilities of the team, but anyone can also take leadership one step further and be willing to take a back seat to others and quietly help them to achieve. If a nurse manager can do this enthusiastically, then the manager can call himself or herself a coach.

2. Cheerfulness and Happiness

Coaches don't walk around like the village idiot, but they are willing to share themselves with others through a display of good spirits. Coaches know that remaining cheerful while accepting responsibility makes others feel good. Happiness and cheerfulness are contagious, and wise nurse managers try to infect the entire unit.

The role of coach calls for an individual capable of inspiring others to achieve, and one of the best ways to accomplish this is to help others face up to the reality of the situation. Good coaches do this by never exaggerating the situation, by being honest—even in the gravest of situations—and by never making light of another's circumstances.

Coaches know that people who are cheerful in the face of adversity inspire their followers and disarm their opponents. A sense of confidence excites and motivates the team to win under the worst of circumstances. A good example is how Coach June Jones behaved when he assumed the position of head football coach at the University of Hawaii in 1999. The team had come off the worst single-season performance of any Division I university in the history of the National Collegiate Athletic Association (NCAA), 0 and 12. The team had not won on the road in over five seasons (another NCAA record) and faced the first game of the season against Pacific-10 Conference powerhouse University of Southern California. Yet in every interview, at every opportunity to show leadership, Coach Jones projected a tranquility that indicated happiness with the situation. Coach Jones communicated an attitude of victory to the University of Hawaii and left a lot of opponents guessing about what he was up to.

3. Honesty

Coaches need to communicate information, and some of this information will not be pleasant. They cannot hem and haw or water down the truth. They know that to do so would be to put their followers at risk by creating a sense of uncertainty. A coach's job is to keep the people to whom he or she is responsible grounded in reality, and to do that effectively, the coach must be, above all, honest.

There is nothing wrong with making a mistake or telling someone that the situation is hopeless, as long as the research that proves it to be true has been accomplished. As a matter of fact, leaders have a responsibility to report failure, improbabilities, and increased need.

Coaches don't sugarcoat the truth. They do not need to be ruthless or coldly blunt, but they must convey unsavory news in one piece. Passing along short fragments here and there in hopes that someone will catch on produces insecurity and distrust in the team and creates a virus that can run through an organization and eliminate its chance of future success.

Being direct is important, and being honest and direct is critical. Managers who are uncomfortable doing this have only a slim chance of being recognized as good coaches. Managers can improve their skills by making notes and using them as an aid when they go to meetings.

!*CRITICAL POINT*

Being direct does not include being belligerent, rude, or unkind. Good coaches never employ these tactics. Being direct simply means talking in an easily understood and frank manner. Nurse managers hold an important position, one that almost always generates respect, even admiration, in the hearts of those with

whom they work. Nurse managers' words have a significant impact—all of the time. Because this is so, they need to make sure that they speak at low to normal voice levels. Managers should never shout, raise their voices, or become emotional. Doing these things only makes managers look bad and almost always has a negative impact on the audience. Nurse managers can never hope to be recognized as leaders if they do not demonstrate self-control at all times.

4. Resourcefulness

Good coaches make effective use of the resources they have available to support their teams—even if the resources are considered inadequate. A coach's responsibilities include obtaining the resources necessary to manage effectively and help the team grow, but sometimes money, people, and physical resources just aren't available. Unavailability of resources, however, does not provide a reason to quit, complain, or defer until the resources do become available. Good coaches use the lack of resources as a tool to motivate, inspire, and achieve. Once again, Coach June Jones provides the classic example of a coach with this quality:

When June Jones, former head coach of the San Diego Chargers of the National Football League, took over as the head football coach at the University of Hawaii, he found that the resources simply were not available to build the type of football team the university was looking for. The personnel he had to work with were, for the greatest part, returning performers from the previous year's 0-and-12 season. The university was undergoing significant funding problems, due in large part to a poor economic climate that had existed throughout the state of Hawaii for the previous 7 years. There were no weight-training facilities and only a marginal practice environment.

But Coach Jones did not see the situation as reason to postpone the building of a football powerhouse. He simply dug a little deeper into his talent bag and, working with his coaching staff, developed methods to overcome the challenges being faced.

Coach Jones led the University of Hawaii Rainbow Warriors to a 9-and-4 season in his first year, capturing the Western Athletic Championship, and took his team to its first postseason bowl in over a decade. Winning is about attitude and perseverance and is not the product of possession.

Coach Jones faced the fact that resources were not available and reworked his plan to take advantage of the resources that he did have. Maybe that meant that everyone had to work a little harder and put in some extra hours. Perhaps it meant traveling to a nearby weight-training facility. Maybe it meant giving more of himself. That is the difference between being in charge and being an inspiration. If nurse managers, in their role as leaders, work with their staffs (coach them) and inform them honestly of the situation, there is good reason for unit members to support them.

5. Ability to Influence (Persuasiveness)

People follow individuals who can convince them that to do so is in their best interests. Either through words or deeds, or perhaps a combination of both, nurse managers must convince people to go where they want them to go, do what they want them to do, and think like they need them to think. Great coaches don't just dream about a better situation, they transform that dream into a vision (with the help of the team) and continually communicate their vision to every member of the team, every time they have an opportunity. Great coaches talk about the vision as if it *has* to be realized and constantly and consistently reinforce the reason the team should follow. They talk about the vision until the team is able to say, "Oh, yeah! Of course that is the way it will be."

How do nurse managers become this type of influential figure? How do they become persuasive?

Nurse managers start by focusing efforts on something that everyone wants. Because of their role as unit managers, this can be a successful nursing unit, because every member of the staff has a stake in keeping the unit thriving. Their jobs are on the line, so it can be made very personal. "Some very respected business consultants say that the position a coach stands for can even be something that people want, but think is impossible to obtain" (p. 176), declared Marshall Loeb,[3] managing editor of *Fortune* and *Money* magazines.

One of the methods used by influential people to get others to listen to them is silence. In the role of coach, the nurse manager can use this technique very effectively by simply not responding immediately to what people say. If the nurse manager thinks that what a person is saying is nonsense, the manager should never fuel that person's enthusiasm by arguing with him or her. Instead, the manager should make the nay-sayer defend his or her position by looking the person in the eye and saying, "Oh, really?" By making the individual defend his or her position in a quiet, reserved way, the nurse manager can take away a lot of the person's enthusiasm and make the person's position just a little bit shaky—shaky enough, perhaps, to give the manager a chance to make his or her own point.

Influential people are almost always easygoing, low-keyed, and reserved. They tend to speak in a moderate voice, but that doesn't mean that they are not resolute in their beliefs or incapable of informing people exactly how they feel. Influential people stand up for their beliefs, even in the face of intense animosity. They just do it in a way that defuses tension, relaxes the opposition, and disarms hostility. Quiet patience and reserve will make an opponent think, "Wow, this may be right. Look at the way in which it is being defended." Even hostile people admire a calm bearing, reserved demeanor, and proper behavior when they see it.

6. Approachability

Many people who have tried to lead and coach a nursing unit believe that an emotional or psychologic distance divides them from the staff or that they possess special knowledge or special burdens to which their individual staff members will never be privy. One can hear such nurse managers remark to members of their staffs, "If you only knew what I know...," as if their position has provided them with special intelligence. At least in the vast majority of situations, this is utter nonsense.

People in leadership positions often do have a better view of the big picture, but they tend not to be in possession of the little details. Good coaches understand that they don't have all of the information and continually rely on their followers and assistants to fill in the gaps in their knowledge.

Being a nurse manager and serving in the capacity of a coach or leader is a privilege. It is not a power trip. The position makes one responsible for others; it does not guarantee that others are, or will feel, inferior.

Competent nurse managers adopt a relaxed, approachable manner in their normal relations with the staff. However, this does not mean that they do not attempt to use every opportunity to persuade others to follow them. The best features the nurse manager has available to influence the situation are his or her physical attributes. A nurse manager can be tall and lithe, short and heavyset, attractive or not so attractive—these things don't really matter, unless they are very extreme. What people enjoy seeing are those people who carry themselves well, who walk straight with their shoulders forward and with purpose in their step, who are enthusiastic, in control, and radiate confidence.

Coaches know that it is easier to induce others to cooperate than to force them to comply. Because the nurse manager holds more cards than does any single member of the staff, giving is easier. Being cooperative instead of confrontational allows a nurse manager to operate from a position of strength. If people perceive the nurse manager as someone who is willing to negotiate, willing to find common ground, and even willing to give up things to make them happy, they will view the nurse manager as a generous individual.

This is an advantage for the nurse manager intent on operating a high-quality nursing unit. People believe that a person who is confident enough to be approachable holds a position of strength. By being approachable, nurse managers create the perception of strength in themselves and in their units.

7. Generosity

Nurse managers, like all good leaders, should place the needs of team members above their own needs. One of the best ways to demonstrate this attitude is to be willing to sacrifice and, if necessary, put aside personal needs to provide for the unit as a whole.

Coaches know that being generous with others is necessary. Generosity lifts mundane execution of a mission to a higher plane. For example, if a nurse manager says that he or she wants the unit to consistently treat the unit's patients as special customers, the team will nod and show other physical signs of agreement. But if the nurse manager presents an opportunity for them, the team will eagerly rise to the bait. "You all know that the organization provides an annual award for the best nursing unit. Starting this year, I'd like to see our unit win that award and use the prestige it will bring to persuade the administration to fund a day care and recreational center for our use." If this is done properly and with sincerity, team members will sit up, lean forward, and aggressively start talking among themselves about how they can win the award. These actions demonstrate not only concurrence but also a willingness to work harder, do more, and be more enthusiastic. People will do more if there is a tangible return, an investment being made for their benefit. Generosity is a tremendous motivator. It makes people feel better about the work they are being asked to do.

8. Courage

The word *courage* usually brings to mind death-defying actions, but in management, courage means the willingness to take risks. As the directors of nursing units, nurse managers enter new and personally uncharted waters. They must know how to keep a stiff backbone, trust in instinct, and move into the unknown even when they are as scared as the people who will eventually follow them. The difference is that nurse managers must not openly display their fear.

Effective nurse managers plan well, and it is the process of planning that helps them overcome their fear. Fear is generated by things that are not understood, and planning prepares nurse managers for most of the likely obstacles that will have to be overcome as the staff moves toward the vision. However, no amount of planning can foresee all of the challenges that might occur, and eventually every nurse manager will be confronted with completely unknown circumstances that will force the manager to make unpopular decisions. This is the point at which courage comes into play. These situations will most likely bring the nurse manager under fire, and a truly excellent manager will stick with conviction to a plan he or she has formulated based on the best information available. The nurse manager must demonstrate courage in confrontation by calmly explaining why the chosen path is necessary and continue to elicit the staff's support.

When nurse managers do not demonstrate resolve or appear indecisive, their staffs may withhold support or, in the most severe cases, rebel outright. Courage is developed from a position of knowledge. The more nurse managers know about a given subject, the less likely they are to make an error in judgment. If nurse managers prepare themselves well, keep themselves abreast of changes, and think through the challenges, being courageous is a great deal easier and their demonstration of courage is much more convincing.

9. Positive Attitude or Assertiveness

Every person in the nursing profession—and in life—has the opportunity to choose how he or she will perceive and react to the challenges that are faced. Each person can choose to withdraw, to be negative, or to be positive. The individual can develop a "can do" or a "can't do" attitude. He or she can be assertive or defensive, action-oriented or reactionary. The choice is up to the individual.

If nurse managers choose the negative approach, however, they will find it to be a significant handicap. People who lead others must think positively and be assertive. Good managers recognize that, once they decide something can be done, they gain nothing by delaying. True leaders know that if planning has been carried out properly, the necessary resources are in line, and the proper personnel are in place, there is no reason to wait. The right thing to do is to get on with it.

Perhaps some criticism of the modern leadership approach is justified. There is a widespread belief that too much time is spent worrying about what people will think and ensuring that leadership positions are maintained. Too much effort is expended in endless committee meetings, and too much courage is sacrificed in the name of caring. Too many of today's leaders focus on these issues. For example, it was far easier to send humanitarian aid to the survivors of the slaughter in Africa than to take the steps necessary to prevent it. Historians[4] believe that the willingness to take the less assertive position is a major contributing factor in the failure of the United States and its Western allies—the strongest powers on the planet—to prevent human misery in many countries needing help.

Nurse managers, at least the good ones, know that they need to be positive in thought and in action. They know that they must take steps to remedy a situation before it gets out of hand, and many times that means dealing with the consequences of their actions after the fact. The willingness to take positive action, or assertiveness, is a fundamental attribute of the effective nurse manager and is paramount for achieving success in the role of leader of the nursing unit.

10. Understanding

Very few people will see things in exactly the same way as one another. People perceive things based on their previous experience and the conditions of the environment in which they were reared. These fundamental differences mean that any two people can look at an identical situation and develop two completely different opinions.

When nurse managers are coaching their staffs, true effectiveness results from motivating the individual members to want to participate, to desire to excel, and to believe in the reasons for their efforts. If nurse managers, as coaches, perceive things differently from their staff members, there is only one way they can accomplish their mission and that is to be willing to understand their staffs' perceptions. Perception is reality. If you do not remember anything else from this textbook, remember this: *perception is reality!* Good nurse managers know that their ability to accomplish depends on their ability to understand how each member of the unit sees things. The closer nurse managers can come to satisfying individual perceptions, the greater the chance that staff members will follow and perform.

Coaching is compromise—not necessarily of ideals, beliefs, and processes, but of perception. Successful nurse managers know that there are alternative ways of looking at the same challenge and work very hard to get those views shared openly. They get the different approaches out on the table and work with the staff—both as a group and individually—to sort through all the different views, selecting a piece from here and a piece from there until an approach is reached that accomplishes the mission and satisfies the perception of the majority.

It is the willingness to understand differences that helps some nurse managers achieve greatness. A great manager knows that being different does not mean being wrong! Such a manager understands that it is okay to be different and accepts people as they are before trying to work with them to become what the manager needs them to be.

The nurse manager must appreciate and understand others. The nurse manager must ensure that individual employees support the excellence of the unit, but it is not the job of the employees to determine what that level of excellence should be. It is the job of the nurse manager to teach and work with the staff members, to be patient, and to understand their differences. If the nurse manager can convince employees that they are valuable, that the manager respects their differences and understands their individual desires, the manager will achieve more than he or she desires. The manager will not only have people who follow instructions, but people who are committed and loyal—dedicated, hard-working, and willing to be there when the going gets rough. When this occurs, the nurse manager will have achieved greatness as a coach.

A PLAN FOR MASTERING COACHING SKILLS

Such a variety of individual skills are necessary to be a good coach that it is impossible to explain them all in this chapter. Similarly, a nurse manager cannot be given a plan of action that will fit every situation and every set of circumstances. To provide a fixed step-by-step plan on how to master coaching skills would be a complex process. The only thing that remains constant in any nurse manager's attempt to become a great coach or an effective leader (two things that are often thought to be one and the same) is that the manager must constantly learn from experience.

Although there is no established plan of action that can be followed to get the nurse manager through every situation, there are some things that, done well and with flexibility, can greatly enhance the opportunity for success. The following sections outline 10 steps considered critical for the would-be coach.

1. Prepare

There is no such thing as being too prepared. Good coaches are constantly looking for new methods, new approaches, better planning tools, and better methods for inspiring others. For nurse managers, being good coaches means making it a habit to draw from the talents of those with whom they have contact. They emulate other good coaches and remain humble enough to learn from those whom they are tasked to teach. Finally, successful coaches prepare for success by learning from the mistakes they have made in the past and from the mistakes they have witnessed others making.

Becoming a great coach, and remaining one, is a continual process of preparation.

2. Choose and Commit

Nurse managers, in their role as coaches, should carefully evaluate a course of action and, once they have made their choice, commit themselves fully to its realization. They commit themselves to the vision, embrace it, and work with staff members to realize it.

3. Keep an Open Mind

The nurse manager's vision for the unit should be a collaborative result of a team action, and once the vision is established, all members should use their full capabilities to work toward its realization. However, this does not mean that once the vision is established the methods used to attain it cannot be altered to meet changes in the environment, new information, new personnel, changes in resources, or other such influences.

No one's method is absolute. Good nurse managers will learn from observation, reaction, and the environment, and use the information obtained to change how they go about attaining the team's vision. Set-in-concrete, my-way-or-the-highway approaches may work, but the chances are very good that they will never achieve the results that an open mind can.

4. Practice

There is an old Hollywood joke that the person who can fake sincerity has it made. That may work in the movies, but in the demanding environment of the nursing unit, it is far less likely that nurse managers will be able to carry off anything by faking it.

Instead of a faker, what is needed in management is someone who is well rehearsed. Nurse managers, in their role as coaches of the nursing staff, must be able to influence other people and validate their causes. This means that messages must be practiced and repracticed to improve the quality of delivery. It is much like giving a speech in public. Many people are very afraid of being in front of an audience. This fear can be overcome—perhaps not easily, but certainly overcome—by almost everyone who really tries. The process involves rehearsing the lines, practicing the delivery, and making clear, valid points. Coaching is much the same, and it is the well-practiced coach who is recognized as the outstanding leader.

Nurse managers also make as much time as possible for their staffs to practice. The practice time is used to uncover and correct mistakes before they can cause real damage. The practice environment should be a "safe haven" for the staff member. Here, mistakes can be made and each one presented as an opportunity to learn. People can learn to relax, work on natural style, and develop the performance process according to their individual skills under the caring eye of a coach who is tolerant of error, concerned for excellence, and willing to assist.

Every job, every action, and every reaction can be practiced. It is up to the creative coach to determine exactly how.

5. Maintain Discipline

Nurse managers, in their role as coaches, must effectively exercise two types of discipline: (1) discipline of the team, and (2) personal discipline. The first type is applied as conditions dictate with compassion and understanding, and with an eye for improving the individual's performance. Personal discipline, however, is an entirely different process.

Exercising personal discipline is the process of consistently telling oneself the truth, evaluating one's actions, and improving one's potential. It is working hard to overcome personal weaknesses and maintaining a willingness to use the talents of others to offset personal shortcomings. It is forcing oneself to be aware of the environment around one, observing others, and being willing to learn and change.

Being disciplined means being careful: careful how the team is formed, careful how the team's efforts are directed, and careful in what is expected of others. Good nurse managers do not allow sentimentality to cloud their judgment. If they find that they have a staff member whom they like but who consistently underperforms, they have the courage to address the shortcomings and work with the poor performer, and if he or she does not improve, they have the common sense to get rid of the person.

6. Meet Deadlines and Be Punctual

Few people are more aggravating than someone who is late or more destructive than someone who can't meet a deadline. *Being* on time, and *finishing* on time are fundamental aspects of responsibility. No one can be a superior nurse manager (a person who influences others) and act irresponsibly.

People form opinions of the nurse manager from his or her actions. Although this should be no revelation to anyone who runs a nursing unit, it seems to be so when it comes to being punctual. The success of the individual nursing unit as a functioning part of the hospital has a lot to do with conveying importance to others: not self-importance but perceived importance. Other units within the organization, for example, must perceive that the nurse manager and his or her staff believe that these other units are important. Nothing can destroy this perception faster than being late, delivering late, or failing to meet a deadline.

There is no acceptable excuse for being late. Telling someone that an earlier meeting ran overtime is simply another way of saying, "Your meeting is not as important as my prior meeting." Being late is rude, unprofessional, and inexcusable—every time it occurs, regardless of the circumstances.

7. Stay in Contact

One of the biggest mistakes nurse managers can make is to allow a perceived gap to develop between the unit staff and themselves. Nurse managers must work hard to close this gap by reinforcing the perception that they, too, are members of their units. This becomes difficult for the leaders of dynamic places of business, because most staff members already hold the opinion that managers are different; after all, they see them first and foremost as the boss.

This is not to suggest that the nurse manager should act like a staff nurse. The coach has a separate role, and attempting to be like a staff nurse may be foolhardy. Staff don't want the nurse manager to fake anything. They want their boss to walk among them, talk to them in their vernacular, listen to their concerns with genuine interest, take them seriously, and provide open communication in a relaxed manner. In some forward-looking hospitals, last names are no longer used, and no one is referred to by tacking Mr. or Ms. or Mrs. in front of the last name. This practice was developed by what is arguably the most successful business of all time, the Walt Disney Company. Until his death, Walt Disney, certainly one of the most creative and successful individuals of our age, was known to everyone simply as "Walt," and today, throughout Disney, every member of the "cast" is referred to by his or her first name, including the chairman of the board.

If nurse managers behave as if they are different, superior, or unapproachable, team members will quickly distance themselves. If they become known as individuals who "kill the messenger," the staff will quickly disassociate themselves, and if they demean any member of the staff, every member will quickly know it.

Exactly how nurse managers should become accessible was never showcased better than through the actions of Tom Melohn, former chief executive officer of North American Tool and Die. In his book *The New Partnership*,[5] Melohn shared the following seven truths he learned from his 37 years of experience:

1. "The mass of men lead lives of quiet desperation" (as quoted from Henry David Thoreau in *Walden* [1854]).
2. Good people really do want to do a good job.
3. People value honesty—very much. Just tell it like it is.
4. The people "on the line" are no different from you and me.
5. Everyone is creative, in some way.
6. In most situations, the trappings of power get in the way of working together.
7. Trust is very fragile, yet we all yearn to trust each other, our company, and our leaders. (p. 18)

Melohn (called "Tom" by everyone at North American) could be found walking through the shop, talking with machinists, discussing the weather with diemakers, talking philosophy with the loading clerks, and even discussing the company balance sheet with the forklift drivers. People saw him as one of them. He didn't try to be—they perceived him that way. More about Melohn's exploits can be found in his book.[5] It is an exceptional read and highly recommended.

Does this approach work? Following are the results of Melohn's leadership at North American Tool and Die:

Sales: up an average of 28% each year for 12 consecutive years

Pretax earnings*: up 2,400%

Return on investment: in the top 10% of the entire Fortune 500

Company stock: up 47% compounded each year

Productivity*: up 480%

Absenteeism*: less than 1% per year

Personnel turnover*: 0.0025% per year (1 person in 400 left each year)

Customer reject rate: 0.01% for all parts, all years, all customers

---

*Areas that are especially important in the healthcare industry. In fact, they are the most critical issues for most healthcare organizations today, and the things Melohn did at North American are applicable to every healthcare organization and every nursing unit therein.

So what is the conclusion? Can this approach be applied to the nursing unit with its technical and dynamic demands? Absolutely! Keep in mind that the demands of the nursing unit require exceptionally high-quality professionals, but so does every other form of business in the world. Being an educated caregiver does not make one superhuman; rather it creates *the opportunity to become superhuman*. Tom Melohn turned his organization into a single group of superhumans, and fewer than 5% of them had the advantages of advanced education. Think what his tactics could do in an environment staffed with educated professionals.

8. Listen

Authority provides no one with the ability to know it all. Good nurse managers listen effectively. They open up their ears and minds, and listen to everything said and unsaid; as coaches, they attend to the nuances. *Listen* to the following story:

> It is the Second Soviet International, and the leader of the Soviet Socialist Republic, Joseph Stalin, is addressing the gathering of Communist leaders from around the world. Trotsky, Stalin's most formidable opponent, is not present at the meeting and has been threatening to disrupt the fight for unified leadership under Stalin's direction. At the plenary session, Stalin addresses the audience by saying, "I have a telegram from Comrade Trotsky. It reads, 'You were right. I was wrong. I should apologize to you. Trotsky.'" There is thunderous applause from the packed assembly hall. Everyone present seems overcome with excitement, except for one small man, who stands up, raises his hand, and says, "Excuse me, Comrade Stalin, but I think you have it wrong. Trotsky is a Jew, and he speaks with a rising inflection. The telegram should read, 'You were right? I was wrong? I should apologize to you? Trotsky.'"

If you noticed the difference between Stalin's interpretation of the telegram and the small man's the first time you read the paragraph, you have excellent listening skills.

Listening also means hearing what is not being said. Not everyone has the courage to approach the nurse manager and come directly to the point. Many people talk indirectly, and a good leader must be able to decipher their meanings. Some people, for example, will ask, "Are you hungry?" This question can be interpreted as, "I'm curious" or "I'm hungry, would you like to join me in eating?" Someone may use the question, "Can I get you a cup of coffee?" as an excuse for taking a break. A good manager learns to decipher these hidden messages before attempting any action.

9. Cooperate

Excellent performance is built on teamwork and teamwork is built around cooperation—with superiors, peers, juniors, those with whom one has contact, and those whom one may never know. Remember that today's adversary may be tomorrow's ally. Consider the following confession of a leader:

> I spent several years as an infantry reconnaissance officer in the Vietnam War. During that time, I used every method at my disposal to ensure that I, and every member of my team, returned from our missions safely. I saw things that no one should ever experience: the ability of man to be cruel to his fellow man in the most horrible sense of the word. I learned to hate at a very young age.
>
> Today, some 25 years since I last set foot in the steaming jungles of Vietnam, I am the President of the Board of Directors of the Vietnamese American Chamber of Commerce in my home town and actively work to find ways to promote friendly relations between our two countries.

Although the carefully buffed halls of the nursing unit don't often approach the intensity of the battlefield, emotions can run extremely high. It is imperative that nurse managers—the people responsible for coaching their units to success—never let their emotions get the best of their ability to act.

10. Place the Needs of Others Above One's Own

Placing the needs of others above one's own is the last recommendation that will be made in this chapter. Although some people are naturally generous and find it within themselves to be generous with everyone, most people have to contend with a selfish streak. Our world plays to that selfish streak and teaches that it is okay to take more than one gives or more than one needs.

Really good nurse managers, in their role as coaches and leaders, learn to resist this selfish streak. They learn that it can be very beneficial to help another succeed. They learn to appreciate the needs of others and help when they can. This they do without expecting anything in return.

The more nurse managers place the needs of others ahead of their own, the easier it becomes to repeat the action. Think for a moment. If you were the coach of a star performer who is desperately needed to assure victory for your team but playing that star performer could cripple the player, would you, as a coach, allow the star player to perform or would you risk losing the game to prevent an injury? The difference in the answers to this question is the difference between being a great coach and being in charge.

SUMMARY

- Coaching is nothing more than the application of leadership.

- The words *nurse manager, coach, leader,* and *boss* have been used interchangeably throughout this text. This has been done not to confuse or muddy the water but to tie these positions together.

- Being the effective manager of a nursing unit that is organized around the team concept requires a special individual, a caring individual, a generous person willing to give of himself or herself, someone who puts others first, and someone who looks for and works with the goodness and the failings in others—someone who knows that authority means responsibility, not privilege.

- Today, in the business of nursing, the nurse manager must be successful as a coach, a leader, and a boss.

- What you are known by has nothing to do with your title, your position, or the size of your office. It has everything to do with how you are perceived and how you conduct yourself.

- Leadership *is* a privilege and a responsibility, not a position *of* privilege and irresponsibility.

- It is important that all nurse managers, leaders, coaches, and bosses remember the words of the late American president John Fitzgerald Kennedy: "A person is not remembered for what he accomplished in his lifetime; he is remembered for what others believe he accomplished."

FINAL THOUGHTS

Some critical issues must be reinforced to truly appreciate the role of the leader and coach. The following points are critical to the success of anyone aspiring to lead others:

- When faced with a leadership opportunity or a management challenge, it is always best first to consider the source and the nature of the issue. Ask yourself whether it involves personal leadership traits, the patient, the family, the physician, or other parties. Then, consider to what degree the issue pertains to the personal styles of the parties involved. Sometimes simply being aware that personalities may be involved will help resolve the issue.

- Never make the mistake of considering being a leader as the opposite of being a follower. Being a follower requires active presence and full engagement with the leader. Recognize that even if you are a designated leader, you will remain a follower in many circumstances.

- When supplying leadership, place your emphasis on the issue, not the participants or combatants involved. Provide positive reinforcement to the disputing parties to the greatest degree possible and plan for the use of constructive feedback.

THE NURSE MANAGER SPEAKS

Traditional approaches to management in the healthcare industry include the use of authority, control, competition, and logic through management behaviors that are autocratic, directive, and task oriented. Today, however, the highly skilled and technically proficient workforce is forcing organizations to focus more on human needs and less on task accomplishment as the driving factors within management.

The rapid change that characterizes today's healthcare environment is another reason why today's nurse managers should focus on the welfare of their staffs as much as the welfare of their patients. Today's performers think more in terms of their profession than of their organization, and managing these dynamic professionals is becoming an increasing challenge.

Today's truly successful leader understands that it is not enough merely to tell a staff member to perform a job. Today, those instructions need to be tempered with respect, professionalism, and mutual regard to cultivate self-confidence and self-esteem within every contributor in the nursing unit.

To ensure success in managing today's dynamic workforce, the nurse manager must understand that, in the long run, leadership and respect will cultivate far better and more professional performance than will authority and task-oriented direction.

REFERENCES

1. Brown PB: *My season on the brink: a father's seven weeks as a Little League manager,* New York, 1992, St. Martin's.
2. Bennis W, Nanus B: *Leaders: strategies for taking charge,* ed 2, New York, 2003, HarperCollins.
3. Loeb M, Kindel S: *Leadership for dummies,* Chicago, 1999, IDG Books.
4. Legro JW: *Rethinking the world: great power strategies and international order,* Ithaca, NY, 2005, Cornell University Press.
5. Melohn T: *The new partnership,* New York, 1996, Wiley.

SUGGESTED READINGS

Allen KR: *Time and information management that really work,* Los Angeles, 1995, Affinity.
Belasco JA, Stayer RC: *Flight of the buffalo: soaring to excellence, learning to let employees lead,* New York, 1994, Warner.
Bennis W, Mason RO: *High-speed management,* San Francisco, 1993, Jossey-Bass.
Benton DA: *How to think like a CEO,* New York, 1999, Warner.

Covey SR: *The seven habits of highly effective people,* New York, 1989, Simon and Schuster.

Edler R: *If I knew then what I know now,* New York, 1998, Berkeley.

Giblen L: *How to have confidence and power in dealing with people,* New York, 1999, Reward.

Hansten RI: *Clinical delegation skills,* Gaithersburg, Md, 1996, Aspen.

Kriegel RJ: *If it ain't broke ... break it,* New York, 1991, Warner.

Laborde GZ: *Influencing with integrity,* Palo Alto, Calif, 1983, Syntony.

McGuffin JA: *The nurse's guide to successful management,* St Louis, 1999, Mosby.

Meyer C: *Fast cycle time,* New York, 1993, Free Press.

Nelson B: *1001 ways to energize employees,* New York, 1997, Workman.

Sherman SG: *Make yourself memorable,* New York, 1996, Amacom.

Tingley JC: *Say what you mean and get what you want,* New York, 1996, Amacom.

Recruiting
and Selecting Staff

LEARNING SYNOPSIS

Upon successful completion of this chapter, readers will possess a fundamental understanding of the proper procedures and practices to follow in the employment process to ensure compliance with federal and state laws.

OBJECTIVES

1. Specify the key to success in the nursing unit
2. Identify principles and methods of job analysis and the development of the job description
3. Describe the procedures to follow and the methods available to identify, attract, and solicit applicants for positions in the nursing unit
4. Outline the procedures to follow when preparing for and conducting an employment interview
5. List steps that can be taken by the nurse manager to ensure compliance with state and federal employment regulations
6. Identify basic federal laws that apply to the employment process and explain they are administered

In virtually every industry, and especially in service-related and labor-intensive organizations, the quality of the personnel employed has the greatest effect on the organization's ability to achieve its goals and objectives. In fact, most professional consultants believe that it is staff quality that ultimately determines an organization's overall level of success. Finding the very best prospects and then hiring only the best of the best is therefore vital to the health of every organization.

The cost of not having an exceptional hiring program within the hospital can result in excessive expense for the organization and a high level of stress for the nurse manager. The importance of a good hiring program at the unit level cannot be overemphasized, as it goes beyond what it costs the organization in terms of financial outlay to recruit, hire, and train a member of the staff, even considering that this can be a major operating expense. The real expense comes from the emotional turmoil that can be caused by an employee who must later be terminated involuntarily. This *hidden cost* may be even greater than the initial investment and can include the following:

- Damage to the reputation of the unit and the organization due to the low quality of work performed by the unmotivated employee
- Disruption and increased tension in the work environment
- Increased patient dissatisfaction, which may make patients reluctant to return to the particular unit or hospital
- Increased workload and overtime in the nursing unit as other members of the staff are required to compensate for the employee's unsatisfactory performance
- Increased risk of medical malpractice or compensatory damages for injuries caused by a poorly performing employee

The road to success for the nursing unit begins with the selection of the personnel who staff it. No task required of the nurse manager is more important than the selection of personnel. Selecting the right person is a process of matching people to jobs and includes the following four elements:

1. *Job analysis:* determination of exactly what is required to satisfactorily discharge the responsibilities associated with a specific position
2. *Recruitment of applicants:* the processes available to assist managers in identifying and attracting the right applicants
3. *Selection techniques:* the interviewing and evaluation processes that measure the applicants' skills, ability, and knowledge and, at the same time, conform to employment law

4. *Legal conformity:* assurance that the selection techniques developed and used conform to legal stipulations

In most hospitals operating today, the responsibility for selecting nursing personnel is shared by the nurse manager, the nursing service (nursing director or vice president of nursing), and the human resources department. The complexity of the laws governing the employment of personnel makes it absolutely necessary that the employment process be conducted in a very disciplined manner. Nurse managers, in their role as front-line supervisors, are frequently the most knowledgeable members of the management team regarding the specific requirements of the job for which someone is being hired. In fact, they play an important part in the entire hiring process. Of course, they are assisted in their efforts by the nursing service and the human resources department, which is responsible for the posting of the job opening internally and externally, initial screening, and perhaps the first interviewing process. Actually, the human resources department has oversight of the entire hiring process to ensure compliance with applicable state and federal employment regulations.

Table 13-1 shows the steps in the typical selection process and offers generally accepted guidelines regarding who is responsible for each step. The table clearly shows the importance of nurse managers' involvement in the hiring process. Through their active participation, nurse managers demonstrate their personal commitment to the applicant and the company during each interviewing session. However, the real importance of nurse managers in this process lies in the following:

1. They are generally in the best position to assess the applicants' technical competency, potential, and overall suitability.
2. They can answer applicants' technical and work-related questions from a real-world standpoint.

Even if nurse managers are not actively involved in the selection of applicants, they have the responsibility to keep those who are involved informed of the needs of their nursing units and any changes in performance requirements for the job to be filled. Because nurse managers are normally the first individuals in the management chain to be aware of changes in the unit, such as potential resignations, requests for transfer, and maternity leaves, they are the best placed to monitor the changes in personnel needs. They are also aware of changes in the work area that might necessitate a change in personnel, such as moving a nursing position from the day shift to the night shift. Making sure that personnel needs are communicated from the nursing unit to the human

TABLE 13-1

A Typical Selection Process

Task	Responsible Personnel
Design, development, and verification of job requirements	Nursing service
Development of employment application	HR, nursing service
Development of selection process (interview guide, questions, potential testing, application form)	HR, nursing service
Recruitment of qualified personnel	HR, nursing service, nurse manager
Review of applicants' résumés and applications	Nursing service, nurse manager
Preliminary interview, screening of applicants	HR, nursing service, nurse manager
Verification of references, employee record	HR, nursing staff
Interview of prospects, applicants	HR, nurse manager
Medical examination (if required)	HR
Gleaning of available information	Nursing service, nurse manager
Comparison of applicants (employment decision)	Nurse manager
Offering of position to best-qualified applicant	Nurse manager, nursing service, HR
Acceptance of offer	Best-qualified applicant
Employment processing, orientation	Nursing service, HR, nurse manager

HR, Human resources department.

resources department promptly and accurately helps ensure effective coordination of the selection process and the proper staffing of the nursing unit.

JOB ANALYSIS

Before any recruiting or interviewing of prospects can begin, those responsible for the hiring process need to ensure that a completely developed job description exists which delineates the duties of the position and the skills, qualifications, and education required to perform the job. The process of determining the responsibilities and demands of a position is referred to as *job analysis.* A job analysis is a research process that determines the following:

- The principal duties and responsibilities of a particular job
- Tasks that must be done to discharge each duty and responsibility
- The personal qualifications (skills, abilities, education, knowledge, and traits) needed for the job

Done properly, the job analysis will produce an effective job description that will delineate the requirements of a specific position in a specific unit and hospital. Fig. 13-1 is an example of a well-developed job description. (The job description in this figure is an example only. The format and content differ greatly from organization to organization. Nurse managers should check with their human resources managers to determine the format to use in drafting a specific job description.)

Job knowledge provides the foundation for almost every human resource function in the healthcare industry. This applies at the level of the nursing unit because a nurse manager cannot train an individual to perform a job unless the nurse manager knows the tasks involved in the job. In addition, before a nurse manager can evaluate an employee's performance in a position, he or she must understand not only the individual requirements of the job but also the standards that each performer must meet. The job analysis provides the basis for carrying out these essential tasks. It is the responsibility of the nurse manager to ensure that an accurate, up-to-date job description exists for every position for which he or she is responsible. Although the manager will certainly consult with his or her seniors (director of nursing, nursing vice president) to ensure that any job description developed complements other similar job descriptions that might be used in the hospital, and the manager may obtain considerable help from the human resources department in drafting the actual document, the responsibility for having one is the nurse manager's. If the nursing unit does not have a job description that satisfactory defines an existing position, then the nurse manager should develop one. After it is drafted and approved, each person filling the specific job it covers should be given a copy.

An important tool in selecting the proper person for a specific position is the job specification, which details the personal qualifications needed. Although education, knowledge, skill, and ability requirements can be inferred from the description of tasks and duties to be performed, tasks and behaviors are not necessarily covered in the same manner. Consequently, a job analysis that lists the tasks to be performed may be more appropriate than one that lists only personal requirements. Typically, job descriptions that specify

The Job Description

Position: Registered nurse (staff)

Supervised by: Nursing manager

Department: Nursing service

Section: Various nursing areas

Job Grade: 62   **Job Code No:** 1678-1

Overview of Position: Provides professional nursing services and patient care in a variety of inpatient and outpatient settings under only infrequent supervision. Follows established nursing process, including patient assessment, nursing diagnosis, planning, intervention, and evaluation. Ensures compliance with hospital, department, and organizational policies and accepted nursing procedures, standards, processes, and practices.

Duties and Responsibilities

1. Provides direct, professional nursing care to a specified population of patients in both inpatient and outpatient environments.

2. Prepares equipment and assists physicians during examinations and treatments.

3. Performs evaluations of new and existing patients to determine priority and suitability of treatment and/or the necessity for modification.

4. Administers prescribed medications, applies sterile dressings, performs phlebotomy, and monitors vital signs.

5. Maintains confidentiality with regard to patient records.

6. May perform specialized nursing procedures related to the unique needs of a particular patient population.

7. May oversee and guide the work of other nursing and support staff.

8. Performs miscellaneous job-related duties as may be assigned.

Minimum Education and Experience Required: Bachelor's degree in nursing; 6 months of experience directly related to the duties and responsibilities specified.

Licenses/Certifications Required: CPR certified; licensure pending, as documented by temporary license or designation by state licensing agency as licensed registered nurse. Successful candidate must submit to postoffer, preemployment physical examination/medical history check.

Required Training: *In addition to the following, all new employees are required to attend new employee orientation* and training in safety (annually), blood-borne pathogens (annually), hazard communications (area-specific), infectious waste, tuberculosis, and back injury prevention.

Knowledge, Skills, and Abilities Required

1. Ability to plan, implement, and evaluate individual patient care programs.

2. Knowledge of nursing theory and practice.

3. Knowledge of accreditation and certification requirements and standards.

4. Knowledge of clinical and/or surgical facilities, instrument, and equipment.

5. Knowledge of clinical operations and procedures.

6. Knowledge of appropriate procedures and standards for the administration of medications and patient care aids.

7. Skill in preparing and maintaining patient records.

8. Ability to make administrative and procedural decisions and judgment on sensitive, confidential matters.

Fig. 13-1 ■ Example of a job description for the position of registered nurse. *CPR,* Cardiopulmonary resuscitation.

Working Conditions: Work is normally performed in a typical interior office work environment.

Physical Requirements: Moderate physical activity. Requires handling of objects up to 25 pounds or standing and/or walking for more than 4 hours per day.

Environmental Conditions: Work environment involves exposure to potentially dangerous materials and situations that require following extensive safety precautions and may include the use of protective equipment.

Revised Date: 06/05/04

Fig. 13-1—cont'd ■ Example of a job description for the position of registered nurse.

the required tasks for a given position are not available from commercial sources.

Today, many different techniques are available for performing job analysis.[1] Although these options vary greatly in complexity and in their applicability to different kinds of jobs, they do have many similarities. Among these techniques are the following:

- *Supervisory conferences:* In this approach, the person charged with conducting the analysis (job analyst) brings together executives, supervisors, and first-line managers (as applicable) for the purpose of identifying the critical tasks or duties required in a specific job.
- *Critical incident technique:* This method requires managers to effectively identify employee behaviors that have contributed to particularly successful or unsuccessful job performance. This method usually consumes a great deal of time and may not provide a complete picture of the job because only very positive or very negative behaviors will be identified.
- *Work sampling:* In this approach, the analyst actually performs the job in order to define its requirements. This process is rarely used because it is both extremely time consuming and very expensive.
- *Observation:* This is one of the most common methods employed by job analysts. It is most often used for jobs that consist largely of repetitive, short-cycle, manual operations.
- *Interviewing:* In this commonly used method, actual position holders provide information about tasks associated with the job or personal attributes required to perform it.
- *Questionnaires and checklists:* This approach also relies on the input of current or past jobholders to develop the description of tasks and personal requirements. The typical checklist tends to be more structured than the average questionnaire and may consist of hundreds of specific items;

the individual respondent checks off each task he or she performs on the job. The collected data are then analyzed to determine the tasks performed by the majority of persons currently in the job. Questionnaires can be constructed using either a closed-ended or open-ended format depending on how much detail the analyst needs or wishes to collect about the position. A wide range of commercially developed questionnaires are available, but if no suitable questionnaire can be found, then a good human resources department can provide excellent assistance in creating one. When a checklist is used as the basis for job analysis, input from a large number of current and past jobholders is generally required to develop a comprehensive database.

Nurse managers are frequently asked to participate in the development of a job description, usually through a supervisory conference, interviews, or questionnaires, because of their knowledge of different performance requirements.[2]

Assuming that they are free of error, job descriptions and specifications are like photographs of the jobs they describe, but they accurately represent only what the job was at the time the job analysis was performed. Job descriptions are used to develop performance appraisal instruments, training programs, and personnel selection procedures. Fig. 13-2 shows an outline that can be used to develop a job description.

RECRUITMENT

Recruitment is the activity that links the requirements of staff planning with the personnel selection process. Its purpose is to locate and attract qualified applicants in sufficient number so that a pool of potential applicants is available from which qualified individuals can be selected. Although the human resources

Job Description Development Outline

Department:_____ Name of person completing form:_____

Position title of respondent:_____

1. Main purpose or objective of the job:_____
   _____
   _____

2. Title of position being reviewed:_____
   _____
   _____

3. Does position supervise others? ☐ Yes ☐ No
   If so, complete the following:

   Job Title   **Number of People with This Job Title**
   _____   _____
   _____   _____
   _____   _____

4. In the order of importance, list the primary responsibilities of the job (e.g., *"Ensure medications are administered on time"*).
   A._____
   B._____
   C._____
   D._____
   E._____

5. Describe (in the same order of importance as in Question 4) the steps taken to perform each responsibility listed in Question 4, (e.g., *Check with pharmacy to ensure medication is ordered on time*).
   A._____
   B._____
   C._____
   D._____
   E._____

6. List, in order of importance, specific duties that may need to be performed periodically.
   A._____
   B._____
   C._____
   D._____
   E._____

Fig. 13-2 ■ Example of an outline used to develop a job description.

7. Whom does the position contact on institution-related matters (e.g., outside vendors, central supply, laboratory, radiology)? (Do not include supervisors.)

Internal	External
A. _____	A. _____
B. _____	B. _____
C. _____	C. _____
D. _____	D. _____
E. _____	E. _____

8. What special equipment is used by this position?

To Perform Job	To Train Others
A. _____	A. _____
B. _____	B. _____
C. _____	C. _____
D. _____	D. _____
E. _____	E. _____

9. Describe the environment in which work is performed—noise levels, travel, traffic, high pressure, and so forth.

A. _____

B. _____

C. _____

D. _____

E. _____

10. What are the good and bad points of the job?

Good Points	Bad Points
A. _____	A. _____
B. _____	B. _____
C. _____	C. _____
D. _____	D. _____
E. _____	E. _____

11. What is the minimum education required for this job? _____

Why? _____

_____

_____

_____

12. What is the minimum experience required for this job? _____

_____

Why? _____

_____

_____

Fig. 13-2—cont'd ■ Example of an outline used to develop a job description.

Continued

13. Is additional training required for this job (training not available in school)? ☐ Yes ☐ No   If so, what is required?

Additional Training Programs	Why Training Is Needed
A. _____	A. _____
B. _____	B. _____
C. _____	C. _____
D. _____	D. _____
E. _____	E. _____

14. If any, what is the anticipated probation period for this job? (how long will it take for a new hire to perform this job acceptably without supervision?)
Why?

_____

_____

_____

15. What are the minimum physical requirements for this job?

Physical Requirement	Reason
A. _____	A. _____
B. _____	B. _____
C. _____	C. _____
D. _____	D. _____
E. _____	E. _____

16. What special skills and knowledge must be possessed for this job?

Special Skill/Knowledge	Reason
A. _____	A. _____
B. _____	B. _____
C. _____	C. _____
D. _____	D. _____
E. _____	E. _____

17. Additional details concerning this job:

A. _____

B. _____

C. _____

D. _____

E. _____

Fig. 13-2—cont'd ■ Example of an outline used to develop a job description.

department will carry out the majority of the recruiting efforts, nurse managers have an important role to play in the process.

The best way to recruit effective members of the nursing staff is for nurse managers to create a positive work environment that will help retain a higher percentage of the existing staff. When an opening does occur in one of these units, it will generally be filled by highly qualified personnel who have access to the organization's informal channels of communication (i.e., competent people will hear about the opening and apply for the position). In contrast, managers who are unable to maintain a positive work environment will more than likely have higher turnover rates in their units and will be less likely to attract highly qualified replacements in numbers sufficient to supply their units. The efforts of nurse managers to build an environment of trust, professionalism, and cooperative performance pay huge dividends in keeping turnover low and in facilitating the recruitment of replacement personnel.

If formal recruitment becomes necessary, however, nurse managers will recruit replacement personnel using the basic strategies outlined in the following sections.

Where to Look

For most organizations, personnel will be recruited from within the institution's own geographical area; however, limited availability of nurses may require recruitment on a wider scale. A large number of unemployed nurses will seldom be available in any geographic area. Inactive nurses are a potential pool of applicants, particularly in difficult economic times.[3]

Obviously, the physical location of the organization plays an important part in its recruiting efforts. For example, if the organization is in a major metropolitan area, the recruiting effort may be relatively easy, because the city it supports will have a large population from which to draw. In the final analysis, however, all organizations recruit where experience and circumstances indicate they will find people with the necessary skills. Thus, most hospitals adopt a progressive strategy in which they first recruit in the local market and then, if insufficient applicants are available, expand their search in wider and wider circles until a large enough applicant pool is obtained.

Proximity to home is a key factor in a person's choice of a job. This means that nurses living near a hospital represent an inviting opportunity for recruitment.[3] One method of identifying those who comprise this market is to work with the state board of nursing to obtain the names of registered nurses living in zip code areas surrounding the hospital. Another method is effective networking with local businesses. The hospital can ask the assistance of the human resources departments in local industries in targeting spouses of their employees who are nurses. Finally, students at a local school of nursing are an excellent pool of potential employees even before they graduate.

One source of new nurses that is frequently overlooked is inactive nurses. Survey statistics show that between 27% and 40% of the registered nurses in any geographic area are not working in the profession and that approximately 70% of these inactive nurses would consider returning to nursing if things such as improved management, refresher training, and continuing education were made available.[3] Most inactive nurses look at the following elements in considering reemployment in nursing (listed in order of priority):

- Proximity of the job to home
- Management support
- Quality of management
- Salary
- Opportunity to specialize

Finally, there are retired experienced nurses who might consider reentering the job market on a volunteer basis if they are offered the opportunity to learn new skills.

How to Look

Many different options are available to the organization in searching for applicants, including the following:

- Referrals from current employees
- Advertising—in newspapers and journals, and at professional conventions
- Outreach at educational institutions—career days, career counseling services, etc.
- Employment agencies
- Professional recruiters
- Temporary help agencies
- Internet

Most applications are received from individuals who walk into the organization and post their own applications or who respond to some form of advertising; however, acute nursing shortages have forced many hospitals to offer recruiting bonuses for employee referrals. Direct applications and employee referrals are normally quick and relatively inexpensive ways of recruiting people, and many of the best applicants are located using these strategies. These methods are not without their challenges, however. For example, they tend to perpetuate the racial or social mix of the existing workforce. In addition, indirect problems are often created when current staff members refer applicants who are graduates of the same educational institutions.

Advertising is another frequently used method of looking for applicants. It may be as simple as taking out classified advertisements in the local newspapers or posting a web advertisement via the Internet, or it may involve more complex and expensive advertising in medical or nursing journals and recruitment activity at professional meetings. Although advertising is typically a very effective recruiting tool, it tends to be expensive and usually requires the assistance of technical personnel.

Today, a good deal of evidence indicates that the method used in recruiting is related to the subsequent tenure of the individual who is hired by the organization.[4] Research has found that applicants who are located through informal methods, such as those recommended by friends, walk-ins, and rehires, tend to remain with the hiring organization longer than applicants recruited through formal methods (advertising and employment agencies).

The recruiting source has also been shown to be directly related to the subsequent productivity of new personnel. For example, nurses who are recruited by informal methods generally possess realistic information about the job and the institution before they are hired. This inside knowledge helps shape their expectations so that these more closely match the reality of the job, and thus much of the cultural shock typically associated with a new job is eliminated. Individuals who do not possess this inside information and who come to the job with unrealistic expectations tend to have them violated quickly, which increases their dissatisfaction with the job. This results in a higher level of turnover of new hires when the job market is open. If the job market is closed because of tough or difficult economic times, then these individuals will tend to stay with the organization even though they are dissatisfied because they need the job, but they will not perform at the level of the informally recruited employee. This supports the contention that where the organization looks for applicants may have significant consequences for the organization at a later date.

When to Look

The timing of the recruiting effort traditionally has not been a major concern in the healthcare industry because, except for brief periods, there has been a continuing shortage of nurses. But suppose that a situation does exist in which the timing of the recruiting effort could become important. How long does it take from the time a need is identified until a new hire is actually available for work? Generally, the time required for the hospital's recruiting advertisement to begin producing applicants is approximately 10 days. Once prospects have started to apply, an additional 4 days elapse while invitations to interview are issued. Then it generally takes an average of 7 days to arrange for and conduct interviews, and an additional 4 days for the organization to decide whether or not to employ a given individual. Once an offer is made, it takes an average of 10 days for the selected applicant to make up his or her mind to accept the position and an average of 20 more days for the individual accepting the offer to report to work.

These data suggest that vacancies should be advertised almost 2 months before they are expected to occur. In a critical market, the required time can be much longer. These time lines, although only estimates, offer an excellent guideline to use when planning a search for personnel.

How to Sell the Organization to Applicants

The style of communication used by an organization can have a dramatic effect on the success of the recruiting effort. Every contact with applicants requires a professional approach, and each interview must be conducted on time and in a friendly and organized manner, whether it is the initial interview carried out by the human resources department or the final interview performed by the nursing director. In every instance, the organization must be responsive to the applicant's needs.

It is never good business to oversell the organization. Such conduct not only borders on unprofessional but almost always leads to the creation of unrealistic expectations in the applicant that may later lead to dissatisfaction and turnover. Instead, the professional approach is to realistically present the job requirements and rewards. This tactic almost always leads to enhanced job satisfaction, because the applicant learns what the job is actually like and is better prepared to make an intelligent decision about accepting any offer made. For example, it would be unprofessional of a nurse manager to promise an applicant that he or she will have every other weekend off and only a 25% rotation to nights if the opening is on a severely understaffed unit. If the reality of the situation means that the new employee is off only every third weekend and has a 75% night rotation, there is a good chance that the nurse, especially if he or she is highly competent, will resign. Management has the responsibility to represent the conditions of employment honestly. Covering up the gray areas never helps eliminate a shortage of personnel; such an approach perpetuates it. It is far more professional to represent the situation honestly and describe the steps that are being taken to improve it. The applicant will then be in a far better position to make an intelligent, informed decision about a job offer, if one is made.

Expectancy theory suggests that applicants are motivated to apply for those jobs that they believe are attainable and that offer a package of rewards that they find attractive. This knowledge does not help pinpoint precisely the factors that influence beliefs and perceptions on the part of the applicant or the role that recruiting practices play in shaping them. However, it *is* known that job seekers are influenced by the tone of the communications they receive from the organization. Therefore, attention must be given to both the medium used and the message it conveys.

The medium is the method of contact the organization uses to attract potential applicants. Obviously, the medium used should be the one that provides the widest exposure at a realistic price. Unfortunately, most of the media that meet both of these conditions also tend to be inefficient and low in credibility. The more influential methods tend to be the more personal ones (e.g., referral by present employees and identification through professional recruiters). Employees who refer a friend for a position usually enjoy a high level of credibility with the applicant and they usually to communicate far more information about the organization and the job than do other media. The referral process is almost always the most effective means of selling the organization.

Developing an effective recruiting message is often difficult. Although the initial tendency might be to sugarcoat the message or make the position or organization appear more attractive than it actually is, that approach is not considered professional, nor is it in the organization's best interest. Professional nurse managers insist on presenting a balanced message, one that includes honest communication supplemented by personal contact.

Although the nurse recruiters and the organization's human resources department are primarily responsible for recruiting, nurse managers play an important role in the recruiting process. Recruiting is made easier when nurse managers work to create a positive, nurturing atmosphere in their units so that current employees can spread a positive recruiting message, which reduces the need for expensive advertising and reward-based referral. As noted earlier, high-quality management in the operating nursing unit is by far the organization's most effective recruiting tool.

As noted earlier, recruitment is the process used to generate a pool of applicants from whom selections for employment can be made. The primary purpose of any selection procedure is to compare an applicant's abilities and motivation with the requirements and rewards of the job so that the best possible selection can be made. To the extent that these matches are made effectively, positive outcomes such as high job satisfaction and high-quality performance will result.

INTERVIEWING

Many selection methods are available in today's modern nursing environment. However, the most common method used by nurse managers continues to be the personal interview. This is a process of information exchange between the individual applying for a position (applicant) and the manager responsible for the actual hiring (interviewer). Initial screening is usually conducted by the human resources department to ensure that each applicant meets the criteria for education and experience established for the job before an interview is scheduled. If

an interview is granted, it will typically involve a distinct process for each participant, as follows:

The interviewer is representing the organization and has the responsibility to evaluate information gathered from the application form and elicit additional information that may be needed to make a hiring determination. If performance tests were given earlier in the screening process, the interviewer may discuss them during the interview.

The applicant is representing himself or herself and is focused primarily on gathering information about the job, the working environment, performance expectations, and the institution in general.

Nursing supervisors and nurse managers are the individuals most frequently chosen to conduct employment interviews with applicants for staff nursing positions. This responsibility has been delegated to nursing management because human resources personnel typically lack the technical expertise necessary to conduct an interview effectively. Historically, when human resources personnel have attempted to conduct these employment interviews, mistakes have been made because the human resources staff are almost always unfamiliar with specific job dimensions in the nursing field.

The purposes of the interview are the following:

- To obtain sufficient information regarding the applicant to determine whether he or she is suitable for employment for the particular job under consideration. This includes ensuring that each applicant meets the employment standards of the organization.

- To provide the applicant with information about the organization as a whole, the job specifically, and the people employed so that an informed decision can be made by any applicant offered the position.

- To create goodwill between the organization offering the position and the applicant seeking it. Goodwill is generated by the manner in which the interview is conducted and by the professionalism shown by the applicant.

To become effective interviewers, nurse managers must learn to solicit information efficiently so that relevant data can be gathered. Interviews vary in length, sometimes greatly, and, as shown in Table 13-2, generally include an opening, an information-gathering period, and a closing. The opening is important because this is when the applicant is put at ease and rapport is established. Relaxing the applicant will help ensure that the interviewer obtains the information being sought. The information-gathering portion is the core of the interview, because it is here that the

TABLE 13-2

Time Schedule for the Interview

Scheduling time during an interview is at best a subjective process. However, nurse managers must establish some parameters before entering the interview. If nothing more, this step will provide a checklist to ensure that no portion of the interview is inadvertently omitted.

Event	Purpose	Time Allotted
Opening	Break the ice so that applicant will relax	7 minutes
Outlining of process to be followed	Indicate how the interview will proceed	3 minutes
Identification of applicant's interests	Gather personal information	5 minutes
Review of educational history	Establish applicant's qualifications	20 minutes
Discussion of prior performance history	Learn about the applicant's experiences	20 minutes
Discussion of future plans	Identify future goals	10 minutes
Provision of information about the job and organization	Provide information that applicant can use to make an intelligent decision if the position is offered	20 minutes
Question and answer session	Gather and provide additional information	5 minutes
Effective closing	Wrap up on a positive note and provide the applicant with a positive perception of the organization	5 minutes

interviewer collects the information needed to determine the applicant's suitability for the job. During the last step of the information exchange, the interviewer provides information to the applicant. This step is important, because during this period realistic expectations are relayed to the applicant and the interviewer sells the organization as a good place to work. Experienced interviewers keep the interview elements arranged in this order so that both the organization's needs and those of the applicant can be presented thoroughly.

Principles for Effective Interviewing

ADVANCE PLANNING

Before an interview is scheduled, the interviewer should examine a blank application form and identify the specific job requirements. Next, it is a good idea to outline the specific areas that will be covered in the interview and then develop pertinent questions that will provide information about the applicant. The interviewer will want to collect information that measures the applicant against the requirements of the job and the standards of the organization. It is best to conduct interviews in an environment that will be free from interruptions.

Because the personal characteristics of the interviewer, both as an individual and as a representative of the hospital, may influence the applicant's decision, it is imperative that nurse managers prepare themselves for each interview. They should be especially concerned with areas that create first impressions, such as tone of voice, eye contact, appearance, grooming, posture, and gestures. Nurse managers should make sure that professionalism and a positive bearing is maintained throughout the interview and should ensure that each applicant is provided with a positive last impression of the organization. It is this final part of the interview that the applicant will most readily remember when he or she thinks of the experience.

RESPONDING TO THE APPLICANT

Nurse managers must remember that the interview is building an impression of the organization in the applicant. Interviewers are responsible for projecting a professional and concerned attitude. It is recommended that nurse managers express concern for the applicant's feelings as often as possible without losing control of the interview. They should respond in a positive and confident voice to the applicant's comments, questions, and nonverbal behaviors, and if they do not know the answer to a question, they should not say anything that cannot later be regarded as fact. Instead, nurse managers should let the applicant know that they don't have the requested information but will provide it to the applicant at a later date. Nurse managers must create the perception that they are genuinely interested in each applicant, and that is best accomplished by ensuring that an atmosphere of warmth and trust is established through the effective use of encouragement and positive statements throughout the interview.

ELICITING INFORMATION

Open-ended questions (ones that cannot be answered with a one-word response) should be used to elicit pertinent information. Every incomplete answer given and any problem area identified should be carefully probed without endangering the atmosphere of trust. The interview should be structured so that there is time to explore the answers provided to questions posed by both the interviewer and the applicant.

PROVIDING INFORMATION

Appropriate and accurate information should be communicated about the hospital and available jobs for which the applicant might qualify or in which the applicant has expressed an interest. All of the applicant's questions should be answered truthfully without prejudice or animosity. The interviewer must never lose control during an interview process. The interviewer should not tell the applicant about his or her personal problems.

EVALUATING INFORMATION

The information gathered in the interview should be integrated and analyzed so that it can be compared to the information gathered in other interviews. All personal characteristics of the applicant should be compared with the job requirements.

Staying Within the Law

The Equal Employment Opportunity Act, codified in Title 42 of the U.S. Code, was passed in 1972. The court actions that have followed the enactment of this law have caused the following two indelible changes in the hiring process:

1. Organizations have been increasingly careful to use predictors and interviewing techniques that can be shown not to be discriminatory (i.e., that can stand up in a court of law).
2. Organizations have reduced the use of proficiency tests that either implicitly or explicitly show any form of built-in bias. Instead, they are relying heavily on the interview as a selection device. It should be remembered, however, that Title VII of the Civil Rights Act of 1964, which will be discussed more extensively in relation to hiring later in the chapter, applies to interviews as much as it does to tests.

Since the late 1970s many interviewers have become annoyed with what they perceive as the restrictions imposed by equal employment opportunity (EEO) legislation, but the employment act does not, and never has, restricted any employer from asking about or measuring job-related characteristics.

The legislation simply says that it is illegal to make an employment decision based on a person's race, color, sex, religion, national origin, or any other characteristic that might be added by a specific state law. Table 13-3 presents sample employment inquiries that are considered to be appropriate and inappropriate for interviews.[5] The basic rule of thumb in interviewing today is, if any doubt exists about the legality of an interview question, don't use it. If an interview is called into question, the interviewer will have to prove that only job-related questions were asked and that EEO law was not violated. To consider EEO law as a deterrent to professional conduct is a huge mistake. In fact, nurse managers must view EEO regulations as having a positive influence on the working environment at all times. The best way to understand this is to consider what possible relevance sex or race, for instance, has to job performance. If the objective is to identify the best person for employment in the nursing unit, and specifically for a particular job within that unit, EEO legislation is never restrictive.

Preparing for the Interview

Effective preparation for the interview is one of the most important elements of the interview process; however, very few nurse managers adequately prepare themselves. Yet it has been proven over and over again that far less time is required to prepare for an interview than will be squandered in an interview that is not conducted properly. Moreover, beyond the time that might be lost in the interview itself is the far more critical matter of the time that might be spent later trying to correct the performance of a poorly selected employee.

Before the meeting, the interviewer should carefully review the job requirements, the application, and the applicant's résumé. Using these as guidelines, the nurse manager should write down specific questions that will be asked of all applicants to be interviewed, devise a method of tracing responses to those questions, and prepare the interview setting. The closer nurse managers can arrange their planning process to the actual interview, the greater opportunity they will have to enhance the process. Planning ahead will give the nurse manager time to relax and unwind from the pressures and distractions of the job before moving into the interview room, instead of rushing to complete last-minute details concerning the interview. Proper planning will also allow sufficient time between interviews to ensure that the interviewer displays his or her best professional demeanor when interacting with each applicant.

If the nurse manager does not prepare adequately, the result may be a lack of sufficient time to conduct

TABLE 13-3

Solicitation of Preemployment Information

Component	Appropriate Information to Request	Inappropriate Information to Request
Name	1. Applicant's full name 2. Whether applicant has ever worked or undertaken education under a different name	1. Maiden name of married woman 2. Change of name or original name of an applicant whose name has been legally changed
Residence	Place and length of residency and previous addresses	Whether applicant owns home, rents, boards, or lives with parents
Age	Whether applicant is over the legal age of employment	1. Date of birth or age 2. Age specifications or limitations that may bar an applicant who is over or under a specified age
Birthplace or national origin	None	Any question about place of birth of applicant or applicant's parents, grandparents, or spouse
Race or color	None	1. Applicant's race 2. Color of applicant's skin, eyes, hair, distinguishing physical characteristics, scars, or markings
Sex and marital status	None	1. Sex or marital status or any question that could be used to determine same 2. Number of dependents or children 3. Spouse's occupation
Creed or religion	Unions or professional organizations of which applicant is a member, as long as request does not violate the National Labor Relations Act	1. Applicant's religious affiliation 2. Church, parish, or religious holidays observed by applicant
National origin or ancestry	None	Applicant's lineage, ancestry, national origin, descent, parentage, or nationality
Disabilities	Whether applicant has a disability that would prevent him or her from satisfactorily performing the job	Whether applicant has any physical or mental disability or has contracted acquired immunodeficiency syndrome
Photograph	None	1. Photograph with application 2. Photograph after interview but before hiring
Language	Language(s) applicant speaks fluently	1. Applicant's mother tongue 2. Language used at home 3. How applicant acquired the ability to read, write, or speak a language
Relatives	Name, address, and relationship of a person to notify in case of emergency	1. Name and address of any relative 2. Name and address of a spouse or dependent children
Military service	1. Information regarding services rendered while applicant was a member of the armed forces, rank applicant attained, and branch of service in which applicant was involved 2. Whether applicant has received a draft notice	Information regarding service in any armed forces outside the United States
References	Names of persons willing to provide professional and/or character references for applicant	Name of applicant's religious leader or pastor
Arrests and convictions	Convictions that bear a relationship to the job and that have not been expunged or sealed by a court	Number and kinds of arrests
Height and weight	None	Height or weight of applicant, unless justified by business necessity

the interview properly, interruptions, or a failure to gather important information. Other problems associated with poor planning include losing control of the interview because of a desire to be courteous or because a particularly dominant interviewee is encountered and continuing the interview past the point at which a positive impression can be left.

Where to hold the interview is very important. To provide a relaxed, informal atmosphere, a neutral setting away from the demands of the nurse manager's office should be chosen. Both the nurse manager and the applicant should be seated in comfortable chairs and as close together as comfortably possible. If possible, the interview room should not include a table or desk that can put a physical obstacle between them. If an office must be used, the interviewer should arrange the chairs so that the applicant is either on the same side of the desk or, at a minimum, alongside it. There should be complete freedom from distracting phone calls and other interruptions. The applicant should be seated so that he or she cannot look out a window, and the nurse manager should be positioned so as to discourage drop-in visitors.

A selection interview should be planned just like any other critical task in the nurse manager's job. All necessary materials should be on hand, and the interview site should be quiet and pleasant. If other personnel are scheduled to see the applicant, their interview times should be confirmed so that they will be available at the appropriate hour. If coffee or other refreshments are to be offered, advance arrangements need to be made.

Unstructured interviews should be avoided, because they tend to present problems that are difficult to deal with in a carefully orchestrated analysis (and in court). One of the most frequently observed results of a poorly planned interview is the interviewer's failure to ask the same questions of every candidate. If the manager does not ensure that identical questions are asked of every applicant, how can the manager possibly hope to compare the answers received in an analytical manner?

When any human skill or trait is evaluated, it is important to remember that there is no standard or definitive score that can be used as a basis for rating applicants. One can only compare people against other people and against the requirements established for a given job. To ensure that similar questions are asked of all applicants so that their responses can be effectively compared, it is recommended that the nurse manager conduct a structured interview, preferably one based on an interview guide. The notes made about the applicant can be written and retained on the same sheet. The interview guide can prove extremely

beneficial in supporting the job-related reasons for the hiring decision.

Developing a Structured Interview Guide

An interview guide is a written document containing questions, interviewer directions, and other pertinent information that enable the interviewer to follow the same process in each interview and gather the same basic information from each applicant. It is usually specific to a job or job category and may include such instructions as:

- Perform a job analysis to determine the specific tasks required by the job.
- Use the identified tasks to determine personal characteristics (skills, abilities, knowledge) required to satisfactorily perform the job requirements.
- Write interview questions and develop behavioral simulations to determine whether or not the applicant has the personal characteristics required. A behavioral simulation differs from a test in that it is designed to capture actual behavior, not what individuals say they would do. A behavioral simulation is composed of exercises that are designed to elicit specific behavior by placing the person in a controlled situation similar to the job. Examples are typing tests and work-related tasks such as administering medications. To be legal, simulations must meet the following five requirements:
  1. They must be administered in a standardized way.
  2. They must be administered to all applicants reaching the same level of the selection process.
  3. They must require skills that cannot be provided through training.
  4. They must be job related.
  5. They must provide the applicant with appropriate time for preparation.

To help nurse managers develop an effective interview guide, the following tools are provided:

- Fig. 13-3 shows the process used to identify tasks, define required personal characteristics, and devise questions for the interview guide.
- Fig. 13-4 provides a sample format for an interview guide. This figure can be used to construct individualized interview guides, but managers should not copy the questions verbatim. Instead, they should develop their own questions based on the specific categories relevant to the job description of the open position.
- Box 13-1 (p. 261) provides examples of job-related scenarios that might be used when

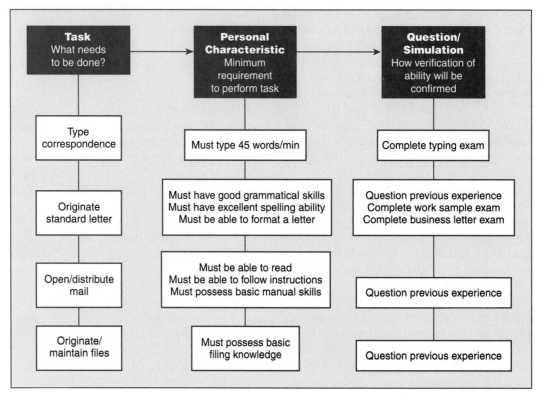

Fig. 13-3 ■ Example of the process used to identify tasks, personal characteristics, and questions to guide an interview.

interviewing an applicant for a position on an oncology unit. These scenarios would be included in the section of the interview guide labeled "Performance-Related Situation."

■ Box 13-2 (p. 262) is an example of the type of information that would be presented during an interview as part of a realistic description of the job environment.

The use of interview guides reduces interviewer bias; provides standardized, relevant, and effective questions; and reduces the potential for leading questions. It also ensures the creation of a database that allows realistic comparison of all applicants. Space left between the questions on the guide provides room for note taking. Finally, and possibly most important of all, the guide provides a written record of the interview.

Nurse managers must learn how to develop questions that elicit information about the skill level, experience, and knowledge of an applicant. It is far easier to design the interview to detect excellence or the lack of it before hiring than to terminate a non-performing employee. Fig. 13-4 provides examples of questions that might be used to ascertain the quality of an employment applicant. Although it is constructed primarily to identify experience levels in an

oncology unit, these questions can easily be adapted to fit almost any work situation.

Conducting the Interview

The nurse manager conducting an interview should make sure that he or she is available and ready to start at the agreed-upon time. The manager should greet the applicant warmly and clearly, and introduce himself or herself. It is strongly recommended that the nurse manager ask the applicant his or her name and if there is a nickname that the applicant prefers to be used. The manager should try to minimize his or her status and position on the management team and should try not to patronize or dominate the conversation. As was stated earlier, it is recommended that the nurse manager not hide behind his or her desk but move the interview to a neutral location; the objective is to create an open atmosphere so that applicants will relax and reveal as much about themselves as possible.

The importance of establishing a good rapport and maintaining it throughout the interview cannot be overstressed. The interviewing process intimidates almost every applicant; therefore, every effort must be made to relax the hopeful individual. In addition,

Format for an Interview Guide

Instructions

1. Note applicant's response to each question used during the interview.

2. After the interview has been completed, immediately record reactions to the response given by the applicant to each question.

3. When interviewing, ask only appropriate questions; for example, education questions might not be appropriate for an applicant who has not attended school in the past 10 years but who has extensive experience in the field.

Complete the Following Information on Each Applicant

Applicant's name: _____

Interviewer's name: _____ Interviewer's position: _____

Date of interview: _____ Position interviewed for: _____

Did interviewer review the actual application form?   ☐ Yes   ☐ No

If so, what were the items of major interest on the application?

_____

_____

_____

Relax the Applicant — Begin the Interview with Small Talk to Establish Rapport

Things for the interviewer to perform/remember:

   ☐ Provide a positive greeting—use a warm and friendly voice, and smile genuinely

   ☐ Use the applicant's name—pronounce it correctly

   ☐ Provide your name—first and last (titles are not normally effective at this point)

   ☐ Establish rapport by taking the time to engage applicant in small talk

Outline the Topics of Discussion for Interview

   ☐ Education level

   ☐ Experience and work history

   ☐ Preview of the job being applied for

   ☐ Miscellaneous topics

Applicant's Education

   ☐ Highest level of education completed: _____

   ☐ Graduation year: _____ Major: _____

   ☐ What courses interested you the most? _____

   ☐ Which courses did you find to be least important? _____

Fig. 13-4 ■ Sample format for an interview guide.

Continued

☐ Were you involved in extracurricular activity?   ☐ Yes   ☐ No

Did the activity pertain to your major?   ☐ Yes   ☐ No

Which activity did you enjoy the most? _____

☐ What nursing school did you attend? _____

☐ Did you graduate?   ☐ Yes   ☐ No   If so, what year? _____

☐ Did you complete additional college work after graduation?   ☐ Yes   ☐ No

If so, what postgraduate work did you do? _____

_____

_____

☐ Did you receive any additional or advanced degrees?   ☐ Yes   ☐ No   If so, what are they? _____

_____

_____

☐ If you could begin your education over, what changes would you make? _____

_____

_____

☐ What are your best memories of your school years? _____

_____

_____

Applicant's Experience and Employment History

☐ What was your last job, or what is your current one? _____

_____

☐ What are/were your primary duties? _____

_____

☐ What types of decisions did/do you routinely make? _____

_____

_____

☐ What do you enjoy the most about your current/last job? _____

_____

_____

☐ What did/do you enjoy the least? _____

_____

_____

☐ At which aspects of your work did you excel? _____

_____

_____

Fig. 13-4—cont'd ■ Sample format for an interview guide.

☐ What areas do you feel you were/are weak in and need to improve? _____
_____
_____

☐ Is there anything about your present/last job you would like to see changed? _____
_____
_____

☐ Why are you leaving/why did you leave your current/last job? _____
_____
_____

☐ What do you see as important in a job? _____
_____
_____

☐ What type of supervisor do you prefer working for? _____
_____
_____

Personal Evaluation

☐ What do you feel are the most important changes you have made in the last 5 years? _____
_____
_____

☐ What do you see yourself doing in the next 10 years? _____
_____
_____

☐ What do you think you can improve about yourself that will help you get to your goal faster? _____
_____
_____

☐ What do you like to do with your off-work time? _____
_____
_____

☐ What do you consider your strongest asset? _____
_____
_____

☐ What do you feel are your other assets? _____
_____
_____

☐ What have you done in your life that you are most proud of? _____
_____
_____

Fig. 13-4—cont'd ■ Sample format for an interview guide.

Continued

☐ Why do you think you will do a good job in this position? _____

_____

_____

Performance-Related Situation

☐ Tell me how you would handle this situation. (Interviewer to put situation here.) _____

_____

_____

Response: _____

_____

_____

Shift Preference

☐ What shift do you prefer?   ☐ Day   ☐ Afternoon   ☐ Night

☐ Will you agree to work a rotating shift?   ☐ Yes   ☐ No

☐ Will you work a night/weekend rotation?   ☐ Yes   ☐ No

Overview of Open Position and Organization

☐ Organizational structure (Human Resources)

☐ Unit structure

☐ Duties involved in open position

☐ Performance standards of the organization and the unit

☐ Available shift   ☐ Days   ☐ Day/evening   ☐ Evenings   ☐ Nights

☐ General discussion of nursing care and unit expectations/goals and objectives

☐ Tour of unit (time permitting)

Closing

☐ Are there any questions that I can answer for you?   ☐ Yes   ☐ No

_____

_____

☐ Date available to start: _____

☐ Follow-up date: _____

☐ Express appreciation for time and close with a thank you

Fig. 13-4—cont'd ■ Sample format for an interview guide.

the applicant is meeting with an individual who has sufficient authority to determine the next step in his or her future, and thus the applicant has a good reason to be hesitant to talk and share. The professional nurse manager eliminates this hesitancy by talking about himself or herself in low and unassuming tones, by sharing neutral and mutual interests such as hobbies or sports, and by using good body language and nonverbal techniques such as maintaining eye contact and sitting up straight in the chair.

When the interviewer feels that the applicant has started to relax, it is time to take the interview forward. One good way to start off in a positive direction is to outline what will be discussed and establish the time frame for the interview.

During the interview, the nurse manager must be careful not to form hasty first impressions of the applicant and should avoid, under any circumstances, making an equally hurried decision. Most people are influenced by their first impressions of an applicant;

BOX 13-1

Developing Job-Related Questions

Instructions: Describe how you would interview and what you would do in the following scenarios.

CASE 1
A patient who has been admitted with a diagnosis of lymphoma is going to begin chemotherapy and you are preparing to administer the first dose. When you enter the room, the patient says, "You know, I just can't believe I have cancer. I realize that is what the doctor says, but I just can't believe it."
Response: _____
_____

CASE 2
The spouse of a patient has overheard some of the doctors who are caring for her husband say that he has received the incorrect dose of chemotherapy. You are the nurse charged with this patient's care.
Response: _____
_____

CASE 3
A young adult has been diagnosed with acute leukemia and often expresses his anger and frustration in the presence of his wife. You have witnessed his frequent outbursts and have become aware of the increasing level of hopelessness that he and his wife are experiencing.
Response: _____

CASE 4
"No code" orders have been posted for a patient who has lung cancer. On the night shift, the patient develops dyspnea, becomes uncomfortable and anxious, and screams out periodically. The patient is receiving 100% oxygen, but the spouse insists that something more be done.
Response: _____
_____

CASE 5
A physician making rounds notices a discrepancy in your patient's intake and output. The weights indicate that the patient has gained 10 lb, but there is no documentation in the record to account for this substantial change.
Response: _____
_____

CASE 6
You are on the night shift and are caring for an extremely ill patient who is receiving platelets and antibiotic therapy. The patient's blood pressure is continuing to drop, and you have discussed the situation with the resident on call twice by telephone. His orders were to continue the current treatment. The patient's condition continues to decline. What would you do?
Response: _____
_____

---

for example, if the applicant has a limp, sweaty handshake, an impression can be made before a word is uttered. Judgments based on first impressions often lead to poor decisions and can easily work against the purpose of the interview (i.e., information collection). This "coloring" of the issue occurs because a nurse manager who works with first impressions also tends to search for information that justifies these impressions, both good and bad. If a manager makes an employment decision based on a first impression, one of the following three things will happen:

1. *He or she will hire the right person:* This is not likely if the decision is based only on the first impression but is certainly a possibility. As the saying goes, it's better to be lucky than good.
2. *He or she will lose a potentially good employee:* If the first impression is negative and the interviewer does not hire the applicant based on it, then the organization will lose a potentially good employee. This is much more serious in an extremely critical labor market, when good people may be hard to find.

3. *He or she will hire the wrong person:* This is certainly the worst of all outcomes, because this one just doesn't go away. Once the wrong person is hired, removal from the job can be extremely difficult and expensive, and can involve litigation. This problem can plague a nursing unit for long periods and can lead to severe difficulties.

SOLICITING INFORMATION

Instead of relying on impressions, the nurse manager should use a structured interview guide, ask pertinent questions, and take copious notes. The nurse manager should ask the applicant for permission to take notes and explain that these will be used as a recall aid and a means to fairly compare all applicants. There are two basic types of questions: (1) open ended and (2) closed ended. An open-ended question is one that requires a substantive answer from the applicant and cannot be answered with a simple yes or no. Such questions are generally used to elicit information about the applicant. Closed-ended questions are those that can be answered with yes, no, or another one-word answer.

Preview Information for Staff Nurse: Anders Burn Unit

The information shown here is intended to be shared with every applicant interviewed for a position as a staff nurse in the Anders Burn Unit at Good Saints Hospital. The information should be shared by a qualified manager of the Anders Burn Unit or senior hospital administrator with knowledge of the unit.

THE NEGATIVE REALITIES OF EMPLOYMENT

There is a down side to employment in the Anders Burn Unit. This critical information should always be presented in an honest, straightforward manner and must not be omitted from any employment interview.

1. Patients, because of the nature of their injuries, are often difficult cases.
2. The unit cares for patients of all ages; elderly and young children are mixed.
3. Each nurse must be able to cope with the psychologic effects on the patient of being burned; this can be especially difficult with children and their parents.
4. The work is emotionally demanding and can be extremely stressful.
5. To be successful, the assigned nurses must perform physically demanding work.

THE POSITIVE ASPECTS OF EMPLOYMENT

The following are some of the positive aspects of employment in the Anders Burn Unit. The information should always be delivered in an honest, straightforward manner and should not be substituted for or presented as compensation for the negative aspects of service in the unit.

1. There is extensive opportunity for the provision of high-quality bedside nursing.
2. Anders is a learning environment.
3. All employees are able to assist with important research.
4. Anders is a small unit with a close-knit and extremely professional staff.
5. Work is performed with both critical and recovering patients.
6. There is a great deal of opportunity to render important decisions in an unsupervised arena.
7. The Anders unit is staffed entirely with the top professionals in burn treatment.
8. The opportunity exists to work with children as well as adults.
9. A large variety of problems (burns and other existing difficulties) are encountered.
10. Patients are physically present for long periods of time, so there is extensive patient and family teaching.

Closed-ended questions (what, where, why, when, how many, etc.) should be used only to elicit specific information when probing. Regardless of which type of question is used, the interviewer should ask questions with a little flare. This means that the interviewer should not fire off questions in rapid succession; instead, the interviewer should allow the applicant a reasonable period of time to formulate his or her response and should always behave as if he or she is interested in the content of the answer. Questions have a tendency to disarm the applicant and they often make people feel vulnerable, so the nurse manager should proceed carefully but deliberately and never be afraid to ask tough questions.

It is highly recommended that the nurse manager use as many work situation–style questions as possible during the interview. Such questions are used to determine the applicant's knowledge of work tasks and ability to perform the work by hypothetically placing the applicant into a real-life situation that can be addressed properly only by someone familiar with the duties of the job. It is easy to ask a nurse if he or she knows how to draw blood. The applicant may say yes, but this doesn't necessarily prove the ability. Instead, it might be more informative to ask the applicant to describe the procedure. Another method would be to ask some very specific questions about drawing blood that only a nurse familiar with the procedure could answer.

Leading questions should be avoided because the "correct" answer is implied in the question (e.g., "The nurses on this unit work a lot of overtime. Do you mind working overtime?") An applicant who wants the job would be a fool to respond with an answer like, "I hate overtime." Although applicants for nursing positions may later prove to be many different things, it is rare to find one who is stupid.

The interviewer may also want to summarize what has been said, use silence to elicit more information, reflect back the applicant's feelings to clarify an issue, or indicate acceptance by urging the applicant to continue.

PROVIDING INFORMATION

An important part of the interview is the provision of information about the job, the unit, and the hospital. This is the interviewer's responsibility, and this presentation should always demonstrate the following three characteristics:

1. *Honesty:* The manager should never tell an applicant something that is not true and verifiable. If that person is eventually hired, the person will certainly find out that the manager was less than forthcoming and this will have a negative effect on future relations between management and labor.

2. *Comprehensiveness:* The manager should tell the whole truth, not just the highlights. No one should spend excessive amounts of time boring the daylights out of an applicant, but the manager should provide enough information to allow the applicant to make an informed decision once the job is offered.

3. *Professionalism:* The manager must never use the interview as a place to grind his or her axe. If a manager must talk about an individual who is not part of the interview, he or she should keep the responses positive and, at all costs, avoid being drawn into a negative "he said, she said" situation. Remember, the nurse manager is a representative of the organization. The manager must fulfill this responsibility by speaking positively or not speaking at all. The manager should never bad-mouth the organization during an interview; it makes both manager and organization look bad.

The nurse manager should decide in advance what kind of information will be provided to the applicant. If the nurse manager fails to present realistic information about the job, both negative and positive, the applicant may accept employment with unrealistic expectations. It has been proven over and over again that it is these early misunderstandings that create dissatisfaction and, ultimately, increases in job turnover and decreases in unit productivity.

Before this part of the interview is reached, the nurse manager should have already formed an initial opinion of the applicant. If the candidate seems promising enough to warrant time's being spent in providing detailed information about the job, then this should be done. If not, then it should not be done. If the manager's earlier questions have revealed that the individual lacks the experience to discharge the fundamental duties of the position, then the manager will simply be wasting his or her time by continuing the interview. The nurse manager should know what information he is is responsible for delivering and what is best provided by others. Human resources personnel usually answer specific questions about benefits or compensation; however, a direct question should not be avoided, and ignorance should never be feigned. If the nurse manager doesn't know the answer, he or she should say so. This is not a time to provide false or misleading information. State and federal regulations must not be violated by relating information about which the interviewer is unsure.

CLOSING

In closing the interview, it is imperative that the nurse manager not present any information regarding the possibility for selection or make a misleading statement that could be wrongly interpreted as a job offer. It is a good idea for the nurse manager to go over the positive points that were developed during the interview and let the applicant know that someone will be following up. The applicant should be given the opportunity to ask any last-minute questions, and the session should be ended on a positive note. It is recommended that the nurse manager walk the applicant out of the building, or at least to the elevator, and, before departing, express appreciation for the applicant's time and willingness to sit through the interview. Remember that it is the last 15 seconds spent with the applicant that will provide the impression of the organization the applicant takes home. Last impressions, unlike first impressions, are critical to the retention of a positive perception.

After the nurse manager has thanked the applicant, the manager should return to the interview room and complete any notes that were begun during the interview.

MAKING THE DECISION TO HIRE

The time the nurse manager takes to make the hiring decision is critical to the selection process; therefore, this time should be spent productively. The manager should keep in mind that the nurse manager's job is to obtain maximum performance from employees and ensure a high level of service quality throughout the nursing unit. This cannot be accomplished if the wrong people are hired to perform the work. The manager must hire professionally by eliminating bias, favoritism, and prejudices from the decision process. Only the best of the best should be hired for the unit, not the best of those who show up for an interview. If no one was interviewed who meets the job requirements or the standards of the unit, no one should be hired. The manager should go back to the human resources department and ask that more applicants be found. The manager should remember that it is extremely difficult to undo a wrong hiring decision. Consider the following story:

Several years ago, as I was finishing my first year as a nurse manager in a large Midwestern hospital, I hired a nurse to fill a position on the day shift. The woman had seemed bright, eager, and very professional in the interview with only minor shortcomings, but I felt I could deal with those and that she would be an excellent performer once she saw what we expected.

Boy, was I wrong. On the second day after her probation was over, the staff started noticing her being absent from the unit, and some of her assignments were not completed. After I discussed these shortcomings with her, she withdrew from the rest of the team, and her performance barely met minimum expectations.

One day, out of frustration and after cleaning up an assignment our wayward nurse had botched, I asked one of the other staff nurses, "Do you suppose this will ever get better?"

The nurse, a longtime associate and trusted professional, looked me in the eye and said, "Don't ever let me hear you complain about her again. She wouldn't be here if you hadn't hired her."

When a manager is hiring, the manager should act as if his or her professional reputation is on the line, because it is. The manager is the one who lets the new hire become part of the unit, and the manager should be very sure that this person is the one who will give the manager what he or she needs. It is far easier to pick up the slack caused by an open position than to undo mistakes made by a bad hire. The person coming in the door has the potential to complement or to disrupt the team, and it is always the nurse manager who bears the responsibility of ensuring that the proper person is hired.

Spending time selecting is always preferable to spending time coaching, disciplining, and evaluating a poor performer.

Interview Reliability and Validity

Over the past two decades, numerous research studies have investigated the reliability and validity of employment interviews. Using extremely wide parameters, these studies have shown that, in general, *intra*rater reliability (reliability of multiple interviews by the same individual) is fairly high, *inter*rater reliability (reliability across different interviewers) is rather low, and the validity of the typical interview is very low. The data gathered by these research studies have also shown the following:

- Well-structured interviews are consistently more reliable and valid than those that are not.
- Interviewers who are under pressure to hire in a short period of time or meet a recruitment quota are less accurate than other interviewers.
- Interviewers who have detailed information about the job for which they are interviewing exhibit higher reliability. However, the interviewer's personal experience does not seem to be related to reliability and validity.
- There is a significant tendency among interviewers to make quick decisions that result in lower accuracy.
- Interviewers develop stereotypes of ideal applicants against which interviewees are evaluated, and many aspects of the stereotype are interviewer specific, a fact that acts to decrease the reliability of the hire and the validity of the process.

- Race and sex have been found to significantly influence interviewers' evaluations (even though consideration of these characteristics in making employment decisions violates federal law).

Possibly the biggest single weakness of the interview process is the interviewer's tendency to attempt an assessment of an applicant's "basic character" during the short time the interviewer spends with the interviewee.[6] Subjective judgments are frequently made regarding an applicant's personality characteristics as well as his or her knowledge and skill levels. To entirely eliminate this type of prejudice from the interviewing process is extremely difficult, if not impossible. Nevertheless, it is disturbing that many evaluations are far more subjective than they need to be, especially when interviewers attempt to assess personality characteristics. This type of subjectivity should not be part of the interviewing process. In fact, the information sought during an interview should be limited to what is necessary to answer the following two fundamental questions:

1. *Will* the applicant perform the job?
2. *Can* the applicant perform the job?

The best predictor of the applicant's future behavior in these two areas is his or her past performance. When interviewing, the nurse manager should be concerned primarily with the applicant's previous work and nonwork experience, educational level and training, and current behavior. The nurse manager should avoid making assessments of personality characteristics, which even highly trained psychologists have difficulty measuring accurately.

Testing

A test is defined as any standardized procedure for obtaining information from individuals that is systematically administered to all applicants for a specific job. To comply with federal employment law, any instrument used as a test must be designed to gather only information pertaining to the abilities, skills, motivation, or knowledge necessary to perform a specific job or aspect of a job. Tests are routinely administered to assess such things as aptitude, personality and interest, and skill, and fall into the following broad categories:

- *Aptitude tests* measure those individual characteristics that are likely to lead to the acquisition of knowledge or skill; they therefore indicate what tasks the applicant might be able to perform in the future, given the opportunity and/or training. Aptitude tests are more accurate in predicting an individual's ability to complete training assignments than in predicting job performance. These tests are not generally considered an accurate employment predictor.

- *Personality and interest inventories* attempt to measure a person's motivation or personality characteristics, but they are not used to any great extent in employee selection. They are not typically considered accurate employment predictors.
- *Work sample tests* are quite literally samples or simulations of the work that the applicant will be expected to perform on the job. The underlying assumption of this type of examination is that an applicant's performance in doing a representative sample of the job will predict actual performance on the job. Work samples fall into the following groups:

    Behavioral: These tests require an applicant actually to perform behaviors involved in the job; a typing test is an excellent example of a behavioral test.

    Knowledge: These tests measure the knowledge required to do the job; an example is a medical terminology test for an applicant for the position of unit clerk.

Testing is usually conducted by the human resources department or the nursing service staff, and nurse managers seldom, if ever, become involved in it. Their exclusion is usually based on the following two factors:

1. The legal requirements associated with these kinds of selection instruments
2. The necessity to comply with policies for standardized administration

Education, Experience, and Physical Examinations

Educational and experience requirements for nurses have traditionally played an important role in staff selection in the healthcare industry. How well applicants meet these requirements is most frequently determined using criteria that substitute for work sample tests. The establishment of minimum educational standards is similar to a job knowledge sample because it tends to ensure that all applicants have at least a minimal amount of the necessary knowledge. Experience requirements are very much like behavioral samples because the inherent assumption is that a nurse with a given number of years of experience will have performed a certain number of required tasks.

References and letters of recommendation are other means used to assess an applicant's past job experience, but there is little hard evidence that these items have any real validity (very few people will write bad letters of recommendation), and when applicants are almost invariably described in positive terms, one really does not know their potential for success in the job. In those rare instances when candidates are described in negative terms, there is substantial reason to presume a potential for future problems. Typically, however, any criticism that is registered will be very mild and is generally apparent in what is *not* said rather than what *is* said. Letters that reflect any criticism should be treated as a significant warning.

In almost every hiring situation, the prospect fills out an application form that requests information regarding previous experience, education, and references. Most of these application forms also ask for the applicant's medical history and may even request specific personal data. The fact that the information is requested does not, however, guarantee the accuracy of the information provided. The obvious question is whether applicants will either intentionally or unintentionally distort their responses on an application form. Most studies of this subject have found that there is actually very little distortion, at least not of the easily verifiable information. Although it is generally accepted that applicants may embellish, rarely do they enter complete falsehoods on application blanks. Compared with other predictors used in the employment process, the application form may be one of the more valid; its validity parallels that of work sample exercises.

The preemployment physical examination serves a number of selection purposes. It screens out applicants who may have major physical or obvious mental impairments that would seriously impede successful job performance. It may also identify applicants who have chronic physical ailments that may lead to unfavorable attendance records or who may have excessive future claims against health insurance. The interpretation of the results of a physical examination should be left to the human resources department because of employment regulations and the potential for litigation associated with them. Also, great care should be taken not to violate the applicant's rights under the Americans with Disabilities Act.

Assessment Centers

In the past two decades, many organizations outside the healthcare industry have turned to assessment centers, or professional consulting firms, to identify personnel for specific jobs, especially supervisory and managerial personnel. This remains a relatively new and very isolated practice for healthcare institutions, however.

An assessment center is not necessarily a place. Instead, it can be, and generally is, a process used for identifying individual strengths and weaknesses for a specified purpose such as selection, promotion, or development.[7] Individuals engage in a series of exercises that have been constructed to simulate critical behaviors related to success on the job. Participation is both individual and group based. The assessment center method is particularly appealing to organizations because judgments are far more objective and are based in the applicant's overt behavior during the assessment, which parallels the exact behaviors required on the job. The likelihood of predicting future job performance is enhanced by the use of multiple assessment techniques, the standardization methods of making inferences, and the pooling of the judgments of multiple assessors.

Assessment centers have especially proven themselves in the evaluation of candidates who are being considered for jobs that are quite different from the ones they currently hold, such as promotion from a technical to an administrative position—performer to manager. Experience has taught that it is very difficult to evaluate how proficiently a staff nurse whose experience centers on clinical skills will perform when asked to focus on managerial behaviors, and therefore this type of promotion is often the most difficult to make. The fact that an individual is an excellent clinician does not prove that he or she will be an excellent manager. Many a hospital has lost a good clinical nurse only to inherit a poor manager because its senior management attempted to judge managerial ability by evaluating clinical performance. In this case, an assessment center is an appropriate method for evaluation because it has the capability to simulate managerial behaviors.

The essential elements of the assessment center process are as follows:

- The analysis of relevant job behaviors to determine the characteristics, skills, abilities, and knowledge that requires evaluation
- Identification of the techniques or exercises necessary to provide information that can be used in evaluating job-related characteristics, skills, and/or abilities
- The provision of multiple assessment techniques, at least one of which is a behavioral simulation
- Assessment along multiple dimensions that describe the skills, abilities, and knowledge required to do the job
- Use of multiple assessors (nursing service supervisors and directors) who receive comprehensive training that will prepare them to process information in a manner that is both fair and impartial
- Judgments resulting in a hiring or promotional decision, which are based on a pooling of the information from the different assessors and techniques and are made by consensus

Common evaluation tools used in assessment centers include interviews, organizational games, leaderless group discussion (staff meetings), presentations, role playing, and occasionally paper and pencil tests.

VALIDITY AND LEGALITY IN HIRING

The selection process should include the use of valid selection predictors. These are instruments (e.g., application forms, tests, interviews) that can be used to forecast an applicant's potential effectiveness as an employee on the job. The validity of a predictor should never be assumed but must be investigated scientifically (i.e., by statistically measuring the connection between the score on a given predictor and some measure of success on the job). This type of analysis will help the organization develop both the predictor and the measure of success. The use of valid predictors is not only desirable in choosing the best employee for a specific position but also satisfies many of the legal requirements that typically must be met. Staff activities have been subjected to considerable scrutiny with regard to discrimination and equal employment opportunity as a result of the passage of Title VII of the Civil Rights Act of 1964, the Equal Pay Act of 1963, and the Age Discrimination in Employment Act of 1967. In many instances, the use of valid predictors has provided justification for the hiring decisions that have been made.

Title VII of the Civil Rights Act specifically prohibits discrimination in any employment decision on the basis of race, color, sex, religion, or national origin. "Any employment decision" includes not only selection but also entrance into training programs, performance appraisal, termination, provision of benefits, and so on. Title VII is applicable to employers who have more than 15 employees, with a few exemptions. Business necessity and bona fide occupational qualification (BFOQ) are examples of two grounds for exemption.

An employer may discriminate on the basis of national origin, religion, sex, and age, for instance, if that discrimination can be shown to be a BFOQ or is necessary for the operation of a business. An example of a BFOQ is a gender requirement for a female role in a theatrical production.

Business necessity can be claimed in cases in which not discriminating would put the organization out of business. For instance, hospitals employ a very small proportion of male nurses and hence can be considered as "discriminating" against male nurses. However, because few male nurses are available in the job market, the high ratio of female nurses in the average hospital is actually a business necessity. Examples of claims generally not sufficient to prove a BFOQ or business necessity are assertions of "customer preference" or qualifications based on gross gender characterizations such as "women cannot lift over 30 pounds." BFOQ claims that have been supported include the refusal to hire women as correctional counselors at an all-male prison.

Title VII is a complaint-oriented law; that is, any person who feels that he or she has been discriminated against may file a complaint with the government against the employer. When a complaint is filed, the Equal Employment Opportunity Commission (EEOC) or the applicable state agency created to enforce the EEO law will send a notice to the employer and initiate an investigation of the complaint. The EEOC has broad investigative power and access to all relevant employment records and documents. If it finds there is reasonable cause to believe that illegal discrimination has taken place, it will notify the employer and attempt to settle the complaint through mediation. If this attempt fails, the EEOC or the individual who initiated the complaint may file a lawsuit against the company. Legal action can result in reinstatement, the issuance of up to 2 years of back pay for the suing party, and even, in the worst cases, criminal liability of the organization and individual managers in that organization.

When an individual files a complaint alleging discrimination in hiring practices, he or she needs only to prove unequal treatment or the hiring of fewer minority members than nonminority members (adverse impact). The burden of proof then shifts to the organization, which must demonstrate that its decision was not related to the individual's race, color, sex, religion, national origin, or other categories that state laws may add such as handicap or national ancestry. There are two possible methods of justifying hiring in response to a discrimination claim:

1. Indicate that the organization did not have the information on race, sex, and so forth in the first place and therefore could not have used it. This is a very difficult claim to make because most applicants are interviewed or are seen in a healthcare organization before the hiring decision is made.
2. Prove that the decision to hire or not hire was based on some job-relevant criterion and not on race, sex, color, religion, or national origin.

The EEOC is charged with enforcing and interpreting the Civil Rights Act and has issued Uniform Guidelines on Employee Selection Procedures. These guidelines specify the types of methods and information required to justify the job relevance of an employer's selection procedures. These guidelines will not be described in detail here; however, the methods

of selection discussed in this chapter do follow the specifications set forth in this document. Nurse managers must remember that the law *does not say* an organization cannot hire the best person for the job or that the organization must hire so many minority individuals. What is says is that race, color, sex, religion, and national origin must not be used as selection criteria. As long as the decision is not made on the basis of minority status, one is complying with U.S. EEO law. Canada and many other nations have developed their civil rights law so that they parallel U.S. law; however, these laws differ from country to country, and this topic is far too complex to cover in this text.

Validation refers to the procedure used to gather evidence that a predictor is truly job related. The outcome of a validation study is information indicating the degree to which the predictor is related to job success. The following are the two major types of validation study possible:

1. *Empirical validation* is the most rigorous, costly, and time consuming. In empirical validation studies, scores on both the predictor and the criterion measures are obtained from job applicants or employees. If employees are used, both predictor and criterion scores are obtained at the same time (concurrent validation). Empirical validation studies are almost always performed by the personnel office or by consultants because they are so complicated and require precise collection of data. Not only do nurse managers rarely become involved in such studies, few hospitals actually use them. Unless adverse impact—underutilization of a protected class—can be proven, the government will not scrutinize any part of the selection system. Therefore, if the number of minority members in a given job classification such as staff nurse or unit clerk is representative of the community at large, then there is no purely legal reason to do validation studies. However, content validation (because it is a logic-based approach) can always be ensured and should be used in most situations, regardless of whether or not a hospital believes that there may be adverse impact in given job categories.
2. *Content validation* is considerably easier because it is a logical rather than an empirical approach, but it may not always make the strongest case that a predictor is job related. Content validity is based on the logical argument that (a) the predictor is a representative sample of the tasks and duties required of a job incumbent, and (b) every measure used in the predictor is an actual part of the job. Content validation is most often used for work sample or job knowledge

predictors such as interviews, typing tests, and assessment center evaluations. For instance, a typing test used to select secretaries does not have content validity because a secretary does other things in addition to typing. However, it does have content validity for the job of clerk-typist. To ensure content validity, one simply has to take from a task list or job description of behaviors a relatively small but representative number of tasks for the applicant to perform during the selection process.

It is important that nursing services examine the validity of their selection procedures, even if the only procedure used is interviewing. Only then can they know if the selection of applicants is being accomplished effectively.

SUMMARY

- The selection of staff is a critical function that involves matching people to jobs. Responsibility for hiring is often shared with nurse managers.
- Selection methods most often include screening application forms, résumés, medical examinations, reference checks, and interviews but may also include tests and assessment center evaluations.
- Job analysis is the key to all selection because it defines the job. Selection procedures are designed to elicit information about applicants. Then people can be placed in positions for which they are suited.
- Recruitment is the process of locating and attracting enough qualified applicants to provide a pool from which the required number of new jobholders can be chosen. Poor-quality applicants and/or a small pool will result in less accurate matches between jobs and applicants.
- Selection interviewing is a complex skill and is intended to obtain information about the applicant and provide the applicant with information about the organization. Nurse managers, if they participate in selection, will be involved in interviewing candidates for jobs in their areas of responsibility.
- Principles for effective interviewing include the following: plan and structure the interview, respond to the applicant to encourage rapport, elicit information through questioning techniques, provide realistic job information, and analyze the information obtained to make a final placement decision.
- Developing a structured interview guide is critical in selection interviewing because it helps the interviewer stay on track and provides a mechanism for taking and storing notes about the applicant.
- Tests and assessment centers are complicated, standardized mechanisms for gathering application data that are sometimes used in selection. Nurse managers are not always involved when these selection techniques are used. Assessment centers are most often used in hiring managers.
- All selection systems must be job related. Job relatedness is confirmed by validation studies. If selection systems are job related, they will not discriminate on the basis of race, color, sex, religion, or national origin, which is a requirement of the Civil Rights Act of 1964.

FINAL THOUGHTS

The acquisition of qualified personnel is one of the most important tasks that nurse managers perform, because it is critical for the unit, the organization, and the quality of the care that is delivered to patients. Therefore, active participation in the recruitment process is important for all nurse managers.

Recruiting is where the success of the organization actually begins. If this function is successful in locating and attracting highly qualified, dynamic individuals to join the organization, then many of the problems that traditionally beset most healthcare organizations (e.g., absenteeism and turnover) can be avoided or at least sharply reduced.

The best form of recruitment occurs when a current employee refers an individual to the organization. Because there is personal risk in recommending anyone to the organization, most highly skilled and professional individuals will not do so unless they are confident that the applicant will be an excellent employee. No one wants to be the person who recommended the unit lemon for a job. If a trusted and professional employee comes forward with a recommendation for an open position, the nurse manager must pay close attention. The same close attention should be paid if a marginal employee recommends an associate. Remember that birds of a feather *do* flock together.

Nurse managers must be very careful, however, about hiring friends and relatives into the workforce. This practice often fosters relationships that are difficult to manage and may even violate equal opportunity hiring requirements.

The employment process is a highly regulated part of the nurse manager's job. There are many state and federal regulations that must be observed during the process. These laws cover everything from equal employment opportunity to discrimination and the rights of the handicapped. These regulations are very stringent, and compliance is required by nearly every organization that employs more than 15 people. There is no room for ignorance in the compliance requirements of these laws, and ignorance is never an acceptable excuse for violating an applicant's rights; neither is lack of intent to discriminate. Although it may not be an employer's intention to violate the law, if this should occur, then the law is clear: a violation is a violation, regardless of the circumstance.

The legal ramifications of poor hiring practices can be severe for both nurse managers and the organizations for which they work. Make sure you are familiar with what you can and can't do before entering into the employment process. Hire carefully, hire objectively, and hire quality. It is easier to hire intelligently than to fire a poor performer.

THE NURSE MANAGER SPEAKS

The employment process shifts into high gear the moment the new hire reports to work on the first day. If it is the intent of the nurse manager to retain the highly qualified and professional individual that he or she has just hired, then some important things must be done on employment day 1.

The first thing that needs to be accomplished on the first day—and, according to many people, the most important thing—is to make the new hire feel welcome and important. This is critical to the well-being of the new employee and gets the individual off on the right foot. The first step is to ensure that time is made available to spend with the new person. It is the manager's job to help a new hire adjust and fit in; it is not the job of the staff nurse whom it is most easy to do without for the day. The professional nurse manager does not ask someone else to perform this important task.

To help the new hire get oriented on that first day, take the new person around the unit and introduce him or her to the staff. At each meeting, introduce the new and resident employees and make sure that something positive is said about what the old employee does in the unit and that at least one of his or her accomplishments is noted. This reference to the excellence of the longer-term employee lets the veteran feel good and raises the standard for the new hire. Never, never, never, delegate this responsibility, because it is critical to getting the new employee well adjusted to the unit.

After the tour of the unit is complete, make sure that time is allocated to sit down with the new employee to go over the job expectations once again and outline the standards of performance in the unit. Discuss initial objectives and work with the new employee to establish several goals for the first month of employment. This is critical, because people remember things and react to stimuli far differently after they're hired than they did during the employment interview. Make sure that the new staff member understands what is expected and what he or she is to accomplish.

Talk once again about what life is like in the unit. Make sure to dispel any misconception that might still be held. Informed people are far happier than those who are continually surprised. Happy people make long-term employees; those who are not increase turnover.

REFERENCES

1. Cascio WF: *Applied psychology in personnel management,* ed 3, Englewood Cliffs, NJ, 1987, Prentice-Hall.
2. Bouchard TJ: *Handbook of industrial and organizational psychology,* Chicago, 1976, Rand McNally.
3. Decker PJ, Moore RC, Sullivan E: How hospitals can solve the nursing shortage, *Hosp Health Serv Adm* 27(6):12, 1982.
4. Decker PJ, Cornelius ET III: A note on recruiting sources and job survival rates, *J Appl Psychol* 64:463, 1979.
5. Poteet G: The employment interview—avoiding discriminatory questioning, *J Nurs Adm* 14(4):38, 1984.
6. Goodale JG: *The fine art of interviewing,* Englewood Cliffs, NJ, 1982, Prentice-Hall.
7. Moses J, Byham W: Applying the assessment center method. In *Pergamon general psychology series 71,* ed 2, New York, 1992, Pergamon.

SUGGESTED READINGS

Bouchard TJ Jr: *Handbook of industrial and organizational psychology,* ed 8, New York, 2000, Rand McNally.

Douglas LM: *The effective nurse leader and manager,* ed 5, St Louis, 1999, Mosby.

Ellis JR, Hartley CL: *Managing and coordinating nursing care,* ed 2, Philadelphia, 1995, Lippincott.

Ertl N: Choosing successful managers: participative selection can help, *J Nurs Adm* 14(4):27, 1984.

Guion RM: *Personnel testing,* New York, 1965, McGraw-Hill.

Loveridge CE, Cummings SH: *Nursing management in the new paradigm,* Gaithersburg, Md, 1996, Aspen.

Marquis BL, Huston CJ: *Management decision making for nurses,* Philadelphia, 1998, Lippincott.

Minor MA: Ten- and six-hour nursing shifts solve staff problems, *Hosp Prog* 52(July):62, 1971.

US Congress: *Federal regulation 38290-315,* Washington, DC, 1978, Author.

14

Managing Budgets and Resources

OUTLINE

LEARNING SYNOPSIS

Upon successful completion of this chapter, readers will possess a fundamental understanding of the critical importance of the budgeting process and effective management of the approved budget to the successful operation of the nursing unit.

OBJECTIVES

1. Be able to identify terms used in the budgetary process
2. Explain why the process of planning and control is so vital to budget development and nursing unit operation
3. Describe various types of budgets and budgeting processes used in the healthcare industry
4. Define variance reporting and explain its potential impact on the management of the budget
5. Identify the various aspects of the budget planning process
6. Describe methods used and processes for developing the supply and expense budget
7. Describe methods used and processes for developing the personnel budget

The dramatic changes that have occurred in the healthcare industry over the past three decades have led to economic uncertainty in the industry as the availability of operating funds has become severely restricted due to ever-increasing competition for available resources. This financial tightening has placed enormous pressure on the average nursing department to increase efficiency and effectiveness simply because of its high operating costs and overall impact on the financial well-being of the host organization (in many cases, the nursing department accounts for about half of the institution's total expenses).

If nursing departments are to meet the demands being placed on them by the extremely difficult financial environment, then all nurse managers must clearly understand their responsibilities regarding the budgetary process. Although many of the more experienced of these professionals have gained moderate levels of proficiency in this area, nurse managers as a whole show an appalling lack of the skills necessary to project costs based on current and anticipated needs. The challenge doesn't stop there, however; most nurse managers also show an almost total lack of understanding of the monitoring aspects of budget control. Correcting this situation is critical for the future success of the healthcare industry, because no one is in a better position than the nurse manager to predict trends in patient census and acuity levels, and in supply and equipment needs. This chapter presents the conceptual framework of budgeting to provide the reader with the knowledge necessary to understand the relationship between available resources, the provision of patient care, and the financial resources required to sustain an effective and high-quality nursing unit.

The topic of budgeting and resource management is introduced here by providing the following definitions of some of the major concepts in this area:

Accounting: A system for recording the financial transactions of a business (e.g., expenses paid and funds received) and organizing this information into reports or statements expressing the fiscal condition of the organization.

Audit: Formal examination and verification of an organization's financial records to determine the financial well-being of the organization, ensure accuracy, and verify that the company maintains its records in accordance with the generally accepted accounting principles.

Break-even point: The point at which the direct and indirect costs associated with producing a product or service equals or is offset by income from that product or service.

Budget: A detailed financial plan that sets forth expectations, serves as a control device, and

allows actual results to be compared with anticipated results. The purpose of the budget is to provide management with a means to project future activities, ensure that the resources necessary to achieve objectives are available at the appropriate time, and confirm that the costs of all projected operations remain within the level of available resources so that the goals of the organization can be met effectively, efficiently, and in a timely manner. Budgets are established as abstract entities and should never be considered to represent actual needs or absolute amounts. The basic structure of the budget indicates the anticipated method of resource procurement and the intended use of resources over a specific time interval. Finally, a budget is used to assist management in its effort to control the expenditure of available resources.

Budgeting: The process of planning for and controlling the use of the resources necessary to ensure anticipated levels of performance by comparing previous results with anticipated needs.

Cost containment: The process of holding costs within a specific or fixed limit.

Costing out: Determining through calculation the cost of specific resources.

Direct costs: The specific and immediate expenses associated with providing a service.

Economics: The study of the production, distribution, and consumption of wealth.

Fixed costs: Costs that remain the same regardless of the volume of business.

Indirect costs: General expenses that are charged to a specific product or service, such as maintenance or administrative costs.

Life cycle: The entire span of time that something exists; for a product, this includes the stages of introduction, growth, maturity, and market decline.

Market: A specific area of commercial activity or group of potential customers in which an organization's products are traded for value.

Marketing: The research and analysis, planning, implementation, and control of programs for exchange of value with target markets to achieve organizational objectives.

Marketing mix: The mixture of techniques used to market a product or service; sometimes referred to as the *four Ps* of marketing—product, price, place, and promotion.

Perception: The sum of a person's beliefs, ideas, and impressions about an object, business, or individual.

Responsibility summary: A formal document generated by the finance department showing budgetary expectations, actual results, and the difference between them.

Segmentation: Separation of the total into subsets; in marketing, identification of specific groups of current or prospective customers within a given market.

Semifixed costs: Costs that are fixed as long as the volume of business remains within established limits.

Semivariable costs: Costs that are fixed at the point of zero consumption and increase within a range of activity.

Stakeholders: The group of individuals or institutions that have an actual or potential interest in or impact on the future success of the organization; sometimes referred to as *publics.*

Variable costs: Costs that change in direct proportion to volume of production.

Variance: The difference between the amount budgeted for a given line item and the actual cost of the item.

Budgeting is a process that is carried out by nearly every business and government. In fact, almost every individual budgets in some manner, although few actually identify the process as such. For instance, everyone who has ever established a plan for paying his or her bills at specific times has created a budget. Although this may be an extremely simple example to introduce the concept of budgeting, such rudimentary personal plans accomplish all of the essential functions of a budget: resources are identified and so are the specific times that they will be needed. What is especially important is the connection between amount (what) and time (when) that is established in even the simplest forms of budget. Resources must be available at the required time or the process is not properly managed.

PLANNING AND CONTROL

One of the primary functions of a budget is to help management plan and control the distribution of resources in the organization. The following sections discuss each aspect of this process separately to clarify the individual elements that go into the establishment of a well-developed planning and management process.

Planning

Planning is an extremely complex process whose basic aim is to review the established goals and objectives of the unit for which a budget is being developed (i.e., the individual nursing unit, the nursing department, or the organization) for a specified period (usually a fiscal or calendar year). Planning is absolutely necessary if the essential financial projections that will ultimately be contained in the operating budget are to be developed proficiently. The planning process actually compels managers at all levels to look outside the day-to-day activities of their areas of responsibility and into the future to identify potential needs and establish a time frame for resource allocation that allows the satisfactory discharge of their responsibilities. This is especially important in resolving potential problems, because it allocates the necessary resources in a timely manner so that corrective steps can be taken before a challenge becomes unmanageable. Planning moves the budgeting process from a disorganized, reactive method of management to a more formal and controlled process. When planning is accomplished well, individual managers will spend far less time reacting to unanticipated problems and more time pursuing important and productive endeavors.

Planning, as part of the overall budgeting process, brings the following two critical elements under control in the organization:

1. *Communication:* Operating budgets are prepared by the individual units in the organization and, after being pulled together (usually by departments and divisions), are compiled into the organization's master budget. This process involves every level of management in the organization and ensures that the established performance goals are well communicated. The process of compiling, reviewing, and revising data for the budget requires open lines of communication between performers, supervisors, managers, and executives at all levels and helps to build strong performance-related relationships between managers in different departments whose operations are related or interdependent.

2. *Coordination:* The preparation of the budget is a well-orchestrated operation in every successful organization. The process of working together to create such a complex tool ensures that the primary goals of the organization will be carried forward into the individual goals and objectives of even the smallest units and that solid lines of coordination will be established between departments. In this manner, the budgeting process eliminates the possibility that a department will operate without considering the efforts of other departments and keeps all departments focused on satisfying the organization's overall objectives. The increased coordination results in organization-wide efficiency and reduced operating expenses.

When the planning process is completed, the individually developed unit plans and their accompanying budgets are rolled into the organization's master plan of action, which reflects the coordinated vision for all levels of management. An effective planning process is absolutely essential for the organization to operate smoothly and efficiently and to meet the specific goals and objectives that have been established.

Control

Budgeting supports another critical function of management: control. It gives management a means of restricting performance so that it remains in line with the available resources. The process of control includes all of the actions taken by management to ensure that the established goals and objectives are met and that all of the individual elements of the organization work in a manner consistent with organizational policies. Management exercises its control by comparing the actual results achieved against the projections contained in the original budget for a specified time period. By continually monitoring these differences, management is able to make necessary modifications and corrections to the plan which ensure that the established goals and objectives are met in a timely and efficient manner without unnecessary expenditure of available resources. Thus, an integral feature of the planning process is that it provides the ability to control the operation of the organization; the possession of a plan gives managers a means to compare actual versus anticipated performance.

It is highly unlikely that any projection made during the initial planning process will exactly match the results achieved if the plan is considered line by line. Variance is an anticipated part of planning, and management routinely establishes limits for its control. If, for example, management determines that any amount up to and including 4% of a line item's budget or a maximum of $500 is an acceptable variance, then only variances that exceed these amounts will be examined. However, this fact does not relieve the individual manager of the responsibility to remain within the authorized budget amount that has been approved for specific categories of expenditure. Most organizations view a manager whose unit or department is consistently over budget as an individual who is not performing to the expectations of the position.

BUDGETARY CONCEPTS AND CONSIDERATIONS

Responsibility Accounting

The budgeting process is based on the concept of responsibility accounting; that is, each manager's performance is evaluated in terms of how well he or she manages those items directly under his or her control. To manage these items effectively and objectively, the individual manager must carefully evaluate and catalogue the costs and revenues over which he or she has control. The effect achieved by responsibility accounting is the personalization of the overall accounting system, something that is absolutely necessary to ensure both effective planning and effective control.

Responsibility accounting is based on the following three fundamental assumptions:

1. Costs can be organized according to levels of management responsibility.
2. Costs that are charged to a specific manager are controllable at that level of performance.
3. Budget data can be generated in a form (a combination of amount and time) that can be used effectively as a basis for evaluating individual performance.

A formal control system designed to ensure budgetary accountability is presented in Fig. 14-1. The form shown should be completed monthly by all nurse managers who have budgetary responsibility using the information they have obtained from the responsibility summary (the finance department document showing budgetary expectations, actual results, and the difference between them). If the responsible nurse managers follow this process, any variances revealed can be systematically reviewed and justified, and all necessary modifications can be made to the budget to ensure that the necessary resources are available when they are actually needed.

The Budget Process as a Motivating Factor

The budget process, when conducted properly, can be an extremely effective tool that nurse managers can use to motivate their unit staffs. This is especially true if the budget has been developed using a teamwork approach. When the members of the staff participate in the planning process, they are far more likely to support the operating budget and also far more likely to view the budget as representing a fair and unbiased standard for evaluating their performance. If the budget process is well managed, staff members can obtain a great deal of individual satisfaction when the goals and objectives outlined in the budget are achieved. Conversely, a poorly developed or poorly managed budget can become a major source of friction between management and staff.

For the budget to become an effective motivational device, nurse managers must recognize that the budget is a tool, not a holy writ, and therefore it is not perfect. In other words, if, at the end of the reporting

Budget Reporting

Units of Service		Current Month Actual			Current Month Budget			Year-to-Date Actual Budget		
Category Code	Account Description	Current Month			Year-to-Date			Average Unit Cost		
		Actual	Budget	Variance	Actual	Budget	Variance	Actual	Budget	Variance
Income										
110	Income from inpatients									
120	Income from other sources									
Total Income										
Salary Categories										
10	Management personnel									
20	Technical specialists									
30	Registered nurses									
40	Licensed vocational nurses									
50	Licensed specialists									
60	Aides and orderlies									
70	Clerical and administrative									
80	Other standard salaries									
90	Vacation time paid									
100	Holiday time paid									
110	Sick leave paid									
120	FICA tax paid									
130	Other professional salaries									
Total Salaries										
Surgical Expense Categories										
300	Sutures and surgical									
310	Needles									
320	Surgical packs									
330	Surgical supplies									
340	IV solution									
350	Other medical care									
Total Surgical Expenses										
Supply Expense										
310	Cleaning supplies									

Fig. 14-1 ■ An example of a formal control system to ensure budgetary accountability. *FICA,* Federal Insurance Contributions Act; *IV,* intravenous.

period, the results achieved do not exactly match the projections, that may not be the result of poor staff performance. The budget should never be used as a club to beat people into performing or as a means of ridding the unit of an undesirable employee. These negative actions will only serve to undermine the importance of the budget and cause other members of the staff to view it negatively. Professional nurse managers use the budget as a tool to motivate, excite, and celebrate, because there is real truth in the maxim, "The use of positive motivators will reap positive motivation."

Differences between actual and budgeted values can be caused by a myriad of problems other than poor staff performance, including the following:

Management may have made mistakes: Errors in both vision and projection may have occurred when the managers created the budget. If not all possible circumstances were accounted for and not all situations were foreseen, there is every likelihood that a variance will occur at some time during the budget period.

Budgets rarely if ever are approved in the full amounts requested: When individual budgets are created, there is an excellent chance that their cumulative totals will exceed the total amount of money available. This means that a budget review must reduce the dollar amounts in many categories. However, this does not necessarily mean that the level of performance required during the year will be reduced. When the level of performance is the same but budget amounts are reduced, a legitimate budget variance will occur.

Whatever the reason, changes and modifications to authorized budgets are frequently necessary. Senior management is ultimately responsible for the proper maintenance of the budget, and that responsibility includes communicating the proper attitude regarding variances to all other levels of personnel. The budget is a tool, and to be effective, it must be considered a working document that permits adjustments when necessary, logical, and justifiable. The proper attitude to have regarding the budget is to consider the budget a serious part of overall management and to make every effort to keep costs within authorized allowances, but also to recognize that it is an imperfect document that can be altered to meet unexpected circumstances.

All nurse managers must share their budgets with the members of their staffs. By doing so, they establish it as a positive part of their units' management efforts. Employees should be able to see how the budget is used to help create realistic operating goals, measure results, and identify and isolate areas that may require more attention than was originally expected.

The proper administration of a budget program requires a great deal of insight and sensitivity from management and understanding and support from employees. Junior managers and employees will not function in a way that will guarantee performance within budgetary limitations if they believe that senior management is not committed to maintaining the budget or if they view it only as a tool for control and intimidation. The ultimate objective of every responsible management team is to develop awareness of the budget and its restrictions and to work together with every employee to use it as a positive tool for achieving both individual and institutional goals.

Budget Performance Periods

The effective period for a budget can vary greatly, ranging from a few days to many years, depending on the objectives of the budget and the uncertainties associated with it. Generally, operating budgets are established annually, and larger high-cost budgets cover several years of performance. For example, budgets that are concerned with major purchases (e.g., land, buildings, and high-cost equipment) have long time horizons and may extend 5, 10, or even 20 years or more into the future. Generally, a characteristic feature of a long-term budget is that it is very broad in content and omits much of the detail seen in an annual budget. Day-to-day operating budgets, however, are established to correspond with the starting and ending dates of the organization's accounting year.

Nursing unit budgets are examples of short-term budgets and are usually developed for the 1-year period corresponding to the organization's fiscal year. Most organizations divide the annual budget into four quarters and then subdivide each quarter into the corresponding 3 months. In this manner, near-term estimates can be projected with a good deal of accuracy, and corrections can easily be made for any variances.

Of course, there are many variations on the standard budget format, including the following:

Continuous or perpetual budget: This type of budget is designed to keep a specific time period under management review. For example, if an operating budget is managed in this way, then as soon as one month is completed, the next month is added, so that there are always 12 months' worth of budget data before management. Such budgets have proven their effectiveness by compelling managers to continually focus on the coming 12 months, which stabilizes the planning horizon.

Multiple-year budget: This type of budget is developed in 3- to 5-year increments that continually replenish themselves; after the end of the first year, a fourth or sixth year is added to the total to keep 3 or 5 years of budget in front of management at all times. This type of budget is generally used in budgeting for large capital items. The benefit is that only 1 year's budget has to be developed annually, which limits the amount of effort required to maintain an effective long-term fiscal process.

Fig. 14-2 shows a formal method of ensuring accountability within the budget reporting system. Known as a variance report, this form is typically completed monthly by the individual managers who are required to administer budgets. The information provided is obtained from their authorized budget and expenditure reports. Unit managers simply fill in the blanks with figures representing their authorized budget (current month budget) and actual expenditures (current month actual). Then they make the required calculations and submit their reports to their immediate seniors, who compile the individual unit

Variance Reporting Cost center _____ Month and year _____					
Budget Categories	**Current Month Actual**	**Current Month Budget**	**Difference ($$$)**	**Percent Difference (%-)**	**Justification for Variance**
Income Generated					
Income					
Expense					
Salaries					
Benefits					
Other professional fees					
Subtotal					
Authorized Expense Categories					
Medical supplies—consumable					
Medical supplies—accountable					
Nonmedical supplies					
Employee uniforms and outerwear					
Equipment					
Maintenance and repairs					
Outside services purchased					
Equipment rental/lease					
Dues and subscriptions					

Fig. 14-2 ■ An example of a formal method used to ensure accountability in the budget reporting system.

reports into an overall report for the division and submit it to the organization's senior management.

Zero-Based Budgeting

Zero-based budgeting is a term applied to a budget process that requires all reporting managers to begin the fiscal year at a zero budget level. This means that all managers must include justification for any first-time expenditures in their reports. A zero-based budget process does not allow balances to be carried forward. This is a significant difference from traditional budgets, which typically start the fiscal year with all approved budget money added into the budget; the manager then adds to or subtracts from it according to projected needs, objectives, and the inflation rate or consumer price index.

Zero-based budgeting puts an end to the traditional system of rewarding managers for exceeding previously approved budget limits, because, unlike in the traditional budget process, the next year's budget is not based on the previous year's expenditures. The traditional method of budget management actually can be viewed as a deterrent to managing the budget

and as an incentive to overspending, because it penalizes economical managers who did not consume all of their allocated dollars during the previous fiscal year by reducing the next year's amount to what was actually used.

Zero-based budgeting operates much more positively by addressing basic issues such as the following in the budgetary process:

- Why does this activity or department exist?
- If the reason for existence is sufficient for retention of the activity, then what should be its specific goals and objectives?
- How does the activity support and assist in accomplishing the established organizational goals and objectives?

Zero-based budget management also requires all managers to maintain assigned productivity levels.

Given its obvious advantages over traditional budgeting, the question is why every organization doesn't adopt a system of zero-based budget management. The answer is simple: zero-based budgeting requires a far greater commitment of both time and money for its implementation, so that many organizations simply cannot afford to use this system. However, most well-funded and well-staffed organizations have come to view zero-based budgeting as an important part of their overall management philosophy in spite of its obvious drawbacks, believing that the additional expense is more than offset by the gains from stricter spending and more efficient management.

Flexible Budgeting

The flexible budget system is one of the most popular styles of budget management because it allows management to modify budget allocations to keep pace with shifts in the market, changes in the activities of the organization and individual units, and previously unanticipated expenditures even after the fiscal year has begun. This form of budget management is highly favored and is widely used throughout the healthcare industry today, simply because the business environment in which healthcare organizations operate is so volatile. Elements such as patient census, acuity mix, and the use of resources are extremely hard to forecast in an environment that can change without notice. By allowing the budget to bend when there are variances with originally forecast numbers, the organization can easily respond to unanticipated changes and still ensure that the budget accurately reflects productivity.

The flexible budget system uses units of service as the basis for all calculations and adjusts allocations based on the number of units of service actually delivered during a given reporting period. All variance amounts are then compared against these computed flexible standards rather than against fixed budget amounts. The following example of supply expenditures in one nursing unit shows the advantages of flexible budgeting.

Assume that the following are the expenditures for a single budget reporting period:

Supplies	Actual	Authorized	Variance
	$2,300	$2,400	$100

Now assume that the unit of service used by the organization is patient-days and that the original budget authorization was based on 600 patient-days per period.

If only 550 patient-days of service were provided during the month, however, the authorized budget for that month would be reduced to reflect the fact that the period was slower than anticipated. Note that the flexible budgeting system establishes a value for expenditures on supplies based on a predetermined patient-day rate. The originally authorized budget amount shown earlier established this rate at $4.00 per patient per day ($2,400 divided by the anticipated 600 patient-days). Viewed in this light, and with the

flexible value incorporated, the actual unit expenditures look quite different, as follows:

Supplies	Actual	Authorized	Flex Authorized	Variance
	$2,300	$2,400	$2,200	<$100>

Unlike in the previous example, which showed unit supply expenditures to be under budget (+$100), the flexible budget calculates expenses incurred in terms of services rendered, and this puts unit expenditures over budget (<$100>). This type of budget is far more accurate in revealing a unit's budget management process than is the fixed-value system shown earlier. However, flexible budgets do have some of the same requirements as other budgetary systems (e.g., individual managers are required to investigate and provide justification for all negative variances). The following are two examples of cases in which a budget variance might be improved:

1. High patient acuity levels
2. Use of high-cost items mandated for specific patient care

The Operating Budget

The purpose of an operating budget is to provide management with accurate information on the cost of maintaining routine operations in the organization for a given period of time (usually a fiscal year). Individual nursing units are referred to as "cost centers" in this process, and each is responsible for generating an anticipated operating budget. The developed budget proposal includes amounts and justifications for the major expense categories in the unit, such as salaries, personnel benefits, supplies, and any other items necessary for the operation of the unit. Each nursing unit, or cost center, represents the smallest functional cost generator in the organization. Individual cost centers may be classified as revenue generators, such as the laboratory, radiology, and pharmacy departments, or they may be considered as overhead units that do not produce a revenue stream. Examples of overhead units in a healthcare facility are nursing, maintenance, environmental services, and administration. Although each nursing unit in the organization is considered a cost center, very few organizations consider the nursing unit a profit center and therefore do not reimburse it for services rendered. Instead, nursing service costs are embedded in the daily room rate charged to patients and are offset as a general cost of business for the organization.

The development of an operating budget is a lengthy process that normally takes place over the last several months of the current fiscal year; most organizations start the budget process in May and finish it prior to the close of the calendar year. Fig. 14-3 diagrams a typical budget development process (periods are months of the current year.)

Units of Service

With few exceptions, hospital budgets are developed from the forecasts or proposals developed by unit managers. For nursing units, these proposals are based on anticipated patient occupancy rates and acuity levels, and on other approved activity standards. These estimates are developed in terms of units of service, or the amount of money required to deliver one unit of service to one patient. The unit of service is the budgetary concept on which almost all approved operating budgets are based. The unit of service varies greatly from operating unit to operating unit depending on the mission of the providing unit; for example, the environmental service department uses square footage as its primary unit of service, the dietary department bases its projections on meals served, and the emergency department uses patient visits.

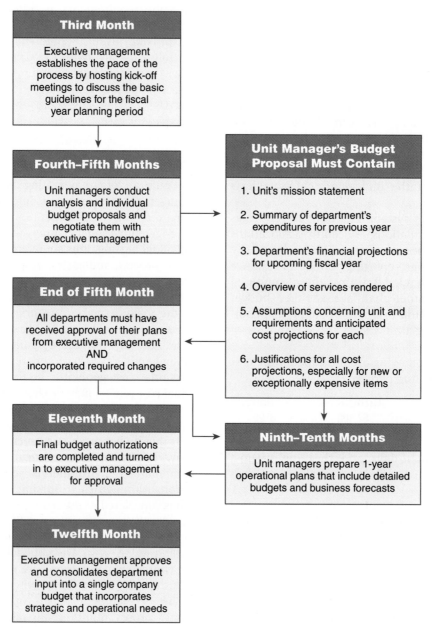

Fig. 14-3 ■ A typical budget development process. (Periods are months of the current year.)

Nurse managers base their units' needs on patient-days, which is determined by multiplying the number of patients assisted by the total number of days available in the budget interval. For example, if the nurse manager envisions the unit as serving 100 patients each day during the 1-year budget period, he or she will multiply the number of patients by 365 to yield 36,500 patient-days. If the nurse manager does not do a good job of estimating the number of patient-days the unit will provide, the budget will not be accurate and variances will be large. If the variance amounts become too large, the usefulness of the unit's budget will be significantly reduced.

! CRITICAL POINT

Almost all organizations consider the development and maintenance of an accurate budget to be a fundamental management responsibility. Those nurse managers who are judged not to be capable of discharging this duty may find themselves candidates for administrative discharge, reassignment, or termination of employment.

The Capital Expenditure Budget

A capital expenditure budget is a special part of the organization's overall budget that specifically manages the purchase of major equipment or real property and the funding of major projects such as facility renovations. The development process for this special budget is much like that for the operating budget in that it typically occurs throughout the fiscal year and culminates in the delivery of the proposed budget for the next fiscal year. Typically, every organization has strict rules regarding the purchase of capital items and limits the authority to approve such expenditures to only a few senior managers. The process of obtaining approval can be as individual as the organization itself, but the one thing that is always required is that every manager keep a chronologic list of all capital items approved, purchased, and maintained for his or her unit. This list should include the original date of purchase, because this information is necessary to determine the useful life cycle of capital equipment.

Every organization has its own particular definition of what constitutes a capital expenditure, but most definitions incorporate the following two factors:

1. *Initial purchase price:* The item must cost more than a preestablished minimum amount.
2. *Life expectancy:* The item must have a life expectancy (life cycle) longer than a set period.

For example, one organization may define a capital expenditure as any item that costs over $1,000 or that has a life cycle of longer than 1 year. Another organization may extend its capital expenditure criterion to include two or more identical items with the same specifications that, if purchased together, exceed a fixed dollar amount. For example, if one mechanical patient hospital bed costs $500, the purchase of two or more can constitute a capital expenditure as long as the combined cost exceeds the $1,000 minimum.

The purchase of capital items usually requires additional steps in the budgeting procedure. For example, almost every organization requires that the originating unit submit its request on a special form (Fig. 14-4). Inspection of this form shows that far more is required than a simple justification and indication of the purchase price; for example, the organization might ask for such things as estimated cost of installation, delivery charges, and price of service contracts. The justification for each capital item is generally far more detailed than that offered for a general budget item and should be well documented. Additional details such as depreciation time span, salvage value, and age of equipment are normally required. This information can generally be obtained from the organization's purchasing and accounting departments. Capital purchase approvals are usually based on urgency of need, criticality of the impact on goals and objectives, and availability of funds. Because institutions usually have a limited amount of hard capital for such purchases, a well-prepared request is essential to obtain approval.

When capital equipment is ordered, the prudent nurse manager also anticipates the impact on the unit's operating budget. For example, if the cardiac unit requests the purchase of monitoring equipment, the cost of electrocardiographic (EKG) paper and electrodes should be determined, documented, and included in the supply budget. In addition, the potential impact of possession of the capital equipment on personnel expenditures should be carefully analyzed. Will use of the equipment require additional personnel? What will it cost to train the existing staff in its operation? Will there be any requirement for increased overtime expenditures or additional nursing hours per patient-day? All such expenses must be carefully quantified and documented, and included in operating budget. If the request for capital expenditure is approved after the operating budget has gone into effect, a special variance request should be sent in to secure any increased funding that will be necessary, with the new equipment purchase and the specific needs related to it cited as justification.

Capital expenditure budgets are not easily developed. For example, rapid changes in technology can make equipment outdated even before the approval process is complete. If nurse managers work closely with their medical and nursing staffs, however, and keep current on technologic changes and future

Capital Item Request Form

Priority listing No. _____

Requesting department: _____

Location: _____

Cost center title: _____

Cost center No.: _____

Type and name of equipment requested: _____
_____
_____

Model No.: _____ Quantity: _____

Recommended vendor: _____

Justification: _____
_____
_____
_____
_____
_____

If more space is required complete on reverse side of form

Reason for Request
☐ Patient care
☐ Nonpatient
☐ Replacement
   If replacement, specify equipment that will be
   replaced: _____
_____
☐ Enhancement for existing equipment
☐ Comply with directive No. _____
☐ Expanding or new program
☐ Increase revenue
☐ Reduce cost

Purchasing department comments: _____
_____
_____

Estimated Costs
Purchase price: _____ R & D cost: _____
Shipping and handling cost: _____
Estimated tax: _____ Other costs: _____

Total Estimated Expenditure: _____

Anticipated Associated Costs
Number of FTEs: _____ Salaries: _____
Nonwage supplies: _____ per _____
Maintenance costs/repair: _____ per _____

Funding Source
☐ Grant No._____
☐ Contract/account No. _____
☐ Special fund No. _____
☐ Other No. _____

Anticipated Date of Purchase: _____
Contact name: _____
Approved by: _____

Fig. 14-4 ■ Sample form for requesting capital items. *FTEs,* Full-time equivalents; *R & D,* research and development.

trends, they can limit this difficulty and be far more effective in anticipating capital needs.

THE SUPPLY AND EXPENSE BUDGET

Developing the Supply and Expense Budget

One of the most critical parts of the budget is the supply and expense budget. This is the tool that is used to manage the funds allocated for the noncapital

equipment and supplies that are needed to operate a nursing unit. The supply and expense budget includes items such as the following:

- Medical and surgical supplies
- Pharmacy items
- Paper, office, and general administrative supplies
- Equipment rental
- Maintenance
- Service contracts

The critical input in the development of the supply and expense budget is the report or statement of expenses, a periodic report generated at the end of predesignated accounting periods (most typical is a monthly report). The standard information contained in the statement of expenses includes the following three items:

1. *Original budgeted amount:* budget line item by line item
2. *Actual amount expended:* again in a budget line item by line item format
3. *Year-to-date total:* a cumulative number that reflects the total amount spent on each line item since the beginning of the fiscal year

The statement of expenses shows every individual approved budget line item for the nursing unit plus the total amount expended in the unit, both in the current month and in the fiscal year to date.

Nurse managers begin the development of the unit's supply budget by analyzing the previous statements of expenses. These reports are used to gather and quantify the information needed in the development of the new budget. Among other things, nurse managers look for the following information:

- Amount of money originally allocated
- Amount of money spent
- Variances
- Causes of variances
- Percentage of the total allocated amount actually used
- Percentages of variances, if any

This information is used by nurse managers to identify any trends that might be significant enough to affect their forecasting efforts for the coming year's budget. For example, a change in the unit's supply requirements or utilization can result from a variety of causes, such as (a) volume changes, (b) a change in patient mix, (c) a change in patient type, (d) installation of new equipment, and (e) changes in procedure. Of course, these are only a few of the many possible changes that can occur during the span of a fiscal year, and each needs to be considered on a unit-by-unit basis and its effects quantified as accurately as possible. Although this is not a glamorous job, it is one of the most important that nurse managers will perform all year. The harder nurse managers work to get this information right, the greater the opportunity for producing an accurate budget that reflects actual needs. The work spent in developing this information will be returned many times over because of the reduced need for variance reporting as the year wears on.

Once the information is collected and quantified, it should be carefully screened to determine if any adjustments are necessary because of factors such as (a) inflation, (b) performance requirement changes, and (c) compliance issues. Most of the information necessary will be supplied to nurse managers either by the accounting department, the human resources department, or the purchasing department. For instance, the purchasing department may predict a 5% increase in pharmacy costs and a 4% increase in all other purchase categories; the human resources department may inform the nurse manager of a 3% across-the-board raise that will go into effect during the upcoming fiscal year; and the accounting department may provide information on applicable taxes and fees.

Assuming that there are no major changes (e.g., in patient census, acuity level, or services provided), then, to develop the budget for the next fiscal year, nurse managers need only to use the numbers from the previous year's report and adjust them for inflation. Pharmacy expenses (medical supplies) can be used as an example. Assume the nurse manager has been given a figure of 5% as the anticipated inflation rate to use in calculating the amount to be budgeted. If the pharmacy expenses for the previous fiscal year were $7,440, or $620 per month, then the budget for the next fiscal year should be $7,812, or $651 per month.

Another classic example of budget adjustment is the following. Using the data from the same annual expense report, let us now assume that an increase in medical-surgical supply expenses is anticipated due to the purchase of several new pieces of monitoring equipment. The extra funds will be used to purchase the necessary EKG paper and electrodes that will be required by the new equipment. This additional cost is anticipated to be $300 per month. If last year's expenses in the medical-surgical supplies budget were $24,981, or $2,082* per month, then to meet the new requirements, the nurse manager will have to budget the previous fiscal year's $2,082 per month plus an additional $300 for the EKG paper and electrodes, plus an additional 5% for inflation, which will result in a proposed budget for the medical-surgical supplies line item of $2,501 per month.

A fundamental part of every nurse manager's role is to become familiar with expense account categories and the specific items contained in each one so that the manager can properly analyze the unit's current expenses and forecast the impact of any future change on the unit's performance, needs, and budget requirements.

---

*In this example, all values have been rounded to the next whole number.

Controlling the Supply and Expense Budget

The monthly expense statements are used as a tool to control the supply and expense budget effectively. Nurse managers begin by determining what, if any, variances occurred and why. This information will help them predict the next year's needs and identify any potential corrective action necessary to get expenditures back within budget allowances.

When the nurse manager is examining the cause for a budget variance, the manager thoroughly reviews the activity level in the unit to determine if it is related in any way to the variance. For example, if research indicates that a variance in supply costs was due to increased use of several items because of an unanticipated increase in patient count, a legitimate reason for the variance exists and there may be no need for corrective action. However, if the research indicates that unit staff have been wasting supplies because of improper technique, then the nurse managers must develop a course of action to return the unit to compliance with authorized budget amounts. Keeping control of expenditures is far easier if nurse managers maintain a professional working relationship with their staffs and can easily ask for staff members' assistance when they discuss the budget with them. The important management element to remember is that the situation must be analyzed carefully so that appropriate action can be taken.

Periodic expense reports are received from the accounting department that reflect pertinent information about the supplies purchased both through in-house ordering systems and from out-of-hospital sources. These reports are critically important to effective management of the budget, because mistakes can be made in the billing process. The prudent nurse manager inspects these reports to make sure that the unit is billed only for the supplies it actually uses. If a difference is noted between the amount billed and the amount used, the nurse manager should contact the purchasing department as quickly as possible to discuss the error. In reviewing the reports, the nurse manager must be sure to make a clear distinction between those charges that are patient charge items and those charges that belong to the unit. It is common practice in most hospitals to charge the individual nursing unit for the cost of patient charge items that are used by the unit but are not, for whatever reason, charged to the patient. These are referred to as *lost charges,* and they can create havoc in the unit's budget management process. Therefore, the nurse manager must develop mechanisms for tracking these charges and, if possible, getting them rescinded if they were not billed correctly through no fault of the nursing unit.

THE PERSONNEL BUDGET

Another critical segment of the overall budget is the personnel budget or, as it is frequently called, the salary or staffing budget. This budget usually accounts for the highest percentage of the overall expense of operating a nursing unit. Personnel costs can easily amount to as much as 90% of the total service budget of the nursing unit. The personnel budget contains the following types of items:

- Salaries (the combined salary costs for all full-time equivalent [FTE* or one 40-hour position] allowances)
- Vacation expenses
- Sick leave expenses
- Holiday costs (including any overtime authorized for payment in labor contracts)
- Overtime
- Salary differentials
- Potential merit increases
- Orientation and education time

Although unit-level nurse managers are the best source of information for determining staffing requirements, nurse managers need to develop their staffing requests using as much objective information as is available.

Relevant Components

A number of significant factors must be considered by nurse managers when they are developing the staffing requirements for their units.

UNITS OF SERVICE

How many units of service are anticipated to be delivered during the next fiscal year? Is this number an increase or decrease from the previous year?

FTE originally meant *full-time employee,* but changes in attitudes and demands have brought about a change in meaning. Today FTE is thought of as full-time *equivalent.* For example, a unit may be authorized for 18 FTEs. This indicates the total number of personnel hours that may be paid each week without incurring overtime costs (40×18). The actual number of physical employees working in the unit, however, may be considerably greater than 18 if part-time and peak-time employees are used. For example, one FTE (40 hours) might be provided by one part-time employee (20 hours) and two peak-time employees (10 hours each).

Remember that the entire personnel budget is based, at least initially, on the projected number of service units. Although this projection is usually the collaborative work of the hospital's financial department and the department of nursing, individual nurse managers must know how it will affect the performance of their units. For example, they must consider the total bed capacity of their nursing units and multiply that by the anticipated percentage of occupancy. Once these data are identified, they must be carefully analyzed to determine if any identifiable trends or patterns are present. For example, a nurse manager might consider a projected occupancy rate of 90% or more to be a stable figure to use with his or her computations, especially if little variation is anticipated from day to day. If a lower occupancy rate is determined, however, the budgeting manager must factor in a larger variation in rate and must look at the available data far more closely for any telltale patterns or trends.

For example, suppose that a nursing unit which holds 30 beds has a 65% occupancy rate. To determine the exact number of personnel that will be needed to service a unit of this size, it is extremely important to understand both the occupancy rate of the unit and changes in that occupancy rate over the days of the week. If there are identifiable patterns or significant variations in the number of patients being served throughout the week, the distribution can have a significant effect on staffing. For instance, if the unit operates with a patient load of 20 patients throughout the week but that number falls to 10 during the weekend, the staffing level requirements will be lower than if the unit operates at the same capacity on all 7 days.

MIX IN PATIENT ACUITY LEVELS

Will the unit be handling patients with more or less serious illnesses? What is the anticipated number of performance hours that will be required to assist the average patient throughout his or her stay? Will the mix of acuity levels require more nursing care or less?

One of the most important tools nurse managers have at their disposal for measuring the complexity of patient care and for categorizing patients according to the level of care required over a specified period of time is the patient classification system. This system can be extremely useful in objectively defining staffing needs and supporting staffing requests. Although there is little doubt that experienced nurse managers can predict staffing needs in the unit fairly accurately, it is very difficult for them to justify specific staffing and budgetary needs without having objective and

reliable historical data. The use of a well-developed patient classification system allows nurse managers to base their decisions regarding future personnel requirements on how much nursing the patients need, rather than on what might actually have been provided in the past. Projections for required personnel levels can then be justified using data that are both objective and verifiable.

Classification systems can vary widely throughout an organization because of the different requirements and different levels of care necessary in specific specialties. Several excellent patient classification systems are available today that are designed to support a variety of management information systems, from the very simple to the most extensive.

REQUIRED HOURS OF NURSING CARE

How many hours of actual nursing care are anticipated to be delivered during the next fiscal year?

The first step in calculating the amount of staffing required in a given unit is to accurately predict the number of patient-days by level of acuity. To show how the required hours can be calculated, let us begin by assuming that a 30-bed medical-surgical unit has an average census of 26 patients per day each month. Using trend analysis, the average daily patient distribution can be determined from objective historical data and classified by level of care required:

Level of Care Required	No. of Patients Assisted per Day
I	5
II	15
III	4
IV	2
TOTAL	26

Next, the number of hours of nursing care required for this particular mix of patients is determined using a patient classification system. For the present purposes, assume that the classification system provided the following information:

Level of Care	Hours Required per Patient-Day
I	5.0
II	6.4
III	8.0
IV	12.0
TOTAL	31.4

To determine the total number of hours of nursing care required for the day, the number of patients needing each level of care is multiplied by the standard hours of care required for that patient category, and the results for all levels of care are totaled. This provides the nurse manager with the information required to draw up the standard labor hours budget, as follows:

Standard Labor Hours Budget
(for the period beginning January 1 and ending December 31)

Level of Care	Patients per Day	Hours per Patient-Day	Hours of Care per 24 Hours
I	5	5.0	25
II	15	6.4	96
III	4	8.0	32
IV	2	12.0	24
TOTAL	26	31.4	177

If the patient census and acuity mix on the nursing unit can realistically be considered to be stable, then the nurse manager can compute the number of nursing care FTEs required (C) by dividing the total required hours of care shown in the previous table (B, or 177) by the total average daily census (A, or 26) to obtain a value of 6.8. The following formula shows the calculation:

$$B \div A = C, \text{ or } 177 \div 26 = 6.8$$

FIXED AND VARIABLE STAFFING

Can the work in the unit be performed using a combination of part-time and peak-time employees? Does the unit have to hire its full complement of FTEs as full-time employees, or can a mixture of part-time and full-time staff meet the objectives? (Money can be saved by employing part-time personnel who do not receive full benefit, vacation, and sick time packages without sacrificing quality patient care.)

If nurse managers choose to employ only full-time personnel, they must be very careful. It is extremely difficult to respond to unforeseen circumstances with a fixed number of personnel, and very few work environments are stable. What really occurs is that the week's work schedule is full of peaks and valleys. One day, there aren't enough beds to accommodate all of the patients requiring care, and the next day, the staff are looking for something to do. A management principle is applicable here: fixed staffing does not change to accommodate demand. There are positions in the typical unit that must be staffed with permanent, full-time employees. The positions of nurse manager, clinical nurse specialist, nurse educator, unit secretary, monitor technician, and a charge nurse on each shift are examples. However, every other position can and quite possibly should be staffed with part- and peak-time employees. Then, as the patient census moves up and down away from what is considered normal, the nurse manager can either call in extra help to cover the peak or reschedule personnel when volume is low. Examples of potential peak-time and part-time

employees are registered nurses, licensed vocational nurses, and nurse's aides.

TECHNOLOGIC CHANGES

Will advances in technology reduce the labor effort in the unit? Or will they temporarily cause an increase in the number of personnel hours needed, especially during training periods? If technology can help the staff work more efficiently, does the unit still require the same number of authorized FTEs? These are serious questions that nurse managers must answer as they build their budgets. Remember this point: Nurse managers are members of the management team. It is their responsibility to effectively manage the assets under their charge. This means that it is their job to be frugal, efficient, and clinical when it comes to making decisions regarding the use of technology. If new equipment has been developed that can reduce the amount of labor necessary to maintain the expected level of quality patient care and the cost of that equipment can be amortized over a realistic period of time, then the technology should be considered.

Technology may also have the opposite effect, of course. For example, if an intensive care unit purchases a new piece of monitoring equipment that has greater capabilities but requires additional staff to aggressively utilize these new features, or if the unit does not have the proper number of registered nurses to manage the new equipment, then an increase in staffing may be in order. Nurse managers should remember that requests to increase the number of FTEs are often difficult to get approved.

CHANGES IN MEDICAL PRACTICE

Are physicians ordering more frequent and increasingly more complex procedures for their patients? How will changes in physician's orders translate into required nursing performance?

When new techniques bring about changes in how medicine is actually practiced, they also lead to changes in the types and quantities of personnel needed. A significant increase in the use of hyperalimentation might increase the demands placed on the nursing staff to the point that an increase in FTEs would be warranted. The same would be true for any change in practice that places greater demands on the staff and thus decreases the ability to maintain the level of services expected without additional personnel.

REGULATORY REQUIREMENTS

Are there new regulatory issues to deal with? Will these regulations create new demands on performance? (It is rare that a new regulation decreases labor requirements.)

The vast changes that have occurred in nursing over the past three decades because of the increasingly complex healthcare services provided to patients, the escalating acuity levels of hospitalized patients, and the growing recognition of the importance of quality of care have led to increasing regulation of nursing requirements in healthcare facilities. It is not uncommon for the standards of the Joint Commission on Accreditation of Healthcare Organizations and a host of different state and federal guidelines to include requirements regarding the number and skill levels of nursing personnel, especially in specialty units.

SUPPORT SERVICES

What is the anticipated demand for new services in the unit, and where will these services come from? What will these new services cost, and specifically who will pay for them? These are important questions to consider before settling on a budget request to cover support services.

Support services include things such as environmental, dietary, radiologic, and laboratory services. Nurse managers should consider what level of support is now being provided, how that support affects staffing requirements, and whether any changes in these services are anticipated.

ORGANIZATIONAL AND UNIT OBJECTIVES FOR THE UPCOMING FISCAL YEAR

What are the specific objectives of the organization for the upcoming year, and how will the unit's specific goals and objectives support their achievement? To accomplish the unit's specific goals and objectives, what, if anything, will need to be done differently? If something needs to be done differently, what is that something, and how will the unit prepare for the required changes? Will training, additional personnel, or increased resources be required? Will these new demands increase the number of people needed to deliver the expected level of quality patient care? If so, in what specific disciplines will more personnel be needed?

Projection of staffing levels should never be attempted until organizational, nursing department, and nursing unit goals have been determined. Any changes brought about by the anticipated goals must be carefully weighed to determine their potential impact on patient care and on the level of staffing necessary.

What has been described earlier is nothing more than a system of realistic strategic planning. When nurse managers spend the time to make accurate forecasts and projections, they will be doing a tremendous service to themselves and their units, one that will carry through for the entire budget period. In their efforts, nurse managers need to coordinate with other departments, with higher levels of management, and with each and every member of their staffs. Adopting a team approach within the unit and with senior management can ensure that the unit remains within budget throughout the entire year.

STAFFING PATTERNS

Experience teaches nurse managers that the peaks and valleys so inherent in patient care actually are somewhat predictable, and therefore so is the workload associated with them. If they start out by using the recommended number of hours of care as a guideline, nurse managers can distribute their available FTE hours rationally over all shifts. Based on their analysis, work schedules are adjusted and an efficient staffing pattern is devised. In developing their plans, nurse managers need to consider such basic factors as what skill mix of personnel is available, what are the anticipated number of work hours, how the workload may realistically be distributed, what delivery systems will be needed, and what each can effectively handle.

PERSONNEL MIX

The personnel mix is the number of employees required and available at each skill level (e.g., registered nurse, licensed vocational nurse, nurse's aide). The mixture of personnel in the unit should be closely monitored to ensure that proper staff are available to handle the type, number, and acuity level of the patients requiring care.

HOURS OF WORK

What are the lengths of the shifts to be worked? By determining whether full-time employees will work an 8-hour, 10-hour, or 12-hour day; how many part-time and peak-time employees will be used; and what their periods of work will be, nurse managers can quickly fill in the staffing pattern for the unit. This pattern, once established, will determine the number of personnel needed.

DISTRIBUTION OF WORKLOAD

What is the workload? When (what shift) are the specific jobs usually performed, and who will be required to do them? These are questions that nurse managers must answer during their analysis of unit requirements. Once they have the answers to these questions, the job of distributing the workload realistically over the different shifts will become much easier. Usually the distribution of labor is centered on the specific requirements of the patient care that is to be provided. Although no magic formula exists for determining the exact number of personnel required on any shift, there are some useful starting points, such as (a) distributing staff equally across all three shifts (usually not an ideal distribution), and (b) assigning a larger percentage of personnel to the day shift, a smaller percentage to the evening shift, and the smallest number to the night shift. Again, the needs of the patients dictate the distribution. However, one major qualifying factor is the sleep patterns of the patients. As a general rule, patients who are awake require greater amounts of care. The key is flexibility. Demands can change from minute to minute; a realistic spread of the labor force cannot be determined unless a minimum of a month's worth of historical data is reviewed.

One thing should be remembered: when distributing the workload, objectivity is the key. Be fair, but be practical.

DELIVERY SYSTEM

What will be the primary method of delivering service in the unit? The method of delivering care (e.g., primary, team, or functional nursing) will affect the staffing patterns established.

Position Control

The list of approved labor positions for the department is referred to as the position control. The available positions are listed by category of personnel (e.g., nurse manager, registered nurse, licensed vocational nurse, nurse's aide). Alongside each of the approved titles is given the approved number of FTEs for that position. An FTE, as explained earlier, is the equivalent of a full-time position or 40 hours of work per week or, in some institutions, 80 hours per 2-week pay period. In institutions that employ nurses on a 12-hour schedule, the FTE is commonly established at 72 instead of 80 hours per pay period.

Exactly how the FTE is computed differs from organization to organization, but federal labor law establishes a full-time position as 2,080 paid hours per year (40 hours per week × 52 weeks per year = 2,080 hours). Paid hours include hours spent in direct performance of work (productive time) plus nonproductive time (vacation, holidays, sick days). The amount of nonproductive time included in each FTE varies with the organization. For the purposes of budgeting, nonproductive time is an expense that must be covered by additional paid productive hours.

THE FULL-TIME EQUIVALENT BUDGET

Exactly how an FTE budget is developed can best be illustrated by the use of a realistic example. Suppose you are the nurse manager in charge of a 26-bed unit.

You have established, and senior management has approved, a distribution schedule that has all of your assigned personnel working an 8-hour shift. Assume that the required number of nursing hours per 24-hour period is 177. Then the number of variable nursing staff required for each 24-hour period can be computed in the following manner:

1. Divide 177 by 8 (number of hours worked by a full-time employee in a specific shift) = variable FTEs required per day, or 22.12.
2. Because each nurse only works one 8-hour shift each day, 5 days per week, additional FTEs (i.e., more than 22.12) will be required to cover the other 2 days of the week, as follows:

177 × 365 (days per year) = 64,605 total hours required per year

64,605 ÷ 2,080 (FTE hours in 1 year) = 31.06 FTEs (total FTEs required for the year)

For a nursing unit staffed entirely by nurses who work 72 hours per pay period on 12-hour shifts, the FTEs required would be higher, as follows:

64,605 (total required hours) ÷ 1,872 (FTE hours in 1 year) = 34.51 FTEs

Once the fixed positions required for the nursing unit have been determined, these are added into the overall position control. Because personnel in fixed positions are not usually replaced when they are not working, each position is simply budgeted as 1.0 FTE.

After unit staffing requirements have been determined, the required FTEs are compared with the available resources. When the FTEs needed do not match the position control either in available numbers of personnel or in necessary mix, the nurse manager must consider requesting new positions or redistributing FTEs among skill levels when the budget is submitted.

Differential and Overtime

Nurse managers determine the budget for any differential paid for evening and night shifts by multiplying the number of hours worked by the differential rate. For example, if the nursing unit requires that four registered nurses work on each evening and night shift, the nurse manager multiplies the differential rate for each shift by the number of hours in that shift (8, 10, or 12) and then multiplies that number by 4 to determine the amount that must be budgeted for the shift differential. Consider the following example:

- If the evening differential is set at an additional $1 per hour, the following calculations would be performed:

$1 per hour × 8 hours per shift per nurse =
$8 per shift per nurse

$8 × 4 nurses = $32 per day differential budget dollars
needed

$32 × 365 days a year = $11,680 per year
differential budget dollars needed

- If the night differential is established at an additional $2 per hour, the following calculations would be performed:

$2 × 8 hours = $16 per shift per nurse

$16 × 4 nurses = $64 per day differential budget dollars
needed

$64 × 365 days = $23,360 per year

- Total annual differential dollars needed is computed by adding the annual evening and night differential figures, as follows:

$11,680 + $23,360 = $35,040 total additional dollars
required for the budget

An overtime budget is created to ensure that adequate funding is available in the budget to cover unforeseen situations that will occur, such as fluctuations in workload or temporary shortages of staff due to illness. Overtime requirements are generally determined by multiplying the historical average number of hours of overtime worked by one and one half times the hourly rate paid to each position. If the historical data indicate that the average amount of overtime worked per week is 8 hours and the average base salary paid to a specific position is $20 per hour, the overtime budget should include $240 per week (8 × $20 × 1.5). Annualized, this figure is $12,480.

If nurse managers elect to use historical data to compute overtime requirements, they must carefully consider whether the amount of overtime worked in the past was actually justified. If overtime was worked when it was not necessary, any computation made using historical data will have to be modified. It is highly recommended that nurse managers use a realistic and objective approach when determining the unit's overtime requirements and begin by looking at possible ways of adjusting the work schedule to cover as much of the overtime requirement as possible. Perhaps a shift from full-time employees to a mix of part-time, full-time, and peak-time employees can alleviate much of the overtime burden by increasing staffing flexibility.

Benefits

The final thing that nurse managers need to consider before they can complete the personnel budget is the cost of employee benefits. In most organizations, this is one of the easier parts of budgeting to accomplish because most require only that managers provide a figure that is a percentage of what they have determined will be the annual salary expenses for the unit. Benefits are those things provided to or for individual employees in addition to personal salary. These include items such as the following:

- Vacation compensation
- Holiday compensation
- Sick leave
- Insurance premiums (e.g., medical and dental insurance coverage)
- Workers' compensation
- Life insurance
- Disability insurance
- Child care

Except for highly compensated employees, annual benefits cost the organization an additional 33% to 40% of the annual salary expenses. For budgeting purposes, nurse managers will usually be provided with a figure for benefit costs by the benefits section of the human resources department or the budget section of the accounting department.

Budget Review

With the final computation for benefits complete, nurse managers can begin to feel that their budgetary forecasting efforts for the year are finished. Before they submit their budgets, however, they must review each line item for accuracy and completeness, and address the following questions:

- Is there sufficient money in the forecast to operate the unit for the entire upcoming year?
- Has a sufficient, realistic justification been provided for each line item of expense?
- If, for any reason, any portion of the budget is reduced by senior management, what can be eliminated in the way of services, resources, or staffing to ensure that the budget remains within authorized limits throughout the year?
- Are the budget projections based on the number of patient-days of care expected to be provided and the anticipated acuity levels of the patients? If so, is the justification stated in the proposed budget in easily understood terms and supported by historical and accurate data?
- Were the daily hours of care required for the projected mix of patients calculated using an acceptable source for standard hours of care?
- Was a staffing pattern developed and used to determine the required variable and fixed FTEs that will be needed to cover the anticipated workload?

- Finally, were costs such as shift differentials, overtime, benefits, and indirect costs added to arrive at the total number of budget dollars needed for operation during the fiscal year?

If nurse managers can answer all of the aforementioned questions with a definite yes, then their budgets are complete and ready for submission. If not, then they need to make any necessary changes or additions to the appropriate sections and verify that all subsequent sections accurately reflect any changes made.

Managing the Personnel Budget

When the budget has been submitted and approved, the actual budget management process is only beginning. Nurse managers must continually monitor their units' expenses so that these do not exceed the resources that have been authorized. This means that managers must complete their units' monthly expense statements accurately.

The nurse manager must carefully monitor each line item of the approved budget to ensure that actual expenditures do not exceed authorized limits. If such an exception is noted, it is extremely important that the manager complete the necessary variance report immediately. When an overbudget variance is identified, the nurse manager must institute correct management procedures at once to ensure that the following month's expenditures are reduced so that the annual budget allowance for that line item is not exceeded. Most organizations don't really mind if a unit remains under budget unless the difference is significant; if it is, however, then senior managers will begin to doubt the accuracy of the budget originally submitted. This doubt very often manifests itself in calls for strict and lengthy justifications for future submissions and a willingness to reduce any future proposed budget for the unit, both of which might later prove to be serious problems for the junior manager.

Budget variances are important, even critical, issues for nurse managers, and the best way to deal with them is to avoid them by giving careful attention to the original budgeting process. Thorough preparation accompanied by logical and verifiable justifications should get the unit the money it needs to operate. Unforeseen circumstances do occur, however, and careful management of the authorized budget will quickly identify variances. Once a variance is identified, justification should be supplied and immediate steps taken to reduce expenditures in that category. Budget management is that simple, and it is a primary and fundamental job of every nurse manager.

If a variance should occur, don't panic. Use the opportunity to learn from the situation. Ask yourself questions that will help you determine the only really important issue: Is the variance due to inappropriate planning or to unanticipated activity that was beyond reasonable expectation and unit-level control? The answer to this question will indicate the direction that must be taken to regain control of the budget.

SUMMARY

- Budgeting is the process of planning future operations and controlling operations by comparing actual results with expectations.
- A budget is a detailed financial plan used to communicate performance expectations and serves as the basis for comparing expectations with actual results.
- The master budget represents a series of interrelated budgets for all the units or activities of the organization.
- Planning and control are two separate functions of the budget.
- Planning involves establishing future goals and objectives and determining the steps necessary to achieve those goals.
- Controlling is the process of comparing actual results with planned or budgeted results. By measuring the differences, managers are better able to make modifications and corrections.
- A total unit budget includes a personnel budget, a supply and expense budget, and a capital expenditure budget.
- The personnel budget is influenced by patient census, acuity level, technologic changes, and changes in medical practice and clinical service.
- A unit personnel budget can be developed by performing the following steps:
    Predicting the number of patient-days for each patient category (level of care)
    Determining the hours of nursing care required for this patient mix
    Distributing the hours required over all shifts
    Developing a staffing pattern that considers the available personnel mix
    Converting hours of care to actual costs

FINAL THOUGHTS

How is the budget managed at the unit level? It is nurse managers who are responsible for meeting their units' fiscal goals. They do this by continually managing the personnel and the supply and expense portions of the operating budget.

Typically, monthly reports of operations are sent to nurse managers, who have the responsibility to investigate and explain any variances they might contain. Each individual unit establishes a limit of overage that is considered reasonable, but even with this allowance, all variances should be considered serious.

There are, of course, many individual factors that can create variances in the unit's budget, but the most common contributors are changes in patient census or patient acuity level; turnover; overtime; illness; loss of time in orientation of new employees, meetings, workshops, and training; and changes in employee mix, paid salary levels, and staffing levels.

Managers are not expected to be able to control all of the potential variances that might occur in the unit. But for those spending categories that are normally within their control, they must make concerted efforts to ensure good management.

There is no replacement for good budget management.

THE NURSE MANAGER SPEAKS

The development of sound financial skills is imperative for today's nurse manager. These analytical skills are rapidly becoming the cornerstone of a cost-conscious nursing environment and are essential for all nurses.

In the manager's development of these analytical skills, one thing is important above all else: the individual's belief that matters such as budget management are as important to the health and welfare of the nursing unit as are the level of professionalism among the staff and the quality of health care that they provide.

Nurses must know and understand that they work in a business and that the successful operation of that business is critical to its survival and to their future employment. Nurses must understand what constitutes profit and why the organization must make a profit to survive; such things are fundamental to financial thinking.

Nurse managers should ensure that each of their subordinates knows what is included in the operating and capital budgets and how these two financial elements interact. Each employee should understand how the budget is developed, how it is administered, and exactly what his or her role is in ensuring that the unit remains within its authorized spending limits.

Management of the budget begins in the hearts and minds of every employee in the unit.

SUGGESTED READINGS

Bailey D: Budgeting skills (continuing education credit), *Nurs Stand* 10(19):43, 1996.

Baker M: Cost-effective management of the hospital-based hospice program, *J Nurs Adm* 22(1):40, 1992.

Caroselli C: Economic awareness of nurses: relationship to budgetary control, *Nurs Econ* 14(5):292, 1996.

Cavouras CA, McKinley J: Variable budgeting for staffing: analysis and evaluation, *Nurs Manage* 28(5):34, 1997.

Cleland V: *The economics of nursing*, Norwalk, Conn, 1990, Appleton and Lange.

Corley MC, Satterwhite BE: Forecasting ambulatory clinic workload to facilitate budgeting, *Nurs Econ* 11(2):77, 1993.

Finkler S, Kovner C: *Financial management for nurse managers and executives*, ed 3, Philadelphia, 2001, Saunders.

Folland S, Goodman AC, Stano M: *The economics of health and healthcare*, ed 4, Upper Saddle River, NJ, 2004, Prentice Hall.

Hall M, Anderson F: Maintaining quality care while decreasing hospice costs, *Nurs Econ* 15(3):157, 1997.

Marrelli T: *The nurse manager's survival guide: practical answers to everyday problems*, ed 3, St Louis, 2004, Mosby.

Moss M: Practical budgeting for the operating room administrator, *Nurs Econ* 1(1):7, 1993.

Pelfry S: Financial techniques for evaluating equipment requisitions, *J Nurs Adm* 21(3):15, 1991.

White SK, Bartug B, Bride W: Supporting nursing innovations in a cost-cutting environment, *Crit Care Nurs Clin North Am* 7(2):399, 1995.

CHAPTER

15

Quality Assurance and Risk Management

OUTLINE

LEARNING SYNOPSIS

Upon successful completion of this chapter, readers will possess a fundamental understanding of the critical importance of quality assurance and risk management to the successful operation of a healthcare organization.

OBJECTIVES

1. Discuss the impact of accountability in the healthcare industry
2. Describe how the concept of accountability has given way to the concept of quality assurance
3. Characterize the quality assurance process and its major components
4. Explain how nursing is monitored in a quality assurance environment
5. Describe the typical structure of a healthcare risk management program
6. Discuss the purpose and composition of the risk management committee
7. Describe the role of the risk manager in the healthcare organization
8. Discuss the role of nursing in the risk management process
9. Describe the process of critical incident reporting, including its major elements and the individual responsible for each
10. Identify major risk areas in the nursing unit
11. Describe the role of the nurse manager in the risk management process
12. Identify effective means available to the nurse manager to evaluate the process of risk management in the nursing unit

Accountability has become an important part of the business philosophy of healthcare organizations and healthcare providers during the past three decades. Because of the large number of highly publicized lawsuits and the exceptionally high amounts awarded in past court judgments, as well as the legislative and judicial actions that have placed the responsibility for patient safety directly on healthcare providers, it has become necessary for every person involved in healthcare management to fully understand the importance of accountability in the organization. In fact, in today's healthcare environment, accountability is a fundamental and primary part of every nurse manager's responsibilities.

The need for accountability in health care has been driven by several landmark decisions. One of the most noteworthy cases, *Darling v. Charleston Community Memorial Hospital*, was decided in 1965.[1] In this case, the Illinois Supreme Court upheld the decision of a Chicago superior court that had found the hospital liable for the care of a patient whose leg had been amputated following complications from a fracture. The decision found the hospital to be negligent in not one but two different areas, as follows:

1. *Failure to inform:* The decision held that the nurse in charge of the patient's care had failed to properly inform the physician, hospital, or any other qualified individual when she first became aware of the onset of complications.
2. *Failure to protect:* The hospital was found to have failed to provide sufficient protection to the patient from the incompetence of the attending physician.

Because this decision was originally upheld, this specific case has been cited time and time again as a precedent for determining a healthcare organization's responsibility to provide a system that monitors the quality of patient care and that has the authority to correct deficiencies in quality as soon as they become known, with or without direct consultation with the attending physician. The situation was made even more acute when a 1969 Supreme Court decision rescinded the immunity of charitable institutions such as hospitals and other not-for-profit organizations. This decision has created an environment in which healthcare organizations have been subjected to an ever-increasing amount of litigation, liability insurance premiums have sky-rocketed, and actual cash settlements have exploded into the realm of the unimaginable.

Negligence, or what is known as an "unintentional tort" in civil law, is today the single largest area of malpractice litigation. Typically, healthcare organizations are held liable for injuries in the following two categories[2]:

1. *Custodial:* falls or other similar injuries sustained as a result of environmental conditions; financial losses from litigation in this category are generally low, although the number of claims has remained very high throughout the past two decades
2. *Professional:* any injury sustained by a patient that is directly linked to the quality of care given or the absence of care after a need for such care had been established

For the past two and a half decades, the healthcare community has held that all injuries resulting from both of these forms of negligence are preventable, and today the industry firmly supports their elimination through demands for advanced training and a higher level of patient care.[3]

One direct result of the ever-increasing willingness of patients to hold the healthcare institution responsible for the quality of care provided is the sky-rocketing cost of malpractice insurance premiums. These now enormous premiums have increased the overall cost of operating a healthcare facility and today have combined with a variety of other factors to push the costs associated with health care to the extreme. In an effort to keep insurance premiums in check, many insurance carriers require healthcare organizations to develop and maintain complex risk management programs as a condition of coverage.

Local state governments began to support the call for a higher quality of patient care when, in January of 1977, the Florida legislature enacted a law that required hospitals, regardless of their size or type, to have an internal program designed to reduce risk to the patient. This law requires that each program maintain an internal incident review committee that oversees patient care and recommends courses of action that support improvements in care. The demands for risk management and quality assurance were further extended when the Joint Commission on Accreditation of Hospitals (now the Joint Commission on Accreditation of Healthcare Organizations, or JCAHO) instituted requirements addressing these issues on January 1, 1980.

Although it is true that the creation of a risk-free healthcare environment is virtually impossible, it is equally true that a viable program designed to implement systematic actions to reduce risks is not only possible but absolutely essential. The quality of health care is every professional care giver's responsibility, and the obligation for quality goes far beyond any laws or regulations, regardless of their severity. Without total dedication to the elimination of potential risk, the factors that have given rise to the current liability challenges to health care will persist and worsen. It is a fact of life throughout the industry that the cost of insurance premiums will continue to rise and the number of record-breaking malpractice settlements will continue to grow, especially with the increasing level of patient expectations, the overall decline in the number of qualified healthcare institutions, and the continual decrease in the number of highly trained specialists. In short, the necessity for a well-developed risk management program in every healthcare organization is not going to disappear. In fact, the continual rise in medical costs and the increasingly active regulatory role being played by the federal government are applying growing pressure to ensure that the treatments provided to patients are both necessary and of a quality that meets or surpasses nationally recognized standards.

This call for higher quality performance is universally accepted by the healthcare industry. Long a vigilant advocate for continually increasing the quality of care provided to patients, many healthcare organizations are close to collapse due to the insistence of the federal government and third-party payers that this higher quality care be delivered at continually lower cost. The demand for lower healthcare costs is today one of the most frequent refrains in the U.S. Congress and in virtually every state legislature. No longer can a healthcare provider treat a patient without keeping a keen eye on the cost of the treatment prescribed. Today's healthcare professional must monitor costs at every possible point of treatment while ensuring that no reduction in the quality of care occurs.

QUALITY ASSURANCE

Accountability, or the obligation to take responsibility for one's actions, grows out of the demand for quality patient care and the requirement for cost containment. These two issues are governed by the standards of performance and regulations that are typically under the oversight of the organization's office of quality assurance. This powerful office develops and/or coordinates all of the internal and external activities in which the healthcare provider engages that relate to establishing, maintaining, and assuring high-quality care for patients, including the assessment of patient care and implementation of corrective action when problems are identified.

The most effective form of quality assurance, however, comes not from an office or a management committee, but from the professionalism that all those responsible for healthcare delivery demand of themselves. Quality assurance based on professionalism can be both voluntary and mandatory. The best examples of voluntary quality assurance in the nursing profession are actions that adhere to the standards of nursing practice of the American Nurses Association

(ANA).[4] Mandatory compliance occurs when a healthcare organization establishes itself in such a manner that it conforms to the regulations of its state board of health. An action that can be considered both voluntary and compulsory is an action a hospital takes to meet JCAHO standards for accreditation. Although such action may be motivated purely by self-interest, a hospital's expenses will not be reimbursed by third-party payers (e.g., Medicare, Medicaid, and health insurance carriers) unless the hospital is accredited.

Quality assurance is the process by which performance (patient care) is evaluated for effectiveness. The system for carrying out quality assurance begins with the establishment of performance standards for appropriate levels and kinds of care. These standards provide the reference point for assessing all potential risk.

After the appropriate standards are established and the baseline or minimum acceptable quality is documented, then, and only then, can actions be taken to mitigate risk. The quality assurance program forms the foundation of every risk management program in operation today, in every sector of the healthcare industry.

The Quality Assurance Program

In the healthcare industry, quality assurance (often referred to as *QA*) is the systematic process used to evaluate the quality of care provided by a particular individual, unit, department, or organization. The process always involves (but is not necessarily limited to) the steps outlined in the following sections: (1) establishing performance and quality-of-care standards, (2) developing and formulating the specific criteria necessary to ensure that established standards are met, (3) evaluating, (4) planning and implementing the changes required to ensure compliance, and (5) following up.

ESTABLISHING PERFORMANCE AND QUALITY-OF-CARE STANDARDS

The healthcare industry and all of the associated professions have developed general standards of performance. Those that are applicable to the practice of nursing can be found in Appendix A of the ANA's *Nursing: Scope and Standard of Practice*.[4] The conduct of every nurse is governed by these broad standards as well as by the more specific standards developed by the particular organization, department, and unit in which the nurse practices. The particular standards that govern the direct care provided to specific patients are developed with consideration for the unique qualities of the unit and its ability to render specific types and levels of care. Together, all of the applicable standards form the foundation on which all quality assurance measures are based. An example of a typical nursing standard is the following:

> Every patient served by a nursing unit will have a written care plan that has been approved by a nurse manager.

DEVELOPING AND FORMULATING THE SPECIFIC CRITERIA NECESSARY TO ENSURE THAT ESTABLISHED STANDARDS ARE MET

After the standards of performance have been established, specific criteria must be developed so that compliance with the standards (whether and to what degree the standards are being met) can be determined. The criteria established to verify compliance must address broad-based standards as well as standards specific to the individual unit. The following is an example of a criterion used to verify compliance:

> For every patient, a nursing care plan is developed and written by a registered nurse and approved by the nurse manager within 12 hours of the patient's admission.

This criterion provides a *measurable* means of monitoring compliance with the quality assurance standard and can be used to measure the degree of performance effectively.

EVALUATING

The third step is an evaluation of the degree of implementation of the established standards; in other words, a periodic review of performance. There are, of course, an almost infinite number of methods that an organization can use to evaluate performance, but the most commonly employed is a review of documentation and performance (e.g., reading patient records, observing activities as they take place, and examining and interviewing patients, families, and staff).

In most organizations, the quality assurance evaluators use patient records to verify compliance simply because of their relative ease of use and availability, even though this practice is not as reliable as direct observation. Although the professional integrity of the average nurse is extremely high, it is quite possible to write treatments in the patient's chart that were never actually accomplished or, for that matter, to forget to annotate the chart with a treatment that was in fact performed. Further, at best the chart can only indicate that specific care was provided; it cannot give any indication of the quality of the treatment given. In the case of the previous examples, to evaluate implementation, patient records would be examined to verify that an individual care plan was written for each patient within the required 12 hours following admission and, if so, that all pertinent standards for such care plans were met.

Still other criteria would be used to r quality of the care plan. For example, th be reviewed to ensure compliance with the follo... standard:

> Every care plan will include patient education appropriate to the patient's medical diagnosis, nursing diagnosis, planned interventions, and discharge planning.

PLANNING AND IMPLEMENTING THE CHANGES REQUIRED TO ENSURE COMPLIANCE

One of the basic rules of quality assurance is that no performance is perfect all of the time; therefore, every program must allow for a process of planning that includes the development of methods for correcting deficiencies. To establish this process, the organization or unit must determine how much deviation from the established standard, if any, is allowed before changes are required. For example, if a nursing unit admits 50 patients in a specific period of time, and care plans are recorded for 45 of them within the required 12 hours after admission and for the remainder within 18 hours, is this deviation acceptable? If not, then exactly what must be done to remedy the situation (i.e., how should the deficiency be corrected)? Are there mitigating factors such as short staffing or perhaps an abundance of inexperienced nurses? Is the admission of 50 patients within the specified time considered an unusually large number of admissions?

The development of plans for correcting any and all noted deficiencies in performance is the responsibility of the nurse manager. After the nurse manager has collected all of the applicable information regarding the incident, including possible causes and any mitigating factors, the manager should consult with the unit staff and/or his or her supervisors and make plans for correcting the performance deficit.

FOLLOWING UP

Follow-up is necessary to confirm correction of all deficiencies noted during performance reviews and to ensure compliance with any new requirements imposed. The process of ensuring quality, like so many other processes, is never fully complete until someone follows up to see how effective changes have been in improving performance. Such follow-up is almost always the responsibility of the nurse manager but also may be performed by the manager's supervisors or even by the vice president of nursing. Regardless of who shoulders the responsibility, the process of follow-up is the final and very necessary step in the quality assurance process.

The lack of proper follow-up is the primary reason that so many quality assurance programs fall short of accomplishing their goal of ensuring quality care. Documenting current care levels and then developing a plan for improvement, no matter how well done or well intended, are absolutely futile unless an aggressive follow-up plan is included. It is follow-up that ensures compliance, not planning. Let us again continue the previous example. If the nurse manager finds that, for all of the next 50 patients, care plans are recorded within the 12-hour standard, then performance can be verified as having improved relative to that standard. If not, then another approach to compliance will have to be taken, or perhaps, under certain circumstances, the appropriateness of the criterion for that unit should be evaluated.

WARNING !

Compliance with a standard should always be the goal of the nurse manager. Attempting to change a criterion should be considered only when very unique circumstances prevail. Failure to abide by a standard all too often gives way to complacency throughout the unit—an undesirable situation in any segment of the healthcare industry.

Monitoring Nursing Care

The delivery of exceptional nursing care to a nursing unit's patients is not the only aspect of quality assurance that nurse managers encounter. As a matter of fact, a truly concerned organization extends the process of quality assurance into every facet of the business, from patient care to employee assistance. However, one of the most frequently encountered aspects of quality assurance, with which all nurse managers are frequently associated, is the continual monitoring of nursing care, something that takes place in virtually every healthcare organization today.

The monitoring of nursing care is a multifaceted process that always includes at least the four elements discussed in the following sections.

NURSING AUDIT

A nursing audit is used to understand exactly what services were provided to a patient, by whom, and to what level of performance quality. The actual audit can be conducted in a variety of different ways and can have a retrospective focus or can occur in parallel with the patient's actual treatment. Typically, however, the nursing audit is performed after the patient is discharged (retrospective). Regardless of when it takes place, the process involves a thorough examination of all the patient's records as well as a careful analysis of a large number of other cases to identify possible trends, areas requiring attention, deficiencies, and possibilities for improvement. The idea is to identify areas in which improvements in patient care can increase the overall quality of treatment provided by the organization.

A concurrent audit is one that is conducted while the patient is receiving his or her course of care. The purpose of the audit is to examine the care being given and to evaluate its effectiveness so that a desirable outcome can be ensured.

Regardless of which type of audit is conducted, the purpose is to discover ways that treatments can be improved and thereby to ensure the provision of high-quality care throughout the organization. These nursing audits are not intended to be witch hunts and should not be viewed as such by the nurse manager or any member of the staff.

PEER REVIEW

Peer review is a form of evaluation conducted by the nursing staff. It is a systematic process of determining the standards and criteria that are indicative of quality care and then assessing performance against them. This form of review considers the members of the nursing profession to be the individuals most capable of knowing what the indicators of quality care are and when this quality care is being provided. This reliance on professional knowledge is most useful when the organization faces a complicated issue, and most often the peer review process involves a number of highly qualified nurses at the same time. The individual opinions given by the nurses are compared to identify trends, areas requiring attention, deficiencies, and possibilities for improvement.

UTILIZATION REVIEW

Utilization reviews are mandated by JCAHO and are required for an organization to maintain its accreditation. They are intended to evaluate the organization to ensure that its current operational procedures are based on an appropriate allocation of resources. Although this type of review does not normally target the nursing department or nursing care, it often uncovers information about nursing practices that requires further investigation.

PATIENT SATISFACTION SURVEY

Today, almost every healthcare organization uses some type of formal method to determine the patient's level of satisfaction with the care received. The most commonly used information-gathering tool is the aftercare survey. This survey consists of a questionnaire that usually is mailed to the patient after discharge, but it can also be administered before the patient leaves the hospital. The patient is requested to complete the questionnaire and return it to hospital administration. This type of evaluation is usually not very effective in identifying broad areas in which the level of nursing care can be enhanced; however, it is extremely effective in identifying individual care providers who have not met the expectations of the patient. Patients tend to be very aware of what constitutes quality service, and most are extremely forthcoming in their evaluation of the level of care they received. However, because of the potential for patients to use the survey as a forum to dredge up personal grievances and provide individual opinion, all patient satisfaction surveys must be interpreted in conjunction with several other indicators of quality.

• • •

Once the healthcare organization has established its standards, published the criteria for determining adherence to those standards, and developed a variety of different methods for evaluating compliance with the standards, it is equipped to effectively evaluate its risk in relation to its accountability. Most organizations accomplish this analysis using one of the following methods:

- Employee and visitor safety review
- Patient-family incident review

Because the nursing profession is centered on the delivery of high-quality patient care, this chapter describes a typical risk management program that focuses on incidents involving patients and their families.

THE RISK MANAGEMENT PROGRAM

In the healthcare industry, the implementation of risk management is part of the on-going process of changing traditional management practices to align more closely with those of nonmedical businesses. In effect, risk management is to health care what prevention of product liability claims is to manufacturing industries. Risk management is the application of a planned program of loss prevention and liability control. The purpose of an effective program of risk management is to enable the organization to identify, analyze, and evaluate potential risks and meet these challenges by implementing procedures designed to reduce the occurrence, frequency, and severity of accidents and injuries. In almost every healthcare organization today, risk management is a process of detection, education, and intervention that is conscientiously carried out at every moment.

To implement a practical and effective program of risk management, the healthcare organization must establish it as a team process that involves every department and every employee. The program must encompass every facet of performance in the organization and enjoy the approval and support of the board of directors. It must couple inputs from the major departments (medicine, nursing, etc.) with the most minute concerns so that solutions can be implemented in a manner that will ensure compliance, cooperation, and cohesiveness among all elements of the organization. Departmental inputs can be received from many different sources; for example, the medicine and nursing departments supply their input through the following channels, among many others:

Annual reviews: the annual reviews conducted by the medical quality assurance committee or the policy procedure committee

Integral reviews: scheduled and unscheduled reviews conducted by the medical and nursing administrative staff

If the risk management program is to be effective, there must be commitment to the program throughout the management team, especially at the senior management level (i.e., the organization's chief executive officer and the director of the nursing service).

Structure

The typical healthcare risk management program encompasses the following activities:

Identification: the process of identifying any and all accident, injury, liability, and financial loss risks. This activity is normally accomplished through an organized process of communication, both formal and informal, and involves all elements of the organization. It also includes an on-going inspection program designed to identify potential problem (risk) areas. Once an area is identified, action is instituted to eliminate the risk on a proactive basis.

Review: an activity normally performed by an organized team of specialists who continually review existing institutional monitoring instruments, such as (a) incident reports, (b) audits, (c) committee minutes, (d) verbal complaints, and (e) patient questionnaires. The purpose of this review is to objectively evaluate all activities or occurrences that might lead to any form of action against the organization. The review committee analyzes all available input for its completeness and identifies any action that must be taken by the institution to reduce potential liability. This group also continually scans the marketplace to identify new systems that can be added to help in collecting factual data essential for risk management.

Analysis: the process of investigating all incidents that occur in the organization to identify potential liability. The focus is on determining the frequency, severity, and causes of previously known and newly identified risk categories, and special attention is given to any incident involving a patient, regardless of the severity. Plans are also developed to implement risk intervention strategies, and a system is provided for estimating the potential liability associated with individual risk categories.

Assessment: the examination of existing procedures to determine if any potential safety or liability issues are present. Most of the effort focuses on the identification and resolution of any form of risk involving current patient care procedures and the evaluation of any proposed programs.

Compliance verification: the process of ensuring that all activities are in compliance with the specifications of the applicable laws and codes that relate to procedures, operations, and patient safety, consent, and care.

Risk reduction: any and all processes that lead to the identification, elimination, and/or reduction of real and potential risk to the greatest degree possible.

Investigation: the aggressive review of all of the efforts of other committees throughout the organization. The primary focus is on evaluating what other committees have produced so that a fair and accurate determination of potential liability can be developed and effective recommendations can be made for actions to eliminate identified risk or, when critical incidents have occurred previously, for corrective actions to prevent future occurrences. This process involves a review of the actions taken and recommendations made by committees such as infection, medical audit, safety and security, pharmacy, nursing audit, and productivity.

Education: the proactive identification of patient, family, and personal knowledge-related needs that may be identified by other risk management actions. Suitable educational activities that can mitigate future risk to the organization are identified and developed.

Evaluation: the process of continually appraising the effectiveness of the risk management program.

Reporting: the development and control of internal reports to the organization's administration, medical staff, and board of directors, and compliance reporting to outside regulatory bodies and third-party insurance providers.

The Risk Management Committee

The creation of an effective risk management program must be supported at the highest management levels.

Failure of management to provide this support will certainly prevent the program from achieving any success. Therefore, the most senior management body of the healthcare organization (the board of directors, in most cases) must be the management element that creates the initial program. To accomplish this, the senior management body can issue an edict that (1) instructs the organization's chief executive to establish the program and (2) authorizes the expenditure of the necessary resources.

Once the determination has been made to create a risk management program and the decree has been received by the chief executive officer, a risk management committee, headed by a senior administrator, is appointed. This committee is responsible for the effective operation of the risk management program, including operational planning, budgeting, compliance verification, procedure development, analysis, and evaluation. Although it may delegate much of the day-to-day effort to subordinate bodies throughout the organization, all responsibility for and authority over the risk management process is held by this committee. To ensure that the program operates effectively and is linked closely with day-to-day performance, the committee appoints a risk manager to oversee the actual implementation of the program.

Typically, healthcare organizations limit membership on the risk management committee to senior managers but make sure that committee members represent a cross section of all operational elements. Interdisciplinary membership ensures that at least one representative from the medicine, nursing, medical records, legal counsel, education, and insurance claims departments will be appointed. The typical membership structure is as follows:

1. Risk manager
2. Nursing personnel: members typically include at least the following:
   - Nursing service administrator
   - Nurse manager representative
   - Staff nurse representative
3. Representative(s) of the medical staff
4. Committee chairs for the following areas:
   - Quality assurance
   - Utilization review
   - Infection control
   - Pharmacy
   - Therapeutics
   - Operating room
   - Legal
   - Human resources
5. Patient accounts representative(s)
6. Legal counsel: many times this is a ex-officio (nonvoting) member

7. Others: a wide variety of individuals may be included, but the education and training coordinator and a representative from the insurance claims department are almost always members

The committee normally elects a chairman from among its members. This chairman is usually the risk manager or a senior member of administration but can be anyone in the group. The responsibility of the chairman (in conjunction with the risk manager, if the latter does not hold this position) is to oversee the actions taken by the risk management committee. These include actions such as the following:

1. Develop and promote appropriate measures to minimize risk to patients and hospital personnel
2. Conduct all risk management activities in the organization
3. Develop risk management policies and guidelines for critical incident management
4. Establish and develop programs that will accomplish the following:
   - Increase staff awareness
   - Improve risk detection
   - Enhance performance through education
   - Ensure proper reporting of risk potential and risk-related incidents

The Risk Manager

The position of risk manager is usually filled by a senior member of the organization's administration. The risk manager is tasked with administering the risk management program throughout the institution. The risk manager executes his or her duties by serving as the primary liaison between the organization's senior administration, the risk management committee, and all other related hospital committees and departments. In addition, the risk manager provides liaison between the organization and insurance company representatives, hospital attorneys, and regulatory agencies. Typically, the risk manager reports directly to the chief executive officer or the organization's senior administrator and has a clearly defined function in the organizational structure of the institution.

During the early days of healthcare risk management, risk managers rarely were defined as such. They were selected from among the members of the senior management committee and came from a variety of backgrounds, including administration, law, nursing, quality assurance, and claims departments of insurance companies. What was needed at the time was someone who possessed effective communicative, analytic, and evaluative skills (such as those learned in designing and conducting research). These early risk

managers were also people who could easily develop positive interpersonal relationships and who were known as good leaders.

Today risk management is such an integral part of the healthcare management process that professional risk managers often staff these positions. Many universities now offer courses of study in risk management, and it is rapidly becoming a profession unto itself. These highly focused and capable managers today lead large multifaceted teams of professionals and play an incredibly important part in the successful operation of the healthcare institution.

Although the specific duties of the risk manager vary from organization to organization, the following duties will always be performed:

Direction of the risk management committee: schedules meetings and prepares agendas for the committee. If the risk manager is not the serving chairman of the committee, these duties will be relegated to the serving chairman, but the risk manager will assist.

Analysis: reviews all incident reports generated in the organization on a daily basis; makes recommendations and ensures the development of corrective action.

Investigation: usually oversees an investigation section that is charged with investigating all incident reports and making recommendations to the risk management committee on the findings.

Response: either takes action on critical incidents or refers them for action to appropriately qualified personnel, such as physicians, nurse managers, or heads of specific committees. Once an incident has been referred for action, the risk manager is responsible for following up on all incident reports with organizational staff, patients, and patients' families as necessary.

Monitoring: monitors the data collection mechanisms such as incident report summaries; oversees the development of specific instructions and standards to ensure accurate and timely collection of relevant data.

Patient liaison: periodically visits with patients at high risk and their families to demonstrate the organization's concern for their welfare firsthand. This practice is extremely important, because the demonstration of concern has been proven to be the single most effective method available to healthcare institutions to avoid or at least reduce litigation. Although there is no accurate method of identifying all patients who are at high risk, this category typically includes those patients receiving long-term care; those admitted multiple times; those admitted into the intensive care, critical care, and cardiac care units;

those coming to the emergency department at night; and postoperative patients.

Litigation management: ensures the preparation of reports that provide periodic summaries of active and resolved litigation. These reports identify the type of litigation, the degree of culpability (if any), the outcome, and the cost.

Reporting: at a minimum, prepares and submits to the board of directors via the senior administrative officer a periodic summary incident report; also manages the development of reports on any special or specific action requested by the board of directors, the chief executive officer, and regulatory agencies.

Administration of the risk management program: acts as the single individual charged with the development, implementation, and administration of the risk management program. This duty is usually discharged with the assistance of specialized personnel from departments throughout the organization, the chair of the risk management committee, the risk management committee members, and staff education department.

Fig. 15-1 shows the typical relationships among the various tasks and personnel involved in a risk management program.

THE ROLE OF NURSING IN RISK MANAGEMENT

The effect of the nursing department on the organization's risk management program cannot be underestimated. It is this department that contributes the greatest risk exposure to the organization through its around-the-clock patient care, and effective risk man-

agement by every member of the nursing department is obligatory if the institution is to have a successful risk management program.

The nursing department, led by the senior nursing administrator, must be committed to the successful implementation of the organization's risk management program. The attitude and dedication of the nursing management team is the single biggest factor in positively influencing the staff and gaining their willing participation. It is the nursing staff, through their continuous patient contact, who will ultimately implement and guarantee the success of the risk management program.

Risk management is critical to the mitigation of liability in the nursing department, because the activities of the nursing staff continually intersect five areas of highest risk in the organization:

1. *Medication:* Errors may be caused by the administration of improper medication, improper administration of ordered medication, and failure to identify errors in the prescription of medication.

2. *Complications:* Complications may occur from diagnostic or treatment procedures. Although typically they are not *caused* by nursing personnel, a high percentage of litigation has placed blame on the nursing team by citing failure to anticipate complications.

3. *Accidents:* Unexpected and many times unavoidable patient accidents, such as falls, continue to be a major risk to the healthcare organization, especially in times of staff reduction.

4. *Perception:* Patient or family dissatisfaction with care, whether the deficiencies are real or imagined, is a continual source of risk to the health-

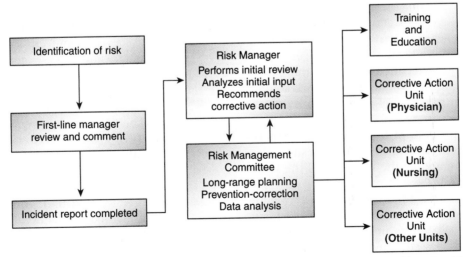

Fig. 15-1 ■ Typical relationships among the various tasks and personnel involved in a risk management program.

care organization. The nursing staff play a critical role in developing the patient's perception of the organization as a caring, professional, and well-operated institution.

5. *Refusal of treatment:* When a patient or a patient's family member refuses prescribed treatment or will not provide consent for a specific treatment, even if it is determined to be life enhancing, the risk to the organization is always significant. The nursing staff play a critical part in explaining treatments and obtaining consent, and it is essential that this aspect of risk be well managed.

Although the five aforementioned risk areas are critical, there is one other area in which nurses have the primary responsibility that must be continually monitored by the risk management program, and that is record keeping. The medical records and incident reports that are generated by the nursing department provide the organization with far more than just the documentation of hospital, nurse, and physician accountability. These records also serve as a first line of defense in cases in which litigation is pursued. At the same time, however, the preparation and maintenance of these records is the single biggest source of risk to the organization. For example, it is conservatively estimated that, for every incident reported, as many as 35 go unreported. Historically, when hospital records have been subpoenaed during litigation and information in them has been found to be faulty, inadequate, or incomplete, the organization has almost always been found negligent in the care of the aggrieved patient, and the judgments awarded have been significantly higher.[3]

Incident Reporting

Throughout the healthcare industry, incident reports are used to analyze the severity, frequency, and causes of unplanned events that fall within the five major risk areas. The analysis of these reports provides the individual organization with a basis for intervention.

It cannot be stated too often or too emphatically that accurate and comprehensive reporting both on the patient's chart and in individual incident reports is essential to the organization's ability to protect itself and its individual care providers from the damaging effects of litigation.

Incident reporting starts on the front line of contact with the patient and therefore is most often the responsibility of the individual staff nurse as he or she is directed by the nurse manager. Although virtually every nurse readily acknowledges the importance of reporting accurately, very few actually aggressively pursue an individual policy of doing so. In fact, most nurses—and this includes most nurse managers—are reluctant to provide accurate documentation, probably due to the historically overzealous reactions received from administration officers. The fear of the consequences of providing this information that is harbored either consciously or unconsciously by most nursing personnel is a major cause of risk in the industry today.

Elimination of the fear of the consequences of accurate reporting is critical to the effective management of risk. Although this is an on-going problem and one with significant complications, most of the issues can be resolved by aggressively engaging in the following two leadership activities:

1. *Educating:* The provision of adequate training is a fundamental part of leadership. An effective staff education program emphasizing the importance of comprehensive, objective reporting that omits inflammatory words and judgmental statements is a critical initial step in developing confidence in staff nurses. This form of training is also highly recommended for all members of the organization's management team, without exception.

2. *Accepting accountability:* The demonstration and professional acceptance of accountability is critical to the development of effective incident reporting. Accountability is taking responsibility for one's individual actions and, in the case of management, the actions of subordinates. The problem that plagues so many organizations is management's historical desire to turn accountability into a witch hunt that omits or overlooks management's responsibility and places the blame on the individual performer. Nurse managers, in their role as leaders of individual nursing units, must demonstrate a clear understanding that the purpose of the incident reporting process is to provide documentation and enable follow-up. This professional group must lead the effort to ensure that incident reports are not used, under any circumstances, for the initiation of disciplinary action.

Exactly what constitutes a reportable incident, as defined by the standards and operational procedures of the institution, varies slightly from organization to organization. However, nearly all organizations agree that a reportable incident includes any unplanned or unexpected circumstance that directly or indirectly affects or may potentially affect any patient or family member.

The quality of the report is influenced by the professionalism demonstrated by the reporting nurse and the suitability of the form used to construct the report. Therefore, nurse managers should focus their attention on both issues (i.e., development of the professional ability required for the staff nurse to write a good report and the adequacy of the form and the data it calls for).[5] A representative form is shown in Fig. 15-2.

Each organization will have its own specific standards of performance for identifying and handling reportable incidents; however, most processes for dealing with such incidents will include the following six basic steps:

1. *Detection:* The discovery of a potential risk can occur at just about any time and can be reported by just about anyone. Reports of potential risk can be received from physicians, nurses, therapists, specialists, other hospital employees, volunteers, patients, or even a member of a patient's family.

2. *Notification:* Once the risk has been identified, it must be reported to the risk management system. This is accomplished by completing the organization's critical incident report form and forwarding it to the risk manager. The report must be filed within 24 hours of the initial identification of the risk. If the incident is significant enough, a telephone call or e-mail may be appropriate to alert the risk management department of the incident so that the department can expedite its follow-up action. This is especially true for extremely serious incidents, especially potentially life-threatening events.

3. *Investigation:* Once the incident report has been received, the risk manager immediately initiates an investigation into the incident. All facts uncovered become part of the permanent file concerning the incident.

4. *Discussion:* Because the risk management department cannot possibly employ all of the technical experts needed to completely evaluate every incident that can occur in a healthcare institution, the risk manager often seeks outside assistance. In investigating most incidents, the manager consults with physicians, risk management committee members, or both.

5. *Response:* Once the facts of the incident have been gathered and analyzed and a resolution has been developed, the risk manager eliminates any misunderstanding of the situation on the part of those involved, especially if they include a patient or any member of the patient's family. The discussion should be brief and should cover the points necessary for resolution of the concern. The risk manager should always refrain from implying fault or responsibility for the incident in his discussion with a patient. If necessary, the patient is referred to an appropriate source for assistance, and compensation for any needed service is offered by the hospital.

6. *Documentation:* The risk manager makes sure that all records regarding the incident are filed appropriately. These include as a minimum the incident report, any records outlining the follow-up procedures that were implemented, and documentation of any action that was taken.

Risk Categories

Although it would be foolish to attempt to list every possible risk that can be present in a healthcare organization, some rather broad categories can be identified that go beyond individual organizational structures and specific missions. Several of these have been mentioned earlier. The following sections discuss four major risk categories that apply to virtually every organization in the healthcare industry.

MEDICATION

Errors in the delivery of prescribed medication, although perhaps not a common occurrence in a specific nursing unit, certainly are encountered frequently enough throughout the industry to be a major area of risk and are significant enough to warrant their own special risk category. Two classes of error that fall into this category are the following:

Errors in the administration of intravenous (IV) fluids: incidents in which a patient is given the wrong fluid, a patient is not given a fluid that has been prescribed, or the correct fluid is given but is delivered at the wrong time or in the wrong dosage

Errors in the administration of prescribed medication (excluding IV fluids): incidents in which a patient is given the wrong medication, the wrong medication is prescribed, a properly prescribed medication is not given, or a properly prescribed medication is given in the wrong dosage or by the wrong delivery method

EXAMPLE A: JONES, M. R.

The risk was developed as a downstream effect of a mistake made when the patient was admitted from the emergency department to a general nursing unit. The admitting clerk transcribed the patient's weight incorrectly from the emergency department sheet, and the dosage of medication that was calculated and delivered after admitting the patient was based on the incorrect weight. The first dose of the medication given was nearly double the amount that would have been proper for the patient's correct weight. The error was discovered after the first dose had been given, and a correction was entered in the patient's chart. The attending physician omitted the scheduled second dose.

Critical Incident Report

Date of incident:	Risk management required? Yes ☐ No ☐

PATIENT

Number:

Risk management officer assigned:

Patient name:

Risk management control number:

Address:

| Ward No.: | Room No.: | Home phone No.: | Age: | Sex: ☐ M ☐ F | Date admitted: |

Reason for admission:

Attending physician: Charge/primary nurse:

List medications administered within previous 6 hours (if applicable)

Adjustable bed height? ☐ Yes ☐ No   Position: ☐ High ☐ Low   Bedrails: ☐ Up ☐ Down ☐ None   Is this a legal issue?

Activity orders: ☐ Restraints ☐ Bedrest ☐ "Close" assistance   ☐ Up assistance   ☐ Yes ☐ No

Type of incident: Medication   Diagnostic procedure   Patient movement   Patient treatment   Patient/family attitude

INCIDENT FACTS

Exact location of incident:

| Day of week: | Date: | Time: | Shift: ☐ Day ☐ Eve ☐ Night |

Description of incident by person preparing report:

Name(s) of persons present at time of incident (include employees):	Address:	Phone No.:
1		
2		
3		
4		
5		
6		
7		

MEDICAL

Was person involved examined by a physician in hospital?   Yes ☐ No ☐   Date: Time: Where:

Name of physician: Any apparent injury? Yes ☐ No ☐   X-rays taken?   Yes ☐ No ☐

Physician's comments:

| Signature of person preparing report: _____ | Title: | Date: |

Printed name of individual preparing report:

Immediate follow-up:

Follow-up at discharge:

_____
Signature of patient care manager

Fig. 15-2 ■ Example of a critical incident report form.

EXAMPLE B: MILES, B. M.

The attending physician ordered that Tegretol (carbamazepine) be given to the patient. When the medex was checked, dosage was found to be listed as "Tegretol 100 mg chewable tab—50 mg p.o. b.i.d." The patient received Tegretol 100 mg p.o. at 14:00 and not the correct dose of 50 mg p.o. as listed in the medex. When the nurse manager checked medications at 14:30, she detected the error, noting that the correct dose was 50 mg instead of the 100 mg that was given. The attending physician was notified, and she instructed the nursing staff to hold the second dose.

EXAMPLE C: BROWN, W. C.

While conducting rounds at 15:30 the registered nurse noted that the bag of fluid hanging was D$_5$ISOM (dextrose 5% in Isolyte M) and not the prescribed D$_5$W (dextrose 5% in water). The patient's chart indicated that the bag was last checked at 14:00. The bag was changed immediately to the prescribed D$_5$W and the attending physician was notified.

DIAGNOSTIC PROCEDURES

Incidents that occur before, during, or after a sample stick, biopsy, contrast radiography, lumbar puncture, or other invasive procedures present another potentially problematic area.

EXAMPLE A: WONG, P. H.

During a normal check of the patient's IV site, it was noticed that the site was inflamed and distended. The IV was disconnected immediately, and when the tape was removed, a small portion of the skin was found to have broken down in the area where the tape had been applied. In addition, there was a small knot on the medial aspect of the left antecubital area immediately above the IV insertion site. The patient's physician was notified and the wound was dressed.

EXAMPLE B: PUNDEL, B. F.

When the patient was being turned, she complained of a burning sensation. Further investigation revealed a rash covering 50% to 75% of both buttocks. The absorbent pad on the patient's bed was found to be heavily saturated with urine. Bed linens were changed and powder was applied to the patient's buttocks.

REFUSAL OR NONCONSENT

Situations in which a patient or a member of a patient's family refuses treatment that has been prescribed or refuses to sign consent papers represent another area of concern.

EXAMPLE A: DIFFICULT, I. M.

Immediately following a visit from his parish priest, the patient proclaimed that he no longer was in need of medical attention and demanded to be discharged.

The patient was asked to wait until his physician could be called. During the personal consultation with the patient, the physician explained the potential side effects if treatment were discontinued. The physician's comments had a limited effect on the patient as he continued to ask for immediate discharge. After several attempts at persuasion, the physician explained the hospital's "against medical advice" form and secured the patient's signature. The patient was discharged without medication.

EXAMPLE B: NOTWELLINFORMED, I. M.

The patient refused to sign the consent form for a bone marrow procedure, stating that he did not understand the potential side effects. When the physician arrived, he reviewed the reasons for doing the test and the possible side effects three different times. After the discussion, the patient still indicated a lack of understanding, so the physician informed the patient that if he did not have the patient's consent in writing, he would be unable to perform the test and offered to have another physician provide the patient with a second opinion, to which the patient agreed. After the consulting doctor left, the patient signed the consent form even though he still indicated a lack of full understanding of the potential side effects.

PATIENT OR FAMILY ATTITUDE TOWARD CARE

Whenever a patient or a member of a patient's family indicates a general dissatisfaction with the care that has been provided and attempts to resolve the situation have not met with positive results, it is imperative that an incident report be filed.

EXAMPLE A: JONES, B. A.

The patient was an 8-month-old infant, and the mother complained that she found the child saturated with urine when she arrived each morning at approximately 08:00. The mother was informed that the procedure was to change infant diapers and bed linens during the 06:00 feedings and before medications were given. The chart indicated that the child's diaper was changed each morning at the prescribed time and a check of the skin on the patient's back, buttocks, and perineal areas showed it to be free of breakdown. The parents were not satisfied with the explanation and expressed their concern that the hospital was not doing enough to safeguard the child's health. Treatment was discussed with the patient's primary nurse, and the matter was referred to the nurse manager.

EXAMPLE B: SMITH, B. B.

The patient appeared to be extremely upset and angry. He informed the nurse that he felt his wife had been mistreated in the emergency department waiting room the previous night. He repeatedly expressed a desire to speak to someone from administration, but when the nurse called, she was unable to reach the on-duty administrator. The nurse told Mr. Smith that she would continue to try to locate the on-duty administrator and offered the patient an opportunity to call at a later time or perhaps the next morning. Somewhat placated, Mr. Smith thanked the nurse for her time and assured her that he would call the administrator the next day.

THE ROLE OF THE NURSE MANAGER

A well-designed and well-functioning risk management system allows the healthcare facility to act proactively in a wide variety of areas; for example, by doing the following:

Focusing on the basic cause of potential liability claims: This is critical because long-term study has shown that most liability claims can be resolved with prompt and purposeful action at the time of the infraction.

Detecting deficiencies early: If operated well, the risk management system will be of significant benefit to the organization in its efforts to identify those employees, units, departments, procedures, and regulations that are not meeting patients' expectations or that could potentially cause harm.

Identifying communication failure: Rapid identification of those situations in which the communication systems in the organization fail greatly enhances the opportunity for the organization to remedy a deficiency before a claim is filed.

The success or failure of any organization's risk management program will be determined by the quality of nursing performance and the attention given to it by the individual nurse manager. Because they are at the management level closest to actual patient care, nurse managers are pivotal to the success of risk management. It is absolutely imperative that nurse managers consider risk management to be one of their most fundamental and critical responsibilities.

Developing the required sense of urgency begins with understanding the importance of the risk management program. Because nurse managers typically work in extremely stressful environments and continually juggle a myriad of responsibilities, it is important that they be well informed. How well the organization's senior management and administration keep the unit managers informed of the critical issues pertaining to them often determines whether individual healthcare managers perform to their highest level of professionalism. Nurse managers make decisions every day, hundreds of them, and they do so based on the known or perceived priority of each. To make

the right decision and ultimately assign the correct priority to that decision, all nurse managers must understand that risk management is critical.

Teaching the importance of risk management is the organization's responsibility. Nurse managers must be taught to consider everyday occurrences as more than the simple events they appear to be. For example, they must learn to see beyond the obvious and identify every patient incident and patient's or family member's expression of dissatisfaction as a serious failing in the level of quality being achieved in patient care. Perhaps even more importantly, however, nurse managers must see these incidents as potential liabilities for the organization. Every time a patient becomes distraught enough to register a complaint, it must be treated as a critical indication of high risk. In addition, nurse managers must understand that apparent satisfaction on the part of the patient is not an absolute measure of low risk, because many people will not complain before seeking outside legal advice. To assist nurse managers in maintaining close liaison with the patients in their charge, with their employees, and with all associated departments, the risk management system should emphasize leadership, managerial skills enhancement, and service quality. Nurse managers should receive extensive training in the emotional as well as the technical aspects of management.

In their position as the manager closest to the actual delivery of patient care, nurse managers are instrumental in establishing the patient's positive perception of the organization. Historically, more litigation has been initiated as a result of poor communication between the organization, its immediate representatives, and the patient than for any other single reason. What makes this statistic difficult to bear is that an extremely high percentage of the legal cases that were ultimately lost by healthcare organizations could have been prevented if, after an incident or bad outcome, the patient or the patient's family had received a quick, simple visit from a well-trained hospital representative. An example of just how effective rapid action by a skilled communicator can be is provided by the following true story:

Rachel had been hospitalized for a tonsillectomy in August, and when she returned home, her mother discovered a needle embedded in her foot. Rachel's mother called the hospital to determine a course of action. When she was connected to the nurse manager of the Pediatric Department, she was given information that was pertinent, helpful, and understandable. The nurse manager requested that Rachel's mother send the hospital the piece of needle so that appropriate tests could be made to eliminate any unforeseen complications, and offered to provide free medical assistance if Rachel should need it.

Several days later, the nurse manager called Rachel's mother to inquire about the child's condition. She was informed that Rachel was fine and received an expression of appreciation from the mother for the follow-up call.

Even though the offer of free medical assistance had been made to Rachel's mother, the nurse manager never heard from her again, until several weeks later when she received a letter of appreciation that formally thanked her for "caring."

In contrast, consider the following situation in which poor communication and poor-quality service was a leading factor in a court action:

While being prepared for surgery, Marks received an overdose of preoperative medication. The side effects were rather severe and the scheduled surgery was delayed until the effects of the medication were under control. When discussing the issue with the parents, the nurse manager explained the facts in a cold, unemotional manner and quickly outlined the hospital's position regarding any potential liability for what she termed "the accident." She did not make herself available for questions, nor did she refer the parents to a physician. Neither did she tell the parents that the hospital had kept the child under close observation by specialists until there was absolutely no possibility of continued danger. In fact, she offered no comforting information whatsoever, and left the parents to think the worst.

Several weeks later, the nurse manager and the hospital's senior administrator were each served with a court summons requiring them to testify in the case of *Marks v. Saint Vincent's;* the suit was litigated for nearly 3 weeks, ending in a mid–six-figure settlement to Marks. The settlement was not awarded for the actual mistake that had been made in preoperative care but for the stress and turmoil that the parents had been put through by the hospital. The fact that Marks had received significant attention from specialists and that extraordinary effort was made to protect his life was never an issue in support of the hospital, because the manager failed to inform the parents of these interventions.

In both of these situations, prompt attention and care by the nurse manager did protect—or could have protected—the organization from a serious liability claim. The divergent outcomes of these two incidents bring home the point that needs to be learned; namely, that recognition of the incident, quick personal follow-up and action, personal contact, and effective, compassionate communication can make the difference between resolving a situation of risk and losing a litigated case. Conservative estimates are that as many as 90% of all patient and family concerns can and should be handled at the unit level. It cannot be stressed enough that the presence of a risk management program and a designated risk manager does not eliminate the need for nurse managers to develop their patient communication skills. When nurse managers cannot effectively deal with these types of challenges to the organization, they are negligent in discharging their responsibility to their patients, themselves, and the organization as a whole. The organization's risk management system and the risk manager are tools of support; they do not eliminate professional responsibility.

Fundamental Behaviors

Working with a patient or a member of the patient's family, especially in situations in which potential risk is involved, can be exceptionally difficult. The handling of a patient's or family member's complaints is extremely important, however, and should never be taken lightly or passed off to another unless that individual can enhance the situation. What makes these confrontations difficult is not the professional explanation that is required but the emotionally charged circumstances that surround them.

Nurse managers need to know how to handle emotional situations involving patients. Many times, these emotional exchanges are simply a release of pent-up emotion, but all too frequently they are the beginning of a long and expensive court action. The more nurse managers can do to defuse these emotionally charged moments, the greater the opportunity to minimize the organizational risk involved. The cardinal rule is that patients and family members must be satisfied. Box 15-1 lists a set of behaviors that can be used to deal with a complaint and ensure satisfaction of the patient or family member. Usually, the resolution of these emotionally charged moments requires nothing more than exercising good old-fashioned common sense.

BOX 15-1

Handling Complaints

1. Listen carefully to the complaint and indicate attention with positive body signals.
2. Do not speak until the complainant has finished talking.
3. Do not react with emotion or become defensive; do not quote policy.
4. Ask the complainant what he or she feels would be a satisfactory solution.
5. Explain what can and cannot be done to solve the problem and why.
6. Agree on specific steps to be taken and specific deadlines.

The first two key behaviors listed in Box 15-1 have to do with *listening*. This is a skill that appears to be relatively simple but is in fact extraordinarily difficult for many people. Nurse managers who have difficulty in this area should try to remember the following three simple rules:

1. *Never argue.* Arguing is never a good approach, because it will only increase the person's anger or emotion. Trying to defend one's position by raising one's voice or disagreeing with another is foolhardy at best and in many cases is like throwing gasoline on an open flame.

2. *Never quote policy.* Telling the patient or family member what the organization's policy is will never improve a potentially damaging situation. In such a circumstance, policy is not a defense, it is a shelter that people hide behind, and that is exactly how the patient or family member will view it. Tom Peters, the business guru who wrote the book *In Search of Excellence*, makes the statement that quoting policy is simply another way of saying "you can't do that."[6]

3. *Don't interrupt.* Nothing will get an angry person excited faster than being interrupted when he or she is trying to make a point. This form of conduct is both unprofessional and reprehensible. The other individual should be allowed to talk and make his or her point. Many times, that is all that is necessary to completely resolve the issue.

After the nurse manager listens carefully, it is time to make a realistic attempt at problem resolution. Often, this can be done simply by asking what the person expects in the form of a solution. After the person's desires have been heard, the nurse manager must be able to negotiate a settlement between the individual's expectation and the realistic possibilities. Carefully, the nurse manager, supported by other hospital representatives if necessary, should explain what, in his or her professional opinion, might be the best approach to resolution. What can and cannot be done and why should be explained. No attempt should be made to negotiate with the injured party until he or she understands the options. The nurse manager should not lie, conceal, or belittle the person's concern. It is important to be as specific as possible and to avoid as much ambiguity as possible. Vague resolutions of problems generally create more severe problems later.

Documentation

Nurse managers must also be sure that all incidents are properly documented. The documentation on the incident form should be detailed and should include all the factors relating to the incident as demonstrated in the previous examples. However, the documentation in the patient's chart should contain only simple, straightforward statements of the *facts* and of the patient's physical response. It is imperative that proper wording be used; no reference should be made to the incident report and no negative words such as *error* or *inappropriate* should be used. For example, if a patient received an improper dose of a prescribed drug, the chart should read, "100 mg of meperidine administered. Physician notified." The remainder of the comments made in the chart should include any patient reaction such as, "Patient's vital signs unchanged." If there is an untoward reaction, a follow-up note should be written in the chart, giving an update of the patient's status. A note related to the patient's reaction should be written as frequently as the status changes and should continue until the patient returns to the status level that existed before the incorrect dose was administered.

When the incident report is completed, every facet of the incident should be detailed. This is the time to be expressive, not reserved. The more accurately information can be related in this report, the better-equipped the organization will be to resolve the incident and protect itself from potential litigation. Note that the sample incident report form shown in Fig. 15-2 contains a section requesting details on the follow-up (the block reading "Immediate follow-up" and "Follow-up at discharge"). Nurse managers are generally responsible for determining the appropriate follow-up, and this section of the form should never be left blank. In the case of the patient with the tissue change around the IV site presented earlier, the nurse manager's immediate follow-up action would be noted and a comment would be included indicating that the nurse manager had referred the matter to the attending physician. A possible entry written at the time of the patient's discharge might be the following: "Discussed matter with attending physician. Follow-up treatment indicated that the skin around the IV site is healing well. Patient's mother was provided with an appointment at the outpatient clinic so the site could be checked and the progress of healing monitored. Patient's condition will be noted and follow-up will continue as necessary."

A strong word of caution needs to be included at this point. Nurse managers are responsible for protecting the organization. That is the bottom line of every manager's responsibility. Charting and completing incident reports are excellent times to remember this basic duty. The patient's chart and the incident report are not places that should be used to indicate fault. These documents can easily be subpoenaed and can be used in litigation against the hospital. Negative comments such as "The incident would never have occurred if Dr. X had written the correct order in the first place" or "This carelessness is inexcusable" are totally inappropriate and should be reserved for other forums.

Although it is no secret that many errors are caused by carelessness and that individuals are practicing in the healthcare field who possibly should not be there, these concerns are better expressed in ways that allow them to be controlled internally, such as before the risk management committee or in the nurse manager's office.

The Proper and Professional Attitude

The nurse manager is the individual who sets the tone in the nursing unit. It is the nurse manager who molds the professional attitudes of all members of the staff, from janitor to senior registered nurse. Therefore, logic decrees that it is also the nurse manager who creates the type of environment that fosters safety and low-risk performance. Studies have shown that, in units in which managers lead by example and display a professional and caring attitude, the incidence of unacceptable behavior resulting in patient-related incidents and legal challenges is minimal. When nurse managers understand that their role as a manager is to develop an environment in which trust, good communication, and quality performance are constantly present, they are far more likely to avoid incidents that place the organization and themselves at risk. In fact, although incidents involving gross negligence sometimes do occur, the most frequent cause of litigation is an unfriendly, uncaring attitude on the part of hospital staff.

The importance of attitude can easily be seen in the following real-life examples. Evaluate the very different outcomes and consider whether both incidents could not have ended properly.

PATIENT A

Upon the patient's return from the radiology department, it was noted that the skin around the IV site was very puffy from obvious leakage of dye into the tissue. After 3 days, the skin sloughed. A note placed in the patient's chart by the physician at the time of discharge indicated that plastic surgery would be required to return the area to a normal appearance. No critical incident report was filed, and there was no indication that the incident had been discussed with the patient. Within 6 weeks following the patient's discharge, the hospital received notification from the patient's attorney of the intent to initiate a suit.

PATIENT B

Upon the patient's return from the radiology department, infiltration was noted at the IV site. A critical incident report was filed as soon as the patient was settled, which indicated that the dye had infused into the tissue. The nurse manager noted in the incident report that she wished to provide follow-up, and the risk manager, after the investigation, returned the incident report to her. Discussion of the incident led to consultation with the patient's physician, and together, the three informed the patient of the possibility of a skin slough. They offered to provide the patient with appropriate referral and treatment, if necessary. Continued follow-up showed that there was an indication of skin sloughing, and the physician determined that plastic surgery might be required. Arrangements for future treatment were made with the patient. The family took no legal action.

It is easy to see from these two examples that it was the nurse manager's immediate and professional action in the second case that made the difference in the final outcome. Professionalism begins with the attitude demonstrated by the manager—in every situation—and nursing is no exception. If history indicates that a friendly, professional, and caring attitude prevents most legal action, then why don't all nurse managers consider it their responsibility to develop this approach? What should be done with nurse managers who have cold and distant relations with their staffs and with the unit's patients? Consider the example provided earlier of the mother who was distressed about her baby's condition when she arrived at the hospital each morning. It is simple to see how the situation easily could have ended up in litigation. Parents, almost without exception, become extremely distressed if their children are not cared for in what *they* consider an appropriate manner. If no personal response or follow-up is made when they register a complaint, they are very likely to react emotionally, and even legally. When the complaint is met with reasonable concern and follow-up, however, there is every reason to believe that the parents not only will not institute legal action but will become advocates for what they perceive as a "caring and professional" organization. It is the nurse manager who creates an environment of concern, compassion, and professionalism. Staff members will emulate the qualities they are shown. In almost every incident investigated, it is attitude and lack of concern that set the wheels of legal action in motion. Think what it could mean for the nurse manager and the nursing unit never to have to face legal action and the results it can bring.

Although nurse managers will be involved in other aspects of the risk management system, such as determining staff educational needs and participating in programs designed to meet those needs, or in establishing protocols for classifying patients at risk, their primary responsibility will always be to create a caring, professional, and compassionate environment in the nursing unit. Regardless of their level of activity, however, nurse managers' positive and aggressive participation is critical to the success of the risk management program.

EVALUATION OF RISK MANAGEMENT

Effectively identifying and reducing the risk inherent in the delivery of health care requires close monitoring and analysis of every incident report filed. The organization should work to develop strong and explicit directives governing the completion of these important documents and should establish a standard of performance that is obligatory for every member of the staff.

It is the organization's management team that will determine whether the risk management program is an effective or an ineffective one. Although every good risk management program needs support and participation by all staff, what it needs far more is direction, support, and active participation by every member of management. This requirement for full and total support by management is absolute, and no manager should ever be allowed to avoid it.

Does management have a track record of support for risk management? Not really. In fact, because risk management programs require funding and personnel resources, it has been the practice of management during lean times when budgets are closely examined to make the risk management program one of the first to be cut. Is this because hospital administrators don't want a low-risk environment? No, it is because they don't believe in paying what it costs to implement and maintain an effective program that, once in place and operating effectively, removes the fundamental reasons it was initiated in the first place. When the litigation dies away because the organization is behaving responsibly, the first question asked about the risk management program is, "Do we still need it?"

Risk management is initiated to reduce those losses that need not occur, and continual implementation is required to guarantee continued success. In fact, this is one case in which it can truthfully be said that it is absolutely necessary to spend money to save it. Management needs to understand that realizing a return on the investment will take time but that, without total commitment, it will be difficult to calculate how much can be lost. What is absolutely true is that, almost without exception, risk management programs have proven to be far more than cost effective; they have proven to be a significant means of *generating* money instead of *losing* money.

A well-developed risk management program can increase revenue because it creates the perception of excellence in the minds of the physicians who refer patients and in the community itself. Given a choice, all doctors and all patients will choose a hospital they think is more professional, more concerned, and more caring than others. Responsiveness to patients' needs will always be seen as a reason to choose one institution over the available competition. The medical profession has had more than its share of negative press in the past, and future incidents will continue to generate the sensationalism that sells newspapers. Most of the time, this is a good thing. Because of this sensationalism and the unbelievably high settlements awarded patients through court decisions, the courts, insurance carriers, and legislatures have demanded that the healthcare industry improve its ability to respond to patient demands. Effective risk management meets this obligation.

Finally, risk management makes good sense for the industry and for every nurse manager working in it. It has proven its ability to positively affect the quality of patient care and, ultimately, to reduce potential liability. In fact, it is one of the best means available for the healthcare industry to showcase the outstanding character and professionalism of everyone involved in the medical professions.

SUMMARY

- The need for accountability in healthcare institutions has prompted the recent development of quality assurance and risk management programs.
- Quality assurance is the process by which patient care is evaluated for effectiveness.
- A quality assurance program is the basis for managing risk.
- The key ingredients of successful patient care–related risk management are an organized method of incident reporting; review and follow-up of reported incidents; a risk management program that includes a risk manager and a committee with well-defined objectives; nurse managers who support the risk management program; and, most important, maintenance of an environment that is perceived as friendly and caring by patients and their families.
- Detection, notification, investigation, discussion, response, and documentation were said to be the steps used in reporting incidents.
- The best methods for handling a dissatisfied or angry patient or family member are:
  1. Listen carefully to the complaint and indicate attention with positive body signals.
  2. Do not speak until the complainant has finished speaking.

3. Do not react with emotion or become defensive. Do not quote policy.
4. Ask the complainant what he or she feels would be a satisfactory solution.
5. Explain what can and cannot be done to solve the problem and why.
6. Agree on specific steps to be taken and specific deadlines.

■ The documentation on the incident form should be detailed, including all of the factors relating to the incident as demonstrated in the previous examples. However, the documentation of the patient's chart should contain only simple, straightforward statements of the *facts* and of the patient's physical response.

■ The organization's management is directly responsible for the success or failure of risk management programs.

FINAL THOUGHTS

Many healthcare organizations are in the process of transforming their internal systems to quality management systems. Historically, this approach to management has been proven to result in a significant increase in productivity and a dramatic decrease in risk exposure. The development of an effective quality improvement program requires the identification of patients' expectations, comprehensive planning (both short and long term), a multidisciplinary approach to management and leadership, careful evaluation of projected outcomes, and modification of the managerial style of the organization to create a working environment that promotes initiative, professionalism, and creativity. The primary principles of quality management are the following:

■ Decisions are based on fact, not desires or political considerations.
■ Quality is defined by the stakeholders of the organization (patients, employees, vendors, and the community at large).
■ Quality management is most efficient in an environment in which inspired leadership and trust are present.
■ For a quality management program to work, both management and staff at all levels must be committed to its success.

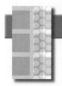

THE NURSE MANAGER SPEAKS

The segments of the healthcare industry that have moved the direction of their organizations toward one of quality management have proven to themselves that quality well managed is an asset with unparalleled impact.

In a quality management environment, the primary functions of every member of the team are the identification of risk and the prevention of error. To fulfill these functions, the quality team plans carefully to achieve realistic and attainable goals. Initially, this effort centers on the expenditure of resources (time and money), but eventually the effort permeates the entire organization, so that the act of providing quality service itself becomes a positive income generator.

The major steps in developing a continuous quality improvement program are as follows:

1. Identification of need
2. Assembly of a multidisciplinary review team
3. Collection and analysis of data to verify and substantiate identified needs
4. Establishment of realistic goals and objectives
5. Creation of performance standards
6. Development of a mission and vision as part of an overall business plan that will achieve the goals of the organization
7. Evaluation of the process
8. Modification of the original plan to incorporate identified strengths and compensate for identified weaknesses
9. Implementation of the modified plan and evaluation of the results

REFERENCES

1. Darling v. Charleston Community Memorial Hospital, 33 Ill 2nd, 211 NE 2nd 253, 326 (1965); appeal denied by 383 U.S. 946, 16 L Ed, 2nd 209, 86 Supreme Court 1204 (1966).
2. Lanham GB, Orlikoff JE: Full coverage of issues reflects importance of risk management, *Hospitals* 55:165, 1981.
3. Dixon NE: *Quality, trending and management: a hospital-wide quality assurance program*, ed 4, Chicago, 1980, American Hospital Association.
4. Ballard KA, Arbogast D, Boeckman J, and others: *Nursing: scope and standard of practice*, Silver Spring, MD, 2004, American Nurses Association.
5. Duran GS: On the scene: risk management in health care, *Nurs Adm Q* 5:19, 1980.
6. Peters TJ, Waterman RH Jr: *In search of excellence*, ed 4, New York, 2004, Collins.

SUGGESTED READINGS

Allen D, Calkin J, Peterson M: Making shared governance work: a conceptual model, *J Nurs Adm* 17(1):37, 1988.
American Nurses Association: *A code for nurses with interpretive statements*, Kansas City, Mo, 1995, Author.
American Nurses Association: Legal developments, *ANA's Labor and Employment Newsletter* March 10-11, 1995.
Anschutz EE: *TQM America*, Bradenton, Fla, 1995, McGuinn and McGuire.

Bailey D: Budgeting skills, *Nurs Stand* 10(19):45, 1996.

Bowles KL, Naylor MD: Nursing intervention classification systems, *J Nurs Sch* 28(4):303, 1996.

Cleland V: *The economics of nursing*, Norwalk, Conn, 1990, Appleton and Lange.

Deming WE: *Out of the crisis*, Cambridge, Mass, 1986, Massachusetts Institute of Technology.

Drucker P: *The frontiers of management*, New York, 1986, Dutton.

Fiesta J: Labor law update—part 1, *J Nurs Manag* 28(1):27, 1997.

Finkler S, Kovner C: *Financial management for nurse managers and executives*, ed 3, Philadelphia, 1993, Saunders.

Flanagan L: *Collective bargaining and the nursing profession*, New York, 1986, Dutton.

Folland S, Goodman AC, Stano M: *The economics of health and healthcare*, ed 4, Upper Saddle River, NJ, 2004, Prentice Hall.

Hillard LS: Risk management: an important part of quality, *Home Care News* 4(1), 1997.

Marrelli T: *The nurse manager's survival guide: practical answers to everyday problems*, ed 3, St Louis, 2004, Mosby.

Marriner Tomey A: *Guide to nursing management and leadership*, ed 7, St Louis, 2004, Mosby.

Managing the Stress of Management

OUTLINE

LEARNING SYNOPSIS

Upon successful completion of this chapter, readers will possess a fundamental understanding of the importance of the effective management of stress to the successful administration of a nursing unit.

OBJECTIVES

1. Properly define stress as it applies to the nursing environment
2. Describe how stress and performance interrelate and how altering the balance between the two can upset the working environment
3. Identify the antecedents of stress and discuss how job tasks and physical environments can be causes of stress
4. Describe how interpersonal and individual factors affect stress in the work environment
5. Discuss the potential consequences of stress in the working environment
6. Identify steps that can be taken by the individual to reduce personal stress
7. Identify steps that can be taken by the nurse manager to reduce stress in the nursing unit
8. Identify steps that can be taken by the organization to reduce stress and improve performance
9. Discuss things the individual can do to reduce stress and maximize personal levels of success

Stress! The word itself causes many people to go rigid and overreact, acting as a sort of negative stimulus. But the truth is that no one passes through this world without experiencing considerable stress in one form or another. From the dawn of human civilization to the very minute that you read this text, each generation and each person in that generation has experienced his or her own individual set of stress experiences.

Stress began somewhere back in the Stone Age when the Neanderthals lived to a ripe old age of approximately 18 while encountering a wide variety of hair-raising stress stimuli, many of which still confront humans today. Although none of the world's current population is outrunning a saber-toothed tiger, some of the remaining stress stimuli still remain foreboding.

What is it that initiates a stress reaction in today's manager? Basically, it is a response to some stimulus. When the brain recognizes, or even thinks it recognizes, a potential danger, it initiates a string of reactions in the body. Chemicals are released that put the nervous system into overdrive. The heart beats faster and breathing accelerates so that enough oxygen can be obtained to power the body after the brain decides whether to fight or flee.

Regardless of whether the decision is to fight or flee, the body still has to draw on its physical resources. In fact, so many different systems in the body accelerate to meet the need at hand that it would take quite a few pages to describe them all. It is enough to say that reflexes get sharper so that the body can react faster. Even the blood is stimulated to clot faster so that if one gets clawed, one won't bleed as rapidly.

Now flash forward to the modern nursing unit. Suppose a new piece of technology is introduced into the unit, and you are tasked with training all of the staff nurses to use it in just 2 days. You're comfortable with the old equipment and really don't want the responsibility of teaching others how to use the new equipment. But the patients need this new procedure, and you really have no choice. What do you do?

You gear up, that's what you do. You put all of your energy and intensity into the effort. This is no simple task, because to do so you must be at your peak operating strength at all times. So for the next 2 days—at work, at lunch, at home, and at all points in between—your internal systems are operating at maximum capability, or at least at inappropriately high levels. You're not terribly excited about feeling the way you do, but to accomplish your goal, you know that you can't simply turn off your internal drive. Therefore, you react. You start with a couple of extra cups of coffee, perhaps an aspirin or a miracle mood modifier, or whatever else is within reach. After your shift is over, perhaps you meet a friend at O'Malley's for a couple of drinks or, if you're a seasoned veteran of these types of dramas, you run an extra couple of laps around the park. Maybe you don't get enough sleep at night, but regardless, the next day, whatever stress control you had gained the day before quickly deserts you. You're back in the nursing unit ready for round two of doing things in a completely different and unfamiliar way. You don't like it, but you know you have to do it. Your body responds by operating in high gear for much too long a period. By the end of the second day, you are stressed out!

Sound familiar? It should, because that is exactly how most of life is in the healthcare industry, and especially in management—too much work, not enough time, and never enough qualified help. The combination adds up to one big dose of stress.

How can you help yourself? Experts say that the best and often the clearly most effective way of helping yourself is to understand what is happening. Amazingly enough, in almost every situation managers will face, at least half of the battle in alleviating stress is simply becoming aware of how to react to the situation. Sound too good? Too simple? Well, it's the truth. In fact, the single most important truth regarding stress is that for most people, most of the time, most of the stress they encounter is self-induced.

Of course, traumatic incidents, cataclysmic losses, and such sometimes occur; but for the most part, stress is self-imposed. The focus of this chapter is the day-to-day, week-to-week types of stress that the nurse manager experiences simply from having too much responsibility, living in a frenetic society, and operating in a demanding career field in which there is little room for error—in other words, the good old-fashioned type of stress that is experienced by everyone in a position of responsibility; the stress that comes from commuting to work, from working for a less than perfect supervisor, and from having others share their grief with you.

UNDERSTANDING STRESS

Stress, for the purpose of this chapter, is defined as the reaction an individual has to any demand placed on the individual by the environment that is perceived as a threat.[1] In fact, this internal reaction can be generated anytime an individual faces more incompatible demands than can be assimilated. Dr. Hans Selye,[2] considered by many to be the father of stress research, wrote that the human body wears itself out in responding to what he called *normal stressors*, or events of stress. This wearing away of the body's capability is increased or decreased in direct relation to the frequency and intensity of the experienced stress and is greatest when the individual is experiencing stress that is greater than he or she is capable of managing.

Selye[2] believed that an individual's response to the stimulus of stress was the same regardless of whether the stress was positive or negative. Thus, moving into a new home or starting a new job can be just as stressful as having a bill collector call for an overdue debt. Selye also firmly believed that all people experience some form of stress and that stress is absolutely essential to sustain life. Everyone recognizes that a small amount of stress can actually enhance performance. Thus stress, in the right proportion, can be good; when it becomes overpowering, however, the individual can easily respond in a physiologically or psychologically maladaptive manner.

One of the best ways to think about stress is as a weight acting on a simple balance scale. Fig. 16-1 shows how maintaining a good balance actually requires a certain optimal level of stress. When the level of stress being experienced is equal to the individual's ability to manage it, the body is in a state of equilibrium, which typically results in high levels of performance and satisfaction. It is normal for the body still to undergo some wear, even from the minutest stress, but it will not sustain real damage as long as the level of stress does not exceed the person's ability to manage it.

On the other hand, when the amount of stress becomes greater than the individual's ability to handle it, a damaging level of pressure can be felt by the individual. This situation is so common that it has produced certain expressions with which everyone in society is familiar (e.g., "she has a lot on her mind" or "he is bearing a real burden"). This negative situation frequently leads to physiologic and psychologic problems for the individual and to problems such as lower performance and higher absenteeism for the organization. An imbalance can also be felt if not enough pressure is placed on the individual. When the amount of stress is less than the person can manage, the result is apathy, boredom, low motivation, poor performance, and increased absenteeism, which often result in the individual's quitting his or her job. This situation is frequently recognized after the fact, when people make comments like, "They weren't using her talent, and she got bored."

Stressors are not universal; that is, the same stimulus does not have the same effect on everyone. What is extremely stressful to one person can be a mundane occurrence for another. How a given stressor affects a particular individual depends on how that individual perceives it. One individual may deal well with a given stimulus, whereas another person with a similar background may be overwhelmed by it.

Stress can be caused by a myriad of different stimuli—an almost infinite number, in fact. In the nursing environment, these sources tend to be similar, regardless of the specific organization. Fig. 16-2 shows a typical model of stress. The model is organized to make it easy to see how the antecedents of stress, the intervening variables of role ambiguity and role conflict, and the consequences of stress interrelate. The factors shown are only examples; actual stressors may be quite different from person to person.

Antecedents of Stress

The stress that results from job tasks and the physical environment actually are caused by things such as too much work (task overload); task-related factors like confusion regarding priority, conflicting tasks, and inability to perform the assigned task; and poor communication of expectations (failure to understand the task or performance requirement). Although any number of things can contribute to role ambiguity, one of the foremost is a lack of proper preparation or training. Poorly trained individuals almost always feel more stress in performing their jobs and subsequently experience lower self-esteem and higher rates of dissatisfaction.

LEVEL OF URGENCY

Nurses, including nurse managers, are often subjected to levels of stress not felt in other occupations simply because they are frequently required to perform their work in life-or-death situations. Nursing is an occupation characterized by intermittent periods of extreme overload brought on by emergencies, and these all-too-frequent occurrences can take an enormous toll on nurses, regardless of their professional capabilities.

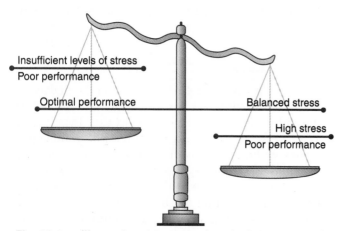

Fig. 16-1 ■ Illustration demonstrating the importance of a good balance in stress level.

EXPERIENCE	OVERRIDING CONSTRAINTS	POSSIBLE CONSEQUENCES
Organizational Factors		**Negative Effects**
Job tasks		Stress
Physical environment	A	Health problems
Supervisor behavior	Stress	Marital problems
Institutional factors	Model	Drug abuse
Change		Low performance
Traditions		Low satisfaction
Self-worth		Low self-esteem
Divisiveness		Absenteeism
		Turnover
	Role ambiguity	Dissatisfaction
Interpersonal Factors		**Positive Factors**
Role requirements		Role redefinition
Trust		Sharing of roles
Respect for others		Integration of roles
Multiple roles		
	Role conflict	Confrontation
		Redefinition
Individual Factors		
Rate of life change		Reorientation
Ability to perform		Reactive coping
Self-esteem/perception		Increased performance
Tolerance		Increased efficiency

Fig. 16-2 ■ A typical model of stress.

MANAGEMENT

A major factor in the amount of stress placed on nurses is the attitude, manner, and level of professionalism of the nurse manager for whom they work. Nurse managers who operate from a position of authority and not leadership often create undue stress in their employees. Close, punitive, and/or authoritarian supervision can have detrimental effects on the performance of the average nurse. Although these qualities certainly have their place in the overall scheme of management (e.g., in emergency situations), nurse managers who rely on them continually or as their primary source of control risk a great deal because of it. The nursing units of such managers will always be characterized by lower job satisfaction, higher absenteeism, and greater turnover, and for the most part these negative outcomes will result directly from the degree of stress that the managers themselves inflict on their employees through their controlling attitudes. In fact, the degree to which nurse managers influence instead of control their employees greatly affects the overall health of the organization.*

THE ORGANIZATION

By itself, the organization can create significant levels of stress in the working environment. Institutional expectations, performance standards, and managerial quality can lead to heightened levels of stress, especially when they conflict with an employee's needs.

STAFFING LEVELS

One of the major factors contributing to stress is the tendency demonstrated in the healthcare industry over the past two decades to run the organization with lean personnel structures. Understaffing and the practice of assigning staff to unfamiliar units to plug existing holes are classic examples of the organization's running amok and leaving stress, anxiety, and poor performance in its wake.

LOYALTY

Another tremendous source of stress is the tendency of organizations to demand that an employee's primary loyalty be to the organization rather than to family, self, group, or profession. When an employee's actions run counter to the expectations of the

*If it seems as though this textbook holds the nurse manager responsible for a great many things that occur in the working environment of the nursing unit, that is a correct perception, because nurse managers are responsible for this environment—all of it, the good and the bad. They set the tone, they create the attitude, and they control the performance. Being a manager makes an individual responsible. Every time a poor manager is assigned to a position of authority, the individual performers will suffer far more stress than if the manager were a positive influence.

organization, the reaction of the senior members of the institution creates enormous stress on the employee.

MULTIPLE LINES OF AUTHORITY

The organization also creates stress by having unclear or multiple lines of authority to which the employee must respond. When multiple lines of authority conflict, the stress on the employee can increase dramatically. This is especially true when satisfying the requests of one authority figure makes it impossible to satisfy those of the other.

CHANGE

The rapidly changing environment of healthcare institutions has also been a contributor to stress in nursing. Rapid changes in technology, increased demand from patients for service, liability issues, increased pressure for efficiency due to competition, and pressure from agencies such as Medicare have made the role of nurses more difficult, conflicted, and stressful.

SOCIETY

Some nursing traditions remain a source of unnecessary stress, although perhaps they are not the major factor they have been in the past. Researchers have pointed out that of all the challenges faced by the typical staff nurse, the problem of personal sense of self-worth is the most basic.[3] Because an overwhelming percentage of nursing professionals are female (estimated at approximately 95%), many of the attitudes toward women prevalent in society are reflected in how nurses think of themselves. The traditional, and very untrue, stereotypes about women still portray them as passive, weak, intuitive, inconsistent, dependent, empathic, sensitive, and subjective. When nurses demonstrate traits that are generally considered masculine (assertiveness, independence, competitiveness, rational thinking, self-discipline, and innovation) they are often considered butchy or non-feminine. No matter how little truth there may be in these beliefs, they are very real to many people. Tradition has always valued the "female" traits of empathy and sensitivity and considered them as high-quality attributes for a nurse, and nurses who have demonstrated assertive, independent, analytic, and competitive traits have been discouraged. Today, the image of nursing as a female occupation still persists, although to a much lesser degree than two decades ago. As the role of women continues to evolve in our society, so will the nursing profession.

Nursing has gone through some of the most dramatic changes ever experienced by a single profession, especially in the past three decades. Today's nursing professional commands a far higher level of respect in the healthcare industry than ever before. Today, one will not see a nurse get up from his or her work to give a physician a chair simply because the doctor has chosen to do some charting. There are still many casualties of times long past, however, and many organizations encourage nurses to participate in continuing education that places emphasis on assertiveness training. Today, the nursing profession is viewed with respect, high regard, and even admiration. Nursing administration has grown into its own specific specialty, with graduate nursing education being offered by most major universities to train individuals in precisely that field. Today's director of nursing is viewed as a peer of most senior hospital administrators at the vice presidential or assistant administrator level.

Interpersonal Factors
PROFESSIONAL DIVISIONS AND MIXED ROLE MESSAGES

The problem of low feelings of personal self-worth is exacerbated by the fact that nurses must continually contend with divisions within their profession. This separation began with the historical conflict regarding education (i.e., level of degree achieved dictates level of work available). The question of education and capability is one that rages hot and heavy throughout the industry, and this controversy has led to stress for many nurses because of the varied role messages that have been sent.

If the question, "What is the current role of the nurse?" were asked of different groups outside the nursing profession, a wide range of responses would be received. The typical role permitted by a hospital administration, which has been shaped by the administration's need to maintain efficiency and limit exposure to risk, often conflicts with what society sees as the nurse's helping and healing role. What is the perception of physicians concerning the role of the nurse? Does the role differ depending on whether functional, team, or primary nursing is employed? Does the role differ with the type of healthcare institution? What are nurses' perceptions of these various role definers? These are all issues that increase the stress levels under which the typical nurse performs.

The nursing profession has grown remarkably in its maturity. Today's nursing professionals are far more likely than their predecessors to join and take an active part in fraternal and professional organizations. Nevertheless, the image of the nurse is still that of someone who performs a job instead of someone who is a true professional. The perception of the nurse as indifferent to major issues keeps professional associations from lobbying as aggressively as they might on issues important to the profession. Specialty nursing organizations such as those for critical care nurses and operating room nurses continue to have greater success in recruiting and keeping active members; however, the lobbying efforts of these specialty organizations have had only a limited effect in improving overall conditions for nursing because they are focused primarily on specific issues that benefit their membership. In fact, many of these specialty organizations have acted as a distancing mechanism between their members and unspecialized nurses and have thereby increased the number of varying messages nurses receive.

MULTIPLE ROLES

The multiple roles that typical nurses play in their lives are also a continuing source of stress in the profession. A primary example is the conflict between home life and professional career. Nurses, like those in nearly every other occupation, perform a number of roles, but in a career field that is heavily dominated by women, this duality is much more stressful because the nurse's role is often in open conflict with society's expectation that a woman will be the major contributor to parenting. The situation is exacerbated by the profession's requirement to deliver care 24 hours a day and 365 days a year. The shift and weekend work schedules required by most nursing jobs put enormous stress on the average employee. Experience has shown that a large percentage of nurses who must work on the evening or night shift frequently experience physiologic problems if their spouses or children are on different time schedules. This already significant problem can become acute if the shift nurse is required to change time slots periodically. The time interval required to reorient to the new shift schedule can cause significant physiologic challenges in an already difficult situation.

ROLE CHANGES

The adjustment required of a nurse who assumes the position of nurse manager can in itself create tremendous pressure, because there are significant differences between performing a task and supervising others as they perform it. Directing the efforts of others is always demanding and at times can be extremely stressful, especially for nurse managers who were exceptional performers before becoming managers. Many would prefer to perform the nursing tasks themselves because they believe they can do the job better and faster than those they are supervising. The transition from performer to manager is an extremely difficult one, and many exceptionally qualified nurses never really make the change completely. In discussing this conflict, one is reminded of the old naval

challenge of the ship's captain instructing the young ensign in the proper technique for berthing a ship: "The captain bites his tongue until it bleeds, but cannot assume command if the lesson is to be learned."

Individual Factors

There is no limit to the number of different things that can generate stress in the working professional's life, and this is especially true for individuals who operate in environments that are often urgent and in which even the smallest error can have long-term consequences. One of the broadest categories of stressors is what have been termed *individual factors*. These are the individual influences to which each person is subject, and what the nurse manager makes of them and how he or she deals with them can have a very real influence on the nurse manager's quality of life.

LIFE CHANGES

Life-changing events, or the positive and negative things that occur in life to which people must adjust, are one of the most significant sources of stress because they can produce a cumulative form of damaging influence on the individual's health and manner of life. The occurrence of many such life changes in a short period of time can lead to the early manifestation of disease, because the associated stress breaks down the body's natural ability to deal effectively with illness.[4] To accurately measure how much stress an individual actually experiences, researchers T. H. Holmes and R. H. Rahe identified 43 common life-changing events and assigned a point value to each indicating the relative amount of stress associated with that event. Using these assigned values, they developed a rating scale that reflects the relative importance of these life changes and their potential influence on future health and well-being (Fig. 16-3). To use the scale, the individual checks off those life events that occurred within the previous 12 months, and the corresponding point values are then totaled to obtain an overall score. The researchers found that, for individuals whose life change scores totaled more than 150 points, the likelihood of developing a serious illness during the following 24-month period was higher than 50%. Individuals who experienced life events with a total assigned value of more than 300 points developed serious illness at a rate 70% greater than individuals who did not experience the additional stress.

PERSONAL EXPECTATION AND EXPERIENCE

Another major source of stress is the difference between the individual's expectations for his or her performance and that individual's perception of his or

Social Readjustment Rating Scale

Life Event	Value Score	Life Event	Value Score
1. Death of spouse	100 _____	23. Child leaving home	29 _____
2. Divorce	73 _____	24. Trouble with in-laws	29 _____
3. Marital separation	65 _____	25. Outstanding achievement	28 _____
4. Jail term	63 _____	26. Spouse begins/stops work	26 _____
5. Death of close family member	63 _____	27. Starting/finishing school	26 _____
6. Personal injury/illness	53 _____	28. Change in living conditions	25 _____
7. Marriage	50 _____	29. Revision of personal habits	24 _____
8. Fired at work	47 _____	30. Trouble with boss	23 _____
9. Marital reconciliation	45 _____	31. Change in work conditions	20 _____
10. Retirement	45 _____	32. Change in residence	20 _____
11. Change in family member's health	44 _____	33. Change in schools	20 _____
12. Pregnancy	40 _____	34. Change in recreation	19 _____
13. Difficulties with sex	39 _____	35. Change in church activities	19 _____
14. Addition to family	39 _____	36. Change in social activities	18 _____
15. Business readjustment	39 _____	37. Mortgage/loan under $10,000	17 _____
16. Change in financial state	38 _____	38. Change in sleeping habits	16 _____
17. Death of close friend	37 _____	39. Change in family get-togethers	15 _____
18. Change in line of work	36 _____	40. Change in eating habits	15 _____
19. Change in arguments with spouse	35 _____	41. Vacation	13 _____
20. Mortgage/loan over $10,000	30 _____	42. Christmas	12 _____
21. Foreclosure of mortgage loan	29 _____	43. Violation of minor law	11 _____
22. Change in work responsibility	29 _____	**TOTAL**	_____

Once you determine the total number of points that you have incurred within the last 12 months, compare your level of stress experienced with the likelihood of becoming ill within the next 24 months according to the findings of Holmes and Rahe:

Total Points Accumulated	Likelihood of Illness
<150	37%
150-300	51%
>300	Serious danger*

Serious danger was identified by Holmes and Rahe as being the likelihood of a seriously stressed individual, if he or she becomes sick, to suffer a more serious malady (i.e., more likely to develop cancer, have a heart attack, or suffer a form of manic-depressive psychosis than to develop warts or suffer menstrual irregularities).

Fig. 16-3 ■ Rating scale for evaluating the influence of common life-changing events. (From Holmes TH, Rahe RH: The social readjustment rating scale, *J Psychosom Res* 11:213, 1967.)

her actual performance. The effects of this form of stress are influenced by the historical ability of the given individual to deal with stress. In fact, most people tend to repeat their previous behaviors when confronted with a similar stressor in a similar situation, regardless of their level of success in dealing with the original stressor. For example, the self-esteem that individuals develop from their past performance determines, to a large extent, their future ability to deal with role conflict and role ambiguity. Those who have enjoyed previous success in dealing with high levels of ambiguity deal more effectively with it in future encounters and therefore are likely to feel less

stress from it. In fact, an individual who has previously dealt successfully with any specific stress will feel less from a future repetition of the same strain.

PERSONALITY TYPE

Competitive, anxious, and driven individuals—who demonstrate what has been called type A behavior—are far more likely to create stress for themselves than are the more relaxed, friendly, and patient type B individuals. However, type A individuals actually deal better with stressful situations. Individuals who perceive the stressful situations in their lives as being external to themselves often experience less stress in these situations, and such individuals are far less likely to react negatively when they feel themselves being controlled by surrounding events.

Role Conflict and Role Ambiguity

Role conflict and role ambiguity are typically experienced by the individual as a result of some form of role-based stress. Role conflict occurs when the role messages being received by an individual disagree with his or her previously formed role concepts; role ambiguity occurs when poor communication results in the delivery of unclear and inconsistent information about the activities an individual is expected to perform and/or the goals the individual is expected to realize. A prime example of role-based stress in the nursing profession is the almost traditional conflict between the demands made on a nursing professional and the personal needs of the individual who fills that role. For nurse managers, such a conflict often develops when they are dealing with those for whom they are responsible (e.g., trying to reconcile the views of management with the needs of a staff member).

Role conflict is one of the most significant stressors for members of the nursing profession. The widely varying influences in the field of nursing affect every nurse's working environment. Things such as the challenges inherent in the profession, the differences in nurses' educational preparation and the reliance on this single factor to determine wages, the rigid structure of the performance environment, and the overwhelming influence of organized labor and professional nursing organizations create an extremely stressful performance environment for nurses. The situation is exacerbated by the physical setting, patient load, interpersonal relationships, the hierarchy of groups making demands (physicians, patients, staff, and management), and widely differing expectations and role perceptions regarding the nurse's job.

When nurses are not being sufficiently challenged by the tasks they are performing (role underload) or are not being asked to perform up to the level of their abilities (underutilization), stress can also develop. For example, if individuals with high self-esteem and/or high need for achievement are not being used to the full extent of their capabilities or have not been given much responsibility, the situation may become very stressful to them. This type of stress often leads to apathy and low productivity.

Consequences of Stress

What actually happens to individuals when they reach their limits? Although the answers to this question can be as varied as the individuals experiencing stress, most will suffer some form of physiologic and psychologic damage that will manifest itself in structural or functional changes, or both. Warning signs of too much stress include the following:

Anxiety: unduly high levels and prolonged periods of anxiety, or a persistent state of fear or free-floating anxiety that appears to stem from any number of shifting causes

Depression: a feeling of extreme dejection or morbidly excessive melancholy; depression can cause people to withdraw from family and friends, to be unable to experience emotions, and to feel helpless to change the situation

Abrupt mood and behavior changes: frequent outbursts of temper or any other unexpected behavior that is not normally shown by the individual (i.e., erratic behavior).

Perfectionism: the creation of unreasonably high standards for oneself and the perception of never quite satisfying these goals; it can place an individual in serious trouble because it subjects the individual to nearly constant stress

Illness: actual physical illnesses such as peptic ulcer, arthritis, colitis, hypertension, myocardial infarction, and migraine headaches that are frequently induced by stress and may be a precursor to the identification of stress as a medical problem

When individuals attempt to reduce the amount of stress they are dealing with, they may bring on more serious problems. For example, the use of alcohol and other mood-altering drugs to relieve stress can result in the development of chemical dependency.

Some individuals deal with their stress by turning into "workaholics." These people often suffer a syndrome known as *burnout,* a condition that results when individuals have consumed all of their available energy to accomplish a goal or assignment and begin to feel that this energy is still inadequate to achieve any level of success. At this point, the typical reaction is to give up and quit or to move on to another area.

In the nursing profession, the most telling indications of stress are increased absenteeism and turnover, and, because of them, reduced quality of job performance. Job performance suffers during high-stress times simply because so much energy and attention are consumed by the nurse's efforts to reduce the stress that little remains for actual performance. This situation is always financially expensive for the healthcare organization and can easily lead to situations in which the lower level of performance affects patient care enough to increase the organization's level of risk, which may ultimately result in litigation.

A Method of Dealing with Stress

One of the most effective methods of dealing with stress in the workplace is to employ some form of role redefinition. In this process, employees are encouraged to share their role expectations with their peers and through this process actually to clarify that role conception. Together, the group then attempts to integrate the various roles group members have identified, which provides a clearer view of the role for everyone.

Individuals can also directly confront those who are creating the roles in their personal lives and at work. Sometimes simply sitting down and talking about the conflicting role messages that are being received can be therapeutic.

If nurse managers simply take the time to request additional information regarding a specific role, they can do a great deal to reduce the ambiguity in the roles performed in their units. If they can recognize their own level of tolerance for ambiguity and avoid involvement in conflicting roles, they will be taking a large step toward coping with the stress inherent in the job.

Finally, if nurse managers make a legitimate attempt to improve their individual performance and through their efforts become more efficient and effective, they will relieve a great deal of job-related stress. For example, nurse managers who work hard to improve their ability to manage time effectively discover that they are able to get far more accomplished and achieve greater results in the same amount of time. This realization reduces their stress because it improves their self-confidence and self-esteem.

MANAGING STRESS

There is absolutely no dispute that stress can play an important part in any individual's success in the nursing profession. The things that induce stress and the stress itself must be well managed if the individual is to pursue a productive life. Quite a few recognized personal and organizational strategies are available for reducing work-related stress. Nurse managers can use these strategies to reduce their own stress levels, help manage their units, and assist their employees. The following is just a sampling of these strategies:

Increased self-awareness: Almost an inherent part of nursing is the feeling of many of the best professionals in the field that they can be all things to all people. Although on a rational level competent managers know that this will never be a reality, on a deep emotional level many in the nursing profession continue to hold this belief. However, once individuals begin to accept the fact that they are fallible and have limitations, they are on their way to greater success, if for no other reason than that they can begin to identify potential problems and plan for dealing with them effectively before these problems get out of control.

Outside interests: Those professionals who keep themselves actively involved in things such as hobbies, social groups, and recreational activities seem to deal better with stress. The diversion, relaxation, and enjoyment that are provided by most outside distractions seem to reduce anxiety and distress.

Exercise: The health benefits of regular exercise have long been known to the medical community, and nurses who maintain a program of regular physical exercise do much to improve their ability to cope effectively with stress. The key here is to remember that any physical activity can be beneficial as long as it does not become an obsession that increases stress.

Vacation: Getting away to recover is definitely therapeutic, and therefore people who work in stressful situations should be required to take regular vacations. The change of scenery involved in a vacation can help a person relax and regain the energy necessary to continue, even if the scenery change is only from the nursing unit to the person's backyard.

Relaxation: Relaxing is not an easy task, especially for the individual who continually experiences high levels of stress. However, the simple act of listening to music, reading, socializing with friends, watching movies, or any other activity that requires little of the participant can help a person unwind and gain strength.

Nurse managers, like all managers, can do much to reduce their own personal stress by helping the members of their staffs to reduce theirs. What, specifically, can nurse managers do to reduce stress in their working environments and in individual staff members? The following are some suggestions:

Identify the level of stress: Work with the staff to identify what types of stress occur in the unit, how much is being coped with, and how close individuals are to reaching a stage of burnout. Make sure there is enough stress in the workplace and do not attempt to remove it all; the presence of some stress is important, because without it, staff will become complacent and unmotivated. The nurse manager should consider assigning additional tasks or setting higher goals for subordinates if they are not feeling a little stressed.

Identify the source of the stress: When a subordinate appears to be under a great deal of stress, the nurse manager must work to identify the source(s) of the stress and create viable means of reducing it to promote motivation and desire in the employee.

Determine the role: If role ambiguity or role conflict is creating the stress, the nurse manager should investigate ways to eliminate the confusion and clarify the role(s) for the staff member. The nurse manager should communicate clearly the precise performance expectations for the activities that are to be carried out and the goals that are to be pursued.

Use the appropriate style of management or leadership: How the nurse manager directs the efforts of others can have a great impact on the stress in the unit and on individual performers. Heavy discipline and demand-oriented management are far more likely to create stress than are inspirational guidance and well-developed leadership. Sometimes the manner in which a subordinate is approached can do much to reduce the stress that is felt.

Provide counseling and training: The nurse manager can provide employees with opportunities to talk through their problems, but in some cases, employees would be better served by referral to professional counseling. The manager should determine if it is actually counseling that is needed and not motivation, and then decide whether he or she has the necessary skills to provide it. If the nurse manager does not have the special training required to adequately assist the employee, he or she should not attempt counseling. Training can help an individual develop confidence and self-worth, qualities that are absolutely critical to reducing the level of stress on the job.

Improve the individual's sense of self: If the stress is experienced because the subordinate has low self-esteem and does not perceive his or her contribution as meaningful, the nurse manager should look for ways to positively reinforce the subordinate's belief in his or her abilities and help the employee gain self-confidence. The nurse manager should identify other sources of support, such as unit team members, and work with them to develop ways for the subordinate to deal with stress.

What can the healthcare organization as a whole do to help its employees deal with stress in a meaningful way? The organization can develop clear and concise standards of performance and clearly understood business strategies so that employees can identify what is expected of them and what they must do to excel. Nurse managers are excellent individuals to work with the staff in the development of many of the ideas necessary for implementation, and if they are unable to do so, then they are in an excellent position to encourage senior management to develop or adopt new methods. Some of the simpler and more wide-ranging institutional strategies are outlined in the following sections.

Hire Correctly

An honest attempt should be made to match job requirements with prospective applicants during the selection and placement process. It is far easier not to hire an unsuitable individual than to develop the required qualities in the wrong person after he or she is hired.

Train Effectively

As much skills training should be provided as the budget will allow. Training should be one of the very few things that are left inviolate during times of reduction because it always returns to the organization far more in savings and increased performance than it costs. Training should be obligatory for all personnel, regardless of how senior they are or their level of individual achievement.

Although the traditional view of training is that it is an expensive process that yields little if any real change, the truth is that good training which is well supported by management is one of the least expensive and most cost-recoverable activities that management can provide to the organization. The challenge is really not whether training can make a difference but whether managers are willing to shoulder their responsibilities to realize its benefits. Typically, managers do an excellent job of researching and identifying training courses that can help develop the behavioral change necessary, but they do an extremely poor job of helping to ensure the success of the training. After the program is selected, it is invariably turned over to the education department for implementation, and although these professionals do an admirable job of presenting the information, they cannot turn information into change, regardless of how proficient they are. Training and training departments dispense information, and that is all they do. For employees to accept the new processes presented in the training course, management must provide a reason to change. The education department cannot provide this reason because it does not have control over the future success of the employees. Only individuals in a direct line of authority over the employees can provide employees with a reason to accept the information and change their performance to the new and desired behavior. Many times, the reason to accept the change can be presented through a reward and recognition process; at other times, the approach is simply "change or else."

Providing training is not enough. Management must provide training that works, that is verifiable, and that provides a method for managers to actively lead the process of change in the organization. If managers don't do this, all they are accomplishing by providing training is creating a desire for change and increasing employees' level of personal stress by leaving the decision to make the change up to the employees.

Because employees rarely want to change, leaving this decision up to them is tantamount to throwing away the training investment. A 1998 study conducted by Fujitsu Limited found that when the decision to accept a change recommended by a training program is left up to the employees, fewer than 4% of them will actually make the change.[5]

Provide Participative Decision-Making

Great companies, and this includes great healthcare organizations, make it a practice to actively engage employees at every level in the decision-making process. The more employees can help to develop expectations through the decision-making process, the less likely they are to be stressed by those expectations, and the greater the likelihood of their participation in their fulfillment.

Encourage the Development of Internal Networks

Employees should be encouraged to develop contacts throughout the organization on which they can rely to expedite performance and reduce the stress created by performance requirements. Industry recognized several decades ago that the informal network is extremely successful in getting the job done on time and under budget. All people involved in health care today would prefer to work with individuals they respect and consider friends than with people with whom they are compelled to work. Friendly agreements do more to expedite work and reduce stress than any other free method available to the organization.

Open the Lines of Communication

By keeping the lines of communication open, both upward and downward, the organization offers a real means of clarifying expectations and identifying performance requirements and standards. Consider the following true story:

> When I was managing a large department, I made it common knowledge that employees were not only encouraged to comment and critique communication, but such behavior was expected. When employees brought things to my attention and offered constructive criticisms and a variant approach to performance I rewarded them lavishly with praise, time off, and notoriety.
>
> What I did not allow, and what always brought the roof down on the heads of the employee, was complaining. The difference, I felt, between criticism and complaining is the presence of an alternative method. Complainers never take time to think of a better way, they simply whine. That was not tolerated, and in the few instances when it did occur, the employee was dealt with by explaining exactly what was expected and by being informed that if they wanted things changed, they had better do more than complain; they had to think. No one ever complained twice, but many, many employees openly criticized. (p. 25)[6]

Organize Shift Requirements

Creativity should be used when establishing shift work. If possible, the number of hours a nurse spends on an alternative nondaylight shift should be reduced, rest time should be increased, distinct and adequate meal times should be provided, and food should be available during these periods. One of the ways to do this is to increase the number of part-time people used in the off-shift hours. The shift should be broken down into three sets so that one part-timer works Monday, Tuesday and Wednesday; another handles Thursday, Friday, and Saturday; and a third works Friday, Saturday, and Sunday. The times and shifts should be kept balanced to coincide with increases in patient load, and time off should not be offered to part-time employees. What will be achieved is a very low level of absenteeism, high morale, and a balance between avoidance of frequent changes in shift assignments and provision of adequate opportunities for work. If this is done creatively, the work of three different part-time employees can be combined to make a single full-time equivalent position.

MAXIMIZING THE LEVEL OF SUCCESS

Every person working in the healthcare industry has the same goal: to maximize individual success while minimizing personal stress. Making the following choices can help you achieve this goal:

- Choose to be dynamic
- Choose to maintain humility
- Choose to be widely acknowledged
- Choose to include others in your success
- Choose to feel good about your level of success
- Choose to capitalize easily on your level of success
- Choose to make full use of your talents and skills
- Choose to perform with the highest ethical standards
- Choose to maintain clarity in your work and in your life
- Choose to help others achieve their desired level of success
- Choose to open new opportunities for yourself and for others
- Choose to praise others for their achievements
- Choose to maintain a relaxed perspective regarding your success
- Chose to acknowledge those who have contributed to your success
- Choose to work with others who can help you overcome your weaknesses
- Choose to acknowledge that professional success is not the same as personal happiness

If you name the stressor that is confronting you, identify the challenges being faced, and understand the goals for which you strive, it is guaranteed that you will be able to create what is necessary for you to feel good, lead others in an appropriate and professional manner, and hasten your progress and success.

Finally, you should keep in mind the following 10 fundamental things about stress and its management:

1. You can choose to reduce stress, to have more balance, and to live life with greater grace and ease.
2. As you begin to absorb your choices, you will naturally engage in behavior that supports your choices.
3. Using key words easily helps boost the power of the choices you make.
4. Avoiding words like *can't* helps you overcome seemingly insurmountable obstacles. Remember, *can't* never did anything and is just another word for *won't*.
5. Controlling your personal environment is important but is not always necessary
6. When you choose to confront your stress and deal effectively with each challenge you encounter, you have made the choice of personally reclaiming the direction in which your life is moving.
7. The goals you set for yourself and for others should be realistic ones, and when these goals are achieved, you should celebrate.
8. If you look for success and enjoy achievement, that is what you will find. If you look for problems and focus on their resolution, that is all you will do.
9. Leadership is not doing for others but enabling others to do for themselves.
10. Management is not the same thing as leadership. One deals with things and the other with people. Keep these two different qualities separated and active in your life and you will encounter significantly less stress in your professional life.

SUMMARY

- Stress is the reaction of the individual to demands in the environment that pose a threat.
- Some antecedents of stress are related to the job and organizational factors, whereas others are related to interpersonal and individual circumstances.
- Stress in nursing often results specifically from the nature of the work, from role conflict and role ambiguity, and from problems of perceived worth and divisiveness within the profession.
- The consequences of stress are physiologic and psychologic problems for the individual, poor job performance, low job satisfaction, and high absenteeism.
- Strategies to help individuals as well as institutions reduce stress include clarifying goals and roles; providing support, including training and education in stress management; using participative management techniques; and practicing personal stress management techniques.

FINAL THOUGHTS

The effective management of stress comes down to the process of self-management. It is a means to achieve a balance between what occurs in your professional life and what is needed to make your personal life satisfying. It is absolutely essential that every working professional, especially those involved in management, achieve this equilibrium in their lives.

One of the best ways nurse managers can achieve balance in their lives is to work diligently to reduce the amount of stress with which they are confronted by learning how to relax and look at the big picture. This means making a practical effort to see each facet of life, both professional and personal, as part of the whole of life. When a serious problem is viewed in this way, it often seems less urgent and less demanding. In fact, the stress associated with it will seem to fall away, and a logical approach to a solution will become far easier to see.

If personal and professional goals are viewed as only parts of a bigger picture, it is easier to develop coping strategies that can help blend these two major facets of life.

If nurse managers work diligently to look for solutions as part of a larger scenario, they can gain a sense of control over the demands in their lives.

THE NURSE MANAGER SPEAKS

During the first 6 months after my assignment as nurse manager, I worked diligently to develop a strong trusting relationship with my staff. I wanted them to know that they could rely on me whenever the pressures of unit life became overwhelming.

There came a day when the patient load was relatively small and my presence on the floor was not really needed, so one of my senior registered nurses suggested that I return to my office and finish the paperwork she knew that I took home nightly. She assured me that she would call if there was a change in patient needs.

That single incident was the start of a new way of life in my unit. Because my staff knew that I could be trusted to be immediately available if I was needed, they were supportive of my leaving the floor to complete administrative work during slow periods. I made it a habit to let them know how much their trust had allowed me to accomplish and readily gave them credit for my effort.

The end result was that my personal stress level was significantly reduced, and I became a far better manager, wife, and mother. Although things are never perfect, and I still frequently take work home, I have far more time for my family and myself.

The caring and trust that is shared by my staff helped me resolve the stress that had previously burdened my life. Today, the nurses who work for me see me as a mentor, and my family sees me as a joy.

REFERENCES

1. Steers M: *Introduction to organizational behavior,* ed 4, Santa Monica, Calif, 1996, Goodyear.
2. Selye H: *The stress of life,* New York, 1956, McGraw-Hill.
3. Brooten DA, Hayman L, Naylors MD: *Leadership for change,* Philadelphia, 1978, Lippincott.
4. Holmes TH, Rahe RH: The social adjustment rating scale, *J Psychosom Res* 11:213, 1967.
5. Friedman S: *Creating knowledge from information,* Honolulu, 2003, The Directions Corporation.
6. Hawkins J: *Leadership in the customer's environment,* Honolulu, 2001, The Directions Corporation.

SUGGESTED READINGS

Barkas LL: *Creative stress management,* Englewood Cliffs, NJ, 1989, Prentice-Hall.
Bassman E: *Abuse in the workplace: management remedies and bottom line impact,* Westport, Conn, 1982, Quorum Books.
Bliss ES: *Getting things done,* New York, 1976, Alpha Books.
Bruss J: *The 80-20 rule: consider it from a number of angles,* Deerfield, Ill, 2004, Tagnito Publications.
Davidson J: *Managing stress,* New York, 1999, Bantam Books.
Griessman BE: *The tactics of very successful people,* New York, 1994, McGraw-Hill.
Hawkins JA: *Quality service in the customer's environment,* New York, 2001, Bantam Books.
Koeske G: The impact of over involvement on burnout and job satisfaction, *J Orthopsych* 65(2):282, 1995.
Maslach C: *The truth about burnout,* San Francisco, 1997, Jossey-Bass.
Weiss D: *Get organized: how to control your life through self-management,* New York, 1986, AMACOM Publishers.
Zales M: *Stress in health and diseases,* New York, 1994, Brunner/Mazel.

PART II

GRADUATE CURRICULUM

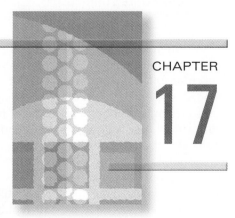

Business Planning for Nursing Management

OUTLINE

LEARNING SYNOPSIS

Upon successful completion of this chapter, readers will possess a fundamental understanding of the importance of writing a business plan, the mechanics of the plan, and its potential effect on the operation of the nursing unit.

OBJECTIVES

1. Describe how developing a personal view of the business plan can assist in its creation
2. Describe the major elements in the writing and construction of the business plan
3. Identify the basic functions of traditional management
4. Discuss exactly what planning is and how it relates to the nurse manager's responsibilities
5. Identify how timing affects the realization of goals and objectives
6. Describe the procedures involved in developing goals, strategies, and objectives
7. Explain the concept of the evolving small unit action plan and describe how its use can benefit the nursing unit
8. Describe effective methods for getting the planning process started
9. Identify the elements of the planning process and explain how they relate to each other and to the ultimate completion of the plan
10. Identify the elements of the SWOT analysis that give it its name and describe the effect of each on the overall planning process

All too often, individuals, nursing units, and entire **organizations** are left to flounder on a sea of luck and opportunity. Needless to say, this is not the recommended method of building a strong and viable healthcare organization or any type of unit or department within one. Leaving the unit's performance and, ultimately, the performance of the organization to chance is almost always an invitation to failure. A healthcare business, like life, requires direction and structure to become all that it is capable of being. To get all of the details, actions, and requirements lined up and heading in a common direction takes a great deal of planning. Planning can add a new dimension to the capability of the unit: *strategic direction*. Effective planning helps to determine *where* the nurse manager wants to take the unit, *what* things must be done to get there, *how* the necessary steps will be accomplished, *whose* help will be needed along the way, and even *when* the unit will arrive at its destination. Without going through a planning process, it is extremely difficult to fully take charge of any unit's future, no matter its size.

Many nurse managers never allow themselves to become involved in the planning process, primarily because, for a variety of reasons, they are uncomfortable with it. This is nonsense, of course, because the things that actually must be done to develop a workable business plan for a nursing unit—or for an entire organization, for that matter—are not very complicated and usually are quite easy to accomplish. The process of developing a plan helps managers learn to think strategically. Even more importantly, it helps managers do the following:

- Develop a mental picture of what they predict for their unit's future. This is most often referred to as a "vision"
- Formulate a statement of purpose that will help them attain what they and their units desire
- Develop specific goals and objectives that will act as a roadmap to help them chart their way toward accomplishment of the vision
- Develop a timetable for the accomplishment of the vision
- Clearly define success in terms important to the unit

Most professional planners believe that it is impossible to plan effectively in one's mind, especially when the object of planning is as complicated and diverse as a nursing unit. Therefore, this chapter focuses on identifying those things that must be accomplished to develop a written plan of action for any type of performance unit. Writing down a performance plan has many different benefits, but the following three are always among them:

1. It provides a tangible instrument to track the progress of the unit.

2. It enables the manager to physically see what the unit's historical actions are and whether or not the unit has completed all of the things that were planned for it to accomplish.
3. It validates the actual performance. Because reality rarely runs true to the plan, having a written vehicle allows the nurse manager to see where deviations have occurred and helps the manager chart a course that will return performance to the desired path.

! CRITICAL POINT

When developing a plan for success, don't rely on memory. The details of managing a nursing unit are so complex and diverse that even the best, most experienced nurse manager can easily lose track of the unit's vision unless it is written down so that it can serve as a constant reminder.

In describing actual planning procedures, this chapter is written with the assumption that you are a nurse manager in charge of a nursing unit in a health service organization. You are asked to respond to any questions in the text and on the forms in the figures as if you were currently filling such a position.

A PERSONAL VIEW OF THE PLAN

For most nurse managers, asking them to develop a plan that will aid them in achieving their units' initial goals is tantamount to asking them for the incredible. The task can be made much easier and far less daunting, however, if every manager learns to develop a simple plan at the beginning of his or her career. One of the best ways to accomplish this is to develop a personal plan for the individual unit. This type of plan is generally much simpler and easier to define than a full business plan because it answers questions that are closer to the individual—things that have been dreamed of, wished for, and formulated in the crevices of the mind over and over again. The development of a personal plan for the nursing unit is no more than taking those dreams, wishes, and formulations and incorporating them into a systematic planning process that will help the nurse manager work toward achieving them in the context of the unit. In addition, creating a personal version of the action plan gives the

Organization is used throughout this chapter to indicate entities from nursing units up through multinational corporations. The planning process and the concepts discussed in this chapter are applicable to organizations of any size—from one with a single employee to one with tens of thousands of employees.

nurse manager experience in the planning process, which will make the development of a formal plan for the nursing unit's business that much easier.

What Is Planning?

Take a minute and place your hand on the table with the back of your hand lying against the tabletop and spread your fingers open wide. Now look down into the exposed palm and mentally trace a path from its center out toward the tip of each finger and thumb.

What you have just done is to look at your goal without a plan. There are five different ways you can proceed to get to the end of your hand, but which is the best? How do you know that the direction you choose will be the safest and most practical?

Now, to illustrate a plan, simply take your hand and ball it into a fist. See how the fingers and thumb close around the palm. Now there is only one direction, straight down the arm to the end of the hand. That is what a plan is—an instrument that clarifies direction and provides impact no matter which direction it is moved.

Similarly, if you think about planning as the process of assembling your thoughts, your resources, and your desires into a fist, you can see how gathering them all together provides better direction to your unit and has the potential to make more of an impression when you implement the plan. This, then, is the essence of planning: the gathering of resources in a systematic manner so that a desired result can be achieved when the plan is used. Instead of the fingers that a fist uses to apply power, however, a plan uses goals, objectives, actions, and strategies to deliver the result.

The venerable sage Casey Stengel cleared up all of the confusion about planning when he uttered the immortal words, "If you don't know where you are going, you may end up somewhere else." That's what planning does—it helps you get where you want to go, much like a road map, so that you don't wind up leading your unit to an unknown destination.

The process of creating a plan is often far more important than the plan itself. The effort required to develop such an instrument forces nurse managers to think about the future carefully and systematically. It demands that they analyze the goals they want to establish and the methods they will use to realize those goals. The creation of such a document requires painstaking thought, responsible action, and personal dedication. Committing the plan to paper forces nurse managers to face their commitment head on. It asks that progress, direction, and timing be checked and verified. It also provides a method of monitoring and adjusting progress as conditions change.

Thus, planning is actually nothing more than an organized method for achieving a goal.

Establishing Goals and Objectives

The development of a list of goals is essential to developing a plan. This process can be expedited by taking a hard and very honest look at the unit and the manner in which it is perceived. What is the unit's purpose? Some may see the unit as a vehicle for providing medical services (wellness), others may see it as a lifetime passion, and still others may see it as the best possible means of avoiding the trap of a boring life. Whatever it is for you, write it down.

Now ask yourself what it is that you expect to gain from your involvement with the nursing unit. What must it deliver to make you happy? Consider the following questions:

- What type of environment do you wish to create in the unit, and what type of external perception of the unit do you wish to produce?
- Who or what is the unit's **competition**, and how do they compete? What are the individual competitor's strengths and weaknesses? How proficient is each? How professional? Which constitute a real threat, and which are just a nuisance? What are the things your unit must do to overcome the threat posed by each challenger?
- What must you do to prepare your unit to compete effectively against its competition so that your unit can achieve its goals?
- What opportunities have you identified for your unit that are not being exploited by others?

Use Fig. 17-1 to develop a clear picture of what you really want to do with your unit and what you will have to accomplish to achieve your goal.

The goals you establish should be taken seriously, and once made, they should not be changed easily. When you are developing these goals, think about them carefully and thoroughly. You should be able to feel the importance of a true goal. Mull the goals over in your mind and bounce them off your subconscious to verify that you really want to establish each of them. This will help you remain consistent in your efforts to achieve every goal that is set. It is strongly suggested that you discuss your goals in your unit with each subordinate or, at a minimum, with someone you respect and trust to provide you with completely honest feedback. This discussion will provide you with validation regarding your objectivity and is critical in establishing high-quality decisions. Use the questions given in Fig. 17-1 to stimulate yourself into

---

Competition or **competitor** is used in this chapter to mean any organization or unit that provides services similar to those performed by the nurse manager's unit. Examples of competitors are two hospitals that both have surgical units and two nursing units that both deliver services to patients.

What Do I Want to Realize from My Unit/Organization?

1. What type of environment do I want the unit/organization to have internally? _____
_____
_____

2. What type of perception of the unit/organization do I want to create externally? _____
_____
_____

3. Who (if any) are the major competitors to my unit/organization? _____
_____
_____

How Do They Compete with Us?	What Are Their Strengths?	How Proficient Are They?	Are They a Threat or Nuisance?	How Do We Overcome Them?
Competitor #1				
_____	_____	_____	_____	_____
_____	_____	_____	_____	_____
Competitor #2				
_____	_____	_____	_____	_____
_____	_____	_____	_____	_____
Competitor #3				
_____	_____	_____	_____	_____
_____	_____	_____	_____	_____

NOTE: Information about competitors can be obtained from industry associations, newspapers, advertising, the Internet, and government registries or by asking customers, talking with fraternal or networking groups, or simple observation. The information is available but effort may be required to dig it all out.

4. What do I have to do to prepare the unit/organization to compete effectively? _____
_____
_____

5. What opportunities has this exercise identified? _____
_____
_____

Fig. 17-1 ■ Sample form used to develop a clear picture of vision and goals for a unit.

establishing the basic goals for your unit. Fig. 17-2 provides a worksheet for more extended planning.

Don't let this list limit you in developing goals in areas that have not been suggested here. The suggestions are made solely to stimulate your thinking and may not be representative of your specific situation. When you make your list, add as many different areas as you think practical. Eliminate those that you do not feel are applicable. Don't underestimate the importance of developing your personal dreams for your unit and/or organization. If you don't understand what you want from the entity for which you are responsible, how can you possibly expect to lead it in a direction that will accomplish the goals you set for it?

! CRITICAL POINT

One of the very best team-building exercises that can be performed in any unit is involving the employees in the actual planning process. Ask every member of your team to supply answers to the questions presented and also ask them about their dreams, wishes, and desires for your unit. When you have collected these data, hold a meeting and discuss these goals. Add them to yours, and together build a vision for your unit to which all its members have contributed.

Extended Planning Worksheet

1. What do you want to achieve with your unit?_____
_____

2. What would you like its capability to be 1 year, 5 years, and even 10 years from now?

   1 year _____   5 years _____   10 years _____

3. What do think needs to be done to improve the health of your unit? _____
_____
_____

4. What other areas of performance do you think your unit could pursue? _____
_____

5. Other than your primary business, are there other areas in which the unit can contribute to, or influence, your
   community or the customer directly? _____
_____
_____

6. What community activities and charities can the business support? _____
_____
_____

Fig. 17-2 ■ Sample extended planning worksheet.

Developing Strategies (Objectives)

Strategies, or objectives, are the things that must be accomplished to achieve a goal. Objectives are always written in the form of an action, and many strategies or objectives may have to be accomplished before a goal can be realized. Unlike a goal, a strategy has a specific time frame associated with it. When developing your goals and strategies (objectives) it is very important to establish realistic time frames for the individual actions, because that will help determine how much effort will have to be exerted to accomplish the required work. Objectives are also important because they break up the larger goal into manageable pieces, and an opportunity is provided to taste a small amount of success on a frequent basis as each objective is accomplished. By celebrating the accomplishment of an objective, you will be able to keep your unit or organization focused on achieving the larger, more complex goal. Individual performers have a way of losing track of what it is they set out to accomplish if they have to wait too long to realize some level of success. The positive feedback generated by a celebration given for accomplishing a specific strategy can do wonders for you, your unit, and your organization.

Fig. 17-3 is a small worksheet that has been provided to help you develop the strategies that you will need to help achieve your goals. As you list your goals, specify several actions that you feel will have to be accomplished to satisfy each goal and write them on the lines to the right of the goal. After you have listed each specific action you think will be necessary, assign a realistic time for its accomplishment.

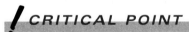

CRITICAL POINT

A strategy should specify the following three elements:
   1. What is to be done
   2. What resources are to be used
   3. What methods are to be employed
When planning strategies, it is important to identify how you will utilize resources to attain goals.

THE STRUCTURE OF PLANNING

Most nurse managers are not involved in the development of large, long-term projects such as building a new hospital wing or designing and constructing a next-generation trauma care facility. Therefore, they should look at the development of their unit's business plan differently than would a manager involved in a larger project such as those mentioned; however, most elements of the planning process are very similar, regardless of the specific situation.

Defining Goals, Strategies, and Time Lines

Goals	Strategies/Objectives	Time Frame
1. _____	A. _____	_____
	B. _____	_____
	C. _____	_____
	D. _____	_____
	E. _____	_____
2. _____	A. _____	_____
	B. _____	_____
	C. _____	_____
	D. _____	_____
	E. _____	_____
3. _____	A. _____	_____
	B. _____	_____
	C. _____	_____
	D. _____	_____
	E. _____	_____
4. _____	A. _____	_____
	B. _____	_____
	C. _____	_____
	D. _____	_____
	E. _____	_____
5. _____	A. _____	_____
	B. _____	_____
	C. _____	_____
	D. _____	_____
	E. _____	_____
6. _____	A. _____	_____
	B. _____	_____
	C. _____	_____
	D. _____	_____
	E. _____	_____
7. _____	A. _____	_____
	B. _____	_____
	C. _____	_____
	D. _____	_____
	E. _____	_____

Fig. 17-3 ■ Sample worksheet for developing the strategies needed to achieve goals.

The Evolving Small Unit Action Plan

Small nursing units generally need to focus their limited assets as much as possible on present-day occurrences. In years past, a 5-year time span for the average plan was considered appropriate, but in today's rapidly changing environment the time frame must be shortened to something more flexible. In fact, changes are occurring so rapidly in the healthcare field that long-term planning has almost been rendered obsolete. A few years ago, a hospital could take

5 years to introduce a new service or treatment and still be competitive enough to achieve profitability. Today, however, units that take 12 months to accomplish this same work are risking the loss of their investment by not being the first into the marketplace with the new service. Small healthcare units that used to take several years after opening to achieve profitability are now being forced to become profitable within 12 months if they are to meet the demands of ever-increasing competition.

Because the demands on performance have increased so greatly, it is no longer possible to plan in the traditional way. Therefore, this chapter recommends that nurse managers create their units' plans using an evolving process. To assist, this chapter introduces the 3-year evolving plan and recommends that nurse managers consider it when laying out the vision for their units' future.

The evolving plan is simple in design. It begins with the development of an initial 3-year plan, and as the first year is completed, that year is removed and the following segments shift forward one slot. Year 2 is now year 1, and year 3 is now year 2. A new third year is then added to fill out the plan. What is nice about this type of structure is that it brings continuity and stability to the plan. Adjustments can be accomplished in the new third year, while the new first and second years can be left virtually intact. This allows continual updating of the plan without disturbing the efforts being made to accomplish the goals that have been established. Fig. 17-4 illustrates the development of the evolving plan.

The 3-year evolving plan allows a small performance unit to keep its plan current without expending tremendous effort. It also provides a means of maintaining plan flexibility, monitoring, and frequent analysis, the three major requirements of any operating design.

When the plan is being updated, prospective changes should be carefully weighed and formulated before the existing structure is modified. Changing any part of a finished plan is not a step that should be taken lightly, but if changes are necessary, they should be made as required. Do not make the mistake of waiting for the entire year to pass before implementing a change. There are times when the rationale for modification is so compelling that the change cannot wait until the third year. When this happens, do not be afraid to break into the 3-year cycle and make the appropriate modifications.

Although nurse managers should consider using the evolving plan, they must make sure to adopt a plan structure that fits their specific needs in the most comprehensive manner. Special circumstances may indicate that a 1-year, 2-year, or even up to a 5-year plan would be preferable, but only individual managers are in a position to make that determination. Managers should use the plan structure that best fits their initial needs and keep it updated as they monitor their market or internal environment and see it change.

WARNING!

Changes to the plan must be weighed carefully, and authority for implementing such changes should be reserved for very senior management. Before any change is made, it should be carefully evaluated for its urgency and potential impact on the unit's overall vision.

The Elements of the Plan

A wide variety of plans may be required to facilitate the operation of any unit, but every type of plan contains similar elements. Regardless of whether the plan is for the overall operation of the unit (business plan), administration, nursing, facilities, emergency, or some specialized function, managers should include the following eight basic elements: (1) vision, (2) mission, (3) goals, (4) strategies, (5) management tools, (6) measurement, (7) analysis, and (8) evaluation.

YEAR OF PERFORMANCE	1	2	3	4	5
		Plan for All 3 Years			
First Year		1	2	3	
Second Year	Done	1	2	Plan 3	
Third Year	Done	Done	1	2	Plan 3

Blue = Years Planning is Actually Accomplished
Black = Years Completed or Planning Accomplished for in Previous Year

Fig. 17-4 ■ The development of the evolving plan.

VISION

A vision is a very concise and clearly articulated statement of what the unit wants to achieve. It may include the unit's philosophy, purpose, beliefs, principles, and industry creed. It is the articulation of how the unit is perceived by those who manage and work in it. If planning is to become a science in the unit, every person working in the unit and every stakeholder should clearly understand the vision that has been established. Enlightened units enthusiastically enlist the help of the entire staff to create the vision.

MISSION

The development of the unit's mission statement should be second in importance only to the creation of the vision. The mission statement should include the unit's major aims, philosophies, and characteristics. The statement is also used to define the type of industry in which the unit operates (health care) and what exactly it intends to accomplish while in operation. The mission statement should complement the unit's vision and should be as brief as possible so that it can be understood and remembered by every member of the unit. (See the example of a mission statement later in this chapter.)

GOALS

A goal defines one of the unit's long-term ambitions. Goals are destinations, not the means of moving toward them, so they should be phrased as simple statements. For example, if the ambition were to build a new trauma unit, the goal would be to build a new trauma unit. The goal should be written as "Build trauma unit" or "Build same-day surgery center." The means that will be used to accomplish the task are not part of the goal and should not appear in the goal statement.

STRATEGIES

Strategies identify the means that will be used to achieve the goal, or what will actually be done to ensure that the destination is reached. Continuing with the example in the previous paragraph, if the goal is to develop a same-day surgery center, then a strategy for accomplishing the goal would be "Identify primary participants within 1 year." Notice that the strategy adds an important element: a time frame. Strategies not only define what will be done but also when it will be accomplished.

MANAGEMENT TOOLS

Just having a vision, goals, and strategies is not enough. Managers needs to devise a means of directing their efforts to ensure that they are leading their units consistently toward the accomplishment of these elements. A management tool that could be used to control the development of a same-day surgery center would be finding space within the hospital where the center can be situated. Its availability for use would have to be determined before it can be planned for and possibly again before remodeling is started.

STANDARDS

Efforts to achieve the goal need to be accomplished in a specific manner. This manner is defined in the standards that are set. These standards establish the parameters for movement toward goal accomplishment. For example, if a same-day surgery center is being created, one of the "standards" that might be set is the specific architect that will be used. Another might be the month that remodeling will start. And yet another might be the interior design of the center.

ANALYSIS

As the unit moves toward the accomplishment of its goal, the manager should review and analyze the data that are made available. The manager should use these data to verify how well the unit is performing and how much of the goal has been accomplished. The data should never be accepted at face value; rather, they should be analyzed to ensure that the things that are being accomplished will achieve the goal that has been set. Sometimes, when the unit is moving toward the accomplishment of a goal, the data that are received indicate that adjustments need to be made to the original strategies or, for that matter, that the goal itself needs to be modified. Changes made early in the progress toward a goal can save money, time, and effort. For example, if the goal is to automate the unit because management wants to improve proficiency and the vendor that was originally wanted moved its headquarters to Atlanta, Georgia, while the unit was working to accomplish its goal, would the goal remain valid? Perhaps. However, if the vendor's move caused undue hardship to the unit, perhaps management should consider changing the goal. If the goal of automation were still important, perhaps the original standard of using a specific vendor would have to be changed.

EVALUATION

After the goal has been accomplished, or at a predetermined time during pursuit of the goal, management should evaluate the efforts made. This evaluation will help to refine business practices and thus to improve the ability to realize future goals. This is a discovery process that provides the unit manager with "lessons learned" and benefits the unit by allowing it to take advantage of experience. For example, during the remodeling for the same-day surgery center, if management had originally asked for marble walls but later discovered that painted concrete walls met its needs and were less expensive, this lesson learned can help the unit save money on the final remodeling.

WARNING !

Changing a goal is a serious matter for any unit and should never be attempted without thoughtful discussion. If the unit used sound judgment and expertise when establishing its goals, then these goals should clearly define the professional practices of the unit. Changing a goal constitutes a major shift in the unit's business concept. Therefore, instead of changing goals, change strategies to keep the unit on the path toward accomplishment. Modify, delete, and add strategies to keep the unit moving toward the attainment of the goal and, ultimately, the vision.

Getting Started

No one should sit down at his or her desk, pull a piece of paper from the drawer, and write down a plan. In fact, very professional managers put a lot of time, thought, and energy into developing their plans. The proper method of development involves needs identification, research, and analysis. These steps are used in the formulation of the plan, and they are constantly being repeated as the unit moves along toward accomplishment. Answering the following specific questions can help the nurse manager begin the process and evaluate progress as the unit moves forward:

Where is the unit now? What is the present situation?

Where would the unit like to be? What is the destination (goal)?

Why is this necessary? What are the reasons that the unit is willing to spend money, time, and effort to achieve this goal?

How will the unit get to where it wants to be? What mode of performance will be used to reach the destination?

When would the unit like to reach its destination? What is the performance time frame? How long does the unit think it will take to achieve its goal?

From whom will the unit require help? What help, if any, will be needed to get the unit to its destination? What abilities, disciplines, experience, types of individuals, and so on, are required?

What is the price? What will the accomplishment of the goal cost? How much is the unit willing or able to spend?

Against what will progress be measured? What are the standards to which the unit will hold itself accountable?

How will progress be managed? What are the tools that will be used to keep the unit on track and focused? Who are the people who will be key players?

From where will help come? What are the areas within the unit whose help will be required to achieve the goal? Will outside vendor assistance be required? Will the unit use consultants?

How will the unit know when the goal has been achieved? What criteria will be used to determine completion (these should be structured by specifying time frames for each strategy needed to accomplish the goal)?

How will the experience be evaluated? What form of analysis will be used?

How will the unit implement lessons learned? What steps will be taken to improve the unit as a result of the experience?

Nurse managers should ensure that every member of the team involved in the accomplishment of the goal, including themselves, is reviewing progress continually. All individuals involved should be asking themselves the previously stated questions over and over again at the appropriate times to ensure that the goal is not only accomplished but accomplished in a manner that is truly beneficial for the unit.

The Path of Performance

The realization of a vision is a strategic path in a nursing unit, and this path should be well delineated. A recommended path for accomplishing the vision is shown in Fig. 17-5. As the figure shows, both the internal and external influences on the unit should be considered, because they may affect efforts to ensure that the resources needed are developed or obtained.

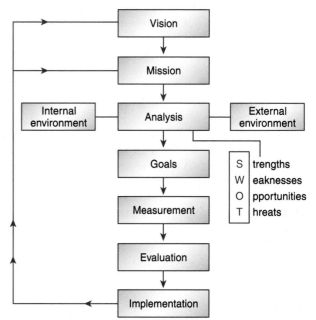

Fig. 17-5 ■ Recommended path for realization of the organization vision.

Unit leaders must develop goals and strategies that are realistically attainable and can be perceived as such by all members of their staffs.

Managers also must consider the needs of their units' service areas (markets) before deciding on what they want to accomplish and then must continually evaluate changes in the marketplace that may indicate that a modification of prepared strategies, or possibly even a goal change, is necessary. (The analysis of market needs is discussed in greater detail later in this chapter.) Managers should not fall into the trap of thinking that because a well-developed plan is available, the planning process is complete. Unit managers should plan continually and view the process of planning as a fundamental part of their profession.

Beginning the Process

After the vision is established and the mission has been developed, the process of planning typically begins with the planner's making assumptions about the conditions, environments, and markets in which the unit must operate. The fact that the process of planning involves predicting the future doesn't mean that managers should drag out the crystal ball and start looking for the correct path. A better place to start is with what has occurred in the past. Historical data are always a good place to sink the unit's roots; however, managers must remember that history does not always accurately predict the future. If they weave a tight pattern of assumptions and historical occurrences, their chances of predicting future events are greatly enhanced.

The process of making assumptions is not—repeat, *not*—the business of guesswork. This is critical, because managers will eventually be making decisions based on the assumptions that they have developed in the planning process. Good assumptions are made by closely examining four factors that influence the unit: strengths, weaknesses, opportunities, and threats. This is referred to as a *SWOT* analysis.

A SWOT analysis is a useful tool for analyzing the unit's overall situation. It is an attempt to weigh the internal strengths and weaknesses of the unit against the threats that may be present from an external source. Managers begin this process by taking a clinical look at the areas of marketing, finance, human resources, technology, production, administration, management structure, service, and any other internal areas or resources the unit has or by which it is influenced.

INTERNAL SWOT ANALYSIS

Investigating the internal workings of the unit takes a clear and analytic mind. This is an important point to remember for small units, because first-line managers

have a tendency to view emotionally those things with which they work on a daily basis. Managers should be careful not to fall victim to this phenomenon when performing their internal SWOT analyses. Fig. 17-6 is a worksheet designed to help novice managers perform a SWOT analysis by identifying critical internal areas they may need to review.

One of the things that is frequently found when conducting a SWOT analysis is that different units and departments interpret the organization's vision and mission differently. Although this is not as common in small units as it is in larger ones, it does become an issue when a unit is growing and expanding. It is imperative that all parts of a unit work toward the attainment of the *same* vision, using the *same* mission guidelines and the *same* goals. A breakdown of these fundamental elements in the unit is a signal that immediate corrective action is required to avoid future trouble.

❢ CRITICAL POINT

The tendency for professionals in the health professions to become biased when thinking about their business is significant. This prejudice, regardless of how well intended, is detrimental to the planning process, and nurse managers should zealously guard against it. It is recommended that the internal SWOT analysis be conducted by an objective third party. The intent of the analysis is to reach an objective understanding of the business. Sometimes achieving that aim takes some outside assistance.

EXTERNAL SWOT ANALYSIS

Most academicians divide the SWOT analysis into an internal segment that considers strengths and weaknesses, and an external segment that examines opportunities and threats. Although no attempt is made here to argue this point, real-world business feels strongly that the entire SWOT process should be applied to each segment. Opportunities and threats exist within the unit just as much as they do in the outside environment, and they can be just as influential. Moreover, it is just as important to understand the strengths and weaknesses of the outside environment as to understand those of the internal environment. This information will help position the performance unit to overcome these external strengths and to take full advantage of any weaknesses that might be identified. Which method the unit uses to implement the SWOT process, however, is an internal management decision.

The external environment is a different sort of entity to deal with in planning. Most if not all of it will be beyond the unit manager's control, and developing controls is not the purpose of the outside SWOT analysis. The purpose is to understand exactly what

Internal SWOT Analysis Worksheet

I. Human Resources

1. Are the goals and strategies used by Human Resources supportive of the unit's vision and mission statement? ☐ Yes ☐ No

   A. If not, how are they different? _____
   _____
   _____

   B. What must be done to allow these goals and strategies to support the vision and the mission?_____
   _____
   _____

2. Are special talents available within the workforce? ☐ Yes ☐ No
   A. If so, what are they? _____
   _____
   _____

3. Does the unit have the necessary leadership to be effectively managed? ☐ Yes ☐ No

4. If leadership is needed, what areas are deficient and why? _____
   _____
   _____

5. What must be done to bring the leadership up to meet requirements? ☐ Hiring ☐ Replacement
   ☐ Skill training ☐ Management training ☐ Increase amount of management ☐ Stronger enforcement
   ☐ Less stringent enforcement ☐ Empowerment ☐ Mentoring ☐ Accountability enhancements ☐ Other
   _____
   _____

6. What is management's relationship with employees?
   ☐ Unsatisfactory ☐ Accepted reluctantly ☐ Accepted ☐ Accepted willingly ☐ Respected

7. If management's relationship with employees is less than "respected," what must be done to enhance it?
   _____
   _____

8. How is management's capability perceived by the average employee? ☐ Exceptional ☐ Excellent
   ☐ Capable ☐ Satisfactory ☐ Below expectations ☐ Unsatisfactory ☐ Unacceptable

9. If the employee's perception of management's capability is less than "capable," what can be done to enhance it? _____
   _____

Fig. 17-6 ■ Sample worksheet for internal SWOT (*s*trengths, *w*eaknesses, *o*pportunities, *t*hreats) analysis.   *Continued*

the unit is confronted by in the marketplace. Managers will want to analyze the outside environment so that they can make adjustments in their units and in their products and services to meet the influences and changes that will originate from this sector.

Although how the unit must work with outside influences and what it will determine to be an outside influence are somewhat different for each unit, there are some common areas that all businesses, including nursing, should analyze. The following eight are among them:

1. Competition
2. Customers
3. Potential customers
4. Social and cultural environment
5. Government regulations
6. Political environment

10. What are the major training issues facing the unit? _____

_____

_____

11. What are the training requirements for the next 6 months? _____

_____

_____

12. What are the training requirements for months 7 to 12? _____

_____

_____

13. What are the training requirements for months 13 to 24? _____

_____

_____

14. How do the pay scales of unit employees relate to those of employees with similar jobs in other companies within the industry? _____

_____

15. What incentives are offered to employees beyond their normal compensation? _____

_____

_____

16. What is the absenteeism rate within the unit? ☐ 0-1 day per year per employee ☐ 2-5 days per year per employee ☐ 6-10 days per year per employee ☐ >10 days per year per employee

17. Is the absenteeism rate considered acceptable? ☐ Yes ☐ No

18. If the absenteeism rate is unacceptable, what is being done to reduce it? _____

_____

19. What is the employee turnover rate within the unit?
☐ 0%-1% ☐ 2%-10% ☐ 11%-25% ☐ 26%-50% ☐ >50%

20. Is the turnover rate considered acceptable? ☐ Yes ☐ No

21. How much of the turnover is from key positions? _____% From management positions? _____%

22. If the turnover rate is unacceptable, what is being done to reduce it? _____

_____

23. Will the turnover rate affect the unit's ability to meet its goals? ☐ Yes ☐ No

24. If so, what critical items must be accomplished to reduce the impact of the turnover rate? _____

_____

Fig. 17-6—cont'd ■ Sample worksheet for internal SWOT (*s*trengths, *w*eaknesses, *o*pportunities, *t*hreats) analysis.

7. Technologic changes
8. The economy

Most of the information managers will need is readily available through a myriad of consulting firms. They can also gather information from trade magazines and from federal, state, and local governmental agencies. They can find many research works at their public library or consult with a local university, because most have research departments that keep these facts readily available. Managers can find information on public companies by reviewing their annual reports, and they can read business publications that cover the health industry and specific service areas. They can go to trade shows, browse the

II. Production and Productivity

1. Are the goals and strategies used in operations and service delivery supportive of the unit's vision and mission statement? ☐ Yes ☐ No

    A. If not, how are they different? _____

    _____

    _____

    B. What must be done to allow these goals and strategies to support the vision and the mission?_____

    _____

    _____

2. How efficient is the unit in delivering its service? ☐ The industry leader ☐ Exceptional ☐ Significantly better than all competition ☐ Better than competition ☐ As good as the competition ☐ Not as good as the best competitor but better than 75% ☐ Not as good as the average competitor

3. If service capability is less than "better than competition," what is being done to enhance it?_____

    _____

    _____

4. Will the unit's service capability adversely affect the attainment of unit goals? ☐ Yes ☐ No

5. If so, what is being done to enhance service capability? _____

    _____

6. Are the quality service controls that are in place sufficient? ☐ Yes ☐ No

7. If not why not? What is being done to improve the controls? _____

    _____

8. Is the unit's resource and purchasing capability sufficient to meet goals? ☐ Yes ☐ No

9. If not, why not? What is being done to improve this capability? _____

    _____

10. Is the unit able to find the best source for service delivery? ☐ Yes ☐ No

11. If not, why not? What is being done to improve professional sources and physician referrals?_____

    _____

12. Is the unit exploring innovation in the development of its service? ☐ Yes ☐ No

13. If so, what is being done? If not, why not? _____

    _____

14. If there are problems with delivery within the unit, to what are they attributable? _____

    _____

Fig. 17-6—cont'd ■ Sample worksheet for internal SWOT (*s*trengths, *w*eaknesses, *o*pportunities, *t*hreats) analysis.   *Continued*

Internet, read trade magazines, and ask questions themselves. Fig. 17-7 is a worksheet to assist in tracking the major influences and developing an external SWOT analysis.

Managers must remember that outside influences are changing constantly and that close attention is required on a consistent basis so that they can position their units to take advantage of each change. If managers do not pay attention to the environment, they may be caught behind in a major shift, and this can pose significant problems for even the most successful healthcare units—possibly to the point of causing them to collapse for lack of a market to serve.

III. Marketing and Sales

1. Are the goals and strategies used in the Marketing and Sales Divisions supportive of the unit's vision and mission statement? ☐ Yes ☐ No

   A. If not, how are they different? _____
   _____
   _____

   B. What must be done to allow these goals and strategies to support the vision and the mission?
   _____
   _____

2. Whom has the unit targeted as primary customers? _____

3. What is the target market? _____
   _____

4. How does the unit distribute its products/services? _____
   _____

5. What is the unit's pricing strategy? _____
   _____

6. What is the unit's primary advertising and promotional medium? _____
   _____

7. Does the unit require a professional sales team? ☐ Yes ☐ No

8. If a professional sales team is used, is it effective in meeting the sales goals? ☐ Yes ☐ No

9. If not, why not? _____
   _____

10. What must be done to enhance the sales efforts and effectiveness of the sales team? _____
    _____
    _____

11. Who are the best customers (those who provide us with 80% of our business)? _____
    _____
    _____

12. Who, and what areas, are not being served? _____
    _____

Fig. 17-6—cont'd ■ Sample worksheet for internal SWOT (*s*trengths, *w*eaknesses, *o*pportunities, *t*hreats) analysis.

IV. Finance

1. Are the goals and strategies used in the Finance Division supportive of the unit's vision and mission statement? ☐ Yes ☐ No

    A. If not, how are they different? _____

    _____

    _____

    B. What must be done to allow these goals and strategies to support the vision and the mission?_____

    _____

    _____

2. What is the unit's cash position? ☐ Extremely good — well diversified ☐ Excellent — good balances and sufficient diversification ☐ Good — sufficient assets — no diversification ☐ Acceptable — good cash balances — no other assets ☐ Poor — marginal cash — no other assets ☐ Unacceptable — insufficient cash flow

3. If less than "good," what is being done to improve cash position and increase diversification? _____

    _____

    _____

4. What has been identified as the unit's break-even point? _____

    _____

5. Is the break-even point well managed, and are sufficient controls in place to ensure that it is attained? ☐ Yes ☐ No If not, what is being done, or needs to be done, to meet these needs? _____

    _____

6. Is the unit attaining the profit margins and goals that have been established? ☐ Yes ☐ No If not, what is being done, or needs to be done, to meet these levels? _____

    _____

7. What part of the unit provides the best return on investment (ROI)? _____

    _____

8. Why is this area the most effective? _____

    _____

9. What, if anything, is being done in this area that can be applied to other areas of the unit? _____

    _____

    _____

10. Does the unit have the ability to borrow money? ☐ Yes ☐ No If so, what is its payback ability? _____

    _____

    _____

    If not, what must be done to develop borrowing power? _____

    _____

Fig. 17-6—cont'd ■ Sample worksheet for internal SWOT (*s*trengths, *w*eaknesses, *o*pportunities, *t*hreats) analysis. *Continued*

V. **What Are the Unit's Internal Strengths?**

Strength 1 _____

How can this strength best be utilized?_____

_____

Strength 2 _____

How can this strength best be utilized?_____

_____

Strength 3 _____

How can this strength best be utilized?_____

_____

VI. **What Are the Unit's Internal Weaknesses?**

Weakness 1 _____

How can this weakness be overcome or compensated for? _____

_____

Weakness 2 _____

How can this weakness be overcome or compensated for? _____

_____

Weakness 3 _____

How can this weakness be overcome or compensated for? _____

_____

VII. **What Are the Unit's Most Significant Opportunities?**

Opportunity 1 _____

How can this opportunity be realized? _____

_____

Opportunity 2 _____

How can this opportunity be realized? _____

_____

Opportunity 3 _____

How can this opportunity be realized? _____

_____

VIII. **What Are the Major Threats Facing the Unit?**

Threat 1 _____

How can this threat be neutralized? _____

_____

Threat 2 _____

How can this threat be neutralized? _____

_____

Threat 3 _____

How can this threat be neutralized? _____

_____

Fig. 17-6—cont'd ■ Sample worksheet for internal SWOT (*s*trengths, *w*eaknesses, *o*pportunities, *t*hreats) analysis.

External SWOT Analysis

I. Competition

1. Who are your top three competitors?

(1) _____ (2) _____ (3) _____

2. What are their strengths and weaknesses?

    A. Competitor 1 _____

        1. Strengths: _____

        _____

        2. Weaknesses: _____

        _____

    B. Competitor 2 _____

        1. Strengths: _____

        _____

        2. Weaknesses: _____

        _____

    C. Competitor 3 _____

        1. Strengths: _____

        _____

        2. Weaknesses: _____

        _____

II. Current Customers

1. Who currently are your top 10 customers? (1) _____ (2) _____

(3) _____ (4) _____ (5) _____

(6) _____ (7) _____ (8) _____

(9) _____ (10) _____

2. What are the major opportunities that these customers represent to your business? _____

_____

_____

3. What are the major concerns you need to have when dealing with these customers? _____

_____

Fig. 17-7 ■ Sample worksheet for external SWOT (*strengths*, *weaknesses*, *opportunities*, *threats*) analysis.   *Continued*

THE ELEMENTS OF THE PLAN

Planning involves considerable thought and preplanning work. It is an almost constant process for those units that take it seriously, and there is plenty of hard evidence that every unit should do so. For example, researchers M. L. Collins and M. J. Porras found that those organizations that planned as part of their fundamental business process performed, on average, eight times better than those that did not. In addition, the stocks of companies that planned well performed an average of 55 times better than the overall stock market.[1]

Planning is an absolute necessity in management, and because far too many managers misunderstand many of the aspects of developing a good plan, some of the key points are repeated here.

III. Potential Customers

1. Who are your top 10 best prospects? (1) _____ (2) _____
   (3) _____ (4) _____ (5) _____
   (6) _____ (7) _____ (8) _____
   (9) _____ (10) _____

2. What are the major opportunities that these prospects represent to your business? _____
   _____

3. What are the major concerns you need to have when dealing with these prospects? _____
   _____
   _____

IV. Social Environment

1. Describe the social environment in which you operate your business. _____
   _____
   _____

2. What opportunities does this environment offer your business? _____
   _____

3. What are the major threats this environment poses for your business? _____
   _____

V. Cultural Environment

1. Describe the cultural environment in which you operate your business. _____
   _____
   _____

2. What opportunities does this environment offer your business? _____
   _____

3. What are the major threats this environment poses for your business? _____
   _____

VI. Government Regulations

1. What are the major regulatory agencies in your industry (include all federal, state, and local)? _____
   _____
   _____
   _____

Fig. 17-7—cont'd ■ Sample worksheet for external SWOT (*s*trengths, *w*eaknesses, *o*pportunities, *t*hreats) analysis.

Vision

Arguably the most important part of any plan is the vision. Many professionals contend that it is impossible for managers to have a plan if they don't know how to visualize themselves and their units in the future. This is so fundamental that it is not even necessary to discuss whether or not managers need a good vision to be effective planners; it should be an understood fact.

There is a practical side to the vision that is worth discussing, however, and this is that *the act of envisioning the business focuses the unit toward a single goal.*

2. What major opportunities do these agencies offer your business?_____

_____

_____

3. What are the major threats these agencies pose for your business?_____

_____

_____

VII. The Political Environment

1. Describe the political environment in which your business operates. _____

_____

2. What major opportunities does this environment offer your business?_____

_____

_____

3. What are the major threats this environment poses for your business?_____

_____

_____

VIII. Technology

1. Describe the major technology changes that may influence your business. _____

_____

_____

2. What major opportunities do these changes offer your business? _____

_____

_____

3. What are the major threats these changes pose for your business? _____

_____

_____

IX. Economy

1. Describe the economical environment in which your business operates._____

_____

2. What major opportunities does this environment offer your business? _____

_____

3. What are the major threats this environment poses for your business?_____

_____

Fig. 17-7—cont'd ■ Sample worksheet for external SWOT (*s*trengths, *w*eaknesses, *o*pportunities, *t*hreats) analysis.

Researchers Collins and Porras argued that this was the most significant reason why, among the companies they studied, those that had a good vision outperformed those that did not by such a wide margin.[1] The act of creating a vision provides a direction for the unit. It tells the staff where they will end up if they do everything well, and it gives managers a focal point to help organize their assets.

By definition, a vision is a way of seeing or conceiving what a unit wants to create or achieve. Although it is considered a fundamental business act to have a vision for the organization, it is also very good business to have a vision for each of the major divisions (as long as each supports the overall vision). Looking at existing vision statements such as the following can help managers get started in creating their own.

THE DIRECTIONS CORPORATION (HONOLULU, HAWAII)[2]

The Directions Corporation shall be the number one source of customer specific, and culturally sensitive, programs within the adult education industry.

UNIVERSITY OF TEXAS AT EL PASO (EL PASO, TEXAS)[3]

The School of Nursing's vision is to become the premier Hispanic-serving School of Nursing in the nation dedicated to improving the health of citizens, particularly Hispanics.

THE JOHNS HOPKINS HOSPITAL AND HEALTH SYSTEM (BALTIMORE, MARYLAND)[4]

To contribute to the science of medicine and the wellness of the public through the education and provision of qualified medical personnel.*

As can be seen, visions do not have to be very long or complex, and the best ones aren't. They are straightforward, simple, and factual. When managers are developing vision statements for their organizations or their major divisions, they should not try to write elaborate ones; it is best to be brief. Every member of the unit should know the vision and be able to recall it from memory. The briefer it is, the greater the chances that all of the unit's employees will remember it.

This last statement brings up an important point about visions: *to be effective, a vision needs to be shared.* If the manager does not share his or her vision within the organization, the manager cannot expect employees to help convert that vision into action. The simple act of sharing a unit vision can have an exciting effect on the members in the unit. It will help every member of the team direct his or her efforts toward attaining the vision, and the manager will be surprised at how effective that can be in helping the unit grow and improving its effectiveness.

A vision should be treated like a valuable part of the organization. If it is to become a tool that creates synergy within the unit, it must be demonstrated by the organization's leadership and accepted by every employee. Accomplishing this will not be easy, and although healthcare organizations are usually more effective in creating a shared vision than are their larger multinational business cousins, doing so still

---

*This was the vision statement at the time of initial research for this book. A revised mission statement (shown later) was found for this institution, but a revised vision statement could not be found. Because all vision statements evolve and change as the organization grows, this may or may not be current.

requires extensive work on the part of each unit's leadership. To create a shared vision within the organization or unit, management should consider the following when developing this vision:

- Design the organizational environment so that it encourages creativity, excitement, and individual growth.
- Include subordinates in the creation of the vision. This is *not* a management function.
- Do not campaign or attempt to sell the vision to the employees. Instead, let them assist in its development.
- Keep the vision simple. Make it a snapshot, not a movie epic, of the future of the organization as management sees it.
- Ensure that every member of management and every single employee—from the janitor to the chief executive officer—believes in the vision and makes it a fundamental part of his or her performance.
- Make the vision an honest, realistic expression.
- Keep the vision in line with the values of the individuals who work in the organization.
- Make the vision a positive source of excitement and never use it as a hammer or club to direct or gain obedience.
- Do not simply pay the vision lip service. It must be aggressively pursued if it is to be effective.
- Continually encourage support for the vision; never attempt to force everyone to be a believer.

It is not the job of managers to be the keepers of the vision. Although certain pieces of information are reserved for senior management's use, the vision is not, and should never be, maintained as a matter of senior privilege. For a vision to become a reality, in a unit of any type or size, it must be understood, shared, accepted, and lived by everyone responsible for realizing it. This means *everyone*, internally and externally. Even the vendors that supply the unit should be made aware of the vision, *and they should be expected to work hard to support its attainment.* If a vendor's efforts are contrary to the organizational vision, it is highly recommended that managers find another vendor. Fig. 17-8 shows those with whom the vision should be shared.

Each group identified in Fig. 17-8 has an influence on the success of the unit, and therefore each should understand what the unit is trying to create. All these groups also serve as a potential source of ideas and actions that can benefit the unit, and the more they know about what the unit is trying to build, the more help they can provide. All the groups shown in Fig. 17-8, especially customers (patients), identify with organizations that share their vision with them. They often begin to feel like a partner with the unit and become much more loyal in their dealings with it.

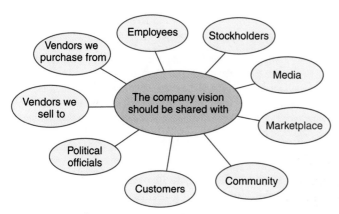

Fig. 17-8 ■ Groups connected to the organization with whom managers must share the vision to make it understood.

Mission Statement

Sometimes known as *company values,* or *organizational philosophy,* the mission statement is the foundation of the unit. It provides the overall reason that the unit exists and answers the question, "What is our business?" If the unit cannot answer this question, it will prove exceedingly difficult, if not impossible, to construct a plan that will help the unit continue to exist, let alone to prosper.

Mission statements are intended to supply abstract concepts of what it is management intends to achieve in the organization. When managers create theirs, they should not specify rigid, inflexible actions. Instead, their mission statements should include the following:

Tone of the unit: the emotional aspect of the unit's business attitude and performance environment

Common purpose: statements that will help managers rally others in support of the unit's initial goals

Unit culture: what it is that makes the unit unique, including beliefs, ideals, and concerns

Inspiration and motivation: the words that encourage and stimulate others to envision and work toward a higher level

Direction: the path toward growth or the way the unit is headed

Philosophy: fundamental beliefs—what is expected and what are believed to be fundamental truths

Feeling of success: statements that enable every performer to feel the energy that creates the potential opportunity

With their mission statements, managers convey an image to all who read them: employees, vendors, patients, and families; therefore, these statements should be positive but realistic; honest but enlightened; and above all, enthusiastic. People get excited when they read stimulating things. Managers want their statements to elicit the stakeholders' enthusiasm, not to bore them with facts. Keep in mind that the mission statement is expressing the unit's values—the fundamental beliefs that it holds in the highest esteem. Managers should talk about these things. They should use words like *honesty, loyalty, quality, fairness,* and *integrity.* Following are the mission statements for the units for which visions were shared earlier:

THE DIRECTIONS CORPORATION (HONOLULU, HAWAII)[2]

The Directions Corporation is committed to the development of unique adult education programs that meet the individual needs of our customers and reflect each client's unique culture. We understand our responsibility to listen effectively, research thoroughly, develop carefully, and provide our customers with an opportunity to approve our work before we deliver our products. We believe that this combination of effort will provide our customers with educational programs that satisfy their unique needs, as only they understand those needs. We are committed to an extraordinary level of service that is designed to keep our customers in control of the development, presentation and management of their training efforts. Finally we believe the provision of these ideals need not be expensive, and that our clients should be able to fully recover their costs within the time span of the first presentation of our product.

UNIVERSITY OF TEXAS AT EL PASO, SCHOOL OF NURSING (EL PASO, TEXAS)[3]

The School of Nursing at the University of Texas at El Paso College of Health Sciences supports the overall mission of the University. In addition, the mission of the School of Nursing is to prepare caring professional nurses to address multiple complex human needs in a binational and multicultural community. Socioeconomic environmental characteristics of the United States–Mexico border region impact health status, healthcare access, and service delivery. In partnership with clients and communities, graduates are prepared to access human and technologic resources and collaborate with local, state, national, and international agencies to improve the quality of life along the United States–Mexico borders, particularly the Texas-Mexico community of interest.

THE JOHNS HOPKINS HOSPITAL AND HEALTH SYSTEM (BALTIMORE, MARYLAND)[4]

- To be the world's preeminent health care institution
- To provide the highest quality care and service for all people in the prevention, diagnosis, and treatment of human illness
- To operate cooperatively and interdependently with the faculty of the The Johns Hopkins University to

support education in the health professions and research and development into causes and treatment of human illness

- To be the leading health care institution in the application of discovery
- To attract and support physicians and other health care professionals of the highest character and greatest skill
- To provide facilities and amenities which promote the highest quality care, afford solace, and enhance the surrounding community

The length of the statement is not important; it is the content that matters. Although some units can say what they believe in a few simple words, others require more. How the words stimulate and motivate is the critical factor. Nevertheless, the mission statement should be kept to fewer than 150 words and no more than two paragraphs.

As with the vision, the mission statement must be shared to realize its full potential. The more the unit can share the mission with its stakeholders, the greater the opportunity it will have to enlist their support for its beliefs and goals.

Finally, the mission statement does not represent a destination. It expresses the ideals and desires of the organization. As the unit grows, these elements can and do evolve and may even take on different forms. When changes occur in goals and strategies, these changes must be reflected in the mission statement as well. At a minimum, managers should evaluate their mission statement each time they update their action plan to ensure that it remains in tune with their new goals.

Goals

Regardless of whether they are called long-range aims, goals, or desires, goals are the things the unit wants to accomplish or the steps that outline the performance required to reach the vision. They are the actions necessary to fulfill the vision.

Goals complement the mission statement by providing the details for its broad views. They define specific areas of work, a clear and distinct direction, and standards of performance. Goals do not specify time frames for accomplishment and are not written with specific performers in mind. Bureaucratic units tend to create their goals through an autocratic process; executive management writes the goals and hands them out. Other, more enlightened units create their goals by working from the bottom up. The key thing to remember about setting goals is that people who have had a hand in creating the goals are far more willing to put forth the effort necessary to achieve them.

! CRITICAL POINT

It is strongly recommended that goals be drafted by the people who are responsible for attaining them. Ownership and buy-in are important determinants in the willingness to pursue goals. The more individuals believe that the goals that need accomplishing are their goals, the greater the likelihood of obtaining their willing participation.

Fig. 17-9 is a form to help managers develop their units' goals. The following terms in the figure require definition:

Strategy/objective: the action that will be performed

Priority of performance: importance in the overall initial strategy for this goal/objective

Individual strategy: the way the unit will go about accomplishing the goal/objective

Person(s) responsible: the name of the specific individual who will be tasked with ensuring that the given strategy is carried out in a satisfactory manner

Anticipated completion date: the date the unit expects to complete the individual strategy; although this should be a floating date, any change to the original should require approval of the senior manager in the unit

Anticipated cost: the amount the unit expects to spend in terms of real dollars to carry out this strategy

Anticipated return on investment: the amount the unit expects to gain from carrying out this strategy; the benefit to the unit

Measurement performed by: the method management will use to measure the effectiveness of this strategy; the name of the individual responsible for tracking the performance can also be included

Senior officer accountable: in addition to the responsible manager, a member of the senior management team who is accountable for the quality of performance in carrying out the strategy

It is no accident that the form has room for only five strategies for each goal or objective. If a goal or objective cannot be accomplished by five steps (strategies), then it has been poorly formulated (i.e., it is too broad).

During the formulation of specific strategies, the goal or objective being developed is frequently found to be unrealistic. Managers should not be afraid to make changes. Managers may even find that those things written originally as strategies can become goals or objectives and vice versa.

The accomplishment of goals must be measured in order for goals to be effective. It is absolutely critical that the unit evaluate the attainment of each strategy, and the overall goal it supports, against real expec-

Goal/objective: _____ Goal No.: _____
Priority of performance: _____

	Individual Strategy	Person(s) Responsible	Anticipated Completion Date	Anticipated Cost	Anticipated Return on Investment	Measurement Performed By	Senior Officer Accountable
1.							
2.							
3.							
4.							
5.							

Fig. 17-9 ■ Sample form for the development of goals. See text for definition of the terms used on the form.

tations. When goals and objectives are established, everyone must clearly understand exactly what is expected as a result before the measurement method is defined.

Once managers have established the correct expectations and developed the monitoring tool, work toward the strategies and the goals and objectives they support must be monitored to determine the degree and direction of progress. Box 17-1 lists several indicators that can be used to evaluate progress. However, managers should endeavor to follow the practices in their own industry as much as possible when determining specific evaluation criteria.

Monitoring tools should be used on an on-going basis, and measurement should be conducted both at regular intervals and when a change in the environment creates a need. The manager must ensure that the unit's progress is measured by someone who is objective. One of the best ways to accomplish this is to have an individual goal monitored by more than one person or by someone who is not a part of or influenced by the actual performance.

When managers are developing goals and objectives and the corresponding strategies that will cause them to take shape, it is wise for them consider what impact the goal or objective will have on the unit.

BOX 17-1

Indicators Used to Evaluate Progress

Sales (patient) volume
Return on investment (ROI)
Return on equity (ROE)
Profits
Market share
Customer satisfaction
Employee satisfaction
Earnings
Adherence to deadlines
Budget
Percentage completion
Attitude toward goal
Employee retention
Internal operating efficiency

■ Are the results that were achieved what was anticipated and projected?
■ Is the goal still consistent with the mission statement and vision?
■ Is the ROI or ROE still in line with what was projected?
■ How do the actual results measure up against those that were projected?

Finally, the following are some basic rules to be followed in developing goals and objectives:

Clarify what is wanted before beginning: Goals, objectives, and strategies have a way of defining the unit. They determine how the unit will be perceived. Be careful that what is created projects the intended image.

Do the right thing correctly, not the wrong thing correctly: Doing something that ends up not benefiting the unit is nonsense, no matter how well it is done. Careful analysis before starting will prevent this.

Establish priorities that make the best use of assets: When determining priorities, also dictate how the unit's assets must be used. Make sure that the resources are on hand, and the importance of their use is understood, in a manner that complements the unit's (and even the manager's) business style.

Define the parameters of performance: Most units, when asked how big they want to be, respond simply, "As big as we can be." A better approach is to define what "big" means to the unit and then plan for attaining that size. If the scope of the operation is understood, it is much easier to establish goals and objectives that are realistic and attainable.

Be systematic: Establish time frames and deadlines that let management take advantage of the unit's personnel assets without depleting, overextending, or disenchanting them. Goals, objectives, and strategies should motivate and excite, not beat down and demoralize. Sometimes too many requirements, or too short a time for meeting them, can have a severe negative influence. Be careful and exercise restraint. It is better to achieve a few good goals successfully than to fail to achieve a large number of goals.

Have fun: Always keep in mind this incredibly important admonition: *work is supposed to be fun.* Managers are asking themselves and others to accomplish things continually. Human beings will always accomplish more when they enjoy what they are doing than when they don't. To help the unit have some fun, build in some celebrations and some time for recognition of achievement. Keeping everyone excited is much easier if what is being asked is necessary, important, achievable, and *fun.* Don't run a sweatshop; run a Disneyland.

WRITING THE PLAN

Let's set things straight right from the start: there is no proper way to write a plan; therefore, managers should use whatever format gets the best results. This chapter presents a specific approach. Nurse managers should evaluate what is offered and, if it works for their units (it will for most), then use it. If, however, they feel that their units can benefit from taking a different approach, then that is the format they should use. For example, if the plan is for a very small group, then a simpler, more straightforward approach might be desired. Managers can ask themselves the following four questions when determining the proper format for their specific units:

1. Who is the plan for?
2. What is the plan for (obtaining financing, gaining approval, guiding implementation, etc.)?
3. Is visual impact important?
4. To what degree will those who receive the document actually read it? Will they skim through it? Will they read the executive summary and then flip through the sections? Or will they carefully read the material?

Sections of the Plan

Well-constructed plans almost always include several distinct sections that are designed to separate the plan's information into critical areas of discussion. It is not likely that a given plan will require all of the sections described in the following discussion.

COVER PAGE

Every plan should have a cover page. The plan's author can be creative and include graphics that reflect the plan's contents, put the unit's logo on it, or use well-chosen words to identify the content. The choice is the author's. Fig. 17-10 provides several examples.

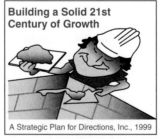

Building a Solid 21st Century of Growth

A Strategic Plan for Directions, Inc., 1999

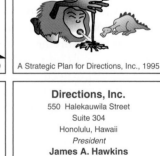

Getting Things Started
A Plan for Developmental Growth

A Strategic Plan for Directions, Inc., 1995

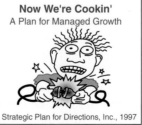

Now We're Cookin'
A Plan for Managed Growth

A Strategic Plan for Directions, Inc., 1997

Directions, Inc.
550 Halekauwila Street
Suite 304
Honolulu, Hawaii
President
James A. Hawkins
A Business Plan
1998

Fig. 17-10 ■ **Sample cover pages for a business plan.**

The cover pages shown in Fig. 17-10 are actual covers used by The Directions Corporation, a Honolulu-based curriculum development company that writes adult education curricula. Notice that the scenes on the front page do not necessarily depict the education industry but rather a topic on which the author wants the reader to focus in the plan. Also notice that the author wasn't afraid to have fun with a serious subject. The exception is the cover page shown on the bottom right, which was designed for a plan to develop operating capital (venture capitalists are not noted for their love of entertainment, and it is recommended that capital venture covers be kept plain and simple).

TITLE PAGE

The first page inside the cover is the title page (Fig. 17-11). This single sheet tells the reader what the report is about. It should contain the following seven elements:

1. The title of the report
2. The time frame that is covered by the report
3. The date that the report was written
4. The name of the responsible officer

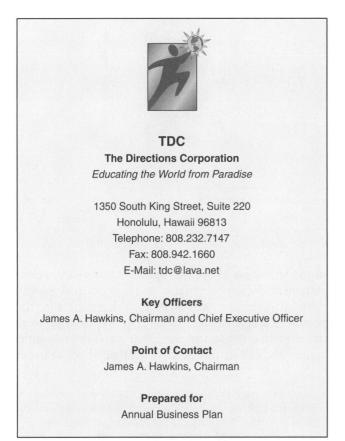

TDC

The Directions Corporation

Educating the World from Paradise

1350 South King Street, Suite 220
Honolulu, Hawaii 96813
Telephone: 808.232.7147
Fax: 808.942.1660
E-Mail: tdc@lava.net

Key Officers

James A. Hawkins, Chairman and Chief Executive Officer

Point of Contact

James A. Hawkins, Chairman

Prepared for

Annual Business Plan

Fig. 17-11 ■ **Sample title page for a business plan.**

5. Contact information (company address, telephone number, fax number, and e-mail address)
6. The name of the unit
7. Either a copyright statement or a level-of-confidentiality statement

TABLE OF CONTENTS

A table of contents is absolutely necessary for any initial action plan. It should appear immediately after the cover page and should supply easy reference to and page locations for the items covered in the plan (Fig. 17-12). Exceptional plans tab the major parts of the plan to make their location easy for the reader.

It is also a good idea to list all of the figures, diagrams, and enclosures in the plan in the table of contents. This helps the reader find a chart or form that has been seen earlier.

EXECUTIVE SUMMARY

There are different schools of thought about whether an executive summary should be included in a plan. One camp argues that including it is an absolute necessity because many busy executives do not have time to read the whole plan, and the executive summary enables them to understand the plan without having to read its entire contents. The other school of thought says that if the reader does not have time to read the entire plan, then it probably has been given to the wrong person. Whether or not to include an executive summary is the writer's decision. Information about it has been provided here to allow the novice manager to make an educated choice.

The executive summary, like the table of contents, is normally written after the plan has been completed. It does not have to be done this way, however. Some people write the summary first and use it as a guideline in preparing the remainder of the plan. Managers should use whatever process works best for them, but they should make sure that the executive summary reflects what is contained in the body of the plan. Those who write the executive summary first have a tendency to overelaborate and change some of the content in the body of the plan, and this is *always* a mistake.

At a minimum, the executive summary should accomplish the following:

1. Identify and define the unit
2. State the unit's vision
3. Give the unit's mission statement
4. Provide a situational analysis of the unit
5. List the goals of the unit
6. Identify the strategies to be used to realize the goals
7. Provide a listing of responsible officers

Business Plan for 1998

Table of Contents

Fig. 17-12 ■ Sample business plan table of contents.

---

8. Establish time frames and **milestones**
9. Provide basic financial information

Remember that a summary is just that—a short version of the body. Fight the tendency to be verbose in this section. Follow the KISS principle (*keep it short and simple*) as much as possible without leaving out key points.

INTRODUCTION OR PREFACE

The introduction or preface is an optional section. There is no set manner in which it has to be written, and for that matter, it need not be written at all. One of the best ways to use this option is to provide a clear statement of purpose; that is, to tell the reader exactly why the document was written. It is also nice for the writer to acknowledge all of the people who were involved in creating the plan. Many enlightened units simply include in this section a single sheet of paper

Milestones are significant events that occur during the time span of the plan. These are often grouped together in a chart or flow diagram referred to as the *milestone chart*.

signed by all of the employees and managers who assisted in the plan's development.

SITUATIONAL ANALYSIS

If the reader needs to be provided with a clear view of the present condition of the unit, the situation analysis section is the place to provide it. It should contain an in-depth analysis of the current market (external) environment, and it should relate this environment to the present condition of the unit. This section should draw its contents from conclusions that were reached when the SWOT analysis was performed. (The actual analysis, research details, and other data can be presented as an appendix.)

CRITICAL CONCLUSIONS

The critical conclusions section should contain the findings of the research that was conducted to develop the plan. These facts should be arranged so as to provide the reader with two things: (1) the knowledge that the analysis generated, and (2) the reason that this plan was developed (why it was necessary).

RECOMMENDATIONS

The recommendations section lists what the unit wishes to do or what it is recommending through the plan. This includes goals and strategies as well as time lines and milestones. In addition, managers should specify how they recommend measuring and monitoring the progress of the plan and how they will know when they have achieved success. (Many managers consider the measurement aspect so critical that they supply this information in a separate section. The choice is individual and should be based on the reasons for writing the plan and the intended audience.)

FINANCIAL PROJECTIONS

The amount of information that managers place in the financial projections section depends on the reasons for the development of the plan. If they are using the plan to develop capital, this section should be more extensive, with at least a 3-year projection. It is best to place only critical (key) information in the body of the plan and to provide the supporting data in the appendixes.

APPENDIXES

The appendixes contain the support material for the plan. They should provide the detailed studies, analysis, and other information that backs up what has been said in the body of the plan. Managers can include reference materials, glossaries, exhibits, diagrams, brochures, financial charts, and any other material that they feel is needed to support the plan.

OTHER TOPICS

The following is a list of other information that may be included in the plan. The complexity of the plan should fit the situation, the purpose, and the audience.

Marketing information: How the unit plans to deliver its products and/or services to the patient. Subsections on advertising and promotion may be included.

Business relationships: Those who know the unit and with whom the unit does business.

List of competitors: The unit's major competitors. Their strengths, perceived weaknesses, and a plan for dealing with each may also be included. Again, the complexity of the presentation is based on the purpose of the plan.

Management: Résumés for and background information on the key managers and team members in the unit.

Pricing strategy: Description of the processes the unit uses to establish the prices it asks for its products and services. This includes the reasoning used in creating the pricing structure, explanations of how the strategy provides the unit with competitive advantage, and so on.

Risk analysis: Identification of the major risk(s) faced by the unit and its plans for dealing with, overcoming, or managing the exposure.

Sales plan: How the unit intends to deal with the individual sale of the product or service. **Sales** is *not* marketing. The sales plan should not be placed in the marketing section.

The foregoing list is by no means all-inclusive. What a manager actually puts in the plan is for that manager and his or her key officers to decide.

Compilation of the Required Information

Figs. 17-13 through 17-23 present a variety of forms that can be used to compile the information necessary for a business plan. The forms presented here have been taken from those used by private, for-profit enterprises and where possible have been modified for

---

Sales involves a one-on-one encounter with a customer; marketing, on the other hand, is the promotion of a product or service to a group. Sales relies on presenting the benefits of the product (how it will help the customer), whereas marketing concentrates on describing the facts about or features of the product (what the product is like and what its specifications are).

Target Customer Profiling Worksheet

Gender (male, female, or both): _____

Ideal age: _____   Income level: _____

Education level: _____   Employment type (white collar, blue collar, self): _____

_____

Average age range: _____   Lifestyle (personality type): _____

_____

Physical location of company (city, state, country): _____

_____

Estimated size of target audience (in round numbers): _____

What percent of total market does customer represent? _____

Is there potential growth in the market? If so, how much? _____

_____

How much will customer pay for product/service? _____

Why will customer pay this much? _____

Major customer buying habits: _____

To what units do customers belong? _____

What publications, if any, does customer read? _____

What events does customer attend (religious, social, fraternal, business)? _____

_____

Preferred method of marketing to customer: _____

_____

Customer turn-on(s): _____

Customer turn-off(s): _____

Topics to avoid: _____

Remarks or special considerations: _____

_____

_____

Fig. 17-13 ■ Sample target customer profiling worksheet.

use in the healthcare industry. All of the questions contained on these forms are applicable in the healthcare industry, but not all may be applicable to your specific unit. You are encouraged to use the material presented as a means to stimulate your thought processes or as an actual support tool for plan development if possible. Don't dismiss the forms as nonapplicable, however, simply because you don't need them at your present level of management. As your career develops, you will find them relevant.

CONCLUSION

Planning is a complex and demanding process. Thought and hard work are required to perform it properly, and there is no sense in planning unless you

Worksheet for Analyzing the Healthcare Industry

What is the total annual sales within the industry? _____

What is your unit's specific field of expertise? _____

What is the anticipated growth in your field during the next 5 years? _____

10 years? _____ Is the industry growing or declining? _____

Who are the top units within your field? _____

_____

Is your unit's most direct competitor a big or small provider? (Small companies are those with annual gross

sales volumes less than $5 million.) _____

_____

What are your industry's major regulatory issues? _____

What near-term effects can they pose on the industry? _____

What long-term effects can they pose? _____

_____

What are the major economic issues facing your industry? _____

What near-term effects can they pose on the industry? _____

What long-term effects can they pose? _____

_____

What technologic changes can affect your industry? _____

What near-term effects can they pose on the industry? _____

What long-term effects can they pose? _____

_____

What products exist within your industry that are similar to yours? _____

_____

_____

What enhancements can your unit bring to your industry? _____

_____

What is the average net profit of a unit similar to yours (annual and per item sold)? _____

_____

What is the average markup on your product/service? _____

What Is the average profit margin for a similar product within the industry? _____

_____

_____

What is your anticipated inventory turnover rate? _____

What is the average turnover rate for your industry? _____

What is your anticipated annual sales amount? _____

What is the average annual sales amount for companies like yours? _____

_____

Fig. 17-14 ■ **Sample healthcare industry analysis worksheet.**

Sales and Dispersal Planning Worksheet

General Sales

1. What sales technique do you employ, or do you intend to employ, in your unit?
   ☐ In-store ☐ Telephone solicitation ☐ Direct mail ☐ Face-to-face ☐ Referral ☐ Cold calls ☐ Warm calls

2. Do you intend to use an active sales force? ☐ Yes ☐ No   If so, what type?
   ☐ Self ☐ Telemarketing firm ☐ Internal sales team ☐ Outside consultants ☐ Manufacturer's representatives

3. If you plan to use your own sales team, how many salespeople will you require (including yourself, if applicable)?
   ☐ 1   ☐ 2-5   ☐ 6-10   ☐ 11-25   ☐ > 25

4. Do you plan to sell via the Internet? If so, how? _____
   ☐ Company website   ☐ Unit mail stops   ☐ Other:_____

Retail Sales

1. What type of sales outlet will you use?
   ☐ Storefront locations   ☐ Catalog distribution   ☐ Internet

2. If you use actual retail storefronts, how many will there be? _____

3. Who are your targeted customers?
   ☐ Women ☐ Men ☐ Men and women ☐ Children ☐ Older generation ☐ Younger generation ☐ All ages

4. What is the availability of your targeted customers? How many are there? _____

5. Where do your customers live in relation to your business location(s)?
   ☐ Within walking distance   ☐ <5 minutes' drive   ☐ 10-15 minutes' drive   ☐ >15 minutes' drive
   ☐ In same town   ☐ Within same state   ☐ Within the United States   ☐ International

6. Will your customers expect discounts? ☐ Yes ☐ No   If so, what type? _____

7. Will you provide credit to your customers? ☐ Yes ☐ No   If so, what type?
   ☐ Internal credit   ☐ Visa   ☐ Mastercard   ☐ American Express   ☐ Other_____

8. How will you service your customers after the sale? _____
   _____

9. Will you accept returned merchandise? ☐ Yes ☐ No   If so, how?
   ☐ Within 30 days of sale   ☐ With receipt   ☐ Without receipt   ☐ Unquestioned   ☐ Other

10. How do you intend to attract customers?
    ☐ Word of mouth   ☐ Referral   ☐ Local advertising   ☐ Specialty advertising   ☐ Other

Fig. 17-15 ■ Sample sales and dispersal planning worksheet.

Wholesale Distribution

1. What type of distributor will you use?
☐ Company-owned ☐ Manufacturer's representatives ☐ Retail customers ☐ Other

2. How many distribution points do you have?
☐ Just your company ☐ 1 in addition to self ☐ 2-5 ☐ 6-10 ☐ 11-25 ☐ >25

3. What payment terms will you give your distributors?
☐ C.O.D. ☐ Net 30 ☐ Net 60 ☐ >60 days

4. Who is responsible for paying the freight cost for distribution? ☐ You ☐ Distributor

5. How do you intend to establish your distribution network? _____

_____

NOTE: The questions asked in this form might need extensive modification to fully fit the actual situation of a healthcare unit. The questions provided here are representative of a typical for-profit business and are meant to stimulate your creative process.

Fig. 17-15—cont'd ■ Sample sales and dispersal planning worksheet.

intend to do it correctly. Following haphazardly prepared plans is foolhardy. Although this textbook recommends that, as a nurse manager, you plan as much as is necessary to develop your unit in a controlled and well-managed way, it is more important that you realize that planning is not something to be taken lightly. It is your unit, and you must protect it by establishing creative, well thought-out, and highly developed planning procedures.

SUMMARY

- The process of developing a plan helps any manager learn to think strategically and perform the following tasks:
  - Develop a mental picture of the unit's future; this is often referred to as a *vision*
  - Formulate a statement of purpose that will help attain what is desired
  - Develop specific goals and objectives that act as a roadmap to help chart the unit's way toward realization of its vision
  - Devise a timetable for the accomplishment of the vision
  - Clearly define success in terms important to the unit
- Most professional planners believe that it is impossible to plan effectively in one's mind, especially when the object of planning is as complicated and diverse as a nursing unit. Therefore, this chapter focused on helping to identify those things that

must be accomplished to develop a written plan of action for a unit. A written performance plan has the following benefits:
- It provides a tangible instrument to track the progress of the unit.
- It allows managers to physically see what the unit's historical actions were and whether or not the unit has completed all of the things that were planned for it to accomplish.
- It validates actual performance. Reality rarely runs true to the plan, and the written vehicle allows a unit to see where deviations have occurred and how it can chart a course that will return performance to its original path.
- A systematic process was outlined for the development of an initial plan, including the provision of a step-by-step method, graphic examples, and forms that can be used in developing the information that must be included.

 FINAL THOUGHTS

Strategic planning has the purpose of clarifying an organization's beliefs and values. It accomplishes this by analyzing the organization's strengths and weaknesses as well as its potential opportunities and threats.

Strategic planning identifies exactly where the organization is going and how it plans to get there. It provides direction, improves efficiency, eliminates poorly

Product/Service Development Worksheet

All Types of Businesses

1. Describe your product/service:_____

_____

2. Now describe your product/service in fewer than 10 words:_____

_____

3. What are the special features of your product/service? (What is it, and how is it structured?)

Feature 1: _____

Feature 2: _____

Feature 3: _____

4. What are the benefits to your customers if they buy your product/service? (What is in it for the customers? How will the product/service improve their lives, increase their convenience, save them time or money?)

Benefit 1: _____

Benefit 2: _____

Benefit 3: _____

5. What makes your product/service unique? (Why would the customer buy your product or use your service instead of those offered by your competition?)_____

_____

Product-Based Business (If your business produces or sells tangible products, answer these questions.)

1. What form is your product currently in? ☐ Development ☐ Production ☐ Ready for sale
2. Do you have a patent, copyright, or registered trademark? ☐ Yes ☐ No
3. How will you market your product? ☐ Intercompany marketing team ☐ Outside marketing firm
4. Will you expand your product to several models or maintain a single version?
   ☐ Single version ☐ Multiple models ☐ Spin-off product lines

Service-Based Business (If your business provides an intangible service, answer these questions.)

1. What "extra value" does your service bring to your customers that your competitor's does not? _____

_____

2. Will you provide a specific service or a broad range of services? ☐ Single ☐ Broad range
3. Will you service a specific type of customer or anyone? ☐ Specific type ☐ Anyone
4. What is unique about your service? _____

_____

5. How will your customers know that they are receiving a good deal? _____

_____

_____

Fig. 17-16 ■ Sample product and service development worksheet.

Price Development Worksheet

Retail Units

1. What percentage will you mark up your services/products? _____

2. How can you justify the price you will have to ask? _____

3. How does your price compare with your competitor's on a similar item?
   ☐ Lower ☐ About the same ☐ Higher ☐ Significantly higher

4. What incentive, if any, will you offer your customer to pay your price? _____

5. What is special about your unit that will draw customers at a higher price? _____

6. Is there any way to lower your price? _____

Service Companies

1. What hourly rate does it cost you to provide your service? _____

2. What percentage will you mark up your per-hour cost? _____

3. How does your price compare with your competitor's for a similar sevice?
   ☐ Lower ☐ About the same ☐ Higher ☐ Significantly higher

4. Why would a customer choose your service over that of the available competition? _____

5. Is there any way you can lower your price? _____

Fig. 17-17 ■ Sample price development worksheet.

designed or underused programs, prevents duplication of effort, concentrates available resources on a priority basis, improves communication and the coordination of activities, provides an opportunity for expansion, allows adaptation to the changing business environment, and sets realistic but challenging goals.

Strategic planning provides a vision of tomorrow for the leader's use today.

THE NURSE MANAGER SPEAKS

It is critical to the success of the healthcare unit that all nurse managers be committed to effective strategic planning. Strategic planning must never be considered busywork. Instead, managers must take it upon themselves to learn the importance of long-range planning and the proper methods for accomplishing it.

Each nurse manager should prepare a vision and a mission statement for his or her unit. The vision is nothing more than a mental image of how the nurse manager sees his or her unit over an extended period of time. What will the unit look like 5 years from now?

The mission states the purpose of the unit. It sets forth the philosophy, aims, and characteristics of the unit in readily understood terms that every member of the unit can easily recall.

Every nurse manager is responsible for guiding his or her unit toward success. Effective strategic planning is how success gets started.

Operations Planning Guide

1. What days will your unit be open?
   ☐ Monday ☐ Tuesday ☐ Wednesday ☐ Thursday ☐ Friday ☐ Saturday ☐ Sunday

2. What will be your hours of operation?
   Monday-Friday: _____ Saturday: _____ Sunday: _____

3. Is there any time when no one will be available during working hours?
   ☐ No   ☐ Yes   When? _____ Why? _____

4. What will be the standard greeting to customers when they enter your unit? _____
   _____

5. How do you want the unit's telephone answered? _____
   _____

6. What forms of payment will you accept?
   ☐ Cash ☐ Check ☐ Credit ☐ Visa ☐ Mastercard ☐ American Express ☐ Other _____

7. What kind of terms will you ask for when extending credit?
   ☐ 30 days same as cash   ☐ Net 30   ☐ Net 60   ☐ Internal revolving charge card

8. Will you accept returns on merchandise sold? Under what circumstances?
   ☐ With receipt   ☐ Within 30 days   ☐ Exchange   ☐ Like merchandise   ☐ Purchase credit

9. Will you close your business for holidays? Which ones? _____
   _____

10. Will your customers come to your location, or will you visit theirs? _____
    _____

11. Who will pay for repairs and services to the products you sell?
    ☐ Customer   ☐ Your company   ☐ Warranty   ☐ Service contract   ☐ Shared with customer

12. Where will you keep your inventory?
    ☐ On site   ☐ Warehouse   ☐ Vendor   ☐ Fulfillment service

13. Where will you produce your product?   ☐ On site   ☐ Use third-party vendor

14. Where will you procure your inventory?
    ☐ Produce it yourself   ☐ Use third-party vendor   ☐ Use fulfillment service

Fig. 17-18 ■ Sample operations planning guide.

Competition Analysis Worksheet

Analyzed Area	1st Competitor	2nd Competitor	3rd Competitor
Company name			
Years in business			
Address/location			
Specific specialty			
No. 1 product name			
Major selling point			
No. 2 product name			
Major selling point			
No. 3 product name			
Major selling point			
Primary market			
Secondary market			
Service quality level			
Major strengths			
Weaknesses			
Reputation			
Major attitude and approach to business			
Strategy to be used in meeting this competitor			

Fig. 17-19 ■ Sample competition analysis worksheet.

Promotion Planning Worksheet

Activity	Budgeted Cost	Anticipated Dates of Performance	Special Considerations
Advertising			
Television			
Radio			
Major newspapers			
Local newspapers			
Trade publications			
Other _____			
Sales			
Introductory offer			
Free samples			
Special coupon			
Incentive program			
Alternative Advertising			
Seminars/presentations			
Special announcements			
Newsletters			
Grand opening			
Open house			
Other _____			
Presentation Media			
Logo stationery			
Business cards			
Brochures/handouts/fliers			
Other _____			

Fig. 17-20 ■ Sample promotion planning worksheet.

Production Development Worksheet

Product name: _____ Date of completion: _____

COMPONENT 1   NAME:_____

Pricing Criteria	Description of Requirement	Cost per Unit	Cost of Assembly
Material			
Special tooling			
Setup charge			
Delivery costs			
Labor costs			

COMPONENT 2   NAME :_____

Pricing Criteria	Description of Requirement	Cost per Unit	Cost of Assembly
Material			
Special tooling			
Setup charge			
Delivery costs			
Labor costs			

COMPONENT 3   NAME :_____

Pricing Criteria	Description of Requirement	Cost per Unit	Cost of Assembly
Material			
Special tooling			
Setup charge			
Delivery costs			
Labor costs			

PACKAGING COSTS

Pricing Criteria	Description of Requirement	Cost per Unit	Cost of Assembly
Material			
Special tooling			
Setup charge			
Delivery costs			
Labor costs			

MISCELLANEOUS COSTS

Pricing Criteria	Description of Requirement	Cost per Unit	Cost of Assembly
Assembly			
Final product setup			
Royal ties paid			
Estimated overhead			
TOTAL COSTS			

Fig. 17-21 ■ Sample product development worksheet.

Required Equipment and Supplies Worksheet

Required Item Name/Nomenclature	Vendor Name	Purchase Price	Purchase or Lease	Date Needed	Special Considerations
1.					
2.					
3.					
4.					
5.					
6.					
Office Equipment					
Telephone system					
Answering system					
Fax machine					
Copy machine					
Computer(s)					
Computer peripherals					
A. Printers					
B. Scanners					
C. Network					
Computer software					
A.					
B.					
C.					
D.					
E.					
Specialized software					
A.					
B.					
C.					
Postage meter					
Filing cabinets					
Size 1					
Size 2					
Size 3					
Bulletin boards					
Supplies Required					
Stationery					
Business cards					
1.					
2.					
3.					
4.					
5.					
6.					
7.					
8.					

Fig. 17-22 ■ Sample required equipment and supplies worksheet.

Vendor Analysis Worksheet

Product Name/Description:_____

Supplier Name	Price	Delivery Time	Sales Terms	Credit Terms	Comments
1.					
2.					
3.					
4.					
5.					

Product Name/Description:_____

Supplier Name	Price	Delivery Time	Sales Terms	Credit Terms	Comments
1.					
2.					
3.					
4.					
5.					

Product Name/Description:_____

Supplier Name	Price	Delivery Time	Sales Terms	Credit Terms	Comments
1.					
2.					
3.					
4.					
5.					

Product Name/Description:_____

Supplier Name	Price	Delivery Time	Sales Terms	Credit Terms	Comments
1.					
2.					
3.					
4.					
5.					

Product Name/Description:_____

Supplier Name	Price	Delivery Time	Sales Terms	Credit Terms	Comments
1.					
2.					
3.					
4.					
5.					

Fig. 17-23 ■ Sample vendor analysis worksheet.

REFERENCES

1. Collins ML, Porras MJ: *Preparing the organization for competition,* New York, 1988, Harper and Row.
2. Hawkins J: *The Directions Corporation: 2005 business plan,* Honolulu, 2005, The Directions Corporation.
3. University of Texas at El Paso: UTEP's vision, mission, and goals, no date, retrieved February 13, 2006, from http://www.utep.edu/aboututep/visionmissionandgoals.aspx.
4. The Johns Hopkins Hospital and Health System: The mission of The Johns Hopkins Hospital and Health System, no date, retrieved January 3, 2006, from http://www.hopkinshospital.org/hospital/mission.html.

SUGGESTED READINGS

Allee V: *The knowledge evolution: expanding organizational intelligence,* Newton, Mass, 1997, Butterworth-Heinemann.

Baskin K: *Corporate DNA: learning from life,* Newton, Mass, 1998, Butterworth-Heinemann.

Bennis W, Nanus B: *Leaders,* New York, 1983, Dell.

Blanchard K: *The heart of a leader: insights on the art of influence,* Colorado Springs, Colo, 2004, Honor Books/Cook Communications.

Brown JS: *Seeing differently: insights on innovation,* Harvard Business Review book series, Cambridge, Mass, 1997, Harvard Business School Press.

Burton EJ, McBride WB: *Total business planning: a step-by-step guide with forms,* New York, 1991, Wiley.

Davis M: *A practical guide to unit design,* Menlo Park, Calif, 1996, Crisp Publishers.

Dettmer W: *Breaking the constraints to world-class performance,* Milwaukee, 1998, ASQ Quality Press.

Dienemann J: *Nursing administration: strategic perspectives and applications,* Norwalk, Conn, 1990, Appleton and Lange.

Dobson P, Starkley K: *The strategic management blueprint,* Oxford, England, 1993, Blackwell.

Douglas LM: *The effective nurse leader and manager,* St Louis, 1996, Mosby.

Economy P: *Business negotiating basics,* Chicago, 1990, IDG Books.

Economy P: *Negotiating to win,* Chicago, 1990, IDG Books.

Greenberg J: *Behavior in organizations,* Upper Saddle River, NJ, 1999, Prentice Hall.

Helgesen S: *Web of inclusion: a new architecture for building great institutions,* Milwaukee, 1998, ASQ Quality Press.

Hersey P, Blanchard K, Johnson D: *Managing organizational behavior,* Upper Saddle River, NJ, 1996, Prentice Hall.

Hill N: *Napoleon Hill's key to success,* New York, 1997, Plume.

Hirschhorn L: *The workplace within: psychodynamics of unit life,* Cambridge, Mass, 1990, MIT Press.

Maister D: *True professionalism: the courage to care about your people, your clients, and your career,* New York, 1997, Free Press.

Marquis BL, Huston CJ: *Leadership roles and management functions in nursing: theory and application,* Philadelphia, 1996, Lippincott.

McCormack M: *What they don't teach you at Harvard Business School,* New York, 1988, Bantam Doubleday.

Muihead BK: *High-velocity leadership: faster, cheaper, better,* New York, 1999, HarperBusiness.

Nelson R: *Fundamental management practices: people, projects and teams,* Chicago, 1996, IDG Books.

Nelson R: *Empowering employees through delegation,* Upper Saddle River, NJ, 1998, Prentice Hall.

Nelson R: *Decision point,* Upper Saddle River, NJ, 2000, Prentice Hall.

Reinman J: *Thinking for a living,* Athens, Ga, 1998, Longstreet Press.

Schon D: *The reflective practitioner: how professionals think in action,* New York, 1984, Basic Books.

Stone D: *Difficult conversations: how to discuss what matters most,* New York, 1995, Doubleday.

Swansburg RC: *Management and leadership for nurse managers,* Sudbury, Mass, 1996, Jones and Bartlett.

Yoder-Wise PS: *Leading and managing in nursing,* ed 3, St Louis, 2003, Mosby.

Managing the Transitions of Change

OUTLINE

LEARNING SYNOPSIS

Upon successful completion of this chapter, readers will possess a fundamental understanding of the importance of managing the transitions that occur in a period of change.

OBJECTIVES

1. Define the difference between change and transition
2. Explain why change itself is not what people have difficulty with when moving from the old to the new
3. Identify what must be done before one can begin something new
4. Describe methods and steps that can be used to effectively manage the transition of change in any situation
5. Identify different strategies for dealing with nonstop change
6. List skills that a nurse manager can use to build trust in a unit during periods of change and transition
7. Describe effective methods for managing oneself during periods of change, transition, and stress

Those who administer change are often confronted with blank stares, grumbling, small acts of defiance, and even subtle shreds of sabotage that can easily turn an incredible idea into an unworkable mess. Change is a constant in everyone's life, however, and the healthcare industry has seen more than its share over the past two decades. It is critical to the continued excellence of the nursing profession that every nurse manager learn to lead his or her team effectively through it.

Although much of the change that affects nurse managers' lives is not earth shattering, many changes that occur in the nursing environment can be and are. Many of the changes that nurse managers will implement will be critical to the quality of the patient care delivered by their team members. These changes do not fall into the category of "It would be nice if we could do it" or "I'll do it the next time I get a chance." They involve the split-second decision-making that separates the exceptional people from the also-rans. These changes may allow a medical care facility to be competitive, to be effective, and to be profitable. Change is not a game for nurse managers or the medical profession; it is survival. Those who can manage it well will prosper; those who cannot aren't likely to last long.

This chapter assumes that most of the time you have been involved in the healthcare field as a professional nurse you have been instrumental in the operation of your unit. As a nurse, when you have seen a challenge, you have developed a means to deal with it and have implemented change, either by yourself or assisted by others. If you have been a supervisor and have had a few subordinates reporting to you, it has been you who have told the team members what to do and you who have ensured that the task was done properly. But now you are taking steps to grow within the profession by becoming a nurse manager. In this new job, you will manage new faces and have new levels of responsibility. You will find out that the old process of "tell and do" may not work quite the same way. Simple, unquestioning compliance will seem to materialize less and less often when you start managing through other supervisors and interacting with more senior managers.

There are many reasons for the changes that will take place in your environment. For one thing, the growth in your responsibilities will turn the management of change into a daily occurrence. So frequently will you be subjected to it that one change won't be completed before the next one is begun. Although you, as nurse manager, might thrive on this type of chaos, the average employee will not show your level of enthusiasm for such a demanding regimen.

Another reason is that growth will cause your responsibilities to spread into different arenas, and these will impose the reality that competition is truly fierce. So intense is the competition within senior management that there is seldom room for error. Misjudgment, or even honest mistakes, can land you in court, sued by the competition—and even by your own employees. The new risks you are about to inherit cover the gamut from personal rights infringement to stress-related disability to you personally! Think about that. An employee can sue you—*and win*—because it is too difficult to work around you.

Now here's the rub. What has gotten you to this level of success within the profession is an ability to perform functional tasks like providing the excellent patient care, delivering the service, and providing the professional advice that your patients and other medical professionals need. Most high-performance nursing professionals are better at doing these things than they are at managing the performance of others. Personnel management is not an area that is generally attractive to today's nursing professional. After all, few are psychologists, and most truly enjoy providing direct patient care. The average professional nurse just wants to obtain excellent patient results and has little interest in dealing with the emotional side of the internal environment. As you advance in the management arena, however, that simplification vanishes. As you assume increasing responsibilities, there is no way that you, the professional nurse manager, can avoid getting into that "people stuff." As your job moves you away from being a performer to being a manager, someone else must now do the things you used to do. This evolution involves change, and there is no way that you can deal effectively with change without being efficient at dealing with people.

Luckily, managing change, and the transitions that create the challenges arising from change, is not all that difficult, especially for a nursing professional with an advanced education. In fact, you have been accomplishing much of what will be required ever since you became a member of the healthcare profession—every time you collaborated with a physician, understood a patient, or presented a tactful compromise during a serious negotiation. What you need to add to these demonstrated skills is not an extensive undertaking. Instead, what you need to learn is a method of making others feel comfortable with their jobs and with the changes they must confront. When you can do that with a high frequency of success, you will have a performance asset no matter where you are or what you are doing.

Managing change will not always be easy, but it will always be essential. This chapter provides you with a few hints on how to get started.

THE CHALLENGE

Change in itself does not produce the difficulty that people experience in moving from one thing to another, nor do the changes that nurse managers must implement as their business grows cause them stress; rather, stress comes from the transition that must be made as one moves from the old to the new. *Change* is positional: the new method, the new boss, the new idea, the new policy. *Transition* is the mental process that people go through as they struggle to accept these new things. Change is a thing that people do; transition is something with which people deal. Change is not personal, it is external. Transition, on the other hand, is highly emotional and purely internal.

Unless managers are able to help their organizations deal effectively with the transition caused by change, they don't have much chance for success. This is why good ideas often don't live up to expectations. For example, a large regional hospital in the Arizona desert thought to improve its efficiency by setting up employee performance "circles." It was felt that the circles would get the employees thinking about ways to cut costs and improve efficiency. The administrative executive placed in charge of the effort later reported that no significant cost-saving ideas were generated in the nearly 2 years that the program ran. The executive cited poor involvement and a reluctance to change as causes for the failure of the program.

At least the hospital realized that employees must go through some form of behavioral change if an idea is going to work. It actually came a long way toward understanding the differences between change and transition. Many people believe that transition is merely gradual or unfinished change. These two concepts are very different. Change represents a destination. It is what a person does—an outcome, such as shifting from a traditional nursing mode to a specialized team effort.

Transition is not change; it does not start after the change outcome has been realized. It involves emotionally letting go of the idea that the old reality is sacred. It is an attitude change, a behavioral acceptance of the new while letting go of the old. Nothing can have a greater impact on the continued success of a healthcare institution than the ability to identify who will have to let go of what to accept the changes that must occur.

Transition, unlike change, starts with an ending. It is the break with what is comfortable and proven.

Think about transition in terms with which you can identify. Look at what you had to do to make the switch from student to professional nurse. You had to let go of the familiar and embrace the unknown. The kind of work that you knew thoroughly came to an end, and each day brought something new to challenge you. The process had endings. It also had losses, some good and some not so good. That is realistic, isn't it?

Imagine the following situation: The hospital in which you work has outgrown it current facilities and requires a new location with greater square footage and easier access. Maybe more parking is needed for the growing number of employees, physicians, and visitors. Perhaps, as nurse manager, you have concentrated your efforts during the change on making the new location better for your growing team. On the first day in the new hospital, all you hear from your nurses is grumbling. People aren't focusing on the availability of parking or the larger patient spaces. The only thing they are talking about is the longer drive they had to make through heavier traffic to get to the new location. Are they being ungrateful? No—simply human.

As the nurse manager, you must begin the process of change by managing the transition that occurs between the old and the new.

Transition starts with letting go and moves quickly into a nether region that lies between letting go and accepting the new. We'll call this the "gray zone." This is the twilight area that separates the old from the new. It is the period that occurs between letting go of the old and experiencing comfort with the new.

Typically, change occurs rapidly. You move into a new house. You get a promotion. You change your hairstyle. Externally, things happen quickly. But internally, your acceptance of these new changes may take a great deal more time. Just because you got a new haircut does not mean you immediately accept the way it makes you look. Negative thoughts lurk in your subconscious: "What if I look strange?" "What if my fellow employees don't like the new style?" You enter into a kind of emotional no-man's-land full of these land mines and wander about until the new becomes comfortable.

Understanding this no-man's-land is important to effecting change in the nursing unit. Employees, regardless of their level of professionalism, often don't understand this transition, and that accounts for the large turnover of personnel during periods of major change. Employees become uneasy as they move through the gray zone, become disenchanted, and abandon the situation for one with which they feel comfortable.

The gray zone is a positive condition, however—or at least it can be if it is managed well. It represents the hospital's best chance for creativity, renewal, and development. It is the period when innovation is most possible and when true growth actually begins. On the other hand, the gray zone can represent a dangerous situation if it is mishandled. Then it can lead to turnover, disenchantment, and lost trust.

DEFINING THE CHALLENGE INTO ACTION

The specific situation described in the following case study and exercise may not be one that is familiar in the nursing profession or in a particular healthcare facility. The situation has been devised to demonstrate the need for managers to carefully plan their decisions before taking action and to demonstrate the difficulties that poor planning can cause in any working situation. When you perform the exercise, evaluate only the situation that is presented in the case study and do not dwell on whether the nursing profession operates in this specific way or not. Demonstrating the effect of change and the need for analytic thought is what is important here.

CASE STUDY

You are the vice president of nursing in a high-technology hospital and you want to make a change in procedure. You are getting some resistance from your employees. They tell you that the implementation is going to take more effort than you originally thought. In your mind you see the change as being a sound business decision and necessary for your unit to retain its competitive advantage. You are having difficulty understanding the resistance. Let's paint the picture in real terms; then see if you can use your basic understanding of transition as it was presented earlier to develop a better sense of exactly what is going on.

Your hospital has traditionally conducted the business of patient care using a division of labor. It has positioned the nursing staff in a number of units in the hospital, provided them with redundancy in terms of advanced equipment, and asked them to administer patient care based on the physical and mental urgency of the patient's request and the technical competence required to perform the care. The hospital has built a culture of professionalism by considering the difficulty of the patient care provided by each level of personnel in conducting individual performance reviews. For all nurses, performance evaluations (and thus compensation levels) are based on documented patient needs, the professional expertise required to provide the required

services, and the efficiency of the individual nurses in rendering that care. Because of the specific categories of professional expertise that have been established, each patient care unit has developed an extremely independent attitude with regard to other units in the hospital and an internal reliance on individual excellence designed to increase the efficiency of that unit. For example, each nursing unit is staffed with employees of a variety of different levels of nursing expertise, and management has grouped patient care tasks by the level of expertise and training necessary to accomplish the required care. All patient calls are directed to a centralized nursing station for action, and a nurse manager at the desk decides which level of nurse will provide the care. The first tier of staff, who are the least qualified, are assigned the responsibility of handling basic requests, such as requests for assisting in walking, helping with the activities of daily living, or changing bed linens. If, however, the patient requires a professional nurse to assess his or her condition or provide specialized care, the assignment is given to one of the available registered nurses (RNs). These highly educated RNs handle the majority of difficult problems and are instrumental in getting most of the patients back on the correct path. When extremely serious problems occur, however, patient care is supported by a third tier of personnel—the nursing supervisors. The supervisors have many years of experience in the nursing profession. They are usually called upon to assist only in major trauma cases and in other emergency situations, but they can, if necessary, reschedule the unit's entire staff to assist in solving a specific problem.

Each level of care is provided by the employee who has the required level of expertise on a rotating basis. The nurse manager remains responsible for ensuring a smooth flow in patient care and for evaluating the performance of each individually assigned nurse. Over the years, this hierarchy of care provision has created many severe internal conflicts and constant tension between the levels of performers. Distrust has built up among the three levels of staff members. Those at each level of expertise feel that they are the ones who carry the majority of the load and that the others are just support people whom they suspect of not pulling their weight. The individual nurse supervisors are very turf conscious and work against the establishment of a cohesive team.

As you can guess, the atmosphere within the individual units is getting rather testy. Personnel at each level are accusing those in the other groups of passing their work on to the next level. The first- and second-tier staff are accused of being "conveniently busy." The third-tier staff are viewed as procrastinators; if they can't get to a problem immediately, they "put it off" and make the patient wait, often for hours, declaring that they were occupied elsewhere.

Outside the hospital, the community that relies on its services is getting furious. Every time someone from a physician's office calls the hospital, he or she is passed from person to person until a staff member can be found who is "trained" sufficiently to handle the problem. Callers are placed on hold for long periods and often never get a response. The level of customer satisfaction is poor, and this is starting to affect attitudes within the community. Faced with increasing competition, the hospital is rapidly losing patients to other area hospitals, and acceptance within the community is declining as private practice physicians send their patients to other institutions.

The hospital's board of directors brings in a business consultant whose thorough analysis leads to a recommendation for a sweeping change within the organization. The three-tier system of patient care will be eliminated, and staff will be divided into teams composed of personnel from each tier. Each request for assistance, regardless of complexity, will be directed on a rotating basis to a nursing team that will have the collective responsibility of providing a solution. Each team will have a supervisor who will direct the requests to the appropriate team member.

The entire nursing department is brought together by the hospital administrator, and the change is carefully explained. Each member of the team receives a new policy manual, and team leaders are given specialized training to assist them in directing the work effort. The hospital administrator asks you, as the vice president of nursing, to meet with each team in every nursing unit to reinforce the importance of the change and to solicit the support of each team member. Everyone agrees that the change is overdue and welcome.

When the change is first implemented, the difficulties that initially surface are dismissed as being those that always occur during times of flux. But after a few months have passed and the problems still exist, senior hospital managers become concerned. They study the situation and observe that the various unit team leaders are not working within their teams to solve the problems but are relying on old relationships that were developed under the earlier care structure. Patients are now receiving care from any number of different teams without any real coordination, regardless of how hard the nurse manager tries to organize the effort.

Senior management now decides that the situation must be resolved and asks you to straighten out the mess in the nursing units. In what follows, you will find a list of actions that can be undertaken in any situation such as this and a scale that you can use to rate the value of each action and the priority that should be given to

performing it. Read through the list and familiarize yourself with what actions you might take; then go back through the list and assign to each action one of the following five ratings:

1 = *Critical:* This action needs to be accomplished immediately.

2 = *Important but not urgent:* Implementation plans for this action should be developed immediately and implemented as soon as practical.

3 = *Potentially good:* The value of this action will depend on how well it is accomplished.

4 = *Not important:* This action may even result in a waste of time and effort.

5 = *Bad:* This action should not be attempted.

Take your time in examining the possible actions that have been listed. Then work through the problem before you continue on in the chapter. This is an important exercise, and it is not an easy one. The problem that has been presented is complicated, and solving it is designed to be a demanding undertaking. Remember that the importance of this exercise is to get you to understand the effect of change and inadequate planning. Use the scenario presented and the list of potential solutions to arrive at your decisions. This is not an exercise in how problems might be solved in an actual hospital nursing unit or how a real unit might be structured. Do not allow yourself to get hung up on the differences between this scenario and the real world. Study the situation given and respond based only on that situation.

Don't worry about making a mistake because there are no specifically correct ratings for any of the actions listed. Select your response as you wish. After the list has been presented, the chapter discusses the recommended value rating for each action. You can always perform the exercise again later.

■ POSSIBLE ACTIONS

_____ 1. Determine exactly what individual behaviors and attitudes will have to change to make the team concept work.

_____ 2. Provide training in teamwork to the entire organization.

_____ 3. Break the change down into smaller stages. Combine the first and second staff tiers immediately and then add the third tier at a later date. Convert the nurse supervisors into team coordinators as the last step.

_____ 4. Determine who stands to lose something by working under the new system.

_____ 5. Modify the compensation system to reward compliance with the new system.

_____ 6. Sell the new policy by describing the problems that brought it about.

_____ 7. Bring in a motivational speaker to provide employees with instruction in teamwork.

_____ 8. Design temporary procedures to eliminate confusion during the changeover to the new system.

_____ 9. Use the gray zone between abolition of the old system and acceptance of the new system to improve the methods by which services are performed in the units. When necessary, create new services.

_____10. Change the physical layout of the nursing stations so that teams are grouped together and divided by glass partitions.

_____11. Scrap the plan and arrive at one that is less difficult to implement.

_____12. Have the team members talk with disgruntled patients. Make them see the situation firsthand so that they will develop some appreciation of the importance of the problem.

_____13. Appoint nurse managers to oversee the change within specific units and give each one the responsibility to ensure that the change progresses smoothly.

_____14. Give every nurse a badge that displays a team logo.

_____15. Turn the problem over to the entire nursing staff and tell them to come up with a solution and a conversion plan.

_____16. Change the individual award system to a team award system and adjust performance reviews to reward team performance.

_____17. Talk with individual employees and ask them what difficulties they have experienced with the new policy.

_____18. Write a memo to all personnel and explain the required changes once again.

_____19. Redesign the nursing stations and locate the team members together in team locations.

_____20. Create a model team to serve as an example for others. Put your best people on the model team.

_____21. Reorganize the staff of the vice president of nursing into a team and designate the vice president of nursing as a coordinator for the change.

_____22. Send team representatives to visit other organizations where service teams operate successfully.

_____23. Bring the staff together and formally instruct them to quit their foot dragging or face disciplinary action.

_____24. Provide a bonus to the team that receives the highest marks for quality of service from the first 100 patient surveys.

_____25. Provide a new organizational chart to everyone.

_____26. Start holding regular team meetings.

_____27. Talk about transition and its effects on people. Provide specialized instruction to coordinators so that they can help with the transition.

■ SUGGESTED RESPONSES
■ Category 1
Critical (This Action Needs to Be Accomplished Immediately)

1. **Determine exactly what individual behaviors and attitudes will have to change to make the team concept work.** A key to getting your employees through any transition is to determine what changes in behavior and attitude will have to be made. It is never enough to tell people what they have to do. All staff members need to know how the new requirement will differ from what they are doing now. They need to understand what they will have to stop doing and what the new policy will require them to start doing. The more specific you can be with each member of your team, the greater the chances that the person will understand what is required of him or her and the greater the possibility of winning that individual's support.

4. **Determine who stands to lose something by working under the new system.** People resist letting go of what they are comfortable with, not adapting to change itself. They cannot begin to grasp something new until they are ready to let go of the old. Resistance can be reduced by spelling out what might be lost if the change is not implemented quickly. In addition, this knowledge will indicate things to look for and prepare you to deal with resistance before it gets out of hand.

6. **Sell the new policy by describing the problems that brought it about.** Don't make the mistake of underselling the problem and overselling the solution. People must have a reason to accept change, and selling the problem will provide them with realistic and sensible reasons that the change should be accepted.

12. **Have the team members talk with disgruntled patients. Make them see the situation firsthand so that they will develop some appreciation for the importance of the problem.** By revealing the patient's point of view firsthand, you are actually selling the problem to your team. As long as individual nurses are not required to field patient complaints, poor service and poor patient care will be *management* problems and will remain so no matter how much effort you put into trying to convince others of the potential ramifications. To fully gain your nurses' support, you must share the burden of patient complaints and help them see these complaints as part of *their* problem. Set up a program in which

your nurses visit patients and have them bring back a "lessons learned" presentation for others.

17. **Talk with individual employees and ask them what difficulties they have experienced with the new policy.** Most managers like to think they know what is wrong when an organization is having trouble with change. But the reality is that very few really do. It is a human frailty to imagine that everyone sees things your way. Many managers expect their employees to view things as they do, and most employees simply cannot. Unless they have previously held a management position, employees have an entirely different perception of the working environment than that held by management, because they haven't had the same experiences. When you are talking with employees, ask the right questions and ask them in a proper manner. An improper or improperly phrased question can create an adversarial situation that will produce a defensive answer. Lead with your questions but be polite. Keep your tone relaxed and your authority hidden.

26. **Start holding regular team meetings.** Even before you start the change, have your staff begin to meet with one another to discuss it. They will become comfortable with one another and less resistive. It is important that these meetings be frequent and productive. Try sitting in on the staff meetings periodically, but never sit in on all of them. Give your employees space to share their concerns without having to worry about what your reaction might be.

27. **Talk about transition and its effect on people. Provide specialized instruction to coordinators so that they can help with the transition.** The more people know about the effect of transition and what it takes to get through it, the greater the chance that it can be navigated quickly. People deal with other people better if they are prepared to anticipate what the other people might be going through. If individual team members are prepared to experience the effects of transition, they will be less likely to imagine that bad things are occurring. Be honest with your team and don't pretend that accepting change or moving through transition is easy. They are not, and it is harmful to believe that they are.

■ **Category 2**
Important but Not Urgent (Implementation Plans for This Action Should Be Developed Immediately and Implemented as Soon as Practical)

5. **Modify the compensation system to reward compliance with the new system.** This is an important idea, because the sooner you reward the new behavior, the sooner you will have it. Be careful and plan well. A compensation system that is implemented without proper consideration is likely to introduce new problems faster than it can clear up old ones.

8. **Design temporary procedures to eliminate confusion during the changeover to the new system.** The gray zone can be a dangerous period. Confusion can block accomplishment and cause failure. The creation of temporary procedures can help you ease into the change and eliminate many of the challenges arising from too rapid a change.

WARNING !

The introduction of temporary procedures can become confusing and disruptive if not handled carefully. Every attempt should be made to roll the temporary procedures into the final procedures. This can be done, even if extensive change in the procedure is required, by involving the employees in amending the procedure. The more the employees contribute to the changes, the less confusion will be caused by temporary procedures.

9. **Use the gray zone between abolition of the old system and acceptance of the new system to improve the methods by which services are performed in the units. When necessary, create new services.** A period of flux can present an opportunity to attempt things that had been put aside because of conflict with established methods. Generally, innovations can be introduced more easily in this period than they could have been in earlier times.

16. **Change the individual award system to a team award system and adjust performance reviews to reward team performance.** You will never get people to accept team performance if you are rewarding them for individual performance. Make this change as soon as you can; however, make sure that you think through the program thoroughly. Do not change your program too quickly, because that may cause more problems than are remedied.

19. **Redesign the nursing stations and locate the team members together in team locations.** This should be done with caution. If you rearrange the nursing stations, you will cause the change to occur on a physical plane. Such an action may break down many of the barriers, but it does not provide team members a comfortable place to "hide" from the change. Physical surroundings are very important to the average person, and altering them (especially if the change is perceived as a reduction in quality or size) can have a negative as well as a positive influence.

21. **Reorganize the staff of the vice president of nursing into a team and designate the vice president of**

nursing as a coordinator for the change. People need to see their leaders in a role that relates to what is expected of them. Leadership by example has a dramatic effect on change. If the employees see the boss participating, they are much more likely to accept the change for themselves.

22. **Send team representatives to visit other organizations where service teams operate successfully.** The more your employees can feel, hear, and touch the change, the quicker they will learn and accept it. Talking to someone who is actually doing what is expected is far more effective than sending employees to a seminar presented by someone who has never undergone the required change. If you can't take your employees to see others, invite others to visit your location and share their experiences.

■ Category 3
Potentially Good (The Value of This Action Will Depend on How Well It Is Accomplished)

2. **Provide training in teamwork to the entire organization.** Training is important because it helps people understand new methods. For training to be effective, however, it must be a part of a larger effort and must not be left to stand on its own.

7. **Bring in a motivational speaker to provide employees with instruction in teamwork.** By itself, this will accomplish nothing. Management has a tendency to believe that once people receive new information they will automatically accept what has been presented. Nothing is further from the truth. People make personal decisions about whether or not to accept new ideas suggested to them. To make this type of presentation effective, you must support it with a comprehensive and well-demonstrated plan that can be followed easily by all personnel.

13. **Appoint nurse managers to oversee the change within specific units and give each one the responsibility to ensure that the change progresses smoothly.** This is an excellent idea if you have a comprehensive plan to follow. Merely appointing someone and telling that person to "make it happen" almost certainly will not accomplish the change. You do not want to create a situation in which someone becomes perceived as either an enforcer or a lackey. This will only weaken your effort to secure the change.

14. **Give every nurse a badge that displays a teamwork logo.** The badge is a symbol, and symbols are powerful motivators. Badges are useless when used alone and must be provided only as part of a much larger effort. Badges will not be effective if they do not actually symbolize your support.

24. **Provide a bonus to the team that receives the highest marks for quality of service from the first 100 patient surveys.** Rewards and compensation are powerful motivators; however, you need to make sure that the customer satisfaction process is handled in a positive and productive manner. Do not allow these first 100 patients surveyed to receive a quality of service that is different from that given to the next 100 just so a team can win the award. Also, it is not recommended that a specific individual be singled out for an award. You want to reward teamwork, so make sure it is the team's effort that is rewarded.

■ Category 4
Not Important (This Action May Result in a Waste of Time and Effort)

10. **Change the physical layout of the nursing stations so that teams are grouped together and divided by glass partitions.** Although this is basically a good idea, it doesn't go far enough. Leaving people in familiar surroundings allows them to hold onto the old relationships. What you need to do is to relocate the individual performers into team groupings so that their proximity to each other helps them accept the change.

18. **Write a memo to all personnel and explain the required changes once again.** There is only one benefit to writing a memo: when you put things in writing, people have a more difficult time saying that they did not receive instructions. However, memos are generally viewed as a means for the senders to secure their own interests and are often looked down upon. Memos are notoriously poor at explaining complex information and represent one-way communication. Memos can rarely deal effectively with emotional matters.

25. **Provide a new organizational chart to everyone.** Organizational charts are designed to identify reporting relationships and the hierarchy of the organization. The problems that need to be dealt with in this circumstance are the employees' attitudes and behaviors. Showing them whom they will be reporting to, although certainly informative, will not help them, or you, face the real challenges.

■ Category 5
Bad (This Action Should Not Be Attempted)

3. **Break the change down into smaller stages. Combine the first and second staff tiers immediately and then add the third tier at a later date. Convert the nurse supervisors into team coordinators as the last step.** If you could have delivered this change in small pieces, the beginning of the project, when smaller changes are usually easier to assimilate,

would have been the time to do so. However, instituting one change after another is unsettling to the group and signals trouble ahead. It may cause you to lose good people who fear working in what they perceive as an environment in constant flux. It is best to deliver a large change of this nature in one complete package.

11. **Scrap the plan and arrive at one that is less difficult to implement.** *Never do this!* It is your job to find a way out of the problems that have been identified. If you give up, you stand to lose the respect of every member of the unit, and you will have failed in your duty to the organization. This action is irresponsible.

15. **Turn the problem over to the entire nursing staff and tell them to come up with a solution and a conversion plan.** Turning over a project of this nature to a group of people who have already indicated that the change is undesirable is inviting disaster. Getting people involved is a good thing and should be a part of your plan from the beginning, but throwing your leadership away signals defeat, and people rarely rally to the flag of a defeatist.

20. **Create a model team to serve as an example for others. Put your best people on this model team.** This is not a good idea for several reasons:
    - It depletes the existing teams of the best people during the process of change.
    - It creates a situation in which less able individuals are asked to mirror the best. This is always difficult and is rarely achievable.
    - It again sets up an exclusive tier and breaks down the team concept you are trying to create.

23. **Bring the staff together and formally instruct them to quit their foot dragging or face disciplinary action.** Threatening your staff is always counterproductive because it is demeaning and takes away one very important quality that is needed if a person is to accept change—self-regard. It is your job to build trust and to gain cooperation, not to deter it. Making your staff feel small and insecure is not the way to attain your goal. You can use a meeting to clear up details and make expectations clear, but do it in a positive manner and solicit help rather than demand it. The respect and cooperation you need to effectively implement change are things that most employees (and especially professionals) give to you. They are not things that can be demanded or that come as an integral part of your job.

As noted earlier, there is no perfect solution to the situation described or correct responses for the actions listed. The thing you should remember from this exercise, in addition to the possible actions that are

obviously valuable, is that when you are dealing with change, it is not necessarily the change itself that is causing the problems or provoking resistance. When you encounter a situation such as the one presented here in your own organization, make sure you deal with the transition between the old and the new. The transition between the old and the new is where you will find the vast majority of change-related problems. People (including professionals, and many times *especially* professionals) deal with transition on a purely emotional level and therefore can rarely be led through the change simply by presenting facts or even logical reasons. Your leadership is critical if you are to help your employees deal effectively with the fears and anxieties they will develop as you lead your organization through a growth change.

RESOLUTIONS

Before you can begin something new, you must bring to an end the thing that is being replaced. Before your organization can grow, it must let go of its current size and the comfort that employees feel through its closeness. Before your team can learn a new way of doing things, its members must accept that the old way will no longer work. Therefore, all growth depends on ending old ways. The problem is that people, even your people, don't like endings.

Change and endings interact. Change ignites transition, and transition starts with an ending. As your organization grows, your team will have to let go of things that they are comfortable with and embrace things that are new and foreign. The following are two examples.

EXAMPLE A

John Derrick, a nurse manager, wants to add a new service and support a different type of patient. He recognizes that the addition makes perfect sense from a growth standpoint, and it will increase the organization's revenue. But he has employees who have specifically decided to work for his unit because it is small and comfortable. His employees enjoy an atmosphere in which they call each other by their first names and fear that the proposed addition will bring in more people and create an environment of tighter control. As the new service is added and new people are brought in to operate it, an immediate rift starts in the unit. Openly, the staff speak of "us" and "them," and new supervisors are unable to bring the two factions together. Investigation shows that the old team usually creates the friction because they are afraid of the new competition. John's challenge is to get the old employees to let go of their feelings for the old unit and embrace the idea of a new, larger unit.

EXAMPLE B

New growth in the hospital has forced the hospital administrator to hire a new vice president of nursing to run the day-to-day operation of the nursing department. Immediately, the new vice president starts appointing nurse managers and supervisors to put a layer of management between her office and the actual nursing staff. It now takes longer for information to get from the boss down to the nurses, and when it arrives it is often distorted. Decisions that were always made on the spot now require committees and long periods of time. As the months go by, the hospital administrator is seen less and less by the average employee and the new vice president tightens her grip on the nursing department. However, the quality of patient care starts to fall off, and even the most dedicated nurses are finding reasons for not showing up for work. When they are at work, they work at half speed and continually grumble and complain about "how it used to be." The new vice president keeps talking about how much better the new structure is, hoping that somehow she can convince people to help her make it work. In financial terms, the hospital is better off, but the vice president fails to realize that financial security for the hospital means little to people who have lost their familiar surroundings, their sense of being able to approach their boss, their personal self-worth, and their positive outlook regarding the future of the organization.

It was not the changes that took place in either of these cases that the employees resisted. They were unhappy about what they felt they had lost and resisted the ending of what they formerly knew to be good. For these reasons, it does little good for management to talk about how great things will or can be. Instead, it is critical that management deal with the losses and the endings being felt by the employees. How can a manager effectively deal with such things? The following sections provide some recommendations.

Identify Who Is Losing What

When you are beginning the process of making a change, you must realize that people will want to resist. There will be a desire to hold onto the old and resist the new. The best time to deal with this is in the planning stage. The following is a structured method of beginning the change process:

Describe the change: Outline the change to your employees in as much detail as possible. Be specific and tell people exactly what you believe will change. Don't speak in general terms, because this will not provide the average employee with an understanding of what is going to be different once the change has been implemented. Don't use terms like *improved performance, higher quality,* or *decentralized performance.* People generally have difficulty understanding these concepts because they are too broad to see at the personal level.

Visualize the change: Think of the change as turning your boat around in the water. If you turn it too fast, it might capsize; too slowly, and you could run it aground. Think of the people and things that might get wet when you are making the turn. Some things are going to get wet because you planned it that way; in other cases, it will be unintentional. Try to identify beforehand as many of the things that might get wet as possible. Look beyond the initial change and anticipate the secondary changes that will occur. With each of these changes, try to describe exactly what is going to be different when the change is complete.

Deal with cause and effect: Making a change creates a chain of cause-and effect collisions. For each one, try to think of the people who will be affected. As you do, try to identify who is going to have to let go of something. What will the employees have to let go of and how much do those things mean to them? The more you can identify the amount of letting go that has to be done, the more you will be able to help each person deal with the transition of change.

Define what will be lost: If you know what people think they will lose through the implementation of a change, you can easily formulate answers and remedies to help ease the transition.

If the change is already under way, it is easier to find out what the perceived losses are. Simply ask your employees the following three questions:

1. What is different now that the change has occurred?
2. When we made this change, what did we have to give up?
3. What is it you miss since the new change was implemented?

Accept the Loss as Important and Real

Your opinion of the reality of a loss is not what is important. If a person perceives a loss, no matter how much you may disagree, the loss is real to that person. You should not try to argue the loss with the individual. Any attempt to make light of what your employees perceive as a loss will only stop the conversation and cripple your ability to learn more. If you demean others' feelings by expressing your belief that their perceptions are not credible, you will simply convince your employees that you either don't understand them or don't care about them.

When you make changes in your organization, your challenge is to obtain commitment from those who are there to help you. Mere compliance with your wishes is not enough. Perhaps simple compliance will get the job done, but cooperation and support will get it done much better, much faster, and with far better results. For your team to make a commitment, its members must believe that you have their best interests at heart when you are making changes. It is imperative that you listen carefully when your employees tell you what they see as being lost. Good managers never indicate or allow their employees to perceive that they do not believe that their employees' concerns are valid.

Don't React to Overreaction

Overreaction, for purposes of this chapter, is defined as "what occurs when one person reacts more than another." Keep in mind that people will react to change. Some will show only a little reaction, whereas others may react severely. The degree of reaction shown depends on what people believe themselves to be losing. You cannot say to someone else, "Stop overreacting." That will not work. People are losing a piece of their world, or they think they are, and for the most part, thinking they are losing it and losing it are pretty much the same thing in the mind of average employees. It is easier for you, the nurse manager, to be reasonable because you are implementing the change and in many cases know that something will be gained from it.

The degree of overreaction that you will see in your employees can also be directly attributable to what type of losses they have experienced in the past and how those losses have been handled. If staff members have dealt with earlier losses effectively, the reaction to a new change will be more controlled. If they have not dealt effectively with past changes, however, the tendency to overreact to new ones is heightened. The combination of the unresolved old experience with change and the new change can give rise to a much stronger reaction than expected.

Overreaction can be triggered when employees perceive that the change will cause a chain of actions that may end up having a direct personal effect on them. For example, if you dismiss someone who is perceived as having job security, perhaps those remaining will wonder if they are going to be next. In cases like this, strong reaction is normal and generally should not be considered overreaction.

You, as the nurse manager and implementer of change, must learn to look for the loss behind the loss and deal effectively with it. You'll be able to obtain much more support if you can convince your employees that loss A is really not related to perceived loss B. Trying to talk them out of reaction to loss A will not, by itself, provide you with a solution to the problems posed by loss B.

Acknowledge the Loss

One of the best ways to deal with perceived loss is to get it out into the open. Simply acknowledge the loss and express your concern for the affected people. When you do this, make your statements straightforward and simple, as in the following examples:

"I understand your concern over these transfers. We have been losing some good people."

"I know that bringing in this new software has made a lot of you feel like beginners again. I feel that way myself and don't much like the feeling."

"I'm sorry that Joanne decided to leave. I will miss her and wish her good luck."

As a manager of others, you must understand that it is not talking about loss that stirs up emotion. It is failure to acknowledge the loss that angers people. Many managers are afraid to address loss because they think it will inflame their audience. Not so! Only when you fail to acknowledge others' concerns do you increase the potential for resentment.

As a manager, you need to know how to handle pain in others. Although this is certainly a difficult part of the job, it is absolutely necessary when helping your team through transition. Bringing things out into the open through direct conversation often has a healing effect on people. Don't be afraid to express your thoughts and even your own emotion, if that will help your employees understand. However, a sensitive approach must be used. Telling the truth can be very helpful to the team, but it can also be extremely detrimental if not handled properly. Be careful to deliver the truth in a manner that allows it to be well managed and accepted by your audience.

Accept the Signs

When you put an end to something, even if it is to start something better, you can expect to see people in a variety of moods, ranging from elation to hostility. People get angry, sad, frightened, and even depressed when they deal with transition. Don't make the mistake of viewing these reactions as a reflection of bad morale—most often they are not. Reactions are natural when people lose something they feel was important or to which they were attached.

Look for and expect these emotions, but don't expect to see them immediately. Generally they don't show up at the very instant an ending is made. That spot is reserved for denial. Almost all people want to deny that the end has occurred, and this is a natural first stage in the acceptance process. Denial is the way that many people protect themselves from the first impact of loss. This is a healthy response and does not warrant action on your part as long as it does not last too long. If your team stays in denial for more than a few days, however, then you will need to address the subject. Be gentle, but be firm. You might try something like the following:

> Many of you are acting like the change we implemented has not occurred. Well, it has, and it is time that we deal with it. I am concerned that you seem not to be accepting the change. Because I would like to get us through this with as little distress and disruption as possible, I think we should move on, and we can't do that as long as we pretend the change hasn't happened.

Other reactions, such as anger and fear, should be considered serious and dealt with effectively. Don't make the mistake of thinking that you caused them, however. If you do, you may be perceived as defensive and hostile. Don't argue your point. Instead, try to deal with these reactions as outlined in the following sections.

Not everyone will feel the emotions discussed here intensely enough to reveal them, and very few people will experience all of them. But within your organization, you can expect to encounter most of these emotions displayed by a variety of employees. You must work with your employees and help them cope with the transition. Simply telling your staff to "deal with it" will not create adjustment. Failure to adjust to change can create significant challenges for the organization, because it will lead to more resentment and deeper emotional responses when you try to enact further change. These cumulative effects can be devastating for even the best healthcare organization.

ANGER

Actions that span the gamut from simple grumbling to rage can lead to defiant acts such as intentional mistakes, deliberately slow performance (foot dragging), and even direct sabotage.

Good managers understand that some of their employees will react negatively when dealing with change, and often this negative emotion will manifest itself as anger. Although it is understandable, it must be dealt with effectively, because strong reactions of this nature can be extremely detrimental to the smooth operation of the medical unit and can manifest themselves in poor patient care.

One suggestion is to meet with the errant employee one on one and, while keeping your voice even but firm, explain that this type of behavior is unacceptable when openly demonstrated. You might explain that, although there may be nothing wrong with having these feelings, the accompanying behavior is totally unacceptable in the workplace.

This is something with which you, as a manager, must deal. Sticking your head in the sand and hoping that it will pass will only make things worse.

ANXIETY

Anxiety can be a fear of the unknown or an assumed difficult future, or even catastrophic fantasies. This is a natural emotion, and care should be taken to avoid making people feel inadequate because they feel anxious. You can deal with anxiety most effectively by keeping the individual up to date with as much information concerning the change as possible. The more that is known, the less there is to imagine.

NEGOTIATION

Negotiation may take the form of unrealistic attempts to be removed from the situation or to make the situation go away. For example, individuals may try to make a deal with you or may promise things that will allegedly benefit you if you will just undo the change.

Efforts such as these are not attempts by your employees to create real problem-solving situations. You should take a realistic look at what is being promised and carefully weigh the employee's ability to produce results. Don't allow yourself to be swayed by unrealistic promises and desperate arguments.

DEPRESSION

Depression is a profound feeling of sadness, and its physical expression can range from withdrawal to tears. The employee can appear emotionally flat, non-responsive, or simply tired. When any of these signs occurs for an extended period, deal with the problem realistically and, above all, calmly. Don't overreact and don't allow yourself to sympathize. Expressions of understanding and empathy are excellent when appropriate, but you should be careful not to reassure the person by providing unrealistic hope.

CONFUSION

People who are confused by change often exhibit forgetfulness or melancholy. These reactions are brought on by insecurity and can be dealt with effectively simply by talking to the individual. Allow the employee to express his or her feelings and offer reassurance that change often brings confusion. Frequently check back with the individual and ask how things are going.

Balance Out the Loss

Change will be required to help your unit or organization grow to achieve the next level of performance. Changes in the workplace are as inevitable as changes in the weather, but that doesn't mean that everyone will accept changes in the workplace with as much indifference as they show to changes in the weather.

Resistance to change in the workplace most often occurs when employees experience only the difficulty brought on by the change. Although all employees may be able to see the benefits for the organization, many of them will directly experience only a personal loss. This is not a situation in which you can simply talk with your employees and expect them to change. Such an action will not usually get you very far. What you need to do is to find a way that you can help employees through their perceived loss. Once again, keep in mind that a perceived loss is as real to the person who feels it as is an actual loss experienced by everyone. Telling an employee that he or she has had no loss is not a solution and will only cause further resentment. Instead, find a way to compensate for the loss. The following sections show what can be done.

LOSS OF PRESTIGE

Suppose that the growth of your organization creates a reason to streamline some of the functions and reorganize job assignments. To facilitate the change, formerly senior employees are to be grouped with junior personnel and a new job title is to be assigned. The formerly senior employees will no longer be responsible for supervising others and will be only performers.

This loss of position can elicit significant resistance from the senior personnel. They may feel that they have been demoted or have suffered a loss of prestige. If this happens, you can count on confronting some significant negative talk, some foot dragging, and even direct resistance to the change.

Deal with this situation by providing something that compensates for the perceived loss. Simply using the talent that is now available to assist you in implementing the change will help. Go to the formerly senior employees and ask to draw on their technical expertise. Put them in charge of implementing certain aspects of the change and give them some additional responsibility. In the vast majority of cases, this will help to restore some of the prestige they feel they have lost and will provide you with time to deal with the effects of the change on these employees.

LOSS OF POSITION

When change, no matter how much it benefits the company, results in the loss of any employee's position, resistance to the change is going to be much higher. One suggestion is to prepare those who will lose their jobs to fill other positions within the organization. You might even help them plan or find other career positions outside of your unit.

Your willingness to help those who will be displaced will benefit far more people than just those who are leaving the company. The employees who stay will witness your efforts. They will see that you cared enough about your employees to help them personally, and this will help the retained employees deal with their loss and with any uncertainty they might have about their own futures.

The principle of compensating for loss, both real and perceived, is basic to all kinds of change, and failure to deal with loss effectively can cause even the most important or beneficial changes to fail.

Communicate

Of all the groups within an organization, managers are typically the least effective at communicating with others. Although everyone recognizes that communication is vital to the success of every organization, the typical management team constantly generates rationalizations for why it doesn't have to engage in it. Examples are provided in the following sections.

IT ISN'T THE PROPER TIME

Managers typically believe that they must have a timetable to inform others of impending change. They want to control when people find out about future plans. They use excuses such as the following:

"They don't need to know yet."
"We'll tell them when the time is right."

Unless your organization is extremely rare, however, your employees have ways of finding things out on their own. Secrets are not easily kept within an organization. The grapevine, although it almost always transmits information faster than management, is rarely as accurate. When management delays its communication to employees, this unofficial knowledge (rumor) is left to mutate. Rumor, no matter how slight, is not beneficial. Delay in communication builds resentment, bitterness, and mistrust.

Management is not a perfect discipline, and often mistakes are made by the most well intentioned. One area in which mistakes occur is the restriction of information. Although there are many reasons why information should not be given out (marketing strategy, competitive backlash, etc.), denying its existence by lying about it is not the way to deal with the problem. If you are confronted by an employee who asks a direct question about confidential information, don't lie and say that it doesn't exist or that an event won't happen. Simply tell the employee that the answer to the question is considered confidential and that you are not at liberty to provide that information yet. Ask for cooperation and inform the employee that you will provide an answer as soon as possible. Never, never, never lie to your employee.

Employees see things in shades of black and white. If you lie to keep restricted information hidden, then the minute that information becomes public knowledge, you have lost trust. You lied. It's that simple. A lie is a lie is a lie.

I TOLD YOUR SUPERVISOR

Don't assume that because you, the nurse manager, told your subordinate supervisors the staff nurses also got the message. They might have gotten part of the message, a garbled message, or even no message at all. Supervisors go through a transition and engage in denial just like everyone else, and this transition can often interrupt their ability to pass along important information. Some people even consider knowledge to be power and feel that, as long as they know and no one else does, they are somehow more personally secure. Never assume that information given to other members of management will get down through the organization reliably or in a timely fashion. Many managers use a procedure for communicating that covers the two layers immediately below their own positions, either directly or through an active practice of checking with the second layer to ensure that those individuals are getting the word. Simply walking around and asking the lower-level employees can accomplish this. The giant electronics company Hewlett-Packard has a program called MBWA, an acronym for "management by wandering around," in which all of its managers are required to actively participate. The program gets managers out from behind their desks and walking through their departments actively talking with their staffs. While they do this, they ask questions, listen to responses, hear what the grapevine is spreading, and generally promote good management-employee relations. Hewlett-Packard believes—as does this textbook—that good management cannot be achieved from behind a desk, especially during times of change.

Providing effective communication is fundamental to quality management. Never withhold information that should be given out, and if you must restrict information—and there are definitely times when you legitimately must—never lie to your employees about it. Substituting half-truths or making up an outright lie will always lower your stature in the eyes of the average employee. Effective management of change involves the same basic principles of management as does the rest of your job. The more your employees trust you, the greater the support they will give. Trust is always undermined when you lie, so don't do it. The effect will always be detrimental.

Treat the Old Methods with Respect

Our growth depends not on how many experiences we devour, but on how many we digest.

Ralph W. Sockman

Although advancing your organization through growth is important, so are the things you did to get your organization to its present position. Many people allow their enthusiasm for the future to overshadow the accomplishments of the past by telling everyone how much better things will be.

Although that may be how you feel, it may not be how everyone else feels, and if it is not, then your continual downgrading of the way things used to be can create resentment and increased foot dragging. Constantly reminding others that things are better now can consolidate resistance to the change for those who identify with the way things used to be.

When the past is discussed, and it will be when change is taking place, try to do it in a nonjudgmental manner. It is perfectly permissible to compare what has been done in the past with what will be done in the future as long as the past is not demeaned. For example, instead of disparaging the past, give it credit for bringing your organization as far as it has. You might want to let your employees make the comparison for you by getting them to point out the improvements made by the change.

Present your changes as new developments that build on the successes of the past. It will help you move forward faster.

Given what has been presented here, you might easily believe that this chapter is recommending that change be implemented slowly. This is not true. Change is a constant part of the healthcare industry, and whether this change is implemented rapidly or slowly is a decision that should be made case by case. What this chapter recommends is that change be well planned and, once it is implemented, that a time for healing be provided. Implement change in your organization in a manner that best fits your unit's needs and that ensures that the job gets done. Try to remember that enthusiasm for the change may vary from employee to employee and that part of enacting change is dealing effectively with the variables.

The single biggest reason that change fails so often in well-meaning organizations is that not enough time is spent planning the implementation or considering the impact on the individual members of the team. Don't let this happen to your organization as you help it grow.

DEALING WITH NONSTOP CHANGE

Today, there is little doubt that change is the only true constant in the healthcare industry. This has been true for decades, and it is unlikely to change much in the future. To be sure, the last three decades of the twentieth century saw more change than at any other time in the history of nursing. One of the consequences of this nearly continual change is that people react to change differently today than they did in the past simply because there is more of it. The nursing profession doesn't talk about change as an *event* anymore; it talks about change as an ongoing process. One change overlaps another, and another, and finally another until the whole becomes blurred.

Up to this point, the chapter has talked about change as a single action, and a lot of information has been provided about how to deal with the transition from one state to another as if it were a singular action isolated in a laboratory. This way of enacting change bears little similarity to the way change is handled in the real world. There is a reason for this approach. The chapter has explained transition in simple terms because many people, especially those who are very experienced and those who have little experience, are easily overwhelmed by it. Also, the transitions associated with change occur around us so rapidly, and are so close to us, that often they cannot be easily identified.

Now you must take a breath and view change as a process with stages, not as a single action. Change is composed of an ending, then a gray zone of transition, and a new beginning. In the real world, each of us deals with more than one of these stages at a time as we struggle with change after change after change.

There is hope in dealing with this constant change, and that hope lies in the basic character of the human psyche. The average person has an uncanny ability to adjust to new and higher levels of change. Although it is true that people who lived in the nineteenth century would have a tremendous problem coping with the speed and amount of change that occurred in the twentieth century if they experienced it for only a brief time, it is equally true that stopping change altogether would itself create problems. As a matter of fact, slowing change can be very disruptive to a healthcare organization as it grows. However,

there will also come a time when, as change evolves, the organization will need time to allow itself to catch up, to create standards, and to put proper systems into place. You will recognize the need to diminish change when you hear comments such as "The fun is gone" or "We have become just another hospital." These reactions, too, must be dealt with effectively by you as the manager. To help you, suggestions are provided in the following sections.

Don't Add Extra Changes

Change is going to occur, and very often many different changes occur at one time. In the real world, there isn't much you can do to stop it. However, you can avoid adding incidental changes that are unrelated to a larger change that you are implementing. Don't piggyback small changes thoughtlessly, because they can disrupt crucial changes that must be implemented. Managers sometimes think, "Because we are changing a lot of things, we might as well throw in these changes too." That makes sense, however, only if the added changes are related to the changes that are necessary.

Although it may be hard to believe, one of the challenges facing the managements of healthcare institutions today is that it is easy to get hooked on change. The new breed of entrepreneurial administrators and nurse managers working in the industry today normally enjoys the adrenaline rush of a crisis situation, and in an environment in which crisis abounds, they can easily become obsessed with it. This is a dangerous situation for a growing organization and should be avoided at all costs. Superior managers initiate change when they need to, not because it makes them feel good.

Plan for as Much as You Can—But Be Careful What You Plan For

Planning and forecasting are an important part of operating a healthcare unit, but they often miss more boats than they catch. Making a change can end up as a huge fiasco for any company—consider, for example, Coca-Cola's adventure with the "New Coke," Ford Motor Company's Edsel, and Sony Corporation's Betamax. Each of these changes was predicted to be a huge success by "experts." If a change like any of these were attempted by the average hospital, the loss of revenue would be catastrophic.

Planning is not a perfect science, but there are ways that it can be of immeasurable help to you in implementing change. These methods are not often exciting and will rarely provide you with an adrenaline rush, but they are very reliable, and you should use them. They are presented elsewhere in this textbook.

Plan for Life Cycles

Although life-cycle planning is normally viewed as something one would do for products and services, it can also be applied to the development of standards, structures, and policies. In life-cycle planning, the process of change is started while you are in the middle of a successful ride with the current approaches. Things like levels of employment, technical expertise, salary structure, management structure, and a myriad of other elements in your organization all have as clearly limited a life expectancy as do the individual techniques used in surgery. Retirement packages, training programs, and succession charts all become outdated. If you use a life-cycle approach to managing these things, you will avoid the obstacles that can arise when a change must be made in a crisis situation. People are less affected by change when it is expected than when it catches them by surprise.

Consider "What-Ifs"

When you are planning, think about contingencies, or "what-ifs." *What if* this should occur, or this, or even that? Planning for the unexpected is critical to the smooth implementation of change and the avoidance of resistance to transition. If you provide your organization with alternative routes, the changes you have to make will be far less disruptive should you hit a snag in your primary course.

Create a Mindset That Accepts Change

It is never enough to preach to your employees that "thriving on chaos" is essential. It is never enough to explain how "continuous improvement" benefits the unit. You must be prepared to manage the movement of employees through nonstop change.

Nonstop change is no different from the change that was described earlier in this chapter, and the tools you use to help your team get through it are no different from those the chapter has already discussed. Every rate of change is deemed nonstop by those who are having trouble with the transition from old to new. People adjust to everything, even chaos. So change after change becomes the norm just as a single change would become so.

The secret to handling nonstop change effectively is to develop in your team a willingness to deal with change as it occurs and not to magnify it into more than it actually is. Little transitions are continuous in any nursing unit as it evolves. Procedures change to help the team meet different patient needs, maximize efficiency, and reduce cost. These are often "temporary" changes that remain in effect until a better way to do things is discovered. It's called *continuous improvement,* and although it requires transition, it also reaffirms the previous practices that have brought the unit success.

People working in the healthcare industry must realize that endurance depends on change. Failure to make change will lead to failure of the organization.

Clarify Your Goal

Keeping your unit stable as it negotiates the changes that are required to grow demands that you let others know how these changes will help them attain the goals toward which they are all working.

When you are implementing change, you must clarify for everyone just how the change will alter the performance of activities. Every unit in your organization has its own specific mission that is designed to blend with those of other units to help the organization achieve its goals. These individual missions must change as necessary to support the growth that the organization is experiencing.

The trouble is that people within the organization tend to identify with things accomplished, rather than with missions. They do this because it is easier to see how things are being achieved on a personal level than to understand how the overall organization is benefiting. Because this is so, you must constantly work with the individual to reinforce the mission of the organization and, when implementing change, identify how that change will enhance the unit's and the individual's ability to work toward mission accomplishment. This takes patience, communication, and sometimes a great deal of explanation.

Constantly Build Trust

Trust is a critical element in making things happen. The more of it there is, the more smoothly things go. When change does occur, trust can be an incredibly important tool, because people are much more willing to support new ways of doing things when they trust the people putting them forward than when they don't.

Change, in itself, can undermine trust. Everyone knows that trust takes time to develop but can be lost in the blink of an eye. Therefore, trust is something to be guarded and nurtured, and never, *never* demanded.

The way to maintain trust in times of change is to remain trustworthy yourself. Don't lie, don't act wishy-washy, don't ignore people, and don't take people for granted. Trust is earned every moment of every day. Although you hear things like "I trust her a little," the truth is that someone who says this probably doesn't trust "her" at all. You can maintain your employees' trust as your unit grows by doing the following:

Do what you say you will do: Don't make promises and fail to keep them. If you say you will do something, you can bet that someone is going to hold you to your promise. There is no such thing as just "making a statement." People don't hear statements; they hear promises. If you say you will do something, that is a promise, not a statement.

Listen carefully and paraphrase your understanding: When people tell you something, listen carefully and then restate your understanding of what was said. If you are wrong, the individual will set you straight. If you understand correctly, the chances are good that you will generate trust through your actions. Trust is built by people who understand one another.

Understand what matters to others: What matters to you may not be what matters to others. People trust others whom they believe have their best interests at heart.

Open yourself to others: Don't be afraid to have a weakness, and don't be afraid to let it show. Pretending to be perfect might shore up an image, but it does nothing to build trust. If you make a mistake, admit it. The act of admitting an untrustworthy action is itself a trustworthy act. When you appear to be unapproachable, you begin to sow the seeds of mistrust.

Respond to feedback: Respond even to negative feedback. Regard feedback as a valuable management tool and use it to build trust. You do not have to accept everything that is sent in your direction; however, you should examine all information closely for any benefit it might contain.

Don't demand trust or expect it: Many management-level individuals expect to be trusted because they hold a senior position. Trust does not come with position, and it is not inherited from your predecessors. Trust is earned, and although it may be popular to say that trust is given until someone proves undeserving of it, *this just isn't so.* People trust those who have proven themselves to be trustworthy. Trust is different from support, which is something you should expect from all of your subordinates and seniors alike.

Trust others first: People who believe they are trusted are far more willing to give their trust. The reason more management people are not trusting is that they are afraid they will lose something personal. That is always a risk, but giving up what can be gained from trusting others is always a much greater loss.

Don't confuse trust with friendship: Acting like someone's friend to gain trust is itself an untrustworthy act. Besides, trust doesn't always come automatically with friendship.

Tell the truth: Never lie, or support others who do. One of the foundations of America's might is its military, and that organization operates largely on trust. Trust is considered so important that it is taught as a fundamental responsibility of every military officer in every service. This can be witnessed in the honor code of the U.S. Military Academy at West Point, which says: "I will not lie, cheat, steal, or tolerate those who do." This is an excellent principle for your growing organization.

No matter what you do to build trust, you can expect some of your employees not to accept it. The foundations of trust go far back in each person's experience, and those who have worked under poor managers, who have been repeatedly lied to or misled, or have endured broken promises will not find it easy to give trust. You deal with this by simply continuing to practice the precepts given here.

By no stretch of the imagination are the things presented in this chapter everything you can do to deal with an environment fraught with change, but they are extremely important. Fig. 18-1 is a checklist to consider using if you operate your unit in an environment of nonstop change.

TAKING CARE OF YOURSELF

Never has it been more difficult to lead others successfully through the process of growth than it is today. You are constantly being caught between a market that demands change immediately and a workforce that typically sees no reason to change what has brought success in the past. At the same time, the changes in the market have forced many healthcare organizations to operate with fewer staff, with less training, with less time to focus on critical matters, and with an ever-increasing need to delegate responsibility to people who do not inspire a great deal of confidence.

If you are like most nurse managers, you have brought your career from a point where you were responsible for well-defined tasks under your direct

Change Checklist

☐ Yes ☐ No   Have I taught my employees that change is going to be an unavoidable reality as we grow?

☐ Yes ☐ No   Have I created a plan that allows for carefully constructing the pattern of change?

☐ Yes ☐ No   Am I carefully leading my employees through the changes by identifying an "ending" here and a "beginning" there?

☐ Yes ☐ No   Am I being careful not to introduce extra, unrelated changes while my employees are struggling to respond to previous transitions?

☐ Yes ☐ No   Am I being careful not to stake my company on the outcome of a forecasted future?

☐ Yes ☐ No   Does my organization build in "what-if" contingency plans when it develops plans to implement change?

☐ Yes ☐ No   Does my organization include life-cycle projections for policies, systems, and structures during the original development process, and do we start the process of change midway through the life cycle?

☐ Yes ☐ No   Do I accept change as the best way to preserve the essential permanence of the organization?

☐ Yes ☐ No   Have I clarified the mission of my organization and helped others do the same thing within the organization?

☐ Yes ☐ No   Do the organization's mission and all subordinate missions support the attainment of the organization's goals and vision?

☐ Yes ☐ No   Am I being careful to do what I say I will do?

☐ Yes ☐ No   Am I listening to other people carefully and paraphrasing what I hear them saying so that they will understand that I have heard them correctly?

☐ Yes ☐ No   Do I make a conscientious effort to work with what is important to other people?

☐ Yes ☐ No   Do I allow my employees to see the real me, openly and honestly?

☐ Yes ☐ No   Do I earnestly solicit feedback and honor those who provide me with honest, straightforward responses?

☐ Yes ☐ No   Do I make an effort to earn the trust of others?

☐ Yes ☐ No   Do I willingly trust others?

☐ Yes ☐ No   Am I careful not to demand trust from others or confuse it with support?

☐ Yes ☐ No   Am I consistently truthful, even when it's difficult?

☐ Yes ☐ No   Do I retrain from telling half-truths when confronted with a question on restricted matters?

☐ Yes ☐ No   Am I conscientious about letting employees know about the organization's problems?

☐ Yes ☐ No   Have I worked hard to create an environment where honesty is appreciated and frankness is encouraged?

☐ Yes ☐ No   Do I refrain from "killing the messenger" when bad news is brought to my attention?

☐ Yes ☐ No   Do I respond to challenges with creativity and innovation and encourage my unit's employees to do the same?

☐ Yes ☐ No   Do I accept responsibility for the level of acceptance of change within my area of responsibility?

Fig. 18-1 ■ Checklist nurse managers can use when operating a unit in the midst of nonstop change.

control to a point where you can no longer stay on top of everything that is taking place. You now have other professionals beneath you through whom you must work, and they are carrying out most of the responsibilities you were so used to shouldering. Your primary focus has turned from accomplishing to managing, and this shift has not necessarily brought with it appropriate adjustments in salary and worry level.

To make matters worse, the requirements of being a manager can put an enormous stress on family life. Not only do you have to manage the emotional challenges brought to you by your employees, you also need to be ready, on a completely different level, to assist those closest to you as your family struggles with your long hours and constant state of weariness. The normally accepted gender roles in your family may have changed as responsibilities in the family shift to make up for your absence.

Your days are filled with change, constant and demanding. Your life, if typical, appears, at least on the surface, as something between a Greek tragedy and a television situation comedy. There are times when you just want to throw up your hands and say, "Is it really worth all of this?"

How do you take care of yourself? This is not a question that is important only to self-centered individuals. All nurse managers must ask themselves this question and then provide themselves with a positive answer. Nurse managers will not be able to give assistance to others if their own well-being is not addressed. An unhappy individual either subconsciously projects these feelings to others, causing poor performance, or becomes so distracted by personal problems that the entire unit's work suffers.

As a nurse manager who is bringing a healthcare unit into and through a growth process, you absolutely must take care of yourself. The following are some things that may help you perform at your best during times of great change.

Figure Out What Really Needs Changing

As you examine the marketplace and contemplate changes to your unit, consider how those changes will affect your situation and your future. It is important to view the changes you are considering in the broadest possible context. The following are some examples:

- The addition of a layer of management may limit or at least restrict how you deal with the average employee.
- Introduction of a "service culture" may create a new role for you as a spokesperson for quality. That can alter the requirements for your appear-

ance, your mannerisms, and even your method of interacting with others.
- Increasing the degree or closeness of management may cause a challenge to your authority.

Although you have focused on the day-to-day management of your unit as you have carefully propelled it from infancy to its present configuration, your actual performance role will change as the unit increases in size. Day-to-day decisions may have to be turned over at least partly to others or you will impair their effectiveness, and that means you will have to assume a new and perhaps strange role in the continuing success of the unit.

The more changes you implement, the greater the impact for you as well as for your area of responsibility. The actual change being implemented is not the only concern. Changes cause other changes, and many times these secondary and even tertiary effects can significantly alter your personal situation. This is another reason why carefully developed planning skills are critical to effective management of growth in any organization.

Deal with Change in Your Role

Many nurse managers simply don't want to accept the fact that their roles alter as they move up the ladder of responsibility. They cling to the belief that they are the sole decision-makers and that it is their role to oversee every action in the organization. At some point, however, the burden of accomplishing the many tasks necessary to manage a growing healthcare unit can become overwhelming. In addition, nurse managers who maintain single-handed control of the reins risk alienating their subordinate managers or forcing turnover of employees unhappy with their individual roles. Micromanagement is also the cause of one of managers' biggest failings: neglecting to teach their subordinates how to grow by allowing them to perform their jobs. If the manager is constantly doing the work, the subordinate has no opportunity to learn how.

You must be willing to accept that your role will change with the growth of your unit or with your personal advancement. As more and more employees perform more and more of the work for which your unit is responsible, you will require help to effectively lead the organization, and you are going to lose some of the practical performance side of your job to others. And this loss hurts. You are going to be bruised emotionally by some of the changes that you initiate in helping your company to grow.

You will need to deal with your loss by channeling your energy into your new role. Don't hang onto what others can and are waiting to do for you.

Take a Break

Although obviously you cannot simply drop out of the operation of your organization, no matter how appealing the idea may sound at times, every manager must take a break from it from time to time.

The growth of your organization, and your assignment as nurse manager, will provide you with something that you may not have had since you entered the nursing profession: someone with whom to share the responsibility. Your new team of subordinate managers, if you have selected and trained them properly, will provide you with sound backup for your management requirements. This, in turn, will give you an opportunity to take a much-deserved vacation or perhaps a day off to go shopping or play golf.

The point is that it is all right to share some of your responsibilities with your junior managers for short periods. It will help them grow and mature, and it will provide you with time out from under the weight of responsibility.

You will also have the opportunity to reevaluate the individual goals and objectives that you have set for yourself. Your new role can provide you the time to do other things that will help you continue to grow and thus cause you to provide even greater benefit to the organization.

Consider Your Contribution in a New Light

Unless you are unlike most new nurse managers, the operation and management of your unit has kept you very channeled in terms of what you have done since you started in the profession.

As you implement change and your unit grows, you will feel that things are slipping away from you, and to some extent, they will be. How you replace these things and develop new behaviors to benefit your unit will have a tremendous impact, not only on you but on your organization as well.

The people who break free of the views they held yesterday usually do so in similar ways. First, they tend to be very curious about their current situation. They ask themselves the tough questions that start with "Why?" when things seem to be a certain way and with "Why not?" when things seem to be unattainable. They know enough not to accept the rationalizations that most often turn up as their first answers but instead continue to look for the real explanations. Professional nurse managers know that by asking themselves these two simple types of question they will be able to uncover opportunities hiding in the most unlikely places.

Second, these managers know enough to break out of the realm of the ordinary and search for the rare and frequently overlooked, even to the point of investigating the ridiculous and outrageous. They know that a given thing, by itself, may not be workable, but that several such things placed together just might provide an incredible opportunity that has previously been overlooked.

A third method is to look for analogies that suggest a new way. For example, the inventor of Velcro, after walking his dog and removing several cockleburs from its fur, noticed their natural hooklike appearance. The 3M Company was trying to improve its acrylic adhesives when it discovered an unusual bonding agent. A product development researcher looking for a way to keep bookmarks from falling out of church hymnals later applied this adhesive to small pieces of paper, developing Post-it notes.

Although not one of these ideas is likely to give you a fully workable approach to the new role you will play in your organization, all of them will help you see alternatives. What they can do is break up the mediocrity with which managers contend most of the time.

Remember That Changes You Implement Place You in Transition

Nurse managers are no different from their employees. It is a fair bet that every one has the same distaste for transition that their subordinates do. A manager may love change and may get a tremendous rush from the challenge of managing it, but losing part of what one has grown comfortable with is still going to be difficult—even for the most professional nurse manager.

You can deal effectively with your changing role if you plan for the changes as you implement them within your area of influence. Truly effective managers think about the overall picture when they consider change—not just the immediate but also the secondary effects of the change. Next, they imagine how the organization will look after the change has been implemented. Then they plan the change carefully. Finally, they make sure that they clearly define their part in the change and their role after it has been implemented.

Fig. 18-2 is a checklist you can use in implementing plans to take care of yourself.

TAKING CARE OF THE UNIT

To quote a German proverb:

A great war leaves a country with three armies: an army of cripples, an army of mourners, and an army of thieves.

Change Self-Checklist

☐ Yes ☐ No   Have I determined how my situation and my future will be changed by the recent, current, and planned changes within the organization? Do I know exactly what will be different for me?

☐ Yes ☐ No   What part of myself will I be losing, or will I be likely to lose, in the transition that is triggered by a proposed change? If something that is important to me is going to end, what is it exactly? When should I let it go?

☐ Yes ☐ No   What occurrences taking place in my private life may be affecting my ability to deal with the transitions on the job?

☐ Yes ☐ No   Do I accept the fact that changes implemented for the benefit of the organization can have a direct effect on my performance and role within the company?

☐ Yes ☐ No   Am I willing to let go of the day-to-day operation of the unit and begin to work through subordinate managers to achieve growth-oriented results?

☐ Yes ☐ No   Have I trained my managers sufficiently so that they can provide me with quality backup that will allow me to take short breaks in my normal routine?

☐ Yes ☐ No   Have I reevaluated my personal goals so that they are more in line with the requirements I will face after the change is implemented?

☐ Yes ☐ No   Do I try to see my role objectively?

☐ Yes ☐ No   Am I willing to allow other members of my unit to have more and more influence over the operation of the organization?

☐ Yes ☐ No   Do I allow myself to consider outrageous possibilities, and do I consider them as viable leads into future opportunities for myself and the organization?

☐ Yes ☐ No   Do I remember that I am subject as much to the difficulties of transition as are those who work for me?

☐ Yes ☐ No   Am I considering the impact anticipated changes will have on me personally? My family? My health?

☐ Yes ☐ No   Do I see the new changes occurring in my growing organization as opportunities for me personally?

Fig. 18-2 ■ Checklist nurse managers can use when implementing plans to take care of themselves.

Although this proverb has its roots in centuries of violent conflict, it deserves mention in this presentation on change. Think of it as a reminder that, when someone gains, another loses. When change is implemented, it too can produce casualties. It can leave behind those who are wounded by the process, those who grieve over their losses, and those who feel that their personal stature has been so gravely diminished by the experience that they turn malicious and disruptive. These three types of survivors will always be mixed with the winners after the typical business change.

The healthcare industry, however, cannot afford these types of victims. They typically extract far too high a cost in the effort required to repair the damage, increased expenses, or delay in implementing the change. Therefore, when nurse managers start to plan for the growth of their units, they must plan effectively to create a flow of change that limits the number of such survivors and maximizes the number of winners.

The typical healthcare unit certainly must think in terms of organizational fitness when it plans for and implements the changes required for its growth. But it also needs to plan for the care and well-being of its employees as they implement those changes. Because the typical healthcare unit has a limited number of personnel available to help the unit grow effectively, the human impact caused by the enactment of change must be handled carefully. The loss of one key player in a small unit can be devastating; the result of foot dragging by one critical individual can be crippling; and the impact of a negative environment is many times greater than it would be in a large organization.

Is there an alternative to change? Can a healthcare organization grow without it?

The answers to those two questions are far more than a simple no. There is no alternative for change because the prescription for the condition is even more change. It is like drinking a shot of alcohol in the morning to cure a hangover (a practice often referred to as taking the "hair of the dog"). But when dealing with change in something as fragile as a healthcare environment, the remedy is even more challenging than the cure for getting rid of a hangover. Because if the first shot of the hair of the dog doesn't work, what is going to be done about the second and third that will follow in rapid succession?

This is the reason that it is critical for nurse managers, and those who help them manage growth in their areas of responsibility, to become effective transition managers. All individuals involved in the management of growth in a healthcare environment will find themselves confronted daily with the aftermath of change. These leaders must be able to deal with survivors who are struggling with change and winners who are working through varying degrees of transition, as well as with their own transitions. Although there are many well-tested and effective ways to bring opportunity out of chaos, most managers simply don't do it very well. The same is true of organizations as a whole. In fact, most of the organizations that make it out of their formative years simply follow a path toward their own collapse because they fail to find a path for growth.

The management of transition is critical to the growth of a healthcare unit. The proper management of change, and the transition it brings, requires a well-orchestrated team effort—a team effort that must begin with intensive planning and end only after every employee is safely through the transition and the change has been thoroughly implemented. This type of coordinated effort requires trust and honesty from management and from every member of the healthcare team.

The things we have talked about in this chapter should not be taken lightly, because if history has taught us anything about the future, it is that the future will go beyond what we consider the limits of possibility today. Whatever is, will change. And where there is change, there is transition. The transition of change cannot be avoided, but it can be managed, and if nurse managers are to realize the continued growth and survival of their nursing units, they must do so effectively.

SUMMARY

- Managing change, and the transitions that create the challenges within change, is not difficult.
- *Change* is positional: the new method, the new boss, the new idea, the new policy. *Change* is a thing that people do.

- *Transition* is the mental process that people go through as they struggle to accept these new things. *Transition* is something that people deal with.
- Transition is not change; it does not start after the result. It involves the emotional letting go of the bond that holds the old reality as sacred.
- Before beginning something new, an end to the something that is being replaced must be accomplished.
- Managers' opinions of the reality of loss are not important. If a person perceives a loss, no matter how much another may disagree, the loss is real to the person who perceives it.
- The degree of overreaction that will be seen in employees can also be directly attributable to what types of losses they have experienced in the past and how those losses were dealt with.
- One of the best ways to deal with perceived loss is to get it out into the open. Acknowledging loss and expressing concern for the affected people can be instrumental in solving the issue before it becomes a problem.
- Resistance to change most often occurs when employees experience only the difficulty brought on by the change.
- Providing effective communication is fundamental to quality management.
- Change is a constant part of the healthcare industry, and how it is implemented, rapidly or slowly, should be determined on an individual basis.
- The single biggest reason that change fails is that not enough time is spent planning the implementation or considering the impact on the individual members of the team.

FINAL THOUGHTS

Often the changes that a nurse manager must implement seem, at least on the surface, to be rather small, but in the larger picture each may be a piece of a change that is critical to the organization's survival. These aren't the "it would be nice if we could do it" or the "do it when you get around to it" kinds of change. They involve the different technologies the organization needs to deliver high-quality patient care and to survive against overwhelming competition and regulation. Change is the name of the game in the healthcare industry today, and nurse managers who cannot deal with it effectively aren't likely to be around long.

All of the discussion in this chapter about helping people with change may strike you as unnecessary. You may see your management situation as one in which you tell people what to do and they do it. These days, it would be truer to say that they used to do it. Simple, unquestioning compliance is found less and less often in today's employees. Or perhaps you are the type that shies away from the difficulties of managing change because the "people side" of things is not your strong suit.

Managing transition may not be easy, but it is essential. This chapter has provided you with simple ways to get started and, even more importantly, has given you methods to stimulate your thinking. You should consider this one of the most important lessons you will receive in school.

THE NURSE MANAGER SPEAKS

Many nurse managers feel they are better at functional tasks—getting the patients treated, ensuring that the necessary medications are available, and so on—than at managing the staff nurses who are supposed to do those things. They feel that they don't have the skills or training to be psychologists and don't want to get into "that personal stuff." What they want is results!

This attitude may be understandable, but working with people will teach the following two very important lessons:

1. *Managers cannot get the results they need without working effectively with people:* Success means that managers must get people to stop doing things the old way and start doing things the new way. They can't do this without dealing with people on a personal level.
2. *Managers don't need a degree in psychology to manage people:* Managers use psychology every time they try to guess a motive, figure out a tactful response to a difficult situation, or find a way to explain something effectively.

Managing people is about helping others, and that is what managers do to get things done—effectively!

SUGGESTED READINGS

Allee V: *The knowledge evolution: expanding organizational intelligence,* Newton, Mass, 1997, Butterworth-Heinemann.

Baskin K: *Corporate DNA: learning from life,* Newton, Mass, 1998, Butterworth-Heinemann.

Belasco JA: *Teaching the elephant to dance,* New York, 1999, Plume.

Bennis W, Nanus B: *Leaders: the strategies for taking charge,* ed 1, New York, 1985, Harper and Row.

Bennis WG, Benne KD, Chin R: *The planning of change,* New York, 1969, Holt, Rinehart and Winston.

Blanchard K: *The heart of a leader: insights on the art of influence,* Colorado Springs, Colo, 2004, Honor Books/Cook Communications.

Bridges W: *Managing transitions,* Boston, 1997, Addison-Wesley.

Brown JS: *Seeing differently: insights on innovation,* Harvard Business Review book series, Cambridge, Mass, 1997, Harvard Business School Press.

Chou-Hou W: *Sun Tzu: war and management,* New York, 1994, Addison-Wesley.

Davis M: *A practical guide to unit design,* Menlo Park, Calif, 1996, Crisp Publishers.

Dettmer W: *Breaking the constraints to world-class performance,* Milwaukee, 1998, ASQ Quality Press.

Economy P: *Business negotiating basics,* Chicago, 1990, IDG Books.

Economy P: *Negotiating to win,* Chicago, 1990, IDG Books.

Galpin TJ: *The human side of change,* San Francisco, 1996, Jossey-Bass.

Greenberg J: *Behavior in organizations,* Upper Saddle River, NJ, 1999, Prentice Hall.

Helgesen S: *Web of inclusion: a new architecture for building great institutions,* Milwaukee, 1998, ASQ Quality Press.

Hersey P, Blanchard K, Johnson D: *Management organizational behavior,* Upper Saddle River, NJ, 1996, Prentice Hall.

Hill N: *Napoleon Hill's key to success,* New York, 1997, Plume.

Hirschhorn L: *The workplace within: psychodynamics of unit life,* Cambridge, Mass, 1990, MIT Press.

Kanter RM: *The change masters,* New York, 1989, Simon and Schuster.

Maister D: *True professionalism: the courage to care about your people, your clients, and your career,* New York, 1997, Free Press.

McCormack M: *What they don't teach you at Harvard Business School,* New York, 1988, Bantam Doubleday.

Muihead BK: *High-velocity leadership: faster, cheaper, better,* New York, 1999, HarperBusiness.

Nelson R: *Fundamental management practices: people, projects and teams,* Chicago, 1996, IDG Books.

Nelson R: *Empowering employees through delegation,* Upper Saddle River, NJ, 1998, Prentice Hall.

Nelson R: *Decision point,* Upper Saddle River, NJ, 2000, Prentice Hall.

Reinman J: *Thinking for a living,* Athens, Ga, 1998, Longstreet Press.

Schon D: *The reflective practitioner: how professionals think in action,* New York, 1984, Basic Books.

Senge PM: *The fifth discipline,* New York, 1990, Doubleday.

Stone D: *Difficult conversations: how to discuss what matters most,* New York, 1995, Doubleday.

Woodward H, Woodward MB: *Aftershock: helping people through change,* New York, 1987, Wiley.

CHAPTER **18** APPENDIX

PRACTICE SCENARIO

One of the great things about being a part of management is that you will be involved in many of the important decisions made within your organization. In your role as leader, you will always wield great power in your area of responsibility. Therefore, you will want to fulfill your leadership requirements to the very best of your ability. One of the best ways to do this is to practice the necessary skills until they have been refined.

One requirement of leadership is to provide inspirational guidance to the members of your team when they are in tough, stressful periods. Employees will look to their manager to develop programs and processes that not only help them adjust to the transition caused by the changes affecting them but also provide them with performance methods to help them move the unit forward in its growth.

This chapter provides you with an opportunity to practice your skills without interacting with real people. This is a practice exercise that is not scored, and no one is going to watch whether you accomplish it or not. It is strongly recommended that you carry out the tasks described here not once but several times. You should go through the exercise completely, compare your responses with the textbook responses that have been provided, and print a copy of all your answers. Then erase what you wrote and put the exercise away for a couple of weeks. When you feel comfortable, pull the exercise back out and do it again. After you are through, compare your first performance with your second, and then compare both of them with the comparison sheet at the end of this chapter.

Begin the exercise by reading the following realistic scenario. Although it was impossible to construct the scenario to address all of the special circumstances you will encounter as you lead your individual unit, it includes a good many of the most common. This is not intended to be an easy exercise. Real life never is. Remember, you can only benefit if you try.

CASE STUDY

You are the nurse manager in charge of the pediatric service in a large Pacific-based hospital. This medical institution currently employs 3000 individuals, of which your section includes 600. You have been the nurse manager of this unit since 1995 and have been largely responsible for bringing it through most of the growth required for it to become the leading pediatric facility in the entire Pacific. You have developed a strong economic base, and in 1998, the Mid-Pacific Pediatrics Center provided 58% of the Pacific area's primary pediatric care.

Since 1998, however, two Japanese hospitals and one Singapore-based pediatric unit have entered the field against your organization, and these pediatric centers are receiving substantial government subsidies that have enabled them to invest huge amounts of money in facilities and technology to support pediatric medicine. To further complicate your company's business future, the U.S. government has passed difficult third-party payment laws and enacted significantly higher medical care standards that have forced your company to revamp the specific procedures used to diagnose, treat, and cure pediatric illness. Your company's competitors, because of their liberal government subsidies and lower medical standards, were not required to spend the millions of dollars your organization had to outlay to achieve the superior level of health care required to meet the new U.S. standards, nor are they limited in what they can charge to recover the cost of the treatments proided. These new requirements have changed your hospital's patient care capability, and these changes have negatively altered the perception of your organization in the community. This, in turn, has caused your hospital to lose its former patient base to the new competition because your organization cannot afford to provide equal cost subsidies. By the end of 1999, your company's share of the market had decreased to 49%, and the 2000 year-end figures showed a further decrease to 38%. Now, in the middle of 2001, your hospital is faced with continued market share losses and ever-increasing costs of producing high-quality pediatric medical care.

The Joint Commission on Accreditation of Healthcare Organizations has been closely monitoring your hospital's struggle and has provided feedback for months that it will have to make massive changes in procedure and structure to regain its world leadership position. It is now June, and just a week ago your CEO was asked for an official statement. He admitted that the hospital was being forced to trim its costs and reduce its workforce, but he felt that these things could be done by simple consolidation of effort and employee attrition. You supported his position by stating that judicious cuts now would get your pediatric service back to its former leadership position by year's end.

_____9. Fire the current CEO for his inability to provide the proper guidance to avoid this situation.

_____10. Plan some all-hands social events at all company locations—picnics, excursions, cocktail parties, and dinners.

_____11. Establish a suggestion program for reorganization and encourage all employees to submit their ideas on how the process should be carried out.

_____12. Alleviate employees' fears by informing them that the stated reductions are the only ones that will take place.

_____13. Give everyone at Mid-Pacific a badge that proclaims the goal to return to the former dominant position in patient care. It should read "#1 or Bust."

_____14. Make it clear up front that the organization is headed into an extended period of change.

_____15. Find ways to stabilize the gray zone and redefine it in terms that are more beneficial to the organization and to each of the employees.

_____16. Bring in all of the nurse managers and supervisors for an extensive briefing by the executive management team. Hold an open forum at which any question can be asked and will receive an honest, straightforward answer. Do not let the managers and supervisors return to their positions until they are convinced that the organization is handling the matter in the best possible way.

_____17. Set new and higher patient care targets for the upcoming quarter. The purpose is to give each person a lofty goal to shoot for and to ensure that if patient count does fall below goal, enough patients will have been assisted to meet all budget requirements.

_____18. Have all nurse managers and supervisors attend a quality improvement training program.

_____19. Set up a crisis hotline that will provide employees with up-to-date and reliable information to reduce rumor and speculation.

_____20. Sell the problems that have forced the changes to all employees.

_____21. Have the CEO prepare a videotape for distribution to all hands that is intended to fire up the employees and garner support for the changes.

_____22. Have the CEO make a public announcement acknowledging the organization's poor response to changes in the marketplace.

_____23. Redo the compensation structure to reward support of the new system.

_____24. Give all nurse managers and supervisors a special training seminar on the emotional impact of change.

_____25. Cut the salaries of senior management personnel by 20%.

_____26. Develop career-planning seminars for those people whose jobs are being lost due to the downsizing and changes.

_____27. Reorganize the leadership team and redefine the CEO's job as a team coordinator.

_____28. Help the CEO develop a statement regarding organizational transition and what it can do to an organization. The statement should be written in an empathic manner with its primary focus on the welfare of people.

_____29 Institute a beneficial suggestions awards program for employees who submit cost-saving suggestions.

_____30. Explain the purpose, picture, and plan of the announced changes and the parts people will be playing in them.

_____31. Appoint a change manager to be responsible for implementing the changes in a smooth, cohesive manner.

_____32. Plan closure ceremonies for the two sites that will be shut down.

_____33. Develop a plan to buy out the smallest of Mid-Pacific's America-based competitors to regain market share and build a strong U.S.-based pediatric care unit.

_____34. Set up a restructuring task force to recommend the best way to consolidate patient operations and determine the relocation procedures for employees at the Singapore and Guam sites.

As noted, there are no right answers for any of these possibilities. What you would plan in this situation would, of course, be your choice. However, to bring closure to this exercise, the following recommendations are made. Please consider them for the benefit they may offer you.

■ SUGGESTED RESPONSES
■ Category 1
Critical (This Action Needs to Be Accomplished Immediately)

5. **Develop a videotape in which the CEO explains the problem and the plan of action that will be developed. Have the videotape shown at department levels throughout the organization and have the department managers lead a question-and-answer period.** You might rate this as 2 (important but not urgent), because proper preparation will take a little time. The videotape should be kept simple: just the CEO and several top executives sitting around talking about the problems and the solutions they have found. If it is kept simple, most of the development time for the videotape can be eliminated and it can be gotten into the field sooner. This videotape goes way beyond a memo because it has the power to communicate the change in a more personal way.

An alternative would be for the executive management team to make a rapid tour of all of the sites and speak to the employees personally. This would be a much better approach and far more effective.

6. **Set up transition management teams in the Singapore and Guam facilities and in all specific units that might be significantly affected by the changes.** The personnel at these locations will require additional communication channels immediately, and the transition management team is an expedient method of achieving this. These teams need to be aggressive and seek out the challenges occurring in the affected areas, not sit back passively and wait for employees to seek them out. Senior management must act on the information gathered by the transition teams and be vocal about it. If management fails to act on the recommendations received, employees are likely to view this as just another management scam.

7. **Rewrite the CEO's memo to convey more sensitivity to the impact on the organization's employees.** Memos are never good methods to convey news such as this, but this one, in particular, is poorly written. The memo does not state that the CEO accepts any responsibility for the current situation, and, by this omission, clearly denies that possibility. Instead, the memo implies that the employees haven't worked hard enough.

14. **Make it clear up front that the organization is headed into an extended period of change.** This is the truth, and it needs to be expressed to repair lost credibility. Although it may be tempting to provide reassurance, that is a dangerous tack because one can only reassure others for a brief period without supporting these words with action. If the improvements are not seen quickly, the restored confidence will be replaced with mistrust. What was said in an attempt to calm people may be viewed as falsehood.

20. **Sell the problems that have forced the changes to all employees.** This sales job needs to start with the CEO. You will have to convince him that transition-related problems do exist, and until he is sold on this, he isn't going to buy the solution, which is to talk openly and publicly about the organization's real problems. Until he can do this, he won't be able to sell any of his planned changes as being the best ways out of the organization's current situation.

22. **Have the CEO make a public announcement acknowledging the organization's poor response to changes in the marketplace.** Whatever the CEO says, his credibility is already questionable. Just a week earlier, he was reported to be telling the *Wall Street Journal* that the company would be forced to trim its workforce but that by the end of the year everything will be great. It is essential that the CEO take responsibility for the past mistakes and repair his credibility as quickly as possible by issuing honest, straightforward statements concerning the real situation of the company.

28. **Help the CEO develop a statement regarding organizational transition and what it can do to an organization. The statement should be written in an empathic manner with its primary focus on the welfare of people.** Your ability to do this depends on the ability of the CEO to understand organizational transition. You may need to administer a little shock therapy to get the message through to him, and it is better to have this message delivered by someone outside the company. In an organization that has hidden from reality as long as this one has, it will be difficult for an insider to trigger the right alarms. Assuming that the CEO will acknowledge the existence of the transition-related challenges, his open discussion of them will set the proper tone for the entire transition management effort that will be necessary to keep the hospital from continuing its slide south.

16. **Bring in all of the nurse managers and supervisors for an extensive briefing by the executive management team. Hold an open forum at which any question can be asked and will receive an honest, straightforward answer. Do not let the managers and supervisors return to their positions until they are convinced that the organization is handling the matter in the best possible way.** The nurse managers and the supervisors are the professionals who are going to have to answer the myriad of questions posed by the rank-and file employees. It is critical that these leaders believe in what the organization will be doing, because it will be largely through their influence that the rest of the personnel will fall in line. It is critical to the success of the organization to get this group on board supporting the changes immediately. Above all, they should be told the truth—even if some of what needs to be said has to be withheld from subordinates for an unspecified time. Make sure that an adequate forum for questions is provided and that honest, responsive answers are given. Finally, don't pull your punches with this group. Give it to them straight from the shoulder, and don't delay talking with them.

31. **Appoint a change manager to be responsible for implementing the changes in a smooth, cohesive manner.** Someone needs to be in charge of a transition this big. Even before the details of the change are clear, one can be certain that it will cross lines of authority and fall into no one's specific area of responsibility. The change manager should be a recognized high performer who is taken away from his or her primary duties and assigned this role on a permanent basis. It is critical that this person be a top performer, not the person who can most easily

be spared. This person's role will be that of a caretaker, not a boss; a facilitator, not a dictator. He or she should be senior enough to put plenty of authority behind the things recommended. Finally, this person should report directly to the CEO.

■ Category 2

Important but Not Urgent (Implementation Plans for This Action Should Be Developed Immediately and Implemented as Soon as Practical)

30. **Explain the purpose, picture, and plan of the announced changes and the parts people will be playing in them.** This is the core of transition management, but most often the time required to do it keeps it from being accomplished immediately. Nevertheless, this action should not be delayed. Start by talking about the purpose for the changes and try to establish a picture. You can begin the third P by developing a plan for the first few steps and then adding to it as further challenges are identified and prioritized.

4. **Analyze the employee structure to determine who stands to lose as a result of the proposed changes.** This is another critical task but one that requires too much time to be rated as 1. In addition, this should not be considered a one-time task but rather a dynamic project that requires updating and modification as the changes move forward. A good place to start is with the CEO and what he has to lose (which could be his job and/or leadership role if he doesn't change and accept his responsibility for the downturn of the organization).

24. **Give all nurse managers and supervisors a special training seminar on the emotional impact of change.** Helping managers and supervisors recognize that losses will be incurred as a direct result of these changes and preparing them to deal effectively with those losses is very important. The more the managers and supervisors know about transition and how it can manifest itself, the less likely they are to make mistakes in judging attitudes such as "bad morale" and anger.

19. **Set up a crisis hotline that will provide employees with up-to-date and reliable information to reduce rumor and speculation.** This is a critical issue and normally would be given a rating of 1, but it has been placed in this category to ensure that you use caution when setting up this service. Take a little more time and make sure that you have positive people, good machinery, and lots of correct answers before opening the line to employees. Communication—good, effective communication—is critical during periods of great change.

34. **Set up a restructuring task force to recommend the best way to consolidate patient operations and determine the relocation procedure for employees at the Singapore and Guam sites.** What is facing the organization is much more than simply closing down two sites and laying off employees. A far greater concern should be keeping everyone focused on running the hospital. People have a tendency to focus all of their energy on what it takes to get through a crisis, and you need to take steps to ensure that this preoccupation doesn't overshadow the work that has to be done. Keep in mind that the organization has allowed itself to slide into financial difficulty by poorly implementing the new government performance standards and third-party payment requirements. If Mid-Pacific is to be saved, its process must be revitalized. That includes patient care concepts, design of its services, and, most important, the performance and attitudes of its management and employees. This is a huge change, and to pull it off properly, it must be led by people who feel that they have to make it work. This task force is critical to the survival of the organization, and it should be staffed with the company's brightest and most analytic personnel. People from patient care delivery points and management should be included, and the task force should be provided with outside consultant expertise. It should be remembered, however, that no outside expert can successfully perform this job without the organization's people and 100% of top management's support and drive.

26. **Develop career-planning seminars for those people whose jobs are being lost due to the downsizing and changes.** The organization has just placed a brick wall in the middle of the career paths of 600 of its employees. Most of them are up against things they never expected to experience and require help to get through this period and to put their careers back on the right track. If you provide help for the displaced individuals, you will be doing far more than just helping employees who jobs have been terminated. You will be helping all of those who are going to remain. You must understand that all of your employees are going to be affected by this change, and every one of them is going to experience transition problems. How you treat those who are leaving tells the remaining personnel a tremendous amount about you and the organization, and will have a long-lasting impact on their continuing support and loyalty. If you don't help those who are leaving, you can expect those who are staying to be increasingly difficult to deal with because of increased levels of frustration, and you also can expect them to spend time undermining your efforts to turn the organization around.

32. **Plan closure ceremonies for the two sites that will be shut down.** Making a ceremony out of the closing

will help those who are departing the organization bring closure to a part of their lives. These facilities played an important part in the lives of those who worked there, and each employee will have a void when they are gone. The ceremony can be a funeral, a wake, or a celebration of life. The recommendation is that it celebrate life and the opportunity for growth beyond the death of the site. If the departing employees have been prepared properly and a genuine effort has been made to helped them adjust, then the closing should be a celebration, not simply an ending. The planning for such an event can take a great deal of time, and if done correctly can be therapeutic in itself.

29. **Institute a beneficial suggestions awards program for employees who submit cost-saving suggestions.** What will be done at Mid-Pacific is far more than cost cutting; the entire organization will be revamped. One of the best ways to develop the support of those employees who will remain is to invite them to help develop ways to operate the hospital efficiently. A reward program that is implemented to develop ideas for saving money will have many effects: (1) it will galvanize employees into thinking about saving money; (2) it will provide people with a sense of ownership in the new organization; and (3) it will challenge people to think in terms of improvement, not the status quo, and that will help in turning the organization around.

   A couple of quick thoughts about incentive award programs: Having one is not what is important. Using it is. If you are going to initiate such a program, you cannot just pay it lip service. It must be set up to respond to the suggestions rapidly, and you must make a big deal out of each suggestion that is a winner. Typically, a portion of the realized savings is paid to the employee who submits the suggestion, and it is highly recommended that you do that. After all, the savings wouldn't be achieved without that individual's effort. If you institute one of these programs and then drag your feet, or become nonresponsive and overly selective in your approval process, you can generate negative feelings toward the program, the organization, and you personally as manager.

15. **Find ways to stabilize the gray zone and redefine it in terms that are more beneficial to the organization and to each of the employees.** Take care of the endings first, but start thinking about what is sure to be a long time in the gray zone. The journey to reach the new path down which Mid-Pacific will go will last for several years, and most of its employees will experience additional fears during this time. It is recommended that you help them understand why they are, and will be, fearful. One method of doing

this is to give a name to the change. For example, you could call it "Mid-Pacific—on a journey to greatness." This sets up a support for employees and, in itself, expresses the idea of embarking on a journey that will last an unspecified period of time.

8. **Use the time the organization spends in the gray zone of transition to redesign the entire business: strategy, employment, policies, and structure.** No matter how bad a thing looks at first, you will find opportunity in it. "Challenge," in the words of the great Yogi Berra, "is just another way to color winning." This is Mid-Pacific's chance, and perhaps the last chance it will be given, to transform the organization from yesterday's Pacific Rim leader to tomorrow's comeback champion. You, as a manager, are in the driver's seat, and have captured everyone's attention. The debate over the change has quieted. Now is the time to seize the initiative and carry your hospital through a complete overhaul. Certainly the effort will take time, but that is no reason to delay. Make the changes that must be made and finish the job. Emerge a champion, not a chump.

■ **Category 3**
Potentially Good (The Value of This Action Will Depend on How Well It Is Accomplished)

2. **Order an across-the-board budget cut throughout the organization.** It is definitely time to pull in the belt, *but*—and this is a very important *but*—you need to be very sure that you cut effectively and proportionately. Make sure that you set the cut depth with a critical eye, high enough to get everyone's attention and to focus their energies on making budget cuts. But don't kill those people who are making legitimate effort but cannot reach your goal. Cuts are important, but different areas have different requirements. If there is an area that doesn't try, get rid of the manager and caution the troops. If an area is legitimately trying and is having difficulty, however, work with the staff and encourage them. You'll build loyalty and support for yourself by giving it.

25. **Cut the salaries of senior management personnel by 20%.** This is a plan that has merit. It will seize everyone's imagination and send a clear message that the organization's leadership is serious about change. When this is done, however, get the leadership to support the action. If this cut is made by edict, it could well generate defiance, disloyalty, and even hostility in the very people who will be needed to help lead the organization through the challenge of change. Get management to understand the problem and the benefits that can be realized through such a positive act. Champion the act your-

self, and solicit others through your actions. Don't be critical if someone allows his or her personal self-interest to get in the way. If someone refuses the cut, then find a way to use this defiance as an example of short-term thinking and press that lesson home to others. Don't punish or even fire the individual, but make it clear that a wiser course of action would be to support the concept.

10. **Plan some all-hands social events in all company locations—picnics, excursions, cocktail parties, and dinners.** Although people are moving through the gray zone of transition, such events have a remarkable effect on rebuilding the team feeling and the solidarity that provides strength. However, events should be timed to correspond with positive junctures in the process of change. Events with no meaning will be viewed as placation and can convert a positive into a negative. Don't turn this opportunity into a bread-and-circus act. People don't want to be pacified with undeserved and ill-timed parties. You need to have something to celebrate, and in the period of change, you will have plenty of good reasons to do so.

21. **Have the CEO prepare a videotape for distribution to all hands that is intended to fire up the employees and garner support for the changes.** Extreme caution must be exercised with this approach. Keep in mind that the CEO is the individual who, at least initially, will be thought of as the bad guy. It is much better not to use a videotape for this type of presentation; and it should never be directed at getting individual employees fired up but rather at developing a fired-up team. People should be able to see benefits occurring from the change before being asked to "get motivated." If you feel it is important to have a motivational presentation by the CEO, do it on a personal basis. Have him move through the company to give short "up-date" talks and carefully, and ever so subtly, solicit support and continued creativity and initiative.

WARNING **!**

Don't use the CEO for this motivational task unless this person is a dynamic speaker and respected by the employees. Sending a dullard to motivate people is as absurd an act as can be imagined. The person doing the requesting must be a motivated individual who can radiate excitement. Just being the CEO is not qualification enough.

11. **Establish a suggestion program for reorganization and encourage all employees to submit their ideas on how the process should be carried out.** It was previously noted that employee suggestions can be extremely valuable in the rebuilding process.

However, there is a limit to what should be expected of them. Opening up emotionally charged situations such as employee layoffs can be extremely painful for the average employee. Keep in mind that any ideas produced by employees may be no better than those management could have devised and might take a longer period of time to evolve, but what employees do come up with is absolutely critical to the reworking of Mid-Pacific, because it represents employee buy-in. Strategies should not be created to which employees will not agree or commit.

9. **Fire the current CEO for his inability to provide the proper guidance to avoid this situation.** This idea certainly has appeal. Because this individual is the CEO of this organization, his inaction and failure to recognize and respond to market changes are tantamount to failing to carry out his responsibilities to the organization and the stockholders. However, the individuals charged with remedying the situation should maintain a professional approach and ensure that cooler heads prevail here. Many, many times, organizations get the leadership they earn, and a crisis is not the proper time to go on a witch hunt and burn the CEO at the stake. Moreover, changing the leader at this point could cast the organization into a sea of additional changes, and there is plenty to deal with at the present time.

WARNING **!**

Listen, Mr. or Ms. CEO, being the senior executive doesn't guarantee you any permanence in a publicly held organization. Unless you own controlling interest, you are nothing more than a well-compensated employee. Take a lesson from Steve Jobs, founder and significant shareholder in Apple Computer. When Jobs's leadership pushed the company toward insolvency and his actions ran contrary to the desires of the board of directors, he was voted off the board and lost his job as the company's president and CEO. The stockholders don't care who founded or who is leading the company, only who can keep it profitable.

■ **Category 4**
Not Important (This Action May Result in a Waste of Time and Effort)

33. **Develop a plan to buy out the smallest of Mid-Pacific's America-based competitors to regain market share and build a strong U.S.-based pediatric care unit.** Your organization is already overburdened. It has been declining for years, and today is in a very poor state. Why would you want to burden it with the potential ills of another company and the confusion that comes with a merger? Mergers don't just happen; they create tremendous stress and strain on even the most solvent and stable organizations.

Right now is not the time to create any more stress within the organization.

In addition, even if the acquired competitor is in far better shape financially, it will not necessarily be sound enough to support Mid-Pacific while you make this change. The history books are full of cases in which a solvent organization with excellent leadership and cutting-edge procedures purchased a weak company only to be dragged down by the weight of the acquisition. Imagine what might happen if a weak organization (such as this one), with its questionable management and archaic leadership methods, were the purchaser. Do you really believe that management and employees are going to accept the new organization's methods and leadership? This is very doubtful.

27. **Reorganize the leadership team and redefine the CEO's job as a team coordinator.** Without question, this idea has some merit. With Mid-Pacific's outmoded management system, it seems, at this point anyway, that almost any change might be helpful. But is this change going to create a different type of management or is it simply going to change a title?

    Unless this change creates a different attitude and operating structure that is geared to a more dynamic and closer relationship between management and employees, then the idea should be abandoned. If this change is being made to placate the masses, then it is best forgotten because it will serve to deepen the mess that is already threatening to sink the company.

23. **Redo the compensation structure to reward support of the new system.** This, too, will probably be a good idea further down the line, after the situation starts to straighten out and a positive direction is well established. Right now, no new roles, attitudes, or behavior can be said unequivocally to deserve special reward. The single exception is the payment of bonuses for valuable suggestions.

■ **Category 5**
Bad (This Action Should Not Be Attempted)

1. **Cancel the memo and all further communications until firm plans have been made that outline the reductions and consolidations.** If communication is stopped, especially early communication, then confusion will turn into chaos. The employees aren't stupid. They realize that something big is going to occur. There is every chance that a pirated copy of the CEO's first memo is now making its way down the ranks through informal channels. Secretaries had access to this memo before management did, and you can bet that someone shared it with someone else, so don't think for one moment that this story can be contained. If you try to keep things secret,

people's imaginations will start to run wild, and the rumor mill will grind out horrific stories of doom that will scare the pants off even the most loyal employees.

A much better approach is to step up the volume of communication. Make it straight from the shoulder and make it completely honest. Don't let your people hear about what is happening from the local newspapers. Seize the communications initiative and keep it. Talk and talk straight.

12. **Alleviate employees' fears by informing them that the stated reductions are the only ones that will take place.** *This is not true!* Why? Because you don't know it to be a fact. As the change unfolds, it may become evident that original plans have to be modified, and if you have promised that this is the end of layoffs and then circumstances require you to let a single additional person go, you have committed the ultimate sin—you have lied to your employees and they will know it.

    A better course would be to say that these are the only changes that have been identified at this point, and stress that if additional changes become necessary you will be the first to let everyone know.

17. **Set new and higher patient care targets for the upcoming quarter. The purpose is to give each person a lofty goal to shoot for and to ensure that if patient count does fall below goal, enough patients will have been assisted to meet all budget requirements.** Only an extremely foolish individual would do this. It is almost certain that patient count is going to fall, and the best you can hope for is that this reduction in required service will be temporary. Increasing goals will accomplish nothing except to increase the level of inadequacy felt by the average employee.

    A better approach is to set slightly lower goals for patient levels so that the hospital can exceed them. This will build a sense of accomplishment and give you a reason to celebrate. "Victory, not defeat, will motivate a willingness to engage in additional battle."*

3. **Develop and circulate an upbeat news release which states that the plan has been in development for several months, that reorganization is not a sign of declining performance, and that these cuts, although severe, are needed for the organization to regain its leadership position, which is targeted to occur by the end of the year. In all further communications, a positive spin is to be applied.** Being

---

*This quote is from the ancient military leadership teachings of Sun Tzu, which are used by today's top business management teams. For more information on Sun Tzu, read Chou-Hou W: *Sun-Tzu: war and management,* Boston, 1991, Addison-Wesley.

positive in the face of doom is not foolhardy, but lying—especially lying to the very people whose support you need to get through this crisis—certainly is. Although it is important to set an example of "can do" for your employees, it is extremely dangerous to give the impression that the road is going to be smooth or that the outcome is certain.

A better approach is to be as realistic as possible. People appreciate honesty and will work toward improvement if they are being told the truth and are encouraged to move forward by the celebration of small victories when they occur.

Don't confuse positive thinking with wishful thinking. Your employees won't do that.

13. **Give everyone at Mid-Pacific a badge that proclaims the goal to return to the former dominant position in patient care. It should read "#1 or Bust."** At the moment, your organization is having trouble just keeping its head above water. Providing a badge or button that proclaims your intent to regain your number 1 position is definitely not positive at this time and is close to being completely irrelevant to the issues you face. Mottos are useful, but only when they capture something that people can visualize. Giving badges out and forcing people to wear them when they do not communicate clear, concise, and truly emerging possibilities only bring home a single point: "Who is the fool who thought this up?"

Well, how did you do? Remember that there are no specifically correct answers in this exercise. The point here is to get you to practice and to stimulate thought. If you did well, then please accept our congratulations. If you did not, then you have just been given a golden opportunity. Use your disappointment as a jumping-off point for self-improvement. It certainly can't hurt to take a hard look at yourself, and it might not be bad to share this experience with other members of your team.

Developing Relationships with Senior Management

LEARNING SYNOPSIS

Upon successful completion of this chapter, readers will possess a fundamental understanding of the need to work well with senior management and physicians as well as the need to build an environment of cooperation, trust, and performance.

OBJECTIVES

1. Describe the traditional structure of the healthcare organization
2. Give reasons why it is important for the nurse manager to identify with the management team and to assume the role of manager instead of performer
3. Discuss why it is important that an organization have standardized expectations for a specific position and how that affects the nurse manager
4. Identify different methods that a nurse manager can use to develop effective relationships with senior managers
5. Cite general rules that the nurse manager should follow when working with senior managers
6. Identify steps and recommendations to follow in presenting problems to a senior manager
7. Discuss the historical reasons why the relationships between physicians and nurses are strained
8. Identify things that a nurse manager can do to improve his or her relationship with a physician

At least up to this point, this textbook has focused primarily on helping nurse managers develop the management skills they will need to manage and direct the efforts of the nursing unit and the subordinate personnel assigned to them. Special attention has been paid to the development and management of the relationships that are so vital to the successful operation of the nursing unit and that devour such a large share of nurse managers' day-to-day activities. There is another plane, however, on which all nurse managers must perform effectively, and that involves the relationship between themselves and the senior management personnel whom they must continually interact with and support. This chapter focuses on the relationship between nurse managers and senior management; however, those relationships cannot be adequately discussed in isolation from the necessary relationships the nurse manager builds and maintains with peers, subordinates, and those in other units.

The bottom line of the relationship between nurse managers and senior management is that both have been given authority over specific aspects of the operation of the organization by the duly constituted board of directors. They are responsible for implementing the directives, policies, and instructions issued by members of senior management on behalf of the board. Although the primary focus of nurse managers is direct management of patient care and subordinate staff, they have the additional responsibilities of keeping senior management informed of issues and problems that occur within their specific areas of authority and working closely with senior managers to gain their support for necessary changes. These overlapping responsibilities are carried out largely through a campaign of well-developed communication that transcends the lines of authority. Nurse managers are responsible for ensuring that effective communication is maintained at all times and in all directions from their positions in the management structure (i.e., up, down, and laterally).

Many times, the position of nurse managers as the front-line representatives of management is not an enviable one. Here they sit, caught directly in the middle between the demands of senior management and the needs of the staff. Subordinates, for example, frequently have difficulty understanding the decisions that are made and the rules and regulations that are created by organizational management, and nurse managers are the ones who must carefully walk the line between obligatory compliance with senior management edicts and the compassionate understanding of specific employee needs. This liaison aspect of the nurse manager's job is critical to the functional operation of the organization. Through their efforts to keep the transmission of organization goals a smooth

and fluid process, nurse managers provide an invaluable service to the organization.

The term *senior management* can encompass individuals holding a wide range of different positions, from senior personnel who are in a direct line of authority with the nurse manager and to whom he or she reports directly, to many others who are considered senior simply because of the level of managerial authority they have been given (indirect seniors). Exactly whom the nurse manager reports to and how the reporting lines are influenced depends on how the organization is structured. The exact arrangement of the organization's management team can be seen in the organizational chart. This chart consists of a series of boxes arranged in a systemic manner to show the lines of authority that run both laterally and vertically. The nurse manager's position, because it is considered a junior position, will appear at the bottom of the various lateral lines. Typically, nurse managers report directly to another manager within the nursing department (supervisor or assistant director of nursing), but they may also report to a nonnursing administrator if the structure of the organization dictates it. Not all organizations are structured in the traditional manner, however, and if nurse managers are employed by an organization that has a highly decentralized chain of authority, they may find themselves reporting to an administrator, a physician, a divisional nursing director, or even a combination of several such "senior" individuals.

Regardless of the type of organization in which the nurse manager works, however, the skills that allow the nurse manager to support and interact effectively with the people to whom he or she is responsible are essentially the same. Although some special professional issues may need to be considered, especially if the nurse manager reports to a physician, the same fundamental managerial skills are required in all settings.

THE STRUCTURE OF AUTHORITY IN THE HEALTHCARE SYSTEM

Every form of business has some type of organizational authority structure that is tasked with establishing and controlling the rules and regulations, the goals and objectives, and the policy for conducting the effort necessary to implement these goals. This is true regardless of whether the organization is a for-profit or a not-for-profit system, and healthcare institutions are no exception. An authority (management) structure is obligatory for smooth, efficient, and fiscally responsible day-to-day operation.

The structure of a healthcare organization is significantly different from one that might be seen in a product-based business, however, because most healthcare organizations have a dual authority arrangement. A typical healthcare organization has both a lay authority structure (nonmedical) and a unique medical authority structure. For example, a hospital administrator, regardless of seniority, usually has only lay authority, whereas a physician, regardless of how neophyte, has professional authority. When a nurse is functioning as a clinician, he or she has a certain degree of professional authority, but when that same nurse is appointed as a nurse manager, he or she automatically receives the degree of lay authority that is inherent in that position. Physicians and nurses who serve in designated managerial positions can have both lay and professional authority and will move back and forth between exercising the two as the situation requires.

Although it is universally accepted in the healthcare organization that those with both lay and professional authority are concerned primarily with the quality of patient care, the ways in which these two groups perceive their responsibilities to deliver that care are often in conflict. For example, the typical hospital administrator is motivated primarily by the need to generate revenue (i.e., the maintenance of an adequate occupancy rate), whereas the medical authority (physician or nurse) is concerned primarily with the quality of health care available to the patients. This duality of authority often places nurse managers in a position in which they must meet the demands of both the lay and medical authority groups. How effectively they are able to move between these two groups and develop quality performance relationships that build trust and confidence is critical to the performance of their units and to their own continued success.

Power and Politics

Being a part of any management team is a difficult and demanding responsibility, even when very clear lines of authority and reporting requirements are established. For nurse managers operating in the dual authority regime of a healthcare facility, these demands are multiplied significantly. Their efforts begin with understanding that they are, in fact, integral parts of the management team. They may well be very junior members of the team, but they are critical to its success nonetheless. When they assumed the position of nurse manager, they inherited some very significant responsibilities that are not shared with non-management personnel, regardless of the latter's technical skill or educational level. Among these responsibilities are the following:

Participate: Nurse managers are obligated to support the activities of management—even if they disagree with policy or practice. They must participate actively in the management group and are held accountable for their actions.

Carry out decisions: One of the disadvantages faced by nurse managers, because they are junior members of any management team, is that most of the time they will be the managers who carry out policy, not the ones who actually create it. This will frequently put them in a position of carrying out edicts that they do not personally believe in or that they do not think represent the proper way to do what needs to be done. Unfortunately, it doesn't matter what they think. As nurse managers, they are responsible for carrying out policy, not openly criticizing it. When they find themselves in this difficult situation, they must put on their managerial hats and deliver the message to the staff as if they themselves had created it. Anything less is unprofessional and, in many organizations, unforgivable. This doesn't mean that nurse managers must be robots and blindly carry out every order that falls from above. What it does mean is that their criticism must be presented constructively and through the chain of authority. In fact, nurse managers have an *obligation* to criticize senior management edicts, but they must be careful how they do so. The cardinal rule is that managers must never criticize their seniors in the presence of junior personnel. If they do, they undermine their senior managers' authority and ability to be effective in the future. This single rule is absolutely critical to the success of junior managers and must never be forgotten. In fact, general business considers this to be the single biggest management secret in the world.

To implement this important management rule, nurse managers must understand how to use power effectively in a political environment and must clearly understand the difference between power and politics.

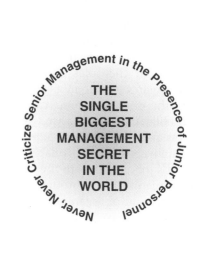

Never, Never Criticize Senior Management in the Presence of Junior Personnel

THE SINGLE BIGGEST MANAGEMENT SECRET IN THE WORLD

Present self: When professional managers present or communicate decisions to their staffs, they do so in a manner that does not reflect negatively on senior management. Regardless of whether or not they agree with the decisions they must implement, they must show a positive and supportive attitude toward these decisions in front of their subordinates. If they do not, they will undermine their ability to support the decisions; will ultimately damage the relationship among themselves, senior management, and their units; and quite possibly will harm the organization. They must convey support for the decision through their personal actions and communication.

POWER

What is power, and how is it used? Power is simply another word for authority, yet it is much more than that. Authority is the right to give orders or enforce rules that is an inherent part of management. Authority is bestowed on nurse managers when they assume their positions. It is given out in measured and tightly controlled allotments, is jealously guarded, and is directly proportional to the level of the management position occupied (e.g., a nurse manager has less authority than does a senior administrator or the vice president of nursing).

Power, on the other hand, has little to do with position and is only partly reliant on authority. Although a certain amount of power is derived from being part of management, its full impact is felt only when it is combined with influence. Influence and authority, when wielded in the proper combination, can truly create immense power, even at the lower end of the management chain. The meaning of power can be easily seen by considering a situation in which a senior member of administration proclaims an edict. Every junior member will act with urgency to carry out the proclamation, simply because the boss declared that it be done. However, this does not mean that the edict will ever become effective or will even be supported to the best of others' ability; compliance is not support.

On the other hand, a very junior person can wield immense power by exercising quiet influence. When a person who is well connected, who is held in high regard, who has a reputation for excellence, and who has earned the trust of others by demonstrating professionalism and integrity merely suggests that something should be done in a certain manner, then people—even very senior people—will notice and listen intently. This ability is seen everywhere and is recognized in comments like, "John (Joan) can sure get things done."

Power should be the ability to influence in a positive manner, but it is often misused and most frequently by people who should not have it. Power gets things done, and as long as the people wielding it remember their responsibility to it and to those it affects, it can be a force for creating magical things in the business world.

Power is most effective when it is not spoken about but simply remains an understood asset. People who wield power most effectively do so quietly and in an unassuming manner. However, power is also a ruthless and uncaring weapon that can maim and destroy wantonly. The only difference between power as a force for good and power as a force for harm is the quality of the individual who wields it. There is real truth in the old proverb, "Good managers never need to remind anyone of their authority."

Power, used correctly, provides nurse managers with the opportunity to influence their subordinates for the greater good of their patients, the organization, and each other. Superior nurse managers understand that there is an awesome responsibility that goes along with having control over the opportunities and future of another, and never abuse power. Most of the highly regarded leaders in the nursing profession believe in the absolute necessity for all nurses to learn how to develop and effectively use power, and for no one is this need more critical than for nurse managers.

POLITICS

Politics is a fundamental reality in any business setting, and nowhere more than in the management sphere. Politics is a powerful, albeit hidden, process permeating every aspect of a manager's life. It is different from the authority that is inherent in the management position simply because it is cultivated and not bestowed. Good managers understand that they have power and rarely use it blatantly. Instead, the truly effective ones rely on their leadership skills and not their authority to get things accomplished. They combine this expertise with things such as compromise to accomplish personal and organizational goals. They also form personal alliances with those who can influence future opportunities and success. This is business politics as it was intended.

Although many of the people who use politics the most have created a negative feeling toward it, politics should not be viewed as a manipulative or dishonest quality or practice. When used properly, it is nothing more than the process of employing circumstances, people, and available resources in an astute manner. Politics and its use does not have to have a negative connotation. What makes it appear harmful and dishonest is a lack of personal integrity on the part of the individual using it and the underlying reason that it is being used.

Although power and influence can be gained by effectively and professionally developing a political network in the nursing field, a large proportion of nurses have been reluctant do this. Traditionally, this reluctance was motivated by the same characteristics that inhibited nurses from dealing with conflict. Today, however, it has little to do with tradition and much more to do with not wanting to be seen as using what so many people consider an unprofessional and manipulative process. The reluctance to rely on politics is far more acute at the junior management level than as one advances up the chain of command. In fact, many senior managers rely heavily on the use of politics to get their jobs done.

A 1985 study confirmed the difference in attitude toward politics that is evident between nursing administrators and first-level nurse managers.[1] The researchers found that the vast majority of administrators, unlike front-line managers, held the following two beliefs:

1. Power is related to political skill.
2. Control over others is necessary to acquire and retain power and autonomy.

Whether these beliefs are actually correct or not is irrelevant; so many administrators believe them to be true that they have become a reality in the healthcare industry. The wide gulf that exists between how administrators view politics and how front-line managers view it is one of the most compelling reasons for the distorted communication, conflict, and lack of unified purpose that exist in many healthcare organizations.

Formal and Informal Power Structures

Every organization in the healthcare industry has at least some unique aspects, but in every one there exists both a formal and an informal power structure. The formal structure is readily identifiable and understood. In fact, it is openly displayed in the organizational chart that is used to visualize the institution's hierarchy of authority. The formal power structure follows the lines of authority shown on the organizational chart and is based on who reports to whom.

Informal power, on the other hand, is wielded in a very vaguely defined and almost indiscernible manner. It is the quiet influence that individuals exercise through a system of networks and alliances that is not part of any official structure.

Within the organization, information flows up, down, and laterally through both the formal and informal structures. Use of the formal structure is the most widely accepted and generally the most effective method of transmitting information. Therefore, the organization's hierarchy (proper channels) is the most common and professional method of communication

used. In this system, there is an unwritten but very binding understanding that problems, should they arise, will be communicated to one's immediate senior *first*. This is the same unwritten understanding that exists between nurse managers and the members of their staffs. This is what is commonly known as *protecting the boss*, and it is absolutely essential to good order and continuing careers in the nursing field.

Nothing ever works completely correctly, however, and there will inevitably be a time when a nurse manager will feel that his or her senior has not handled an issue properly. Differences of opinion occur between managers, and occur frequently, and when they do, the situation can be a minefield of challenges for junior managers. How is such a situation resolved? What must junior managers do to maintain the confidence and support of their seniors? Should they go over their seniors' heads with the problem or should they resign themselves to compliance with something they know to be wrong?

The cardinal rule is this: *Never go over the immediate supervisor's head.* Instead, professional nurse managers will carefully evaluate the situation to ensure that their supervisors have all of the pertinent facts surrounding the issue and clearly know what the potential impact will be. They then request an opportunity to discuss the situation and do so in a calm and reasonable manner—omitting all things personal and emotional. In this way, they can be assured that their concerns will be heard in an unemotional and professional manner. It is imperative that nurse managers (novice and experienced) understand that, although few senior managers would knowingly or willingly create a situation or pass an edict that will cause damage in areas for which they are ultimately responsible, many are very insecure and are not open to criticism. Therefore, every situation of this type must be approached in a very careful and highly sensitive manner. If the nurse manager strongly feels that a situation exists that can be damaging to the unit, or the nurse manager is being asked to do something that he or she simply does not agree with, the nurse manager respectfully and humbly asks to have his or her opinion heard. If, after the situation is discussed with the supervisor, the problem still cannot be worked out, then the nurse manager can ask for an opportunity to discuss it with a senior member of the administration. However, every manager needs to understand that when a junior manager goes over the head of his or her immediate supervisor, the process had better be done professionally, in consultation with the supervisor, and with the clear understanding that he or she is personally risking a great deal. Supervisors, at least the good ones, will encourage their junior managers to openly discuss their disagreements and even to point out perceived mistakes, but rarely will one want a subordinate to carry the problem to a higher authority. Every manager knows that the first thought the senior manager will have is, "Why am I being bothered with this?" and that will be followed almost immediately by, "Why can't these two work out their problems between themselves?"

No managers can afford to have their juniors take problems to their bosses. Just as nurse managers don't want staff nurses going to their supervisors with problems, supervisors don't want nurse managers going to the director of nursing. This is a far more acute problem when managers can't work out their differences, and the situation is always viewed in a negative light. Therefore, good managers make every effort to work things out with their immediate supervisors, and unless it is a grave situation or one that, for whatever reason, they simply cannot bear, they rarely take any problem further than one step in the chain of authority. Instead, they seek compromise with their seniors and do so by using supportable facts and logical reasoning. They leave emotions and personal feelings out of the situation and are always willing to compromise their own positions (Box 19-1).

BOX 19-1

Cardinal Rules for Discussing Disagreement with a Senior Manager

1. Don't go over a senior's head without first trying to resolve the situation with him or her. This is never appropriate and can have severe consequences for you.
2. When discussing a disagreement with a senior, use supportable facts and logical reasoning to present your case.
3. Always seek to compromise and avoid confrontation; arguments are always detrimental to your cause.
4. Be willing to change your position if the senior presents compelling reasons; this includes being willing to admit that you are wrong.
5. Once compromise is achieved or the original edict is invoked, make sure that you support it.
6. Go over your boss's head only after understanding that it is not only you who risks something.
7. Realize that going over your boss's head, no matter how well justified, is not something that any member of senior management supports, and although you might win the battle, there is very good reason to believe that you will lose much in your future.

If the resolution of a nurse manager's problem requires that the manager work with a member of his or her immediate supervisor's peer group, it is vitally important that the nurse manager do this in conjunction with the supervisor. The very first step the nurse manager should take when attempting to resolve an issue with a senior manager is to stop in and discuss the issue with the boss. If the nurse manager does this, the nurse manager will be acting to protect his or her supervisor from a potential surprise from the supervisor's peer or a reprimand from the supervisor's senior, and, at the same time, the nurse manager will be obtaining valuable counsel and possible support. The nurse manager will want to clarify with his or her senior just how much autonomous authority the nurse manager has when dealing with the senior's peer and the best possible manner in which to go about the process.

Just how much authority a nurse manager has in dealing with his or her immediate supervisor's peers varies depending on the hospital's philosophy and the senior's management style. If the senior is the type who prefers to delegate this kind of responsibility, the nurse manager may be expected to handle interdepartmental problems directly with other department heads or administrators. If the senior is a controlling individual, however, the nurse manager must secure support each time he or she needs to deal with another department head, because the supervisor may feel that dealing with peers is his or her responsibility alone. Regardless of the circumstances, the nurse manager must keep his or her senior informed of the purpose and progress of any interdepartmental dealings. This is the age-old practice of supporting the boss and protecting the boss from surprises. For example, if the nurse manager discusses complaints about food quality with the dietary director, the nurse manager should inform his or her immediate supervisor of what was said and make him or her aware of any potential ramifications. If the nurse manager discusses the situation beforehand with his or her supervisor, the nurse manager might be able to strengthen his or her position with knowledge that the nurse manager is not privy to, such as the fact that other units are having similar problems. Keeping the supervisor informed about one's actions with other managers is not only professional conduct, it is politically astute.

A critical element that must be used effectively by managers is the informal structure that exists in every organization. Sometimes known as the grapevine, it can be a powerful ally to the politically savvy manager. This avenue can be used properly only if managers understand that information transmitted in this manner may or may not be accurate, and every piece of information received should be verified before being acted upon. Under no circumstances should this informal process be overlooked or ignored, however, because it may be far more powerful and influential than more acceptable formal channels of communication. When it is used effectively, nurse managers may be able to quietly influence others even though they have little or no authority over them.

Nurse managers must devote time to developing an understanding of the informal structure that exists around them. Part of being an effective manager is efficiently using the resources available. The informal power structure is a very effective one that differs in just about every situation and does not rely on the formal chain of authority in any respect. For example, sometimes a secretary holds informal power; at other times, it is an administrative assistant who reports to the director of nursing service. By knowing who in the organization others take their problems to and who is capable of delivering quality assistance when needed, wise managers can get a tremendous amount accomplished with little effort. Effective use of these informal channels is an imperative and vital exercise of power.

Although nurse managers are given formal power when they assume the responsibilities of their office, they must work hard to develop any form of informal power. They accomplish this by developing a reputation for caring about the needs of others, by demonstrating a willingness to extend themselves personally to help others enhance their performance, and by keeping their ears to the ground and listening to what is really being said in the organization. By improving interpersonal skills and by carefully building a positive and trusting relationship with others, nurse managers can wield a significant amount of influence with those members of the staff who do not report to them, with senior managers, and with other administrators. Through the positive and careful development of informal power, they can vastly improve their ability to beneficially influence the quality of the working environment in their units and the patient care provided.

One last point must be mentioned regarding power and influence, and it takes the form of a strong caution. Power, used correctly, can be an enormous asset augmenting a manager's ability to improve relationships, defuse difficult situations, and improve working conditions. If it is exercised with prudence, care, and concern for others, everyone the manager touches can benefit. However—and this is the important caution—improper use of power as a tool to further the self-interest of the individual manager or the manager's unit can cause irreparable damage to both the nurse manager and those with whom he or she interacts.

Power is a wonderful, exciting, and important tool when used with regard for others and as part of a responsible plan of management, but when used to advance one's own purpose or without regard for the rights, privileges, or well-being of others, it is a very destructive weapon. The ethical and prudent use of power, both formal and informal, is a responsibility that is fundamental to a manager's job and future.

IDENTIFICATION WITH MANAGEMENT

Becoming a manager is a process of change. It doesn't occur overnight and often takes many exceptionally good performers years to complete. Being a manager means that different responsibilities and viewpoints will be held, that what was perceived yesterday as something negative can now be viewed in a positive light because, as a manager, one is privy to the underlying reasons for it. The change that will take place is both physically and mentally obvious to others, if not to the novice manager. What really happens when a high-energy and exceptional clinical nurse becomes a nurse manager, and how is it viewed? The following anecdote provides a representative picture of the change that will occur and the reactions many people will have to it:

> The staff nurses in Joan's unit are quick to remark that she has changed a great deal since she became nurse manager. "She changed. Before she became one of *them*, she would never do that." The refrain was repeated daily throughout the unit.
>
> On the other hand, Joan had never felt so alone. It seemed to her that all of her friends in the nursing staff had turned on her. She thought they were jealous of her promotion and no longer wished to associate with her.

This scenario plays itself out daily everywhere people work when one of the group advances ahead of the others. Why? Because both parties are right: the relationship that formerly existed between co-workers does change when one member of the group becomes a manager. In the example, Joan changed because the responsibilities of her new job forced her to change. After all, she is no longer just responsible for herself and her patients; she is now responsible for the operation of an entire unit. It is her responsibility to ensure that the patients being served by her unit receive the best care that can be provided, that every member of the staff performs to the best of his or her ability and up to the expectations of the organization, and that the resources necessary are made available. To fulfill these new responsibilities, Joan has to adapt her performance to closely coincide with the needs of management, and this shift in effort is what causes her to be identified more as a part of management and less as a fellow nurse. Newly appointed nurse managers must make this shift well enough to ensure that the organizational goals for their units are accomplished on time and under budget. The evolution actually causes physical and attitudinal changes in the new nurse manager ("She didn't act that way when she was one of us").

This change is critical to the success of new managers and of the units for which they become responsible. They must make the change from worker to conductor or they will not be able to accomplish the goals and objectives senior management desires. But beyond that, there comes a time when new managers can no longer do the things that they would like to do or perform the hands-on actions of a member of the staff. At the moment they became managers, their role shifted from doing the work to being responsible for getting it done. If they do not accept this fact and continue to be performers, everyone in their units will suffer, and the organization will not view this as a positive discharge of responsibility.

As new nurse managers start to view themselves as members of the management team, they will begin to see that their problems are interlocked with those of their immediate seniors. When the senior manager makes a commitment, then that commitment will become the new nurse manager's commitment as well. This does not mean that, to be good managers, nurse managers must rubber-stamp every decision their bosses make, but it does mean that managers must be sensitive to the wants and needs of their supervisors. In fact, most good managers are frequently in disagreement with their immediate and senior supervisors. However, they remain concerned about the potential ramifications of their disagreement and carefully disagree with their seniors in private. After these discussion, and when the doors of those private meetings open, these professional nurse managers must rejoin their units firmly committed to the realization of their senior managers' needs. Their follow-though and communication with their subordinates must never reflect any level of dissatisfaction with the mandates of senior management. Although they do not have to agree, it is obligatory that they visibly support and do so with an attitude that says, "*We* want this," not, "*They* want this."

Being part of management is living in a fishbowl. Actions are watched from above and from below with equal attention; some will want to see success and there will be a few who expect and will be very pleased with failure. Everyone will have an opinion as to the quality of performance that is demonstrated, and the truth is that both sides will have an almost equal influence on new managers' ability to succeed.

Nurse managers must support senior management, and they must do so with the best interests of their staffs foremost in their minds.

As the old adage says, for a manager to be successful, he or she must truly want to be in charge.

ROLE EXPECTATIONS

One of the real truths about becoming a manager is that a management position serves as the framework for the performance of a specific role in the organization, and whoever is assigned to that position is anticipated to perform in accordance with the expectations held for it. This standardization of expectations, or the desire that any individual assigned to a given position will perform at the same quality level, is one of the ways in which organizations remain stable over time, even in the face of persistent turnover.

The actual process of management, however, is far different from the rote fulfillment of expectations. In real life, every person who accepts a job brings to it his or her own opinions, talents, and willingness, and this makes the organizational expectations somewhat onerous. It simply is not possible to have different people perform exactly alike; each person is far too unique an individual, and that uniqueness ensures that how different people perceive and perform the job will be different. One fundamental aspect of this uniqueness is seen in the way different people react when other individuals comment on how they should perform. Newly appointed managers might receive one message from their supervisors about the need for long hours and selfless dedication to the job, and another message from their families about the need to be at home more and spend quality time with the children. Mixed messages like these are very common, and frequently the actions they request are mutually exclusive.

One of the biggest challenges faced by organizations as they search for competent employees to fill management positions is that many of the best-qualified staff nurses (clinicians) will not readily accept promotion to such positions, and those who will accept do so only with great trepidation. The primary reason for this, of course, is the natural reluctance of superior performers to leave the occupational fields in which they have excelled to start over in an area that is both confusing and frequently held in less than high regard. This is especially true when professionals are asked to give up their practice of helping patients. Even with its many demands, performing as a clinician is a satisfying and richly rewarding vocation for many. The natural reluctance to abandon this vocation is magnified by the fact that most nurses, regardless of their competence, do little to prepare themselves for eventual promotion to the management level. The most difficult hurdle to overcome in the search for managers, however, is the disdain that most professionals feel for the management process and the overall poor perception of management. Many professionals in the healthcare field actually believe that the primary goal of management is the antithesis of the goal of clinicians (i.e., the delivery of quality care to patients).

One of the most difficult hurdles for most nurses who wish to advance into management positions is that they have not prepared themselves well enough. Although they may be truly gifted clinicians, have demonstrated a significant commitment to the organization, and know the organization well, many simply lack the background in management theory, leadership, research, and performance strategies. Today, personnel who wish to become part of management must prepare themselves ahead of time using educational methods that parallel those that have been used by chief executive officers in industry for decades.

In reality, however, most open nurse management positions are filled by people who hold ambiguous role expectations at best. The ambiguity grows out of their own lack of understanding of what may be needed to perform well in a nurse manager's position as well as to the expectations that senior staff members might have for that position. This same lack of understanding may be true of the positions held by the nurse manager's seniors, the assistant director of nursing service, and so on.

RELATIONSHIPS WITH SENIOR MANAGERS

How do managers go about developing relationships with their immediate supervisors? Developing a close relationship is not necessarily an issue for staff nurses because the chasm that separates performers from managers is often great, but it is very important to nurse managers, because they will rely heavily on their relationships with their immediate seniors. One thing that helps new nurse managers prepare for building long and fruitful relationships with senior managers is that most of the management techniques developed for working with subordinates can also be applied to building relationships with seniors. The importance of building a solid, high-quality relationship with one's seniors cannot be overemphasized. This is a vital association for every nurse manager, and one that needs to be nurtured and worked at consistently. A senior manager has far more influence over the future success of a nurse manager than a nurse manager has over a staff nurse. How well the inter-

action works will largely shape the success of the nursing unit and of the nurse manager.

What makes creating healthy relationships with seniors difficult is the fact that not all nurse manager positions are equal. Just as the reporting relationships in the administrative hierarchy differ from organization to organization, so too do the roles and responsibilities of the various nurse managers differ within a given organization. Because of the differences in overall organizational structure (centralized, decentralized, or matrix) and the influence of the personal philosophies of those in higher management positions, the amount of authority delegated to nurse managers can vary greatly. Some will find themselves with little more authority than that given to the typical charge nurse, whereas others will find themselves shouldering the nearly overwhelming responsibilities of a department manager. The reasons that such differences exist are not germane to this discussion; however, regardless of the scope of the responsibilities taken on by the new nurse manager, the relationship that is built with the immediate supervisor will be the core element. Nurse managers must never assume that, because they have greater responsibilities, they can spend less time cultivating the support of their immediate supervisors. In every situation, there will be a senior and a subordinate manager, and the relationship developed between the two is important to the success of both.

The development of a relationship between two managers is very different from the development of a relationship between a manager and nonmanager or between two performers. Among performers, the close proximity in which the individuals work tends to compel the development of a relationship. As the performers interact, they learn to trust one another and to find different qualities in each other that they admire or at least find pleasing, and from this a relationship and often a strong bonding develops. The relationship between a manager and a nonmanager is more or less like that between a parent and child, in that one is in control and the other is subservient. In this type of relationship, a good deal of restraint is required on the part of both individuals to build trust and reliance, because each is, at least to some degree, wary of the other's intentions and credibility. The most difficult relationship to develop, however, is that between junior managers and their senior managers. Although both are management personnel and for that reason share similar interests and challenges, they rarely work in close proximity, rarely have periods in which they can relax long enough to get to know one another, and rarely start any conversation that does not deal with the solution of problems. Nevertheless, the development of a solid relationship is critical to the success of both, and the process is definitely in the best interests of both.

Although the development of a relationship is typically the responsibility of both parties, many junior personnel behave as if this were not the case. Most allow the senior manager to control the relationship and rarely take an active part, failing to accept their responsibility for the development and maintenance of the relationship. However, all relationships require the active participation of all of the parties involved. Nurse managers have this responsibility, even though it is unwritten and is not a formal expectation. They have the opportunity to develop more out of their relationships with their bosses than casual tolerance; in fact, if they work at securing the trust and confidence of their seniors, they can do much to influence their future.

Obstacles to Relationships

What hurdles are there to overcome in the development of a solid relationship, and what impedes the development of relationships in the management circle? Although many, many hurdles and impediments may be encountered, a few are general enough to apply in almost every situation.

REACTION TO AUTHORITY

One of the primary factors affecting the development of a relationship between a junior and a senior manager is each person's reaction to the authority that he or she holds. Rarely will two managers perceive their responsibilities in the same light. One might consider authority a sacred privilege, and the other may be quite ambivalent about it. The first may perceive this difference in attitude and think that the other is not doing everything possible to discharge his or her duties, whereas the more ambivalent of the two may perceive the actions of the devoted one as being foolish and ill advised. Such differences are overcome by accepting them and not forcing personal expectations or beliefs on another. Junior managers who are genuinely interested in cultivating a positive relationship with their seniors will work toward accepting any differences that exist and will make a serious effort to work within their seniors' value systems as well as maintaining their own. Studies have shown that people who desire to become managers generally harbor very positive feelings about those who are already in authority.[2] In fact, many would-be managers perceive their seniors, and management in general, as people who play a positive role and not necessarily as barriers. It has been shown that how people perceive authority before becoming a part of management is critical to their eventual success as managers themselves.

SELF-ESTEEM

An individual's level of self-esteem has a strong influence on that person's ability to develop relationships in the sphere of management. For example, a manager with low self-esteem may react to another manager in two different but extreme ways[2]:

1. *Unimpressed:* Unimpressed subordinates may harbor strong feelings of inadequacy, which may lead them to think that their own ideas or suggestions are not valuable and possibly that they themselves are wanting. These individuals are not likely to take the initiative or make suggestions, and may even fail to bring important matters to their seniors' attention.

2. *Belligerent:* Belligerent individuals are those who disagree with their seniors as frequently as possible. They argue openly and in sight of others and oppose every action taken by their seniors. People with this type of personality are typically very insecure in their capabilities and believe that finding fault in others bolsters their own image. The reaction to such individuals by other members of the group can be severe, and belligerent individuals can create a good deal of dissension within the group.

Although most people with low self-esteem will present aspects of each of these attitudes in their behavior, all of them tend to exhibit a high degree of sensitivity to any occurrence. For instance, assume that a nurse manager with low self-esteem develops a new staffing pattern for his or her unit and that a higher-level manager rejects the effort. Because of his or her low self-esteem, the nurse manager is likely to take this rejection very personally and not even consider that the senior might have had a solid, objective reason for the denial. But in fact senior managers rarely object to ideas that enhance performance, save money, or reduce effort, and it is extremely rare that quality ideas are rejected simply because of the individual who recommends them.

What, exactly, is self-esteem and what effect does it have on a person's ability to perform? In truth, it is nothing more than individuals' ability to accept themselves for what they are, with all of their assets and limitations. Self-esteem, by this definition, has nothing to do with people's ability to perform well or to achieve high levels of productivity. People are far more complex than that. All individuals have intrinsic worth as human beings. This means that individuals have the ability to view themselves as objectively as they view others, and as long as they continue to do this, they will develop good self-esteem. People who view things objectively understand that events are evaluated based on the facts, not just on personal impact.

UNREALISTIC EXPECTATIONS

When junior managers harbor unrealistic expectations of what their seniors can and should do for them, difficulties arise and impediments are created to the healthy development of a relationship. This is quite common and can easily be remedied through dedication and good communication. The following are three common misconceptions held by subordinates:

1. The senior should always like the subordinate.
2. The senior should take care of the subordinate.
3. The senior should treat the subordinate like a friend.

These are not realistic expectations, and most junior personnel would realize this if confronted about them. Nevertheless, they are the underlying assumptions that many subordinates hold about their relationships with their seniors. Supervisors are managers with difficult responsibilities and nearly overwhelming workloads—they are not junior managers' parents.

DISLIKE

Many people feel that they must like or at least respect the people for whom they work. Although it would be nice if this were the situation, it is not one that materializes frequently. In fact, whether or not subordinates like their bosses is totally irrelevant to the requirement that juniors work in a positive manner with their supervisors, especially at the management level. Whether or not junior managers like their seniors should never affect the level of performance and degree of dedication they provide to their senior managers and should never interfere with the quality of their work. Subordinates are responsible for their performance and for the development of their half of the managerial relationship, just as seniors are responsible for the development their side.

Senior managers need and should demand the support of their juniors. Good nurse managers understand that their overall success and the success of their units are tied directly to the types of relationships they develop with their subordinates, peers, and seniors. They know that every person who works in the organization has the ability to significantly influence other people's level of job satisfaction and future job opportunities. Learning how to effectively relate to his or her senior manager is every nurse manager's responsibility, and the positive extension of self can create a work environment that is far more enriching than one in which conflict and stress constantly exist.

The Junior Manager's Responsibilities

There are hundreds of individual responsibilities that junior managers might have assigned to them.

Nevertheless, a few core elements of management are absolutely critical for novice managers to know and practice well if they are to successfully make the transition from performer to manager. Knowledge of these basics will ensure that new managers develop successful relationships with their seniors and are able to discharge their new duties effectively. The most fundamental elements are described in the following sections.

RECOGNIZE THE LEVEL OF RESPONSIBILITY

All novice managers must realize that the amount of responsibility given them is less than that carried by their seniors. Although this certainly seems like common sense, it is surprising how many new managers feel that their supervisors should be available to them at all times, should be aware of the specific challenges that they are facing daily, and should be ready to assist in the resolution of their problems at any time. When they find that their seniors are not always available, or when they ask questions and the supervisors do not have immediate solutions, they become disillusioned and feel as if they have been left on their own.

The simple truth is that nurse managers' supervisors are just as busy as they are—and in most cases much busier. Just as nurse managers are responsible for the functioning of their entire units, their supervisors are responsible for the functioning of several.

Nurse managers need to remember that they are in charge. They are the ones who must make the day-to-day decisions and who must manage their units. If nursing supervisors had the time or the inclination to run individual nursing units, why would they need the nurse managers?

RESPECT THE SUPERVISOR'S NEEDS

It is absolutely critical to recognize that nursing supervisors are just like everyone else; they need their space to complete their responsibilities, and they all have needs of their own. Nurse managers should make a point of remembering that their seniors are extremely busy and can always use help in completing their work. Providing help does not mean that nurse managers physically lend a hand but rather that they do their own jobs well enough so that senior managers do not have to worry about the nurse managers' jobs or spend more time than absolutely necessary following up on things that they told the nurse managers to do. The best way that junior managers can help their seniors is by being capable of doing the job they have been assigned. The more they can do to ensure that their units operate effectively, the better a relationship they will ultimately have with their supervisors.

Now that we have said that the best thing junior managers can do for their supervisors is to fulfill the responsibilities they have been given, we must talk briefly about working for a senior who is not, shall we say, the best manager around or a type of individual for whom one would want to work. If a nurse manager is one of the unfortunate ones who happens to work for a senior who is less than professional, who has difficulty performing the job, or who is a micromanager, how the nurse manager handles the relationship may change dramatically. In this situation, the nurse manager must remember that the senior is in a position to interfere in the superior-subordinate relationship far more readily than is the nurse manager. Assume that the senior is an individual who has a significant need to feel important and to be needed, and in an effort to satisfy this need, makes a habit of overwhelming the subordinates he or she manages. A classic example is the manager who comes to the rescue whenever a problem faces the unit and seldom, if ever, delegates management of a problem outside of the individual nursing unit. This type of senior will never encourage subordinate managers to development leadership qualities of their own and often will go out of the way to make sure that juniors are dependent on the senior for most of their managerial functions.

The best way for a nurse manager to deal effectively with the controlling or needy senior manager is to let that person know as subtlely as possible that the nurse manager is in control but that he or she welcomes the senior's advice. Confronting the senior or suggesting that he or she is not needed will only damage the relationship the nurse manager needs to develop. This is always an extremely sensitive matter and should never be taken lightly. One of the best ways for the nurse manager to handle this situation is to remain humble and ask for advice on a problem when it is necessary. The nurse manager should use the senior's expertise to improve the quality of the unit but make sure that he or she does not allow the senior to take over the junior's role. Then, the next time the nurse manager calls the senior with a problem, the manager should remind the senior that he or she has wanted to handle a problem himself or herself and remark that perhaps the nurse manager could handle this one with the senior's help. The junior should follow up on this, detail the outcome of his or her problem solving, and ask for advice on other ways to handle similar problems in the future. In this way, the senior remains a part of the process and the junior can develop management skills with assistance.

There is another type of senior manager that juniors must be careful about: those who need to be liked by their subordinates or who perhaps are just not good managers. If the senior manager has an inordinate need to be liked, he or she will have a tendency to continually put personal popularity above the needs of the organization. The senior will most likely be unwilling to make unpopular decisions, even though they may be necessary for the good of the group. Although this type of manager may be exceptionally well liked by subordinates, the quality of his or her work will eventually suffer, and the downslide of that will be that each nursing unit will suffer, as will every subordinate manager and his or her employees. Managers must make decisions, and some of these decisions are going to be unpopular. Managers who fail to recognize this fact are placing their personal needs ahead of their responsibilities; for that, progressive discipline, up to and including termination of employment, can result and is entirely justified.

There is, of course, an opposite type of manager—the type who needs to be disliked or simply doesn't care. This individual often believes that unless he or she micromanages all subordinates, they will not do anything or what they do will be incorrect. The result of this micromanagement is that subordinates become submissive, seldom take initiative and responsibility, and refer everything upward. This is a dangerous situation, because juniors will not become proficient as long as their work is being done for them. The role of a manager is to develop the performance capabilities of his or her subordinates, and as long as the senior manager does the work, juniors will never accept their proper role or—and even more dangerous for the juniors—they will try to do the job they were hired for and run head on into the senior manager's micromanagement and disapproval. The result will be ill feeling, difficulty in cooperating, resentment, and usually disciplinary problems for the junior. Consider the following story:

> After being hired as a nurse manager for a surgical unit at a large regional hospital, I came to know my supervisor, a younger man who was an up and comer in the organization and one who was determined to have things his way; let's call him Dave.
>
> Dave felt that everything accomplished in the units that he oversaw was only done correctly when it was done his way. He personally believed it was within his area of responsibility to make even the most simple of decisions, and that it was his prerogative to tell his nurse managers where they could store supplies, and how to arrange their time schedules. Little, if anything, was left to the nurse manager to decide.
>
> What transpired was that the nurse managers, many of them seasoned, experienced managers who had been in their positions for several years, began to back away from their responsibilities with the attitude that no matter how hard they worked, it would be what Dave decided that would prevail.

To make a long and very ugly story as short as possible, it was not only Dave who ended up paying the price for the sloppy and unprofessional work that permeated the hospital; patient care suffered, each of the nurse managers under Dave had their reputations and careers damaged, and the hospital lost a major lawsuit due to poor risk management.

There are more than just a few effective and very professional ways to work alongside a senior who needs to micromanage his or her junior managers. One of the best is to attempt to ignore the senior's efforts to control and to work with the good that is almost always included in the somewhat heavy-handed directives. If the nurse manager can catch this type of senior actually doing good (and such seniors often do), the nurse manager should learn from what he or she sees, and when it is appropriate, let the senior know how much the nurse manager appreciates what the senior has done and how it helps the manager with his or her job. Also, the nurse manager should remember what it feels like to work for someone who micromanages one's every move and avoid behaving this way toward his or her own subordinates. No matter how much it hurts to continue to work alongside the micromanager, doing so is far better than the situation that will result if the nurse manager tries to confront this type of person and put a stop to the interference. If the junior's efforts to work with the senior are still unsuccessful in changing the micromanaging interference in the unit, the nurse manager may have to consider leaving the institution or at least that particular position. Remember, the nurse manager is only responsible for his or her part of the relationship with the supervisor. The nurse manager is not responsible for the senior's behavior.

GET STARTED

It is very common for a new nurse manager, and even for an experienced manager who is starting in a new position or with a new organization, to feel a little uncertain as the manager contemplates his or her relationship with a senior and the expectations that the senior manager might have for the junior manager. What can be counted on is that the senior has demonstrated his or her confidence in the new nurse manager by selecting him or her for the position. The senior manager would have not selected the new nurse manager if he or she did not believe that this individual possessed the attributes required by the position and had the capability to become successful in it.

The nurse manager should start to develop the working relationship from the first moment in the new position by discussing responsibilities with the senior manager. In these discussions, it is important that both managers come to an agreement on what role the junior is expected to fill, what his or her specific responsibilities will be, and what objectives the senior has for the unit. The new nurse manager must not wait for the senior to have the time to tell the nurse manager what he or she can and cannot do. Managers operate differently than do staff nurses; they can safely assume that they have the authority to proceed with the routine aspects of the job as defined in the organizational job description. Another assumption is that managers are hired to make decisions, implement, plan, and organize, all of which can be done without permission. It is far better for junior managers to go to their supervisors with a basic idea when they need help than to go with nothing and ask for direction. Unless they work for managers with a controlling style, junior managers will be expected to begin on their own. Nurse managers should keep in mind the old saying, "If they didn't want you to do the job or felt that you were incapable of doing it, they wouldn't have hired you." The only exception to the approach described here is a situation in which the manager has a controlling personality; generally, such an individual will tell juniors up front what they can and cannot do.

DON'T WORRY ABOUT MAKING MISTAKES

If mistakes are made, remember that managers must not under any circumstance try to hide them. The professional thing to do is to admit the mistake, accept the responsibility for it, and then use it as a learning opportunity. One of the fastest ways for a junior manager to damage the relationship with his or her senior manager is to make a mistake and hope the senior doesn't find out about it; the senior inevitably will, and when he or she does, the junior can easily lose the senior's respect and, depending on the severity of the mistake and the amount of grief the senior receives because of it, the junior may also lose his or her job. Managers should live by the following simple creed, which will never fail to help a manager achieve excellence:

*I will not lie, cheat, steal, or advance my personal career at the expense of another, nor will I tolerate the presence of those who do.**

MAKE THE DECISIONS

Junior management positions are created because senior managers have found themselves incapable of accomplishing all the work assigned to them. When this situation arises, they gather together comple-

---

*This creed was adapted from the honor code of the U.S. Military Academy at West Point.

mentary responsibilities and delegate them to the new management position. One of the responsibilities that is always delegated, along with the authority to carry it out, is that of making the decisions necessary to ensure good performance, good order, and discipline. Because this authority is always granted to new managers, managers should not be afraid to use it.

In reality, however, a large percentage of new managers do not make good use of their authority and fail to make the decisions that they were hired and empowered to make. The reasons for this failure are as diverse as the individuals who assume these new management roles, but the two primary ones are the following:

1. *They are afraid to make a mistake:* Being new creates a high degree of uncertainty, and many new managers allow this emotion to limit their performance (e.g., they don't make decisions). The reasons range from "I didn't know I could" to "I was afraid I'd look bad." The fear may be caused partly by seniors who have made it plain that they make the decisions, but for the most part, the junior manager is simply afraid of making a mistake. Most senior managers work hard to create a business atmosphere in which people can risk making decisions without fear of punishment if the decisions are erroneous, but whether they do or not, nurse managers are expected make these decisions. Not making decisions because of fear of mistakes is a major mistake in itself. And if junior managers are concerned about looking bad, let them wait until a negative incident occurs that could have been prevented by a timely decision that they did not make, and then they will understand just how grave the situation can be when a manager looks bad.

2. *They are afraid to be held accountable:* Many managers, and many very senior managers, simply won't make a decision because they believe that if they don't, they can't be held accountable. They delay the decision until someone either makes it for them or they trap their boss into making it. Either way, they feel better because they can stand up, when and if a mistake is made, and point their fingers and say, "I didn't approve that."

What managers must understand is that they are accountable for everything that occurs within their area of responsibility—even for decisions that they do not make. If a senior manager makes a decision for a junior, the junior is still responsible for the successful implementation of that decision, and if it fails, the junior is still going to be held accountable.

Accountability is a basic part of management, and there is no way that any manager can escape it. Therefore, it is better to think through a challenge and come up with a decision that is based on fact, the needs of the unit, and the best interests of the organization than it is to avoid an issue or wait until someone who might be less capable makes it.

Very likely the extent of new nurse managers' responsibilities and authority will not become completely clear until they have occupied the new position for an extended period. Although many novice managers are somewhat anxious about this temporary ambiguity, they should never allow it to interfere with the discharge of their duties. In time, and possibly as a result of many collaborative decisions and through a spirit of cooperation, many of the uncertainties will be resolved.

New nurse managers need to accept the fact that almost all senior managers have strengths and limitations. All managers must work with the individuals that they are responsible to and for, so that they can build on each other's strengths and compensate for each other's weaknesses. Developing this mutually supportive relationship is critical to the success of the organization's management team and will help all of the managers improve their effectiveness. All managers should continually try to identify what their associate managers can do well and where they need help. This identification of strengths and weaknesses can be made easy by asking questions such as the following: What can my supervisor do well? What can I do well that can help my senior improve? What does my senior need to know to use my strengths? What can my senior do to offset my weaknesses?

Another absolute certainty is that, regardless of the specific job, juniors will need their senior managers' help and support to do it well. Without supportive senior managers guiding, facilitating, and assisting in their growth, junior managers will never be as proficient at accomplishing their assigned tasks as they must be to be recognized as professionals. Junior managers, to safeguard their own professionalism, must aggressively support the success of their seniors.

General Rules for Working with Senior Managers

Although no sure methods are available that will cover every possible type of nurse manager–senior manager relationship, there are a few general principles that can help all junior managers work more effectively with their seniors. If nurse managers train themselves to use these principles in the daily discharge of their responsibilities, they will improve the part of the relationship they have control over, and this by itself is usually enough to enhance the overall relationship.

Keep in mind that being a part of management at any level is like belonging to a special club that has a limited membership. If the club is to be successful, each member must support the others. Support here does not mean blind obedience or abject compliance but rather working together for the common good. The ancient Chinese used a phrase that is loosely rendered in English as *gung ho,* or "come together." That phrase should describe the individual manager's efforts and the efforts of every other member of the management team. That end can be furthered when every member of the management team accomplishes the objectives outlined in the following sections.

BE PROFESSIONAL

Remember that junior managers are not responsible for their senior managers' conduct, but they are responsible for their own. Regardless of what one's superior says or does, the best way to handle the situation, no matter how grave, is to maintain one's individual composure and personal presence.

Managers should never, under any circumstances, lose control of their tempers or argue with their seniors in the presence of others. They should take whatever steps are necessary to prevent any embarrassment to their seniors and should never ridicule their seniors—not to their faces, in front of others, or out of their presence. Not ever! Using good manners and showing common sense demonstrates professionalism, and when juniors do so, even if their seniors do not, at least the junior managers have done their part.

TAKE TIME TO PRAISE POSITIVE BEHAVIOR

It is a very common observation in management that junior personnel rarely take the time to recognize their seniors' efforts or simply to say "Thank you." Managers, regardless of their level of authority, are first and foremost human, with all the frailties that implies. Every person, regardless of position, needs to hear kind words and to have his or her work recognized by others. When it is prudent, when it can be done honestly and without being perceived as false praise, and when it is warranted, a few words such as, "I appreciate your help," or simply, "Thank you," can make a world of difference in the quality of the relationship that can be built with senior managers.

The opposite also applies. Professional managers do not praise their seniors when it is not warranted. This unsavory conduct is a negative action employed only by the unskilled, unprofessional, and unworthy. It should be considered beneath any professional to toady to his or her senior. If a junior manager attempts

this and his or her senior is a high-quality, professional manager, the junior will find the effort to have been counterproductive, to say the least. Truly professional managers despise subordinates who make a continual effort to ingratiate themselves. Such conduct is not becoming to a professional and should never be attempted.

EXERCISE PATIENCE

Very few managers are without some shortcomings. Some may become upset easily, others may be too directive in their manner, and still others can disappoint. However, it is not the job of junior managers to point out the challenges. As a matter of fact, it is best that junior managers ignore negative behavior in their seniors unless it interferes with the operation of the organization, limits their ability to successfully accomplish their mission, endangers a member of the staff, or serves to reduce the quality of patient care. For instance, if the supervisor shows up during a shift intoxicated, it would be both unsafe and unprofessional to ignore the potential danger of this behavior. The junior's first responsibility is to the patients, the unit, and the organization, and although loyalty to a senior is very important, it does not approach the importance of patient safety or the reduction of the risk faced by the organization due to such conduct. In fact, reporting the incident should be the only thought a professional has, for the good of the organization and for the welfare of the intoxicated senior manager. If the senior has a substance-abuse problem, this act of intervention may save a career and possibly a life.

If the negative acts do not endanger the patients or place the organization in a compromised position, however, it might be wise to ignore as much of the conduct as possible. What seniors do is their responsibility, and if they demonstrate any negative behavior, it most likely is not intended as a personal attack. Senior managers generally make an effort to treat all of their subordinates in a similar manner, and although their actions may be personally unsavory, this may not be a fight worth taking on directly. However, no one is required to accept behavior from a senior that is degrading, dehumanizing, or unprofessional. The fact that the conduct may have been the senior's mode of operation through a hundred different junior managers does not make it right. Every manager is entitled to be treated with respect. The time when a senior manager could get away with treating a junior in a derogatory manner simply because he or she treated everyone that way or made that method his or her hallmark has long since ended. Therefore, it is of no consequence that a senior may have treated a predecessor the same way; if the conduct exhibited toward the nurse manager is considered by the nurse manager to be derogatory, then it should not be condoned.

If such a situation exists, however, it needs to be handled quietly, professionally, and with the utmost decorum. Any challenge to a senior can and frequently will be considered an assault on the senior's authority. If the senior's behavior is unprofessional, degrading, or otherwise interferes with the junior manager's ability to manage the unit and the junior decides it is serious enough to confront the senior, then he or she should do so. But before taking this step, the junior should prepare for the possible consequences of his or her action. If the junior experiences retribution, then he or she might want to talk with the human resources manager or, if that is ineffective, seek help from the union or from the federal labor board. No one has to suffer abuse, and no manager, regardless of the level of authority, has the right to misuse his or her station or fail to comply with state and federal labor law.

LEARN HOW TO HANDLE CONFLICT CONSTRUCTIVELY

The nursing environment is a demanding one, and conflicts do arise. That is a fact of life in the profession, but it does not excuse individual conduct. If a conflict does occur, every manager has an obligation to make a wise decision as to how to handle it. Two approaches are the following:

1. *Take the path of least resistance:* The junior manager might employ the "Yes, boss, anything you say" approach. This is a servile and condescending way of interacting with a senior, however. Although it may be expedient, it is highly unprofessional and is not likely to help gain the senior's respect. It also won't ensure that what is best for the unit is accomplished, and that can cost the junior manager the respect of his or her staff.

   Although there are certainly times when obedience to a senior's desire is necessary, managers have been given the privilege of exception. That is, managers have the right to question their seniors as long as the manner in which they conduct themselves is professional and in keeping with the standards of conduct set by the organization, and their reason for doing so is the betterment of the whole. Confrontation without sufficient reason or justification is foolhardy, but abject compliance is unprofessional.

2. *Be objective:* All managers must, from time to time, deal with those who are perennially negative. These individuals find fault with everything and rarely view things in an unemotional way. Managers have the responsibility to be objective,

not personal; open minded, not self-seeking; and positive, not negative. The best way to ensure that juniors and seniors develop and maintain a healthy and constructive relationship is for both to maintain their objectivity during differences of opinion.

AVOID ARGUMENTS

Management is carried out most efficiently when the managers involved in it avoid conflict with one another. This means that each manager involved in a given situation must work to identify common ground on which all parties can agree. No junior manager will ever win an argument with a senior; at least not totally. Perhaps the junior will win a few battles, but the junior will ultimately pay a price for his or her negative and confrontational manner. Although there will certainly be situations in which differences of opinion will arise, these should never be allowed to degenerate into arguments. It may even be healthy to disagree, but it is never in the best interest of anyone to openly argue a position. Instead, the junior should seek places where a compromise can be made and determine what must be done to allow the junior to aggressively support the senior's position. More will definitely be gained if juniors learn how to disagree without arguing. Disagreements provide opportunities for drawing on assertiveness, communication, and negotiation skills without allowing juniors to fall into the negative conduct of arguing with their seniors, which is always debasing and unprofessional. Smart nurse managers always concern themselves with the senior's viewpoint, even if they themselves don't share it. They use caution when airing any form of disagreement and carefully consider what can be gained and what might be lost by expressing an opposing view.

The junior manager's purpose is to identify efficient and cost-effective means of increasing performance, and because arguing is, at best, a negative exercise, it should not be worth anyone's time. Instead, the junior manager should focus on gentle persuasion and quiet facilitation (i.e., the use of constructive reasoning to identify common ground and effective means of allowing the right thing to be done). It is the junior manager's job to ensure that the performance unit, the senior manager, and the organization will be better off as a result of his or her actions, and the manager must be able to do this without creating dissension.

Complaining and whining about what isn't "fair" is never the conduct expected of managers. Instead, managers should carefully and respectfully talk the situation out in a manner that points out common ground and shared beliefs. Managers should conduct themselves dispassionately and not use the opportunity for compromise as a chance to relieve their tensions and frustration over the problem. If they sense that they need to tell someone about the issue, they should seek out a friend or confidante whom they can trust to provide constructive criticism—not a yes-man but a source of truth and integrity. When they feel better, they can talk with their senior managers and do so with a perspective that they might not otherwise have had.

KEEP THE SENIOR MANAGER INFORMED

One of the things universally disliked in the field of management is the unwarranted surprise. This is what occurs when a senior is reprimanded for something that an immediate junior knew about but chose not to tell the senior. A management position carries with it the obligation to keep the immediate senior informed of what transpires in the junior's area of concern, both the good and the bad—*especially the bad*. Although it is very common for novice managers to feel conflict about following this principle, it is absolutely imperative that they make every effort to do so.

The biggest reason for this conflict is the division of loyalty that a mistake produces. New managers who know about an error are torn between maintaining the confidence of their staffs and fulfilling their obligation to keep their supervisors informed. The situation can be sensitive, and although no one is advocating that managers act as informants for their supervisors, they must represent their seniors' best interests. Most situations of this nature do not involve confidential information, and therefore reporting on them is part of the responsibility that junior managers are trusted to bear. All nurse managers should strive to maintain this trust by keeping their supervisors informed in the following three ways.

1. *Provide feedback on decisions:* It is the responsibility of all managers to supply feedback to their immediate seniors regarding any problems that may result from their supervisors' decisions. They have a fundamental duty to provide a best estimate of both positive and negative outcomes. Managers are obligated to try to negotiate a settlement if they disagree with their seniors' ideas, but if a senior makes a decision against a junior's recommendation, the junior is obligated to implement and support it.

2. *Provide credible information:* Nurse managers are obligated to provide their seniors with the unbiased facts the latter require to make quality decisions. Supervisors need to know what occurs within each of their individual units, and it is the junior managers' responsibility to provide the necessary information. Nurse managers give their seniors inside information about what will be effective at the staff level. This is important input that must be provided to higher managers if they are to develop policies based on reality.

3. *Provide feedback on problems:* Nurse managers are also obligated to objectively inform their immediate seniors when problems occur in their nursing units. They must never let their supervisors be surprised by events in their units, because it is the supervisors who are ultimately responsible for what happens in the units. This information flow is needed so that problems can be resolved as quickly as possible. Many times the proper consultation with senior managers can prevent a small problem from becoming a major crisis, and engaging in such consultation is the responsibility of all managers. If a crisis should occur, it must be handled at once and at the lowest possible management level; however, even if the nurse manager is able to remedy the situation, he or she still has an obligation to inform the immediate supervisor.

There is such a thing as keeping senior managers too informed, however. It is not senior managers' responsibility to conduct the affairs of individual nursing units, and because they have so many responsibilities of their own, they do not need to know every detail of a unit's work. This means that nurse managers should take care of all things within the boundaries of their decision-making authority. In short, all nurse managers should strive to reach a level of proficiency that allows them to make the routine day-to-day decisions.

ADMIT MISTAKES

Being a manager does not endow that person with superhuman powers or make the person able to leap tall buildings in a single bound. In fact, being a manager doesn't really change a person's basic composition one bit; the individual is and remains a fallible human being who makes mistakes. What does change is the fact that a manager must accept full responsibility for his or her actions, without the expectation of support from a senior, especially when those actions result in a mistake. Although it may be human to make a mistake, it is extremely unprofessional to try to conceal it. Managers must be accountable for their mistakes, and if they try to conceal them (an unforgivable error in judgment) or attempt to hide their involvement by focusing the blame on another (a truly despicable act), then they should no longer hold a management position.

Although there will always be a natural tendency for any manager to be embarrassed by a personal mistake, no one should believe that it is wrong to make one. The only thing that is wrong about a mistake is failing to learn from it. If, instead of trying to cover up an error, a nurse manager accepts the responsibility for that error, the nurse manager is likely to gain far more respect from his or her staff and senior manager. Most people do not expect a manager to be superhuman; therefore, little surprise will be shown when managers make the occasional error.

When managers do err, they should try to turn the error into an educational opportunity by asking themselves what they have learned and how they could have done things differently to avoid the error, and then sharing their answers with their staffs and supervisors. This example of selflessness will encourage others to behave similarly and can earn a great deal of respect from others.

MAINTAIN CREDIBILITY

Admitting one's errors is a good place to start to win the respect and trust of others. Another thing that can be done is to work hard to maintain one's credibility. Managers maintain credibility by delivering on promises and maintaining schedules. This means that if managers say they are going to do something, they do it. If they make an appointment, they don't show up late. If they make a commitment, they make sure that they give themselves time enough to deliver on it. All managers will have times when they are asked to bite off more than they can chew, but when that happens they should make an earnest effort to negotiate delivery times that provide them with sufficient time to succeed. If they should start to fall behind, they shouldn't be afraid to renegotiate. If it appears that a commitment might be missed or a schedule delayed, everyone concerned should be informed quickly and as far in advance as possible.

QUIETLY PUBLICIZE ACCOMPLISHMENTS

Doing a good job is good enough only if two things pertain: (1) better is not expected, and (2) someone knows what has been accomplished. It sounds almost too simple to be worth mentioning, yet this is one of the cardinal rules of management: Managers must make people aware of their units' and their own personal accomplishments, and they must be careful how they do it. Although no one likes a braggart, no one will promote a totally humble manager. Doing a good job, even an exceptional one, is not good enough if no one knows this to be so. Guiding a unit to exceed expectations will earn no honor if senior managers don't know about it. Therefore, nurse managers must be the number one champions for their units and must make it part of their job to inform the proper people of their units' accomplishments.

However, and this is a huge however, they absolutely must not allow themselves to appear as braggarts or self-serving individuals while they are showcasing achievements. Good nurse managers know how to make their units' achievements visible, but do so in a subtle and inconspicuous manner. The best way for a nurse manager to do this is to carefully explain the circumstances surrounding the success and let the senior manager draw his or her own conclusions. The nurse manager can simply forward all correspondence received from patients or their families to the senior for review (the good and the bad). Another way is to make the item a part of the agenda for the next meeting with the senior and then discuss it in low tones and as humbly as possible. The key is for managers not to appear as if they are tooting their own horns.

STUDY THE SUPERVISOR'S STYLE

The more a junior manager can learn about the senior manager's style of performance, the greater the junior's opportunity to improve the overall relationship, because little is as destructive to the development of a good relationship as are incongruent work styles. Real misunderstandings can occur when individual work styles are opposed (e.g., an organized, formal style vs. an intuitive, informal one; a task-oriented style vs. a relationship-oriented one; written language preference vs. spoken language preference; group activity preference vs. individual activity preference).

One of the most frequent challenges occurs when one manager is task oriented and the other is relationship oriented. In clinical nursing, a task orientation (i.e., feeling that productivity is measured in terms of accomplishments and results) leads to high esteem for technical skill in patient care tasks; in nursing management, such an orientation leads to high regard for the technical aspects of the job, such as completing reports on time. The relationship-oriented individual feels that interpersonal interactions and abilities are most important (e.g., the ability to intervene effectively in a staff conflict). Most people have a style that is a combination of these orientations but exhibit a preference for one or the other.

If the senior is task oriented and the junior is relationship oriented, their relationship may become very strained and the situation may prove difficult, because it is unlikely that either will fulfill the other's expectations. On the other hand, once both managers recognize this disparity and accept it as a difference in work styles and not a personality conflict, they can turn it into an advantage for both. Juniors can use their strengths to help their seniors make up for the latter's weaknesses and vice versa. If the junior is task oriented and the supervisor is relationship oriented, they can use that information to decide jointly how to divide some overlapping tasks in their respective workloads, and the performance of both will be enhanced. In effect, by working closely, both will be creating a win-win situation.

DON'T IRRITATE THE SENIOR MANAGER

Every nurse manager must learn how to work with the personalities and individual characteristics of his or her senior managers and especially of the immediate senior. Time and energy will not be wasted if the junior manager uses them wisely in an earnest attempt to learn what is necessary to avoid irritating the senior. One might say that the smart thing to do would be to avoid the senior manager's known triggers, but this is not practical because, over an extended relationship, the junior manager will find it almost impossible to avoid tripping over some emotion-laced triggers. But the junior manager can learn to identify what the triggers are; that is, what upsets the senior manager the most. The emotions of people, including senior managers, can be triggered by any number of things, from the use of specific words, to special noises, to unique smells. Just about anything can act as a trigger. The junior manager must learn what these triggers are and avoid them.

If a junior manager does pull the senior's trigger, inadvertently or otherwise, it is almost guaranteed that the discussion with the senior afterward will be negative. Taking the time to learn what it is that upsets the boss is good business, and avoiding these things is important to the junior manager's well-being. Anyone can learn what these things are by being sensitive to other people's verbal and nonverbal communication. The junior manager should take the time to really listen and observe when interacting with his or her seniors and with others. If the junior keeps his or her eyes open and mouth shut, the junior will be surprised what can be learned.

Being sensitive to the senior's triggers, however, should not be construed as giving the junior manager license to avoid carrying information to the senior manager because it might be unpleasant and trigger an undesired response. Intelligent management of self and one's actions with one's senior managers is good business; avoiding issues because they are unpleasant is unprofessional.

DON'T OVERSTAY A WELCOME

The junior manager should not misuse the privilege of the senior's time. Instead, when having an audience with the senior, the junior should avoid lengthy dialogues by summarizing information and emphasizing the critical points. The senior needs to be kept informed but not overwhelmed with the intricacies of an issue; details are the junior's job. When discussing an issue, the junior should be sure that everything necessary has been covered and then emphasize any part of the information that should be left to the senior for action or response. The junior should ask himself or herself, "What does my supervisor need to know to make a decision, to report to his or her superior, to monitor change across units, or to intervene appropriately?" There is a fine line between keeping the senior informed and wasting the senior's time.

Influencing Senior Managers Positively

Most of the information found in textbooks and how-to manuals on the subject of positively influencing another person focuses on the proper techniques for influencing the actions of those individuals for whom one is responsible, not of one's senior managers. In fact, only very rarely is a book written or a course of instruction offered in how to influence one's seniors. But an ability on the part of juniors to persuade and facilitate the actions of their senior managers so that they desire to assist the juniors in accomplishing their assigned responsibilities is absolutely essential. As junior managers, all nurse managers will need to approach their immediate supervisors to ask for support, influence, or approval in dealing with a myriad of different issues. Perhaps they will require their seniors' advice in handling a unique or particularly difficult personnel problem or a union issue. They might need their supervisors' support for the purchase of equipment or supplies, the cost of which exceeds their authorization level. The issue could be almost anything from a request to increase the number of full-time equivalent positions in the unit to help in gathering support for creating a change in procedure or policy.

The issue on which support is required doesn't really matter. What does matter is how the junior manager handles such things as timing the request, providing explanation, and overcoming objections. Even the correct choice of form and the format used in the cover letter are important when preparing to make a request. Whatever the need, the junior manager's chances of influencing a senior in a positive manner will be greatly enhanced if the junior follows the suggestions outlined in the following sections.

CONSIDER THE TIMING

Timing is an absolutely critical issue. The junior manager should carefully select a time that does not interfere with the senior's scheduled tasks (i.e., a time when the supervisor is not overwhelmed by his or her own responsibilities and has a few minutes to spare).

Calling ahead for an appointment will help the senior arrange his or her time so that interruptions will not occur, and that alone will improve the senior's receptivity and frame the mind to listen positively to any presented idea.

PROVIDE JUSTIFICATION

What is the best reason for asking a senior to support the need? The junior manager should be prepared to present the justification for the need concisely and make sure it includes both what benefits will accrue if the request is approved and what is expected to happen if it is disapproved. The recommendation should be based on the facts, and any form of emotion should be avoided. The junior should be prepared to answer questions about the request in a clear and articulate manner. Sound justification answers questions such as the following:

- Why should the senior manager accept the proposal?
- What are the short- and long-term advantages?
- Does the request involve budgetary expenditures? If so, was the item budgeted for? Cost effectiveness is the single most persuasive argument; it should be used to advantage.
- What will the consequences be if this proposed idea is not accepted?
- How will the unit, the division, and the organization be enhanced if the request is approved?
- How does the request affect morale, turnover, or absenteeism? This portion of any justification is critical, because turnover and absenteeism are major expense categories for the organization. If the request can reduce these numbers, the likelihood of approval will be increased.
- How long will it take before promised benefits are realized?

PRESENT THE SENIOR MANAGER'S OBJECTIONS

The manager should think about what the possible objections to the proposal might be and why they might be held. When these objections are understood, it is easy to develop justifications that address each one and thereby to offer the senior a means to provide the approval. Good managers think through problems and requests thoroughly before they present them. They view them from every possible angle and consider many different ways to approach the subject. After they have completed this process, they assign priorities to the different objections and offer solutions.

Ideas, requests, and justifications should be presented in the manner that the organization prescribes or that the senior prefers. This could mean making a verbal request, completing a prescribed form, or submitting a formal written request. In most cases, a combination of these different methods will be used. If the idea or request is presented verbally, the presenter should follow up the initial meeting with a written summary that highlights the decisions that were made and that the approval that was given. Senior managers are very busy people, and they often forget about individual requests. If they have the junior's memo on file when a question is raised, they are far more likely to continue to provide support.

What happens if a senior manager tells a junior no? Regardless of how well the junior prepares, how justified the request is, or how much the organization can benefit from approval, there is always the chance that a request will be denied. Preparation reduces the possibility of refusal, but it does not eliminate it. Therefore, every nurse manager needs to recognize that the senior's answer may be no and to understand what to do if this happens.

EVALUATE THE OBJECTIONS

If the senior denies a request, the junior should think through the objections and carefully evaluate the reasons that were given for the refusal. If no reasons are cited, then the junior should carefully and professionally ask for them. The request should be phrased as an opportunity to learn. "Can you help me understand why the request was denied?" sounds better than "Why did you reject this?" The junior should seek information and never imply disapproval of the request denial or infer an emotional belief in lack of intelligence on the part of the senior. Instead, the junior should ask himself or herself the following four questions:

1. What new information was received?
2. Are there ways the request can be renegotiated?
3. What information is necessary to overcome the objections?
4. Will the supervisor be open to negotiation or resubmittal of the request?

Once the junior manager has the answers to these questions, the junior should carefully approach the senior again with the new data. If the proposal was a high enough priority for the junior to submit it originally, it should be a high enough priority for the junior to submit it again and defend the decision to do so. Many times an initial no is not a permanent denial but a request for additional information and justification. Once that information is obtained, the junior should approach the subject again. The junior should keep an open mind, listen to objections, and make every attempt to respond to the objections with positive justification. The junior manager should never argue with the supervisor or openly proclaim displeasure; that type of reaction will eliminate any future opportunity to resurrect the request. The junior must be professional and learn to use the word *no* to his or her advantage.

Addressing Problems with Senior Managers

There is an expression in business, "Many senior managers have blood on the floor in front of their desks." The saying may be indelicate, but it is figuratively true, and most of the blood that was shed in front of those desks got there because junior managers didn't know how to properly present problems to their bosses. The inability of many junior managers to overcome their fear of reprisal is, by far, a greater cause of this bloodletting than the desire of senior managers to "kill the messenger." Although negative-minded senior managers who *will* kill the bearer of bad tidings certainly exist, they are actually very few in number. Most senior managers want bad news brought to them and would rather hear it from one of their junior managers than be surprised by their own superiors.

The problem is that most juniors don't know how to approach their seniors with bad news and have a very limited understanding of how to avoid verbal barriers. Learning to do so begins with understanding that good senior managers want to help and need to know when something is wrong. In fact, truly professional managers expect their subordinates to bring them bad news. They know that presenting a problem is the first step in getting it rectified. Although some senior managers do demonstrate some behaviors that are ineffective for conveying this message, almost to a person they understand the gravity of problem resolution.

Some methods of approaching a senior with a problem are better than others, and some key behaviors in the process can be identified. These behaviors are designed to facilitate the resolution of problems and, if performed correctly, can significantly reduce the likelihood of retribution. If junior managers abide by the following guidelines, their ability to address negative issues in a positive manner will be greatly enhanced:

State a desire to talk about a work-related problem: The junior manager should not burst into the supervisor's office and blurt this out but rather casually suggest that a problem exists that needs to be addressed. The junior should be firm, polite, and articulate. None of the negatives should be swept under the carpet.

Set a time for discussion: If necessary, the junior should make an appointment to meet with the senior; the junior should let the senior know the level of urgency of the problem (critical, minor, etc.) and estimate the amount of time that will be needed. If the time the junior suggests is not convenient, the junior should ask when and where he or she can meet with the senior.

Address the problem: The junior must explain how the problem is affecting the operation of the unit and provide a best estimate of what its potential consequences are.

Listen: The junior should let the senior restate the problem and make any changes to what is said until both parties are confident that the senior clearly understands what is being presented.

Reaffirm commitment: The junior should never tell the senior that he or she is ready to help. The senior already knows that the junior will assist if the senior desires. After all, it is the junior's problem. What a junior manager can do is reassure the senior of the junior's commitment to the resolution of the issue and state a willingness to cooperate in any solution the senior might offer.

Confirm understanding: The junior must make sure that the supervisor's suggestions and the steps that must be taken to implement them are understood. It is a good idea for the junior to paraphrase them to make sure the supervisor knows what level of understanding is present.

State alternatives: If requested, the junior should state a preferred solution. But if the supervisor overrules this idea and offers an alternative, the junior must be prepared to carry out the senior's desires in a positive and constructive manner.

Agree: The junior should make sure that both the junior and the senior agree on the steps each will take to solve the problem.

Determine follow-up: The junior should ask whether there is a need to follow up on the resolution or status of the problem. If so, specific follow-up date(s) should be planned and recorded. How each person can cooperate and how the two might verify each other's success should be discussed.

WORKING WITH PHYSICIANS

Roots of the Conflict

The conflict that historically has existed between nurses and physicians is related to the following four factors:

1. *Level of education:* Physicians have more education, and this has traditionally been taken to mean that they possess more knowledge regarding diagnosis and patient treatment. This fact

alone has placed the physician ahead of the nurse in the line of authority. In today's society, status is closely correlated with level of education, and physicians have completed considerably more years of education at entry to practice that have nurses. Moreover, the diversity of nurses' educational preparation and concomitant skills baffles both physicians and consumers. Although many people remain opposed to a baccalaureate requirement for entry into nursing practice, increased educational requirements for entry afford any profession higher status. The status of the nursing profession will increase if additional education requirements are imposed for the professional.

2. *Gender:* Traditionally, the vast majority of nurses have been female and most physicians have been male in societies that have espoused male dominance and female subservience. In many heavily industrialized nations, attitudes have changed regarding the automatic subservience of women to men, but much of the success women have had in these countries has increased the conflict between nurse and physician.[3,4] Today, in spite of the changes in legal standing and state and federal laws prohibiting gender-based bias, it is still relatively easy see the effects of gender in many of the relationships that exist between doctors and nurses.

3. *Fear of error:* Typically, physicians fear making an error that could cost a patient his or her life. This fear often manifests itself in physicians' assumption of a self-proclaimed role of unlimited authority. By setting themselves up as the ultimate authority and the only competent source of medical opinion, physicians reduce their anxiety, either conscious or unconscious, over the responsibility they bear in making critical medical decisions that can affect patients' survival. This self-concept of superiority is nurtured throughout the medical education process as the student-intern-resident learns to adapt to the demands of making life-or-death decisions.

4. *Differences in practice:* The obvious differences between the practice of nursing and medical practice also have a negative influence on the relationship between physicians and nurses. Whereas physicians generally have a long-term (possibly lifetime) relationship with their patients and deal with each patient individually, hospital-based nurses have several patients at a time and usually for only a relatively short period. In addition, nurses are concerned with the functioning of their area of responsibility (team, unit, floor) and the way it affects all patient care in the area. Physicians usually have private practices that are their primary concern, and hospital care of their patients is only one component of these practices. Therefore, the focus of care and the structure of work differ greatly in the two groups, although their responsibilities overlap. The significant differences in how the members of each group view themselves and their relationship with patients provide a fertile ground for conflict.

If the career development of physicians is compared with that of nurses, it will be seen that nurses traditionally have been rewarded primarily for obedience, courtesy, and competent task performance and to a far lesser degree for independent thinking or creativity. In many areas, nurses tend to come from lower socioeconomic classes than do physicians. In these environments, male dominance is generally accepted, and that acceptance among nurses encourages dominant behavior in physicians.

Nurse managers should consider adopting the following suggestions in developing their relationships with the physicians with whom they come in contact:

Act as the physician's partner: Both the nurse and the physician are key players on the healthcare team and they share a common goal: the welfare of the patient. The level of the relationship will vary from contact to contact, but there is no reason for a nurse to feel subservient to or less capable than a physician.

Focus on the goal: What is to be accomplished or the problem to be solved should be the primary motivation for both parties. Personality is never more important than patient welfare; therefore, personal differences should not be a factor in establishing good relationships with physicians.

Keep the patient's welfare as the primary focus: If both parties focus on providing quality health care, then very few doctors will fault nurses. Doctors worry that their patients will not receive quality care; if nurse managers develop a reputation for ensuring quality care, the doctors who work with their units will respect their abilities.

Establish clear roles and responsibilities: Managers should ensure that physicians and staff understand what their individual roles are and what duties each will discharge. If managers keep their focus on doing their job well, there will be little time for conflict.

Know the facts: Nurse managers should make sure that they approach physicians with facts, not beliefs. Physicians are trained to be specific, rational, and motivated by facts. They consider feelings and emotions to be lower-level responses. Physicians, or at least most of them, actually are trained to disregard emotion and to focus on facts. For that reason, if for no other, managers should respect their need for facts over feelings.

Respect the person: Physicians are people first, regardless of what they might believe, and they are subject to the same failings as everyone else. An old joke asks the question, "What is the difference between a doctor and God?" The response is, "God doesn't think he's a doctor." This joke is absolute nonsense, but it does indicate some of the strong beliefs nurses hold when it comes to physicians. If managers are willing to put forth a little effort to get to know physicians as people, their effort will not go unrewarded.

Provide the example: Managers' staffs will treat physicians exactly the way their managers do. Subordinates emulate the example set by their managers, and because good order and harmony are part of nurse managers' responsibilities, it is they who must present the desired model of behavior. If nurse managers treat doctors with respect, so will their staffs.

Don't be a doormat: Nurse managers are significant professionals in their own right, and none of them should be less capable in his or her field than doctors are in theirs. Professionals regard each other with respect and expect to have that respect returned. If a physician does not demonstrate professional behavior, the nurse manager should talk with him or her and explain the manager's feelings in a polite but firm manner. Being a physician does not give anyone the right to be rude, obnoxious, overbearing, or unprofessional. The nursing unit is the nurse manager's domain, and he or she establishes the ground rules. If a physician doesn't like the manager's standards of conduct, let the physician go to senior management and complain that a nurse manager asked the physician to be professional and conduct himself or herself in a positive and meaningful way.

Implications for the Nurse Manager

Nurse managers are the keys to establishing positive and professional relationships with the physicians who use the services provided by their nursing units. Through frequent contact with physicians, professional nurse managers can create environments in their units that promote professional interaction between physicians and nurses and that keep the focus of the entire medical staff on delivering quality care to the patients. How do nurse managers proceed in developing excellent relations with doctors? As before, the methods will be almost as unique as the

individual nursing unit and the nurses and doctors who work there, but the broad approaches described in the following sections can serve as a starting point.

ENCOURAGE INTERACTION

Nurse managers should encourage interaction between physicians and the staff nurses in the unit, both formally and informally. Perceived differences between groups of people are reduced when there is increased contact between the individual members of the groups. One very effective way of increasing contact between nurses and physicians is to have staff nurses attend meetings when physicians are present. Institution-wide committees whose decisions will affect patient care should include both physicians and nurses, and if they do not, nurse managers should request the inclusion of nurses.

A 1985 study of medical students[4] showed that they perceived nurses as performing work with which the students were unfamiliar. Because they did not have a comprehensive understanding of the roles nurses play, most medical students envisioned what they felt were logical roles and duties for nurses, and when the students were asked to perform patient care tasks that they believed to be within the realm of a nurse's responsibility, they became resentful. Medical students, in general, believed that nurses' work was less important than physicians' and therefore that nurses did not, in general, deserve equal respect. The research showed that, at best, the perception was that nurses and physicians worked in parallel to each other with only necessary contact and little coordinated effort. When the medical students were forced to work alongside nurses as part of their training, however, they discovered how very similar their roles actually were. Questioned later, the students were able to depict the nurse's role far more accurately and positively. This study seemed to suggest the importance of improving the opportunity for nurses and physicians (and student nurses and medical students) to interact early in their careers so that a positive relationship between the two professions can be developed.

PROMOTE JOINT INVOLVEMENT

Health care in an organizational setting is extremely complex and requires that individuals in a variety of professional specialties act interdependently. In fact, maintenance of relationships among medical professionals is normal behavior throughout the healthcare industry today, if for no other reason than that the accountability for patient welfare is shared. Today's patients believe that everyone involved in delivering patient care is accountable for the quality of the service they receive. This belief is reflected in the significant increase in malpractice suits in the last two decades that include all healthcare participants as defendants.

It is recommended that nurse managers encourage the involvement of their staffs with the physicians who use their services in as many ways as possible, particularly in the problem-solving and decision-making aspects of patient care. Nurse managers must watch for any opportunity to promote this professional alliance, both formally, as in appointment of nurses to collaborative committees, and informally, as by suggestions to either the physician or the nurse that he or she might want to discuss an aspect of a given patient's care with the other.

BE A GOOD ROLE MODEL

As stated earlier, employees emulate their supervisors and so will those professionals with whom a manager interacts. Nurse managers need to become positive role models for their staffs. When individual staff members see their nurse managers collaborating positively with physicians, they will tend to do so as well. If nurse managers demonstrate an attitude of cooperation and collaboration rather than being adversarial and adopting the traditional "we" versus "they" attitude, they will encourage a similar response in staff members.

ACT AS A MEDIATOR

Conflicts will occur, and when they do, the focus should be on preventing them from getting out of control. One of the best ways to accomplish this is for nurse managers to ensure that they maintain objectivity. Sometimes disagreements need a dispassionate person to serve as a referee and mediate the discussion. What is normal in disagreements is that one party is a little bit right and the other is a little bit wrong, but neither is totally either. If the nurse manager jumps to the defense of the staff, the manager may alienate the physician and damage an important relationship. Therefore, the nurse manager should keep himself or herself removed from the emotional undercurrents and focus on seeking a solution.

It is extremely important that nurse managers remember their responsibility to their staffs as they set about to improve collaboration between physicians and nurses. They must perform their fundamental role and protect their staffs from unwarranted harassment and maltreatment. Staff members cannot protect themselves from the onslaught of a determined and upset physician; that is the role of the nurse manager. If nurse managers fail to step up and offer that protection, they risk losing the support of their staffs. Protecting staff does not mean forgiving errors. It means establishing rules for conduct and enforcing

them without prejudice. Nurse managers should never allow a physician to abuse a member of their staffs, just as they should not allow a staff member to belittle, degrade, or defame a physician. Such conduct by either party should be considered reprehensible and should not be tolerated. Establishing and enforcing standards of conduct is critical for nurse managers' success with their staffs and in their organizations.

SUMMARY

- Healthcare institutions have organizational authority structures designed to carry out organizational goals. These structures may be centralized or decentralized depending on the institution's philosophy of control and responsibility.

- The nurse manager is part of the management team, with staff members reporting to the nurse manager and the nurse manager, in turn, reporting to a senior manager.

- An informal as well as a formal structure exists in all organizations; the informal structure is generally considered to exert a great deal of power.

- Roles in organizations define the parameters of a job, remain constant regardless of who occupies the role, and help maintain stability in the organization.

- Nurse managers are responsible for participating actively in the relationship with their senior managers.

- A nurse manager's negative reaction to authority, low self-esteem, and unrealistic expectations of the supervisor may interfere with the development of a positive, growth-enhancing relationship between the nurse manager and his or her superior.

- Characteristics of the supervisor, such as a desire to be needed, liked, or disliked, can interfere with the relationship between the supervisor and nurse manager. The nurse manager can deal constructively with these problems by accepting the senior's need and suggesting changes.

- Basic principles for working with seniors include being courteous, praising positive actions, learning how to handle conflict constructively, keeping the supervisor informed, admitting one's mistakes, publicizing one's accomplishments, and adjusting to the supervisor's work style.

- Nurse managers need to learn how to influence their seniors when presenting new ideas and how to take problems to their seniors.

- Socialization, stereotyping, and the nature of each group's professional work responsibilities account for much of the strain that exists in the relationships between physicians and nurses.

■ Nurse managers can serve as role models exemplifying positive interactions with physicians and can assist their staffs by encouraging interactions in which the focus is on patients and their problems.

FINAL THOUGHTS

Developing effective working relationships with members of senior management can be one of the most daunting aspects of assuming the role of nurse manager. The concept of working in conjunction with managers who, for the most part, are unapproachable by members of the professional staff is a difficult adjustment for the new nurse manager. The need to overcome the personality issues, politics, and demands of management make this difficult process even more demanding. But no matter how difficult, building effective working relationships is obligatory for the nurse manager. There is opportunity, however, because it is also to the benefit of every senior manager to establish good relationships with his or her subordinate managers. The days of the senior manager's being aloof and mysterious are over; today, the focus is on cooperation and teamwork.

THE NURSE MANAGER SPEAKS

When I assumed the role of nurse manager for Unit 6 East of a major metropolitan hospital, I did so with a great deal of trepidation. Although I had been a staff nurse in the same unit for more than 10 years, I was shocked by the degree of difference I noticed when I became a member of the management team. All of a sudden I had an enormous amount of responsibility, and most of it was new for me. However, I made an assessment of my situation and approached my immediate supervisor, and we had the first of many frank and open discussions about how we could work together to help each other become and remain successful. I found that my success was more than just important to my boss; it was essential. I was assured that if I kept my focus on achieving quality patient care and took care of my staff that I would receive all of the help my supervisor was capable of giving.

Today, I am the supervisor and share the same words of wisdom with my new nurse managers—stay focused and in step; I'll be there when you need me. Being in management doesn't mean you are alone—just part of a different team.

REFERENCES

1. Heineken J: Power: conflicting views, *J Nurs Adm* 15(11):36, 1985.
2. Hegarty C: *How to manage your boss*, Mill Valley, Calif, 1982, Whatever Publications.
3. Morgan AP, McCann JM: Nurse-physician relationships: the ongoing conflict, *Nurs Adm Q* 7(4):1, 1983.
4. Webster D: Medical students' view of the role of the nurse, *Nurs Res* 34(5):313, 1985.

SUGGESTED READINGS

American Healthcare Association: *Healthcare's agenda for healthcare reform—PR3 25M*, Kansas City, Mo, 1991, The Association.

Angelini DJ: Mentoring in the career development of hospital staff nurses, *J Prof Nurs* 11:2, 1995.

Ashley J: *Hospitals, paternalism and the role of the nurse*, New York, 1976, Teacher's College Press.

Bassman E: *Abuse in the workplace: management remedies and bottom-line impact*, Westport, Conn, 1982, Quorum Books.

Booth RZ: Power: a negative or positive force in relationships? *Nurs Adm Q* 7(4):10, 1983.

Campbell-Hider N: Updating nurses' bedside manner, *Image J Nurs Sch* 25(2):133, 1993.

Christman L: Nurse-physician communications in the hospital, *JAMA* 194(5):539, 1965.

Curtin LL: Power: the traps of trappings, *Nurs Manage* 20(6):7, 1989.

Friss L: *Strategic management of nurses*, Owings Mills, Md, 1989, AUPHA Press.

Grainger RD: Self-confidence: a feeling you can create, *Am J Nurs* 90(10):12, 1990.

Griessman BE: *The tactics of very successful people*, New York, 1994, McGraw-Hill.

Roberts SJ: Oppressed group behavior: implications for nursing, *Adv Nurs Sci* 5(4):21, 1983.

Stewart BM: An evolutionary concept analysis of mentoring in nursing, *J Prof Nurs* 12(5):311, 1996.

Developing the Superior Performance Team

LEARNING SYNOPSIS

Upon successful completion of this chapter, readers will possess a fundamental understanding of the methods that can be used to develop a superior performance team in the nursing unit, the level of effort required, and the impact such a team can have. Readers will understand the special role that the nurse manager plays in developing the superior team and the potential effect of the manager's leadership.

OBJECTIVES

1. Describe the qualities of teamwork and leadership
2. Identify reasons that a growing small organization should depend on teams
3. Describe seven steps that can be used to develop a team in a growing organization
4. Identify critical issues and procedures to use when a team won't obey instruction or follow the leader

The concept of leadership as promoting teamwork and building success through consensus management is substantially different from the concept of leadership that was taught to nurses and nurse managers just a single generation ago. In today's demanding healthcare environment, effective nurse managers know that success depends on their ability to get others to *want* to do the things that need to be done, rather than simply ordering people to perform. They know that their ability to do so begins with placing the needs of the individuals they lead ahead of their own needs. This means that the mission, from its creation through its realization, must include the staff members at every step of the way. A mission that is simply goal driven, with no concern for the individual staff member, is a recipe for failure.

Obviously, the most expeditious method of accomplishing anything in the nursing unit is simply to order someone to perform what must be done. But that procedure is seldom truly effective and is not what is needed in health care today. Today, nurse managers will have difficulty finding anyone who will tell them that leading their units will be easy or that dictatorial direction is the most efficient method of management, because those things simply aren't true. In fact, developing and leading a team of professionals in today's healthcare organization is far more difficult than simply giving orders to the staff. The extra effort required to accomplish the process is worth the price, however, because the effect that a well-organized and motivated team can have on the success of a nursing unit is incredible. In virtually every performance area known, team performance has proven itself to be far superior to individual accomplishment. The hard work and effort that nurse managers put into developing and managing their teams will pay off in increased production, higher-quality patient care, lower turnover and absenteeism, lower risk, and improved staff loyalty.

The effort required to build a team of professionals, regardless of the specific environment in which it is developed, starts with the leader, but every member of the staff must participate. In fact, there can be no team if the person in charge decides that he or she will assume the responsibility for everything accomplished by the group. Performance must be a team effort, with both the leader and the followers accepting responsibility for their individual actions and the accountability that goes with it.

Leadership is critical in today's healthcare environment; it is not something that is nice to have, it is imperative. Every healthcare organization, and every nursing unit functioning within it, must have leaders who possess the skills, abilities, and attitudes that will enable them to inspire the average staff member into performing at a level of quality that exceeds the requirements outlined in the job description.

There is no quick or simple way to develop nursing leaders or the teams of performers that will follow them. It is a process of learning, trusting, supporting, and, above all, caring. It requires managers and individual members of their staffs to continually extend themselves toward improvement and never to allow themselves to be above gaining new insights or studying innovative procedures and methods.

THE QUALITIES OF TEAMWORK AND LEADERSHIP

As the leader in the nursing unit, the nurse manager has the responsibility to teach his or her staff the basic qualities of leadership and teamwork and to provide each employee with the opportunity to develop his or her individual capabilities. Today the nurse manager must look for the qualities of innovation and initiative in every applicant and teach teamwork and leadership to every employee so that these individuals will have the opportunity to develop into the healthcare leaders of tomorrow. The nurse manager, serving in his or her capacity as unit leader, must reinforce the qualities of leadership and teamwork in all staff members so that the manager may skillfully assist them in accomplishing the goals and objectives assigned to the nursing unit as part of the overall organizational effort to realize the institution's vision. Every member of the organization, both employee and manager, must possess, in addition to individual skills and talents, the essential qualities discussed in the following sections. It is the responsibility of the nurse manager, as the unit leader, to cultivate these qualities in every member of the team and to provide an environment that encourages their development.

Loyalty

Above all else, every individual in the healthcare organization, down to the members of the smallest team or unit, should be encouraged to be loyal. Loyalty, for the purposes of this chapter, is defined as a concern for the welfare and enhancement of the team. It does not require blind obedience but encourages a professional level of disagreement. In an environment built on teamwork, disagreement should not be construed as a demonstration of disloyalty, and staff members who disagree in a professional manner and with the best interests of the team in mind should be listened to by their leaders. On the other hand, staff members or managers who actively participate in or encourage actions that are counter to the continual improvement of the team or that undermine the ability of another to perform at his or her optimum level are disloyal. It is recommended that, when a disloyal staff member is identified, he or she be expeditiously removed from the nursing unit. The negative influence that disloyal employees have on others is like a contagious disease in the human body; it can infiltrate the very fiber of the organization and destroy it.

In those few cases in which a nurse manager is not able to stop the disloyal actions of a staff member or an individual's attitude cannot be changed, the manager should consider harsh action to be appropriate. The nursing unit staff members must stay focused on developing and moving forward together, and because a single disloyal and subversive employee can ruin the efforts of even the most effective team, discipline, up to and including job termination, is warranted.

Those who demonstrate that they are concerned with the welfare of the nursing unit, who continually provide high-quality patient care, and who work diligently toward the improvement of the team, however, should be given every opportunity to succeed. Loyalty is a virtue in the business world, and when it is demonstrated, it should be recognized, encouraged, and used to enhance the combined effort of the team. As leaders, nurse managers must be able to identify their loyal employees and encourage their growth.

WARNING!

Questioning the instructions of a leader is not a sign of disloyalty as long as the dissent is well intended, professionally displayed, and based on a genuine concern for the enhancement of the team. Nurse managers should never discourage members of the staff from questioning their actions, directives, or leadership. In fact, superior managers encourage subordinates to question. Subordinates who question, however, have the responsibility to include in their dissent an idea for improving what they are questioning. To question without intending to improve is not a positive action. Professional nurse managers encourage positive dissent and disagreement, but do not tolerate complaining and whining.

Courage

Nurse managers who want to lead a team as well as the individual staff members who comprise the team must each possess a certain measure of internal fortitude. Leaders, especially in the healthcare industry, must recruit and train staff to work under less than ideal conditions and even under stress to successfully complete the assignments given them. Nurse managers should encourage their staffs to have the patience to accept leadership, not to balk at the sight of obstacles, and not to become discouraged in the face of adversity.

The role of the nurse manager as leader of the nursing unit brings with it periods of loneliness, despair, challenge, and even rejection. A good leader accepts these things as part of the job and suffers them in silence. The leader must not display emotion or personal dissatisfaction to the team, and every member of the team must support the leader through difficult times. The real test of teamwork, in fact, comes only during a period of challenge.

Every member of the team, including its leader, must be encouraged to have the fortitude to act with confidence in times of uncertainty. It is not a measure of professionalism to be able to perform well under ideal situations; anyone can do that. The qualities of teamwork are best evidenced during times of urgency and under conditions that are less than perfect. It is when each individual contributor in the team has to face difficulty that the true benefit of working together for a common purpose is seen.

Desire

Few teams will sustain themselves unless their members possess strong personal desire. Every individual team member, and especially the team leader, should have a strong commitment to support and influence other people, processes, and outcomes. A team member who rebels against the team membership weakens the entire nursing unit.

Nurse managers must be careful not to place into positions of responsibility individual staff members who do not wish to be there. Although such assignments are inevitable, considerable thought must be given to the delegation of responsibility so that the adverse impact generated by a misassigned individual can be minimized. Team members need to remember that not every job they are asked to fill will be exciting and challenging; in fact, the majority will be routine. But every job in the nursing unit is important and should be accomplished at the highest level of quality possible.

Emotional Stamina

Each successively higher level of responsibility in the team will place increased emotional demands on the individual who fills it. Nurse managers, as leaders of their units' performance teams, must assist their employees in developing the stamina to recover rapidly from disappointment. Leaders must encourage their team members to bounce back from discouragement, carry out the responsibilities of their jobs without changing their views when disillusioned, and maintain a clear perspective on their individual roles and the roles of the other team members. It is critical to the success of the team that each member help every other member to develop the emotional strength to persist under seemingly difficult circumstances.

Empathy

Every member of the nursing team, and most assuredly its leader, should be encouraged to develop empathy. Empathy provides the foundation for an appreciation for and understanding of the values held by others and a sensitivity to others' cultures, beliefs, and traditions. If each individual performer attempts to understand the perspectives of the others, the total performance of the team will be enhanced.

Empathy must not be confused with sympathy. Sympathy may result in unwise consolidation in the team (a focused concern for the goals of the team as more important than those of the organization) during times when the good of the organization and the welfare of the patient must be pursued above all other things with skillful diplomacy or direct action.

Decisiveness

Team leaders and individual team members must be decisive. They must know when to act and when not to act, taking into account all facts bearing on the situation and then responsibly fulfilling their individual roles. Waiting to be told what to do is not the manner of the professional, and the team certainly should not condone this behavior. It is especially important for nurse managers to possess the quality of decisiveness as they lead their teams toward the accomplishment of their units' goals.

Leaders and individual performers need to know that vacillation and procrastination confuse and discourage others and open up the organization to needless exposure and risk.

Anticipation

Nurse managers should encourage all members of their staffs to learn through observation and to sharpen their instincts through practical experience. Professional staff members should be encouraged to anticipate thoughts, actions, and consequences, and to accept the level of risk inherent in the act of anticipation. It is through the acceptance of risk that people excel; those who shun it and turn instead to the comfort of personal security are easily surpassed.

Sense of Timing

The timing of recommendations and actions is essential to success. There is no magic formula for helping others develop a sense of timing. As a matter of fact,

and as inappropriate as it may seem, most individuals gain this important skill by applying the lessons they have learned through failure.

Knowing with whom one is dealing and understanding motives, characteristics, the involved politics, priorities, and ambitions is critical even when seeking approval for the simplest recommendation.

Competitiveness

An essential quality of leadership and team building is an intrinsic desire to win. It is not necessary to win all of the time; however, the important contests must be won. Nurse managers must stress to their team members that competition inside and outside of the nursing unit will always be strong and should never be taken lightly. A competitive desire drives those who make it their personal ambition to win, both at work and in situations of personal strife. If the individual members of the nursing unit do not possess a sense of competitiveness, the unit will remain weak and will continually be overcome by the slightest challenge.

Self-Confidence

Proper training and experience develop within team members and team leaders a personal feeling of assurance with which to meet the challenges of everyday performance. Individual team members who show a lack of self-confidence in their efforts to carry out assignments send out subtle signals that the things they are being asked to accomplish are beyond their capabilities. These individuals generally serve to weaken the overall success of the team, which causes them to be identified as the least accomplished members of the team.

Confidence is a sense of knowing that what is being delivered is what is expected; it is not the arrogant swagger of an overly active ego. There is a very discernible difference between the confident demonstration of performance and example, and the overbearing effrontery of the conceited. The quality of self-confidence is especially important for nurse managers, because they cannot elicit a willingness to follow in their staff members if they do not continually project a humble aura of self-confidence. People may follow arrogant leaders, but not for long, not with their full capabilities, and never if they are given a choice.

Accountability

Members of the nursing staff, and especially their leader, must be held accountable for their performance. This is a fundamental part of team building. In the nurse manager's position as the team leader, he or she must remember to praise others for their contributions to the unit's success and must be willing to accept personal responsibility for the failures of the team. Leaders who continually spend their time conducting witch hunts for the guilty during times of adversity are undermining their future ability to function as leaders.

This does not mean that nurse managers should not hold the members of their teams accountable for their performance. In fact, if they do not hold their staffs accountable, they risk losing control. However, holding performers accountable does not mean holding them up to ridicule or in any way demeaning them if they should fail. The creation of a willingness to accept accountability begins with the knowledge that mistakes are permissible—not necessarily excusable, but certainly within the normal realm of performance. If a leader demeans or ridicules any staff member, especially in front of others, the leader reduces that person's confidence and self-regard and, ultimately, his or her ability and willingness to perform at peak efficiency.

Holding staff members accountable means giving them the responsibility and authority to win or lose. If they win, they have earned and deserve all of the credit for their success. Wise leaders never try to openly share the credit that is given for a job well done, even if they did the work themselves. If the team loses, wise nurse managers and proficient leaders thoroughly investigate their own actions to make sure that they provided the team with every opportunity and every means to win. If they did, then their role becomes one of coach and facilitator as they help the participants through the failure and into the process of turning failure into opportunity. Leaders focus their energy on looking for the reasons that success wasn't achieved, and when they have found them, they analyze each reason and create methods for overcoming similar obstacles in the future. In short, nurse managers work with their staffs to ensure that every failure is turned into a learning experience.

People of just about every level and capability are willing to accept accountability for their actions when their leaders view failure as a learning opportunity and not as an excuse for hunting down the guilty and fixing blame.

Being accountable means being willing to stand up and say, "I am responsible." Accountability for one's own actions, and for the outcome of a delegated task, is fundamental to performance.

Responsibility

It is the role of the leader to act as a facilitator whose focus is on teaching the elements of teamwork to every member of the staff. Part of that responsibility is accomplished by ensuring that every member of the staff who has been delegated responsibility for a specific task is provided with the necessary resources to ensure his or her success and by following up to verify that the actions expected are carried out and the directions provided are followed. Staff members at all levels must be taught how and when to perform, with or without direct supervision. Staff members should be expected to accept full responsibility for their actions.

Credibility

Every member of the nursing unit must be credible (i.e., worthy of confidence). In other words, their individual words and actions must be believable to other members of the team, to the patients, and to those individuals who interact with the unit. Professional nurse managers give their trust to all members of their staffs, because they know that, to produce at their optimum levels, staff must be trusted to possess the intelligence and integrity to provide correct information. On the rare occasion when a staff member proves that he or she is not credible, that person should not be allowed to remain in a position in which he or she can influence the team. It is recommended that such an individual be removed from a position of responsibility as quickly as possible (after appropriate opportunities for improvement have been presented).

A large portion of nursing is accomplished by trusting in the capability and professionalism of the individual performer. It is rare that nurse managers have the time to follow staff nurses around as they perform their duties. If nurse managers do not extend their trust to these individuals, they are hampering the success of the team and, ultimately, of the organization.

WARNING *!*

The extension of trust is a necessary risk that must be taken; however, it is not a risk that must be taken blindly or in the face of doubt regarding the individual performer's ability to live up to that trust. When managers extend their trust, they extend themselves, their reputations, and their personal well-being. If they trust another to perform, that does not mean that they give up the ultimate responsibility for all of the actions that are taken. Even if managers delegate responsibility, they do not relinquish their individual accountability. The leader of the team is always responsible for the actions of the group and every individual in it. Although it is essential that team members be trusted, it is not essential for managers to do so without reserving the right to verify the quality demonstration of that trust.

Tenacity and Persistence

Unyielding drive and the stick-to-itiveness necessary to accomplish assignments are desirable and essential capabilities that should be developed in every member of the team. One of the realities of the working world is that weak people persist only when the road is smooth and unchallenged. Strong performers, however, persist and move through temporary moments of disappointment, discouragement, deception, and even feelings of abandonment, and continue until they succeed. Tenacity is often the key to overcoming difficult assignments and achieving challenging goals. The late U.S. president Calvin Coolidge believed in the power of persistence and expressed his commitment to its necessity as follows:

> *Nothing in the world can take the place of persistence.*
> *Talent will not; nothing is more common than unsuccessful men with talent.*
> *Genius will not; unrewarded genius is almost a proverb.*
> *Education will not; the world is full of educated derelicts.*
> *Persistence and determination alone are omnipotent.*

Dependability

If a nurse manager determines that a staff member cannot be depended on to carry out the roles and responsibilities assigned to that person, that team member's responsibilities should be taken away and support should be provided until the person's accountability improves. If, after the staff member receives special assistance, his or her performance continues to be undependable, progressive disciplinary action should be taken to begin the process of replacing the person. Most of the time, nurse managers cannot observe each and every action of their individual subordinates; therefore, they must depend on every individual to perform those things that must be done. Novice nurse managers must understand that the employees working under them as well as the senior managers serving above them are depending on their ability to lead the nursing unit successfully. There is no room in management or among leaders of others for someone who is not dependable. Accomplished leaders and individuals at all levels must understand and accept this fact and take pride in their ability to act dependably.

Stewardship

Each member of the team, and especially the team's leader, must develop the quality of stewardship, or, more simply, the willingness to be a caretaker of others. Every nurse manager should expect all members of his or her team to perform in a manner that encourages confidence, trust, and loyalty on the part of those with whom they come in contact or for whom they may be responsible. Team members must never abuse a patient, a subordinate, a peer, or the leaders above them. Each member should perform in a manner that guides, develops, and encourages excellence and growth in others.

There are few people who can acquire these qualities in a short period. Developing performance of this nature takes time, exposure, and experience and requires patience on the part of the nurse manager. There are few shortcuts, and rarely can one's individual competence be accelerated. If an individual is not willing to pay the price to develop these characteristics, that person limits his or her value to the team and its potential and future success. Even more importantly, that type of individual weakens the overall quality of the team, and for that reason alone, such a person should not be tolerated. As the leader of the nursing unit's team of professionals, the nurse manager must cultivate these qualities and exhibit them consistently. It is the obligation of every nurse manager to provide the team with a personal example of excellence and to encourage these qualities in every employee. Only then will the nursing unit achieve the level of performance expected by the senior administration.

WHY THE NURSING UNIT SHOULD DEPEND ON THE TEAM

A nursing unit that is built on the team concept will always be superior and will always outperform a unit that is based on a command system of management (i.e., the top-down leader is responsible for everything). The primary reason for this fact is astounding in its simplicity: the collective intelligence and capability of the many are *always* superior to the intelligence and capability of the individual. In the nursing environment, where most projects are very complicated, no one person can hope to master all of the details that might be required for success, no matter how well educated, intelligent, or capable that individual may be. The nurse manager may retain ultimate responsibility for the success or failure of the nursing unit, but the team-oriented leader knows that it is best for the individual team members to "lead" the portion of the work in which they are most proficient.

The individual who knows everything there is to know about nursing and patient care is a scarce entity in the healthcare industry. As the demands of the profession increase, even the most experienced and professionally adept nurse managers will move farther and farther away from the responsibility of day-to-day performance. Therefore, it is imperative that the "expert" on the team be given the responsibility for the areas in which he or she holds the greatest amount of expertise. The level of proficiency of a nursing unit run by a team-oriented manager will always surpass that of a similar unit led by a command-oriented manager. When individuals are given responsibility and are held accountable for their actions, their individual capabilities and collective level of success far exceed those of individuals who simply respond to command or instruction. Table 20-1 shows how a teamwork structure differs from a command structure.

Differences Between Command and Team Structures

Significant differences exist between a command structure and a team structure, regardless of where they are used. Many of these differences occur in the areas of vision, planning, mission, and accountability and praise.

VISION

In the healthcare organization or nursing unit operated under a command structure, leaders are individually responsible for developing the vision. It is managers alone who determine where the entity is going, and when they are satisfied that they can drive people successfully toward the realization of this vision, they will make a detailed announcement enlightening the rest of the staff. Subordinate managers (if any) and every member of the staff are forced to accept the leaders' vision of the future or risk alienation, progressive discipline, or outright dismissal. In the command structure, the wishes of the senior are binding, and the capabilities of the many are suppressed.

Life in the team-oriented organization is far removed from the totalitarianism of the command structure. In the team-oriented group, the leader makes the creation of the vision a team action. He or she oversees the development of the vision and stimulates involvement by asking questions. The leader gathers information from all levels of the organization, listens to every team member carefully, and then, working with members of the management team and perhaps even representatives of the labor force, oversees the creation of a vision that can be easily understood and accepted by every member of the team. Once the vision is crafted, the team-oriented leader works to develop a consensus among the team to commit to the vision, carefully modifying and shaping it so that it is as inclusive as possible.

PLANNING

In the command organization, planning is the sole responsibility of the organizational authority. Generally, the senior manager and his or her most trusted and immediate juniors share in plan development, with the right of final decision reserved solely by the boss.

The command group often accomplishes its planning effort in secret and behind closed doors. The results are presented to the organization, if at all, as a take-it-or-leave-it plan of action.

In the team-oriented unit, planning is a task shared by representatives of all performance levels. The unit manager ensures that members of the planning team are selected for their ability to contribute overlapping layers of knowledge and capability (i.e., one's strengths will offset another's weaknesses). Selection for the planning team is based on possession of the necessary skills, not on the position occupied. The leader's role is to encourage initiative and creative thinking, and together the planning team members gather as much information and insight as possible from each other. Once the planning team is convinced that a good collective plan has been developed, the leader acts as a performance facilitator, encouraging staff at all levels of performance and authority to work together to help the plan support the unit's mission. The leader is also responsible for selling the plan to the general

---

TABLE 20-1

Differences Between a Command and a Teamwork Structure

	Command	*Teamwork*
Vision development	Inspirational input (i.e., that which is inspired by the commander)	Performed with substantial input from team
Planning	Performed by management	Performed by team
Mission definition	Performed by leader	Performed by team
Responsibility	Retained solely by leader	Shared by team members
Recognition	Claimed solely by leader	Shared by team members

members of the organization, a task that is accomplished by sharing, not by dictating.

MISSION

In a command-style organization, defining the mission of the organization is the sole responsibility of the manager. The basic belief is that the general members of the organization will not be able to accomplish a mission unless they are told when, where, and how to do so. In the command concept of mission development, the paradox of economics is held to apply: that is, if each performer must decide individually whether to fight or flee, all performers will choose to flee, because no one will trust the next person to fight. The purpose of the command structure is to see that no one flees by providing a severe penalty for desertion in the face of challenge.

In a team-based organization, every one of the team members feels as though he or she is sharing the same things as the rest of the team members. Because of this feeling of sharing, it is easy for the individual team members to work with one another to fashion a mission that the entire team will support. The leader's role is that of a coach or facilitator who suggests strategies that the team can use to shape the mission and then guides the team through obstacles by sharing experience, tactics, and ideas. The paradox of economics mentioned earlier does not hold: the team does not flee in the face of challenge, because everyone knows that success depends on the ability of the team members to perform well together.

ACCOUNTABILITY AND PRAISE

In the command-driven organization, accountability (responsibility) and praise (credit) are the sole domain of the manager. When things go well, all of the accolades are swept into the head office. When things go badly, one of two things is likely to occur: (1) the leader falls on his or her sword, or (2) a witch hunt is undertaken to uncover the guilty parties (and it's likely that plenty of the second will occur before one ever sees the first, because in this type of organization, the leader is seldom considered to be wrong). This is very much the way it has been throughout history, regardless of the profession involved, and nursing is no exception. In this type of environment, it is the manager who is remembered, not the followers (except when the results are negative), and only the manager enjoys a place in history.

In the team-oriented organization, the situation is reversed. Members of the team are expected to accept the responsibility for their actions. Members of the team are credited with the success and held accountable for the failure of their part of the mission. There is no need for witch hunts because the leader bears the ultimate responsibility for failure. However, in this environment fault and guilt are not the motivating factors behind success. Instead, the team-oriented organization is far more interested in learning from its mistakes than in burning the responsible parties at the stake.

Benefits of Teams for Team Members

Individual team members, through their acceptance of the responsibility that comes with being part of a team, gain certain rights and privileges that do not exist in a command structure.

TEAM MEMBERS GAIN OWNERSHIP

Individual members of a team gain ownership of their work. This ownership is generally one of the following two basic types:
1. *Literal:* The team members are the sole beneficiaries of the outcome of their work.
2. *Representative:* The individual team members take great pride in the accomplishments of the team, even though the larger organization benefits.

Ownership is another way of describing acceptance of responsibility, and taking ownership includes receiving the benefits of success and the penalties for failure. A team member who owns his or her work becomes, by definition, a leader even if that person is not given the title or the commensurate salary.

TEAM MEMBERS GAIN ACCOUNTABILITY

Ownership is not the only benefit gained by team members; another critical benefit is accountability. In a team environment, accountability is a two-way street; if the leader holds the individual team members accountable, then the leader must accept his or her own accountability to the team. This type of sharing can be understood easily by thinking about two escaped convicts chained together and running. If one of the convicts stops, the other has to stop. If one of them jerks on the chain, the other person lurches. That is precisely what it is like to be part of a team. Jerking the chain is like making preemptive changes to an established plan that force members of the team to undertake new actions. The team will at least temporarily lose its natural flow, and it will become harder to accomplish the mission. Likewise, when the members of a team decide that they need to compensate for a real or imagined difficulty by slowing down their performance, it is a good bet that project deadlines won't be met.

TEAM MEMBERS GAIN PERMISSION

In a command organization, orders (instructions) are given from the top down, and all of the subordinate employees are expected to obey. In a team-based organization, however, things are different. The team structure forces a high percentage of decisions actually to flow *up* the organizational chart toward the leader, who retains the ultimate authority. In this type of system, the leader is actually giving permission, not orders.

In a team situation, the leader must be a good listener, because many people will approach the leader asking not for straightforward permission to contribute but for encouragement to do so, and a good leader must be able to understand the difference. When team members come to the leader with a proposal, the leader has the responsibility to give them a good hearing. In the hearing, the leader must ask questions and should feel entitled to honest, straightforward responses. This form of management provides the group and its individual members with confidence, because they are able to gain knowledge and experience by actually working through what must be done and how. When the leader gives permission, the leader is actually encouraging the team members to go forward and perform what they believe they can do. The effect of this request-permission cycle is extraordinary. Individual team members are far more willing to contribute to the full extent of their capabilities simply because they believe it's *their* idea. No manner of persuasion or dictatorial direction can substitute for the desire and willingness to perform that is created when a person believes in his or her own ideas.

TEAM MEMBERS GAIN ACCEPTANCE

For individuals to gain acceptance by the team, they must be willing to give up some of their autonomy and allow themselves to become part of a larger entity. They are compensated for this loss by active participation in an effort that will always be more dynamic and more effective than that normally achieved by a single person, regardless of that person's individual capability.

Belonging to a team provides emotional satisfaction to most people. Each person has the right to feel good about being accepted as part of the team, because each person realizes that he or she has been chosen and is being retained for more reasons than simply the possession of needed talent. Team members come to know of the careful review process that is conducted every time a new member is needed and the way the decision is ultimately reached, and through this knowledge, they understand that to become a member of the team every applicant must possess the desired attributes that complement those of other members of the team, including personality traits. Being a member of a team involves much more than possessing specific talents.

Once accepted by the team, the new member has every right to feel a sense of pride in this achievement.

TEAM MEMBERS GAIN FORGIVENESS

Nothing is more destructive to effective team management than the persistent human need to place blame when things don't go as planned. In a command structure, lengthy and expensive witch hunts that track down the culprit and a dictatorial management system that metes out disciplinary action satisfy this need. Nowhere can this be seen more clearly than in the ancient practices of the Roman army. In the Roman legions, if a single legionnaire acted in a cowardly way, every tenth man in that person's century (group of 100 legionnaires commanded by a centurion) was put to death as a reminder to all. (The word *decimation* comes from that practice.) Today, the penalty for failure in most command-oriented organizations is being fired or, at a minimum, ostracized.

In a team environment, the price of failure is very different. Unless a team member willfully fails to perform or intentionally performs in a negative manner, failure within a team is a group event. Failure, like success, is shared by all of the team members (i.e., winning and losing is a team consequence).

Good team leaders understand that a mistake is an opportunity for a quick review of the situation and a chance for the entire group to grow. Smart, capable leaders ask themselves the following questions when their team has not met expectations:

- Why did the mistake happen?
- Did I provide clear and precise instructions?
- Was the mission understood and did it make sense?
- Did I provide adequate tools, resources, and motivation?
- Was I demonstrating the required performance through my actions?

If the leader can answer yes to all of these questions, then and only then should the leader take action against the team or a specific team member. Even then, the action taken should be corrective. Discipline, although sometimes necessary, is used as a last resort in a team. If the same mistake is repeated, clearly something is wrong, perhaps with the individual committing the errors or perhaps with the way the task has been designed. Such a search for excellence is not a means for the truly incompetent person to escape, however. In fact, the internal actions taken by team members will be far more severe than those that management is allowed to mete out.

CREATING A WINNING TEAM

The feelings experienced through winning and success are extraordinary. These feelings alone should provide a natural incentive for leaders to create the best possible teams, but that is not always the way things occur. In fact, a tremendous amount of effort, perseverance, and insight are required to create a winning team. The leader must employ an understanding of human nature as well as demonstrate an ability to carefully align skills and personalities. It is the effort put into the creation of the team by the leader that ultimately determines the team's ability to succeed.

Although most people in leadership roles will be quick to acknowledge the importance of the team, few really understand what needs to be done to create, nurture, and guide such a unit. As the complexity of health care continues to grow, the practice of effective team creation will become more and more critical to future success; therefore, it is important that every nurse manager understand what team building is about. If nurse managers implement the procedures outlined in the following sections, they should be able to develop effective teams that will satisfy the growing demands of the nursing unit.

Step One: Hire the Right People

Anyone who has ever watched children pick teams for a game of baseball can understand the fundamentals necessary to select the right people for a team. The leaders will carefully select the most capable, the most proficient, the fastest, and the smartest from among those available. Gradually, the group members will be divided into teams until only the perceived poor performers are left.

In the business of health care, it is the individual unit leader who is responsible for choosing the members of the team. Even when a new leader inherits a preestablished team, there is usually an opportunity to reshuffle and realign until the leader feels the maximum potential has been developed out of the raw material that has been inherited.

A successful team, regardless of its size or complexity, is created through the combined efforts of the people who comprise it. The individual staff members are joined to form a performance team that ultimately becomes the foundation of the nursing unit. It is through the actions of the individual staff members that the patient perceives the quality of care provided. Because the judged quality of the unit is based on the perceptions of the patients, obtaining the proper people to make up the nursing team becomes one of the most critical parts of running the performance unit. To put it in very simple terms, the best way to avoid problems in patient care is to hire only the very best of the available high-quality personnel (people who meet or exceed the performance standards set by the unit).

The process of hiring employees consists of the following:

1. Identifying the requirements of the position that is open

2. Hiring the correct person who meets the criteria based on those requirements

These two things, on the surface, seem to be relatively simple tasks. At first glance, it would seem that anyone capable of occupying a managerial position should be able to accomplish both as minimum performance requirements. However, these tasks are not easily accomplished, and as a general rule, most people with hiring authority do not perform them well. As a matter of fact, these basic functions are two of the most misused and ill performed of the entire set of essential managerial responsibilities.

The knowledge and skills necessary to do an effective job of hiring employees are not covered in any university curriculum, nor are they automatically acquired when one rises to a managerial position. For a nurse manager to develop the skills necessary to become an effective hiring agent requires extensive work and commitment, and the effort involved should never be taken lightly. The manager starts by carefully analyzing the needs of the team and the special requirements of the unit and translating them into an accurate description of the position requirements. This type of analysis is absolutely essential if the nurse manager is to be able to find the special individuals who will bring success to the unit. If the manager conducts the hiring process carefully, the individuals who are brought onto the team will meet the requirements of the job, suit the needs of the patient, and complement the other individuals on the team.

In most healthcare organizations, the human resources department performs much of the recruiting and initial interviewing of applicants. Nurse managers can work directly with human resources personnel to communicate their exact needs in order to attract the best-qualified applicants. Human resources personnel are trained specifically to prepare job descriptions, place personnel advertisements, establish employment policy, and ensure compliance with state and federal employment law. They are usually the nurse manager's best source of information on these subjects.

If hiring quality team members were as simple as filling an open position with almost any warm body who applies, then total reliance on emotion and gut reaction might be sufficient to find the correct applicant. Unfortunately, a team leader's responsibility is not simply to hire warm bodies but to hire highly qualified personnel; therefore, reliance on personal methods will not get the job done properly. It is the leader's responsibility to hire applicants who are motivated, enthusiastic, positive, hardworking, and, to the greatest extent possible, compatible with the other members of the team. Leaders must look for and identify individuals who possess the special qualities needed by the team if they are to ensure high-quality team performance. A cardinal rule in hiring is never, never to hire someone just to fill an open position. Hire only those people who are capable of contributing to the continued success of the team.

Hiring the wrong person only makes the team's and nurse manager's jobs more difficult. If the manager hires the wrong person, the work doesn't go away; it becomes even more demanding, because it is far more difficult to correct the errors made by a poor performer than to accomplish the work correctly the first time. Also, if the new hire is not compatible with the other team members, the working environment can become a tense and stressful one in which it is both difficult to perform and extremely challenging to lead.

Nurse managers, in their role as unit leaders, have a tremendous responsibility to the team when they seek to employ a new staff member. That responsibility should remain paramount in their minds during the hiring process; however, they must often satisfy the broader desires of the organization. These two sets of requirements can be, and often are, in direct conflict with one another. To satisfy both sets and, at the same time, ensure that they hire properly, nurse managers must be able to blend the necessity for complying with company policies and procedures with the requirement of meeting the team's unique needs. Only by accomplishing this blending process carefully will they satisfy their responsibility to ensure that the organization receives optimum performance from the nursing unit. If, by hiring the wrong person, nurse managers inadvertently reduce the effectiveness of the team, they have failed in their obligation to the organization, the nursing unit, the new staff member, and themselves.

As the leaders of their nursing units, nurse managers must keep themselves and the members of their units extremely concerned with exactly whom they *allow* to become new members of their teams. The reason to be extremely careful is easy to understand; the people who are allowed to join eventually will become the very individuals who help shape the continued success of the unit and ultimately of every individual team member. The people who are hired become part of the only real tool nurse managers have to carry out the mission they are given. Keeping this thought in mind makes it very easy to see just how critical it is for managers to put the right person in the right position at the right time. Failure to accomplish this fundamental process correctly is more than simply wrong; in fact, such an error can have broad ramifications. The bottom line is that nurse managers who do not make it their policy to hire only the most qualified applicants are acting to directly harm the organization, their nursing units, their team members, themselves, and, of course, the individual who is hired. As noted earlier, one of the rules of management is that it is better to keep a position open than to hire the wrong person.

If the nurse manager's primary motivation during the hiring exercise is to simply fill the position, the chances are that he or she will hire the wrong person. Instead of concentrating on getting the open position filled, professional nurse managers put their energy into finding high-quality individuals—people whom they and the members of their teams will be proud to have as contributing members, who can bring strength to the unit and, through their efforts, help all team members improve their individual talents. Although, realistically, the optimal individual may not be available, this does not excuse the nurse manager from making every effort to find such a person.

The process of hiring high-quality individuals is not easy. Not only will nurse managers be burdened with increased workload while a position remains open, but their efforts to find that special individual will be hampered by pressure from their teams. Team members will be working extra hours and performing more tasks while the position remains unfilled, and there is every reason to believe that they will not like that situation. Intelligent nurse managers act to reduce this pressure by keeping the existing team members aware of their concerns about hiring just anyone and their effort to find high-quality individuals. By sharing their concerns with the team and keeping the members informed of the continuing effort, nurse managers are accomplishing several important things: (a) they are reinforcing their support for their teams; (b) they are reminding their teams and each of their members just how important they are to the managers (by insisting on hiring high-quality, complementary personnel, they indirectly communicate to team members that they are special). If nurse managers work hand in hand with team members and keep them informed of the progress being made, they can always count on their teams' support.

Nurse managers should resist the natural impulse to allow the availability of qualified personnel, or lack thereof, to influence their determination to find superior employees. It will be far easier to maintain this resolve if nurse managers remember the following while they continue their search:

1. *The amount of work that can be created if the wrong person is hired:* If the nurse manager hires the wrong person, there will always be more work to do than if the position were to remain open. Not only will the tasks originally assigned to the position have to be accomplished, but the team will also have to correct the errors made by the marginal performer.

2. *The difficulty in explaining why performance does not improve when the team is at full staff:* The team actually has a better reason for lower produc-

tivity while the position remains open than after the new hire is on board. The impact of open positions on performance is usually understandable to senior management, but few will excuse the hiring of the wrong person. The nurse manager must remember that he or she has a responsibility to satisfy the needs of senior management as well as those of the team, and most of the time senior management will be far more demanding. If the position is kept open while a superior candidate is sought, the nurse manager will be addressing both sets of needs.

Another major concern in the employment process is the fact that it is an emotional procedure. Although most managers realize that the hiring process is difficult, not everyone who rises to leadership responsibility possesses the ability to make good initial assessments of people, and many can be swayed by exaggerated claims, smooth talking, and out-and-out fabrications. Experienced nurse managers reduce the potential for such misjudgment by following a consistent procedure when hiring. The system outlined in the following sections exemplifies what many professionals do to avoid these hiring pitfalls.

USE AN EXISTING POSITION DESCRIPTION

Nurse managers should use an existing position description (or develop a new one) that accurately identifies the major responsibilities that will be assigned to the new hire. This document should reflect the needs of the organization as well as the special needs of the team (to the greatest extent possible) and must comply fully with federal and state employment laws and internal company policy. As a minimum, the description should include the following:

- Title of the position
- Reporting responsibility (to whom the position reports)
- Broad statement identifying the scope of the position
- Principal areas of responsibility (it is best to list these in bulleted form)
- Performance requirements for each principal area of responsibility
- Associated responsibilities (other duties of the position that may not fall into a principal area)
- Special skills required, as desired by the organization and the team
- Special team requirements (overtime, rotation of shift, weekend work, travel, etc.)

The best way for a nurse manager to begin the employment process is to ensure that he or she knows *exactly* what type of individual is wanted and what the manager will expect from the position. An accurately

developed job description is an invaluable tool to the nurse manager.

BE OPEN-MINDED

The nurse manager should not prejudice the decision with preconceived expectations and opinions, such as by prejudging a candidate in the following areas:

- Smoking habits
- Ethnicity
- Sexual preference

Not only do such prejudices violate federal employment laws and those of almost every state, they severely limit the nurse manager's range of possible candidates. Instead, the nurse manager should establish guidelines that will allow the potential new hire to mix well with the present team members and focus on these. There is no room in the hiring process to accommodate anyone's personal desires and prejudices. For example, placing an individual who smokes on a team comprised of militant nonsmokers might unbalance the team by creating dissension, but the fact that a person smokes should not be sufficient reason to disqualify that person. Small challenges such as smoking are things that the nurse manager should work out with existing team members before beginning the employment process.

Discrimination based on ethnic background, sexual preference, and the other characteristics enumerated in federal law have absolutely no place in the hiring process. Prejudice of this nature needlessly places both the nurse manager and the organization in an extremely difficult situation. As the individual charged with hiring, the nurse manager is personally responsible for compliance with every aspect of employment law. In fact, in most states, the individual doing the hiring is held personally accountable for his or her actions. Claims of prejudice during the hiring process are made frequently enough that every manager should be careful not to place himself or herself or the organization into such a vulnerable position. Such cases are extremely difficult for the organization to defend and often result in substantial settlements, even if actual wrongdoing is never proved.

BE OBJECTIVE AND FAIR

As professionals, nurse managers must remove their personal feelings from the hiring process. This is not easy; in fact, it is far easier to discuss it than to do it, because everyone has individual likes and dislikes. Human nature is a part of the employment process that must be dealt with in a professional manner. Just because team leaders prefer to be around people with whom they feel comfortable does not mean that leaders should try to satisfy these feelings at the expense of their teams. Objectivity is best created and maintained when nurse managers judge all prospects for the job against identical and impartial criteria. For example, if they ask one applicant seven specific questions, they should ask all other applicants the same seven questions. If they give a test to determine qualifications, they must give the same test to each and every one of the prospects. If possible, it is a good idea to have members of the existing team complete all screening tests *before* these tests are used in hiring. This will help determine whether the contents of the tests are truly applicable to the position and what the acceptable results are.

BE PREPARED

The nurse manager's job is to evaluate all applicants in terms of their potential and against the standards of the organization and the needs of the unit. To accomplish this effectively, the nurse manager must prepare for the interview. The manager can start by working with the members of the existing team to develop a standard set of questions that relate directly to the performance requirements of the position. Based on the applicant's responses to the standard questions, the nurse manager can objectively "score" each applicant and compile an objective comparison of all applicants. The following should be considered in carrying out this process:

Selection criteria: Individual behaviors in the job description and any special skills that may be required to perform the job (which should also be listed on the job description) are pulled out. These are used to define the specific actions the applicant must be able to accomplish in order to perform satisfactorily once hired.

Weighting scale: Each behavior is weighted according to its importance to the performance of the job. Although all of the behaviors listed in the job description should be important, not all will be critical; some will be less important and some will even be categorized as simply nice to have. The assigned weight becomes a number that can be used as a multiplier. When used in conjunction with the actual score given, it can determine the total points earned by the applicant. The recommendation is to use a weighting scale of 1 to 5, with 1 identifying the least critical and 5 the most critical behaviors.

Acceptable level: Not every applicant will score well in all of the areas that are considered important. Nurse managers should know in which areas they are willing to compensate for and which areas are absolutely essential. Also managers must determine the minimum score required to

hire. (If all applicants fail to obtain this score, then no one gets the job.) The minimum score is calculated by multiplying the score given the applicant for each behavior (skill or attribute) listed by the weight assigned to that skill or attribute and then adding up all of the minimum scores to obtain a total minimum acceptable.

Use of a job applicant worksheet will help nurse managers turn their hiring practices into objective processes (Fig. 20-1). Although following standardized procedures will not totally eliminate subjectivity, if done carefully it can help significantly to avoid potential legal problems caused by inconsistent hiring practices.

INVOLVE THE CURRENT TEAM

Teamwork is something that all organizations talk about but few actually implement well. For an organization really to be team oriented, teamwork must be something that is practiced *all* of the time. Quality organizations are committed to *real* teamwork, not *professed* or inconsistent displays they refer to as teamwork. The difference is that a real team attempts to accomplish the important things together, not just the routine or easy things. Hiring team members is one of those important things, and, sad to say, it is one of the things in which the self-proclaimed "team-oriented" organizations never actually allow the team to participate. The vast majority of organizations feel that hiring a new employee is the sovereign domain of management and are very restrictive in whom they allow to engage in this process. Although there are many very good reasons why hiring should not be a general free-for-all, and this text does not advocate that form of conduct, truly team-oriented organizations work hard to develop methods that will allow them to include team members in the hiring process and, at the same time, control the risks that such an action could present. In fact, truly team-oriented organizations and managers would never consider hiring a new team member without consulting the existing team members. It is highly recommended that as many members of the nursing unit as practicable be involved in the hiring process. They can help write job descriptions, assist in developing standardized questions, and even conduct interviews.

Why? For quite a few very good reasons, as follows:

The team has to work with the new hire; the leader does not. After the hire is made, each member of the team has to work *with* the new person—down in the trenches, day after day. The leader does not necessarily have to do that. The new hire will work *for* the leader, and good leaders understand that there is a world of difference between *with* and *for*.

Job Application Worksheet

Specific Behavior Necessary	Score					Weight 1-5	Minimum Acceptable	Total Points	Remarks
	1	2	3	4	5				
Attitude toward nursing					X	5	20	25	Very positive
Knowledge									
Education level					X	4	8	20	MSN
Special training				X		4	8	16	Cardiac, EMT
Attitude toward teamwork					X	5	16	25	Very professional
General nursing experience			X			4	12	12	4 years
Cardiac nursing experience		X				5	10	10	2 years
Positive attitude					X	4	12	20	Exceptional
Computer skills				X		2	4	8	Knows all programs
Interpersonal skills				X		4	12	16	Good reputation
Professional appearance					X	3	9	15	Exceptional
Image projection				X		4	12	16	Professional
Ability to develop rapport				X		4	12	16	Likes people
Articulateness				X		4	12	16	Speaks well
Verbal communication					X	4	12	20	Very articulate
Written communication					X	4	12	20	Understands risk
Desire for position					X	3	9	15	High desire
Ability to work independently					X	5	20	25	Good reputation
Judgment					X	5	20	25	Exceptional
Value at current position					X	4	12	20	Very valuable
Previous performance					X	4	12	20	Outstanding
References					X	3	9	15	Very good
Supervisory experience				X		2	4	8	3 years
TOTALS							257	383	

Position interviewed for: __Staff Nurse__

Name of person being interviewed: __Martha Newbetter, RN__

Current position held: __Staff Nurse in Emergency Department__

Date of interview: __August 8, 2004__

Robert L. Anders   Robert L. Anders, DrPH, RN

Signature of interviewing manager   Printed name of interviewing manager

Fig. 20-1 ■ Example of a job application worksheet. _EMT,_ Emergency medical technician. See text for explanation of weights.

The team is nurtured by the hiring process. Hiring is one of the most important activities performed by an organization. Taking part in the hiring process adds a huge boost to every team member's morale, self-esteem, and perception of self-worth. It also helps the individual performer grow and mature by enabling that person to understand the proper procedures to follow in the hiring process and the reason things have to be done in special ways.

Teamwork is developed. The biggest benefit that can be obtained by encouraging staff members to participate in the hiring process is the interaction that occurs between the team members. As each member of the team argues in support of his or her individual opinions and is required to justify those convictions to the other team members, the process brings the individual team members closer together and helps each member understand that it is okay to have different viewpoints within a team as long as they are examined for their value in improving the unit.

A negative reaction to the new hire is avoided. "Where did they find this person?" "I don't want to work with the new nurse." Almost every nurse manager has overheard such comments in a group of team members. The comments infer that a poor selection has been made and that the boss was wrong in making the selection. Not only does the leader not need to have his or her worth demeaned by team members behind the leader's back, but this type of conduct is not good for the team. The leader must ensure that team members possess and profess confidence in the leader's ability and hold an absolute belief in the leader's concern for the welfare of the team *at all times*. The hiring process can provide individual team members with tangible proof of their leaders' confidence in and concern for the welfare of the team.

If the leader uses a team hiring process, then every time the leader hears one of the team members grumbling, the leader can simply call that person over and gently remind him or her that *the leader* didn't hire the new person, *the team did*. This action, done gently but firmly, will also impress on the team the fact that the privilege of hiring someone carries with it a responsibility (i.e., ensuring that the new hire becomes successful) and that energy spent grumbling would be more productively spent helping the new team member improve performance.

The new hire is helped to succeed. The new team member, by virtue of being selected to join the nursing unit's team, earns the right to be assured of a fair chance to succeed. The hiring process should firmly place the support of every existing team member behind that right. People are much more willing to help a new person if they have been involved in the decision to hire in the first place.

The reality of being hired into just about any healthcare organization in the world is that the new hire is a stranger starting in a strange environment, regardless of how experienced the person may be. On that first day on the job, few existing employees go out of their way to ensure that the new person is comfortable and starts off on the right foot. If they are involved in the hiring process, however, the old team members will feel an obligation to the new person and will be much more willing to extend themselves. Also, the new hire will know some of the people with whom he or she will be working. This combination of willingness and comfort goes a long way toward ensuring that the new hire gets off to a positive start.

Personal stress for the nurse manager is reduced. The pressures of leadership are such that few nurse managers can spare the time necessary to screen all of the people who apply for positions in a dynamic nursing unit. Every moment the nurse manager spends in the employment process is a moment that is not spent managing the operation of the nursing unit. The individual team members, if well trained, can provide a willing and capable support group to help select the new hire; and because the existing team members feel a sense of responsibility, the manager can have the luxury of picking and choosing the areas in which he or she will give personal assistance.

The applicant learns enough to say no. Unless the leader is truly an exceptional individual, the people interviewed for team positions rarely will ask the leader the questions that are most important to them personally—questions like, What is it really like to work here? What is the boss really like to work for? Am I going to be treated fairly?

These questions are held back for obvious reasons. First, applicants don't want to offend and risk not being hired. In addition, applicants may feel that the answers given by the leader would be, to say the least, biased and opinionated.

However, if applicants don't have the opportunity to ask these questions and receive answers that they perceive as truthful, they will not learn enough about the reality of the organization to make an informed decision if they are offered the position. This leads to erroneous conceptions of the job on the part of applicants, which ultimately results in higher turnover than necessary.

If, however, applicants can feel free to ask members of the team these questions and receive only honest, straightforward answers, their ability to make an educated decision will be greatly enhanced, and any misconceived opinions of the nursing unit can be put to rest immediately. The long-term result will be happier staff members and lower than normal turnover.

This benefit alone can save the team from selecting someone whom it may later regret hiring. An even bigger benefit of this form of team hiring is that the team will be in a position to prevent an applicant from accepting a position that the applicant really doesn't want or will not fit into well and then later regretting his or her decision.

How does the nurse manager get the team involved? Slowly and very carefully at first. The manager should start out by having the team participate in creating position descriptions and writing standardized interview questions. Then the manager should make sure that each member of the team receives training in employment law. Once the nurse manager is confident that the existing team members will not make a mistake that can put the organization at risk, several of them should be invited to drop in while the nurse manager is conducting an interview. When they do, the manager explains that he or she wants the applicant to meet some of the people the applicant will be working with if he or she is offered the job. The manager then excuses himself or herself from the meeting, but not before offering the applicant the opportunity to ask questions of the staff. When the manager leaves the interview, he or she should make sure to stay well out of earshot and visual range. The existing team members should make small talk and visit with the applicant. While they are doing so, the team members should ask predetermined questions (which have been written on small index cards and given to the team members) and answer any questions the applicant asks as honestly as they can. (Applicants will almost always ask questions about the work environment and the quality of the boss.) After the interview is over, the nurse manager meets with the participating team members in a neutral location (not the manager's office) and discusses each applicant. The worksheet and standard questions devised before the interview process began are used, and the team members are encouraged to justify their opinions of the applicant. Then, through a group consensus, the person everyone considers to be the best is hired.

Later, as the team's sophistication grows, the nurse manager should create "employment teams" and have regular hiring periods. At least two teams of no more than three people each are recommended. One team should come from the immediate area in which the applicant will work, and the other team should be selected at large from various other unit sections or shifts. After the initial interview, the applicant is invited to visit with a few members of the team and is taken to the first group. This group talks with the applicant and, as they are doing so, members of a second preselected team casually drop in. After that, the process remains the same as described earlier. The selection process should be fun. Individual team members should argue for and defend their selections, press home their choices, and defend their reasons.

If a simple majority of team members vote nay on a specific applicant, that individual is no longer considered. Once the team hiring decision is made, a team consensus must be reached and everyone must agree to support the decision. All personal preferences must be forgotten, and everyone must work together to make the new hire as welcome and ultimately as successful as possible.

The three big questions are as follows:

1. Does this type of hiring procedure work?
   Yes! Emphatically so. Team-oriented companies typically enjoy a lower turnover in personnel than do command-oriented organizations. The proof of the practice is improved confidence, self-esteem, and belief in the effects of teamwork among the team members. Real teamwork pays off by producing loyal and dedicated employees and an extremely productive work environment.
2. Is it worth the effort?
   Yes. The value of the process can be measured by counting the smiles on the faces of the team members. Today, everyone works under tremendous deadline pressures, against performance guarantees, and under enormous personal stress. Creating situations in which employees get to enjoy each other's company and perform an invaluable service to the organization is worth whatever it costs to build a solid team base.
3. Is this elaborate form of hiring applicable to entry-level employees?
   Yes. Every member of the team is critical to the success of the organization, regardless of his or her position or level of authority. When entry-level employees are being hired, the seniority of the individual team members who participate in the process should be commensurate.

Whatever hiring practices are used, *preparation* and *consistency* should dominate. The nurse manager should work closely with the team and stay up to date on state and federal employment regulations.

WARNING!

The process described here of using employment teams to assist in finding the very best employees has proven incredibly valuable to the small unit manager, but it is a procedure that requires considerable managerial leadership.

Although individual team members must be given latitude to develop the skills needed to assist effectively in hiring, the employment process is an area in which the organization can easily be placed at risk. Therefore, every person involved in the employment process must be well trained before being allowed to participate and must be continually updated on any changes in employment policy. This requirement cannot be stressed strongly enough.

Step Two: Make the Team Diverse

Diversity is a word that means different things to different people. In today's business world, diversity generally means the process of incorporating people who are culturally different from the traditional Caucasians who dominated the American business scene for most of the twentieth century. For the purposes of this course, however, let's focus on a narrower meaning of the word.

When the nurse manager is building a team, it is important that the manager not create it in his or her own image. The team should not be a reflection of the leader. The team should perhaps complement the leader's style and beliefs, but for the most part the team should be composed so as to provide the following:

Compensation for the shortcomings of the leader: No one can do everything well or can do all of the things that a team will have to do. Therefore, leaders should look for people who have skills that they themselves lack. Truly professional managers understand that they need expertise that both complements their talents and offsets their shortcomings. Failure to select personnel who are capable of meeting these needs is unprofessional. (Some managers actually hire people whom they feel comfortable with and who they don't feel will offer a challenge to them. If you are one of these managers, you are doing yourself, your unit, and your organization a severe disservice.)

A wide range of views: Nurse managers will want people who perceive things differently than they do. Although it is certainly more difficult to manage people who view things differently, it is also an invaluable asset to have different outlooks available. Such people can provide managers with ready information about market diversity, with information on the potential impact of actions, and with different opinions, all of which are invaluable to the leader of a dynamic performance unit.

Different skills: When hiring different members of the group, nurse managers should look for people who possess varying skills. Some might be technically oriented, others might be good administrators, and still others might have exceptional bedside nursing skills. The mix will provide the nursing unit with resident expertise and the in-house ability to cross-train the members of the team.

Although most managers generally prefer to lead a team composed of seasoned veterans, it is often far more productive to have a good mix of experience and youth. The rookies will force management to sacrifice a little in the professional categories, but they bring a fresh perspective and significantly different attitudes. Part of the problem with hiring elite professionals is that too many of them believe that they have "been there and done that"—some of them too many times before. Although experience provides benefits, a developing unit needs enthusiasm, energy, and a willingness to try new approaches and concepts. If nurse managers load their teams down with too much experience, they may create a situation in which the flexibility they need most will be sacrificed to those who are unwilling to deviate from traditional roles and approaches.

The benefit of a team is that it is the combination of differences: different approaches, different thoughts, different viewpoints, different attitudes, and different beliefs. In a true team environment, the leader uses his or her skill to create an atmosphere in which difference is respected and in which team members feel free to express themselves and use their imagination and creativity, and know that they will be rewarded for doing so. It is the leader, taking his or her job seriously, who makes order out of what may be perceived as chaos.

Diversity is what the leader should strive for in establishing the team. A word of caution is in order, however: the leader should not try to make the team too diverse. Diversity can also work against a leader. For example, if the nurse manager looks into the talent pool and selects nothing but newcomers with new, untested ideas, the manager will run the risk of having to spend his or her time acting like a fireman, running from place to place putting out blazes. A classic example of bringing in too many young, talented, and creative people and not enough seasoned veterans is the situation that occurred in the Clinton White House during its first 90 days. During that period, it was observed by several Washington insiders that whereas the new president and his closest advisors were extremely creative and intelligent, few of them actually knew anything of practical value.

That is to say that intelligence, desire, and imagination are not all that is needed to run an organization. These things need to be tempered with experience and common sense. The leader's role is not to be a mother hen to the team any more than it is to be a drill sergeant. The presence of too many inexperienced team members will force the leader to spend a disproportionate amount of time solving their problems instead of working on the team's goals.

The recommendation is that the team be a blend of talents as well as a blend of experience and youth. By carefully assessing the team's skill levels, managers can form individuals into subgroups—sort of internal partnerships—that pair the experienced with the inexperienced. They can create teams whose members can assist in developing each other. For example, combining an experienced clinician with a younger, less-experienced nurse will force the younger team member to remember that real life in the nursing unit is far different from what is taught in college and teach the older clinician about new, up-to-date theories and methodology.

Step Three: Limit Team Size

The successful team starts to take shape long before the first team member is placed. A superior nurse manager will begin developing the team on paper by building a perfect model: what would the team look like if the organization could provide the nursing unit with unlimited resources (money, material, and people)? After the "dream team" is constructed, a good leader will immediately start to restructure it so that it fits the reality of the current nursing unit environment. To do this, the nurse manager asks questions such as, Who or what can I do without? Who or what can be eliminated without degrading the potential performance of the team?

Believe it or not, having a team that is "traditional" in size means very little in terms of its effectiveness or ability to contribute. For example, a "traditionally sized" professional softball team has 9 starting players and a roster of approximately 25 support players. People throughout the sport use the number 34 as the "required" size of a ball team, in the belief that fewer players would not provide sufficient depth to get the team through the season. During much of the first half of the twentieth century, however, a softball team composed of just five players and no reserves toured the country playing other professional ball teams. There was a pitcher of incredible talent, a first baseman, an infielder, an outfielder, and a catcher. These five players studied softball as a science. They could tell, for example, from the specific way a batter placed his legs when facing the pitcher where the ball would most likely be hit. This five-man team, known as the King and His Court, rarely lost a softball game and played nearly 100 games each year. A modified King and His Court softball team continues to play today—now using only four players.

Although the nursing unit is a far cry from a baseball field, good ones are built around a team concept that involves very similar ideas, and if it is developed correctly, a small well-honed team not only can but will always outperform a large unprepared one. It is not size that matters in softball or in nursing—it is quality. As the developers of their nursing units' teams, nurse managers should always focus on "right-sizing" their teams. In fact, a primary responsibility of management is continually to look for ways to reduce costs and overhead expenses, and if nurse managers are not taking hard looks at the

sizes of their units and developing methods of getting the work done more efficiently and with fewer personnel, they are not doing the complete job. If they are doing these things, however, their efforts should be governed by the following two basic concepts of team management:

Don't overwork the team: Reducing the size of the team and then forcing the remaining members to pick up the workload of the departed team members can succeed only if there is a balance between workload and team members. This means that the workforce should not be reduced on a whim, or because it is fashionable, or even because immediate seniors wish it to be done (the nurse manager may have to do so in this circumstance, but then he or she must advise the senior managers of the potential ramifications of such an action). Although it is important to keep team members challenged by ensuring that each has a full complement of responsibilities, loading them down so much that they can no longer perform well, have little or no time for creativity, or make mistakes is foolhardy. If management causes the team to become so burdened, they will create an environment that no one wants to work in, and absenteeism and turnover rates will exceed acceptable norms.

Don't put the team in danger: Increasing workloads can have severe mental and physical consequences for the individual members of the team, and this includes the nurse manager. Overworked and highly stressed performers who don't have the time to balance their responsibilities with relaxation and diversity can quickly find their health failing. Unhealthy people do not make quality decisions, maintain enthusiasm, or continue to work in the same job. The end result is that the quality of patient care provided by the unit will decrease and absenteeism and turnover will skyrocket off the chart. Team members will take the time to care for themselves, and increased absenteeism will make the nurse manager's job exceptionally difficult. A smart manager never puts the team or any of its members at risk.

When looking for ways to reduce the size of the team, the nurse manager must remember that, if the team was constructed properly in the first place, each team member brought special skills to the group. Through a program of cross training, other team members can learn many of these specialized skills. One of the results of a well-developed cross-training program is the creation of redundancy (i.e., individual team members' skills overlap to the point that several people in a given unit can perform the same functions). When this situation occurs, it presents the nurse manager with the opportunity to reduce the unit's overhead by promoting the best performers or arranging a cross-department transfer of an exceptional performer to assist in the growth of a sister unit. If a reduction in head count is accomplished as a result of cross-training effectiveness, the wise nurse manager makes sure that the loss of personnel is perceived as a benefit of the training. If the staff feel that their efforts to enhance their capabilities through cross training will result in further negatively perceived cuts in staffing, they will stop learning from one another.

When nurse managers are actually working to reduce the size of their teams, they must continually look to the welfare of their units while doing so. They can ensure that neither their units nor any of the individual performers are harmed if they consider the following:

Automation: Can any of the individual skills be automated? If so, will the automation eliminate the necessity for certain personnel? If it does, what will be the impact on the unit and what must be done so that the individual team members perceive the reduction as a positive measure?

Outsourcing: Can any of the required tasks be outsourced without reducing the quality of patient care? If the work is outsourced, can performance standards be maintained? Will the cost of the outsourcing be a burden on the unit's budget? If so, can senior management provide additional funds? How will the cost be recovered?

Substandard performance: Is any team member not carrying his or her share of the responsibility? If so, should that person be counseled, reprimanded, progressively disciplined, or merely let go? Keep in mind that team members will also observe the performance of each other. If they observe that an individual is not carrying his or her share of the workload and they believe that the nurse manager knows about it and has failed to correct the situation, they can become extremely difficult to manage. Such a failure will cost the nurse manager the team's respect and loyalty, and perhaps their presence.

Outmoded and unnecessary functions: Are there functions that have become unnecessary over time, such as charting by hand after a computerized system with charting software has been installed? If so, then the workload needs to be evaluated to see if an opportunity exists for a reduction in workforce.

Step Four: Establish an Agenda

As the team leader, the nurse manager has the responsibility to determine the team's agenda. An agenda is a step-by-step delineation of how work flows through the group. The leader is tasked with deciding what

individual task priorities are, where resources and effort should be concentrated, where the opportunities lie, what is worth taking advantage of, and what is worth passing on. The leader's job is to bring discipline to the hydralike work group that is the team.

As the leader of a dynamic performance team, the nurse manager has a job that isn't as clear-cut as it would be if he or she were manager of a baseball team or a military commander. Those leaders live and work in very structured environments, and their individual team members perform very well-defined roles. In nursing, the job isn't that easy. Staff nurses are well educated and individually capable professionals who want to perform their jobs with little or no supervision and who, on their own, frequently handle difficult assignments that do not fall into the realm of what is considered normal. Therefore, setting the nursing unit's agenda isn't a straightforward process. For one thing, day-to-day operations have no fixed body of rules. For another, what constitutes winning and losing is not always clearly defined. Finally, the individual performer's role can actually change as the circumstances demand it. Therefore, the astute nurse manager must identify different methods of establishing the team's agenda than would be used by a baseball coach or military officer. The approach described in the following sections is offered for consideration; however, if it is used, its contents should be modified to fit the unit's specific circumstances.

HAVE REGULAR TEAM MEETINGS

Meetings often provide an inexpensive method of keeping the team's agenda in front of all of the members. It is the leader's role to maintain a sense of consistency in these meetings, a job that can easily be done if the leader establishes and follows a standard format each time the team gets together. A variety of methods can be used, but whichever is chosen, the manager should stick to it and keep the meetings germane to team business.

WARNING *!*

Meetings have a way of being perceived as social gatherings and time off unless they are kept short and to the point. Good leaders will ensure that meetings are not held unless (a) there is no other way to disseminate the intended information, (b) there is a specific agenda of topics to be discussed, and (c) a definite time period is established for the meeting. Meetings should be run from an agenda, and once the agenda items have been covered, the meeting should be immediately adjourned and the attendees instructed to return to their work.

Convening a meeting just to get the individual members together is not a good idea. Only under rare circumstances should a get-together be held in the guise of a business meeting. The difference between a meeting and a get-together is simple: business meetings have agendas, get-togethers don't. For even the smallest meeting, an agenda should be available before the meeting is convened and minutes should be taken during the meeting. Otherwise, the meeting doesn't need to be held. There is no sense in holding a meeting if it is not planned or if the information discussed is not recorded.

REVIEW THE GOAL AND MISSION

Agenda setting goes beyond controlling meetings. An agenda also relates the mission and goals of the unit to the day-to-day challenges faced by the team, which the manager must discuss with the team and then take action to overcome. It is the job of the leader to keep the unit's vision, goals, and objectives in the forefront of each team member's mind. An agenda can be an effective tool for doing this. The nurse manager must simply make sure that each line item of the agenda is directly linked to a specific goal or objective and that the vision is clearly printed on the paper. The nurse manager goes over the vision quickly and, when each agenda item is discussed, makes sure that the goal to which it is linked is identified. This is referred to as *communicating the vision.*

REVIEW PROGRESS

The establishment of an agenda provides the nurse manager with an effective means of bringing the team's behavior in line with the vision. The nurse manager must continually reinforce the concept that the team's purpose is not simply to perform day-to-day functions but to achieve higher goals. Team progress should always be measured against the unit's established goals. The progress toward those goals is what the leader uses to motivate and reward the performance of the team.

Teams, no matter how well developed, often reach a point at which they are content to continue their performance in a mode that is both comfortable and not very challenging. This behavior (complacency), although certainly common enough, is a death knell for the dynamic nursing unit. As the leader of the unit, the nurse manager must keep the team motivated and excited. It is extremely important that the nurse manager keep every team member reaching toward a new goal and never be willing to accept the mediocrity that complacency produces.

The nurse manager can keep the tempo exciting and the individual team members motivated if the manager rewards performance by recognizing excellence and never tolerating mediocrity. When team members understand that they will excel only if the team excels, then the team will move forward.

Step Five: Create a Learning Environment

All members of the team must learn from one another. The opportunity to share experiences, talent, opinions, creativity, attitudes, and concepts is the biggest advantage of working with the challenges presented by the team concept.

Teams learn as they perform, and maintaining a record of successes and failures is important. The team leader should ensure that an accurate record of team accomplishments is kept and that it is continually updated. The membership of the team is rarely permanent, and the collective learning that can be developed through team effort must be passed on to new members as they come on board—or even to a new team leader, for that matter. Suppose that the administrative demands of the nursing unit grow to a point where it is physically impossible for the nurse manager to take an active daily leadership role in the operation of the team and an assistant is appointed to help. The nurse manager spends more and more time in his or her office performing other duties and has direct contact with the team less frequently, whereas the assistant spends most of his or her time interacting with the team. What must not occur is a situation in which team members argue with the new assistant that they have already done what the leader wants and have failed. The smart manager will prepare the assistant to assume the clinical side of the nurse manager's role, and one of the best ways to do that is to provide a record of what has been done and why it failed or succeeded.

KEEP A RECORD FOR THE TEAM

The great surveying team of Lewis and Clark kept a diary as they explored the West. Many professional researchers keep journals when they are working to solve a problem. If nurse managers maintain files that contain copies of reports and analyses, observations of team behavior, records of disciplinary concerns, comments on morale issues, personal notes and opinions, internal correspondence, and hard copies of all email related to specific work issues, they will have a comprehensive turnover portfolio to hand to new leaders or assistants as described earlier. This material can also serve as a means to bring new members up to speed on team history if nurse managers separate personal information from team issues.

REQUIRE THE TEAM TO SHARE INFORMATION

If the team develops any materials, whether through group or individual activity, the developed materials belong to the entire group. Failure to share should be considered detrimental to the best interests of the team, and the offender should be subject to the appropriate disciplinary action.

Every team member should be expected to share information with the rest of the group. This means that individual and team skills should be shared to the greatest extent possible. The actual form that teaching takes can vary to fit the specific circumstances of the nursing unit and the material that is to be shared. Some teaching venues can be informal, such as a team meeting (if appropriate notes of the meeting are taken); others are more structured, such as a formal training session.

MAKE GOOD BEHAVIOR LEARNED BEHAVIOR

One of the hardest things for a team to do is to make their good behavior routine. Therefore, as the leader of the team, the nurse manager should make it a requirement that the team work toward a goal of embedding its best practices.

If a member of the team develops a better way to do something, a competent authority should review it, and if it is approved, the new method should be shared with the entire team and thereafter should become part of the team's day-to-day practice. The nurse manager should write the procedure down and make sure that each member sees this description, then follow up to ensure that all members of the team are using the new procedure. When the manager sees the new procedure being practiced, he or she should offer congratulations and recognition; when the manager does not see it being used, he or she should ask why not and correct the situation immediately.

Every nursing unit can take team learning and embed it into its operational procedures. The organization should keep a listing of best practices and update it frequently. When a new, better method is discovered, it should supersede the old. Nurse managers should include in this document their performance tools, analytical reasoning processes, reporting requirements, performance methodologies, and processes for measurement and qualification, presented in a format that allows everyone to be made aware of them and permits easy updating and changing as necessary.

Step Six: Fix the Problem, Not the Blame

Two important parts of team building are absolutely critical to the success of a nursing unit:

1. Acceptance
2. Forgiveness

The team needs to keep its focus on moving forward toward the accomplishment of the goals and mission of the organization. Nothing can interrupt this focus more than an overzealous attempt to place blame (i.e., a witch hunt).

Things will go wrong. That is a part of nursing that is as predictable as change. Great organizations use these unfortunate occurrences as learning opportunities and not as excuses for persecution; the nursing unit should be no exception. This process of learning from adverse events, or at least a process very close to it, is used throughout the healthcare industry to examine why certain medical procedures give the results they do, and the knowledge gained is shared freely. Why should the day-to-day functioning of the individual nursing unit be any different? After all, the goals of both are identical—the improvement of patient care.

Problems are eliminated by building into the team a system of checks and balances. These checks and balances are part of a monitoring system that the leader can use to measure performance on a continual or at least a regular basis. If a leader does not incorporate a system for monitoring the performance of the team into normal business practice, then what goes wrong is the leader's fault and no one else's. The team leader's job is to find ways to anticipate problems and to correct them before they become critical (or actually to prevent them from occurring). If the efforts of the team are brought to a halt by a problem and the individual members are busy pointing fingers and accusing each other, then the blame is always the leader's and never anyone else's. Therefore, there is never a need for a witch hunt.

Those teams that have achieved significant renown in their fields often have been found to practice a technique for fixing problems instead of blame that has been dubbed the *loose construction method*. This phrase refers to a loose interpretation of the U.S. Constitution, and it means, "Anything that is not expressly forbidden is permitted." Nurse managers can apply this technique in their units by letting it be known that any team member is free to complete assignments any way he or she wishes as long as nothing is done that has been expressly forbidden. For example, if the unit cares for cardiac patients, then expressly forbidden job practices might be the use of treatments that are out of date and failure to comply with proven quality treatment standards. How team members actually care for a specific patient, as long as they don't violate these mandates, is the team's decision, not the nurse manager's. By not handicapping the team's performance by requiring a myriad of specific procedures, the intelligent nurse manager is actually encouraging team members to develop, on their own, solutions to problems that occur.

Of course, there is an opposite approach, known as *strict constructionism*. Sometimes the application of this more rigid technique is just the thing that helps a team get moving in the proper direction. Strict constructionism is another constitutional law term. It means, "Only what is expressly permitted can be done." This approach forces the team to follow rigid performance practices, and if the team's goals require attention to close tolerances, tight adherence to rules, and even a focus on appearances, then this is the way to operate the team. Managers will find this type of leadership applied in many nursing units in which little deviation is allowed from established rules and regulations.

Step Seven: Delegate

One of the most effective methods of helping the individual performer, and consequently the team, to grow is to pursue an aggressive program of delegation and cross training. Although, realistically, not everyone can be expected to perform proficiently at all work levels in the organization, each team member should be flexible enough to lend a hand in at least one performance area that is different from his or her primary focus. To facilitate this learning, the nurse manager must provide the opportunity and the motivation to learn. All too often, some team members will be reluctant to share specific skills, and other team members will be reluctant to take on additional responsibilities. Providing the motivation for this exchange of knowledge is the team leader's responsibility. One of the best ways to accomplish this without creating dissension is to delegate.

Delegation is one of the most frequently overlooked responsibilities of the team leader. Although individual team members must be allowed to perform their distinctive work, the unit's growth will be enhanced if each staff member can take on a larger portion of the overall performance requirements or act as a backup to another team member. Nurse managers, as team leaders, cannot do everything, regardless of their personal skill and dedication. If they try, experience says that their overall efficiency will be significantly reduced, and this will have a detrimental effect on the future success of their nursing units.

This is a tough lesson for people who manage nursing units and have put their hearts and souls into developing them. But it is a reality of growth. Sooner or later, the nurse manager's job will grow to the point that he or she can no longer do it all. The manager who continues to feel that he or she must do everything or must closely direct the efforts of others to ensure quality performance is missing the essence of leadership. Leaders are responsible for seeing that the job gets done and for ensuring its quality. It is not the responsibility of managers to perform all of the actual work. To the contrary, a major portion of leaders' responsibility is teaching others to be proficient. Historically, literally thousands of truly gifted entrepreneurs have failed to develop their businesses because they did not trust their subordinates to do a good job. Leaders of virtually every type of enterprise and in every vocation, including nursing, are included in this category. These individuals, as their responsibilities grow, will see a change in their primary obligation from actually doing the work to overseeing, guiding, directing, and motivating others as *they* do the work. Leaders in growing organizations should perform work only when it cannot be accomplished by others, when qualified junior personnel are not available, or when they are demonstrating what is expected. The typical military nurse provides a good example of this understanding of responsibility. As an officer, he or she will not perform a menial task that can be accomplished by hospital corpsmen (enlisted personnel). In the military, not behaving in this way would be considered detrimental to good order and discipline.

An important question is what happens when qualified junior personnel are not available. Does what has just been said about separation of responsibilities mean that leaders should not have things to do? Of course not. Team leaders have specific performance functions, and those functions are inherent in the leadership position as functions that either cannot or should not be delegated. The nurse manager, as the team leader, must decide what tasks cannot be delegated, and the list will differ from team to team, based on the quality and experience of the team's membership. If the nursing unit is blessed with an extraordinary group of highly skilled performers, then the nurse manager will have the opportunity to delegate a wider range of responsibilities. If, however, the team is full of inexperienced newly graduated nurses who are still in an elementary learning mode, there will be less delegation, and those things that are delegated will be less complex and require more follow-up. Regardless of the experience level of the team members, however, nurse managers must always force themselves to delegate.

Many leaders resist delegation. These nondelegators believe that they can perform tasks better and faster than other people. Senior administrators and highly experienced managers come by this belief honestly, through past experience, and should not be ridiculed for holding it. Most successful healthcare organizations got that way because their administrative leaders had a history of being great individual performers.

Great performers develop more than just their individual skills; they develop a belief in their own ability. Truly outstanding performers are absolutely confident that they can accomplish whatever has to be done, quickly, efficiently, and at a lower cost than can another individual. Why? Because outstanding performers have proven their ability to do so over and over again. Their confidence comes from success, and the more successful a person has been, the greater confidence that person will possess. It is natural, then, for outstanding performers to want to rely on what they have confidence in—themselves.

As responsibilities grow, however, performance becomes more complex. More and more of the manager's time is spent in new roles, and additional skills are required to get the entire job done. The responsibilities of directing a nursing unit are just too complicated and varied to allow the manager to continue in the previous performer mode. The responsibilities of leadership dictate that a highly qualified and motivated manager will be forced to give over part of his or her work to others and assume the role of facilitator of another person's success.

It is natural that highly motivated leaders should experience frustration when work is done more slowly than they themselves are used to doing it. Some even get irritated when errors occur that need correcting. In addition, almost every person who has built a successful career as a high-quality performer will be amazed, at least initially, when someone new uses a different approach to perform a specific task. In short, it is difficult to give up what one really enjoys accomplishing.

The process of delegation is critical to the continued growth of every organization, however, and those people who don't, can't, or won't delegate create real problems in their institutions. When leaders continue to insist on either performing themselves or micromanaging the performance of others, they run the risk of infuriating and demoralizing their subordinates, which is a primary reason for labor problems (e.g., strikes, union difficulties, turnover, absenteeism).

What, then, is delegation? And what is the leader's role in the process?

Delegation is simply the act of assigning both the authority and the responsibility for performance. Another member of the team is given the authority to perform a certain task and the responsibility to ensure that it is done correctly. This means that the team member who is doing the work has the right to make choices, make decisions, use discretion, and employ personal methods. In addition, the team member must be held accountable for the actions used to complete the work and for the quality of the performance. Although the team member should be free to

decide how the task will be accomplished, he or she must ensure that the method used allows for the completion, accuracy, and timeliness; is approved and of high quality; and is centered on providing quality patient care at low risk to the unit.

What is the team leader's role?

The team leader's role starts with the actual delegation. Superior leaders make sure that they delegate both elementary jobs and difficult ones—work that brings high return and work that provides no return at all. Good leaders don't keep the high-reward jobs for themselves and give the subordinates the **scut work**. Giving the team all of the difficult or thankless work is commonly referred to as *dumping*. When a leader dumps assignments on junior personnel, delegation will do little to enhance team performance. To the contrary, this type of action will only serve to reduce overall team performance.

The simple act of delegating the work and the authority and responsibility for its performance does not reduce the leader's authority or overall responsibility for the success of the team. The team leader always retains the authority to ensure accurate and timely completion of the delegated task. The difference lies in how a leader applies this authority when working with subordinate personnel. A good leader exercises this authority through a monitoring process that allows the leader to observe progress, offer suggestions for improvement, make recommendations for change, and assign more help to the project without interfering with the direction or actual performance itself (Table 20-2).

Good leaders are careful to channel their leadership through the person who has been delegated the authority for the project. This means that the team leader should not go to anyone other than the person who has received the authority and responsibility for the job to monitor the progress of the work. The job has been delegated; therefore, the team leader should offer suggestions for change and any alternative ideas he or she might have only to the person who has the delegated authority. In addition, the reward for and recognition of success should also come through the delegated junior or, if the leader wishes, at least in the physical presence of the delegated junior.

Scut work refers to the type of work that people of a certain status do not want to perform. For instance, in a hospital nursing unit, the typical registered nurse would consider scrubbing the floor to be scut work. Although he or she realizes the importance of a clean floor to the good order and discipline of the unit, it is not a job that a nurse would accept without considerable pressure from a supervisor.

TABLE 20-2

Leader's and Performer's Responsibilities in Delegation

Action	Leader's Responsibility	Performer's Responsibility
Identify the job to be performed	Give clear instructions	Ask pertinent questions to clarify
Decide course of action	Outline expectations	Lay out and design performance
Perform work	Check and guide for accuracy, timeliness, and quality	Ensure accuracy, timeliness, and quality
Review for accuracy	Perform interim and final review	Perform interim review
Analyze for quality	Perform interim and final analysis	Perform interim analysis
Submit criticism	Deliver to delegatee only	Deliver to assisting personnel
Give recognition and reward	Deliver to delegatee and individual performer in presence of delegatee	Deliver to assisting personnel
Submit final project	Deliver to senior management	Deliver to manager
Receive credit	Pass on to delegatee	Accept if task accomplished without help; otherwise, pass on to assisting personnel

The team leader's role in the delegation process is one of tolerant facilitator or coach. The team leader gives out the assignments, guides the performance, and ensures accurate compliance. Throughout the time the delegated task is being completed, the team leader reviews the work for accuracy and timely progression. It is critical that the leader perform this follow-up, because it is the leader who is ultimately responsible for the completion of the task. Failure to follow up may mean that the project will be done wrong or that the necessary deadline will not be met. If the team leader has not periodically checked on the project while it is in progress, he or she is responsible for any failure that may occur, and no part of this responsibility can be laid at the feet of the performer. (This is separate from the fact that the leader always retains ultimate responsibility.)

The purpose of delegation is twofold:

1. To accomplish the work
2. To improve the performance capability of subordinates

Team leaders can realize the benefits of delegation if they (1) exercise discretion when they delegate, (2) ensure clarity when they outline the project, (3) exercise patience when they guide performance, (4) use sensitivity when they offer suggestions and corrections, (5) are enthusiastic when they recognize excellence and, finally, (6) reward noteworthy performance.

Reluctance to delegate is evident when a team leader asks the question, "Do I just give 'em the ball?" The answer of course is, "Probably not." If team leaders use sensible management practices, they will be careful when passing the ball; that is, team leaders will not give out the work and disappear. Instead, they will be available to provide assistance when requested and will periodically check on progress. In other words, they will follow up. When this follow-up is performed correctly, the team and its individual performers will truly believe they are controlling the project and the team leader will be comfortable with how the work is progressing. Delegation provides an excellent opportunity for the team leader to practice **management by wandering around**. The mere act of **wandering** will put the team leader into contact with the team to ask gentle, persuasive questions that will

Management by wandering around is leadership practice in which the manager turns his or her casual movements through the business environment into a leadership opportunity. As the leader passes through the unit, he or she will talk to one person, thank another, remind someone of an upcoming event, let drop important information, casually follow up on a subject, and so on. By keeping the contact informal and low-key, the leader can verify, affirm, motivate, and encourage others without creating the perception of micromanagement. Hewlett-Packard is credited with first using this method, and it gained popularity in the 1980s when it was showcased in the book by Tom Peters and Robert H. Waterman, Jr., *In Search of Excellence* (New York, 1982, Harper and Row).

Wandering is moving in a manner that appears to be casual and nonpurposeful. The word is used deliberately here in place of the word walking, which is defined as "movement of purpose, or in a direct and intended manner."

quietly steer the team onto the desired course without providing the perception of micromanagement.

One last word about delegation: The team must perceive that the leader is delegating work that will enhance the team's capability or that is for the good of the unit or organization. The team leader must never be perceived as delegating work that he or she simply doesn't want to do. Dumping unwanted or undesirable work is *not* delegation, and such a practice can be disastrous to the team. Team leaders need to make sure that they delegate most of the good jobs and keep the undesirable work for themselves.

WARNING !

Not all work in the nursing unit can or even should be delegated. Nurse managers are responsible for ensuring that the subordinate being asked to perform the work has the training, education, and skill level to fulfill the task satisfactorily. Much attention is being drawn today to the delegation of nursing tasks to nonnursing personnel. It is not the purpose of this text to determine what should be delegated; that is for individual organizations. But all managers should use appropriate professional judgment when assigning tasks to subordinate personnel.

WHEN TEAMS WON'T FOLLOW

In ancient days, leaders had very direct methods of dealing with resistant followers. As was noted earlier, Julius Caesar made it a standard procedure in the Roman army to put to death one legionnaire in ten if a single soldier acted cowardly. Genghis Khan immediately executed any challenger to his authority, and even Queen Elizabeth I of England routinely used the Tower of London's headsman to eliminate dissension. The historical right of discipline sets the stage for the natural tendency of people in charge to overreact when their requests are met with resistance or defiance.

The propensity of leaders to want to have things their way is described in many stories of rebellion found in literature. Great literary works such as *The Caine Mutiny* and *Mutiny on the Bounty* have as their theme the consequences of failed leadership.

These historical and literary chronicles, however, actually deal not with leadership but with command. As has been discussed earlier, the difference between leadership and command is significant, and in today's healthcare environment the command method of directing the efforts of others, although still frequently employed, is losing acceptance in every circle. Today's nursing leaders need a new way to look at the dynamics of interaction between leader and follower and the things that can go awry between them.

The Foundation of Responsibility

If one thinks of the relationship between leaders and followers as similar to the relationship between parents and children, it is easier to understand the special relationship that leaders and followers share. This statement should not be construed to mean that leaders should assume a parental approach in managing their teams. Rather, it is simply a statement that good leaders, like good parents, recognize without even thinking about it that they are responsible for nurturing those who look to them for guidance. Except in cases of willful disobedience, when the team doesn't perform, then just as when a child misbehaves, the fault lies with the leader who is failing to properly communicate his or her values and expectations to the followers (absent, of course, some psychopathology in the follower).

If you accept this analogy, then you must accept that the first questions good leaders ask themselves (just as do good parents) are the following: What am I doing wrong? Why don't the team members do what I want them to do? Have I properly explained the reasons I want the team to do this thing? Have I given mixed signals, acting one way and telling them another? Have I acted in an exemplary manner, so that the team members will have a model to emulate? Have I let them go too far or given more latitude than the team has earned? In short, have I been lax in assessing the team's ability, and the ability of the individual team members, to make decisions and judgments?

These questions are important to successful team building, and leaders need to pose these questions to themselves when things go wrong. Even before asking themselves these questions, however, leaders should be asking themselves another, more important set of questions that fall under the heading of "What kind of failure is this?" Failure can come from different directions. Understanding what kind of failure the manager is dealing with is critical to getting the team back on the right path.

FAILURE OF A VISION

When a vision is conceived, it must be compatible with what is achievable given the resources of the organization, the motivational ability of the leader, and the talents, capabilities, and enthusiasm of the team. If these factors are not properly considered, a failure of vision may result. Some of the special conditions in which this kind of failure can occur are the following:

The vision is not motivating or challenging: A vision must be capable of providing motivation to those who are tasked with achieving it. If the vision is too narrowly conceived, the team is likely to lose its motivation and enthusiasm. This will cause the team's most talented members to look elsewhere for the challenge they desire.

The vision is overshadowed: It is extremely hard to keep team members motivated if they feel they are working on something that will only earn them second place. Even the best vision becomes difficult to manage when the team knows that someone else has developed a better idea.

The vision is perceived as being unachievable: If the vision is too grandiose, the effect it has is not motivational; to the contrary, it can be discouraging. Team members can come to believe they are wasting their time on something that will never be realized.

FAILURE OF A MISSION

The failure of a mission is almost always caused by a failure in planning. Good leaders are supposed to know where the group is to end up and why. It is not uncommon for leaders to develop a sense of mission that blinds them to larger considerations. For example, even if the team is able to complete the mission, the cost to the team may be so high that the team may be irreparably harmed. The individual team members may come to believe that the mission was unnecessary and the cost to the team unwarranted. This type of failure will cause the team to lose confidence in the team leader.

Good leaders know why and what they are doing and how the mission fits into the larger context of the organization, so that they don't squander resources and lose the trust and confidence of the team. This requires leaders to develop and maintain good communication links with other groups within and outside of the organization, so that they can adjust the mission.

One of the best methods for maintaining communication with other groups is credited to Wall Street analyst Craig Gordon, director of OTA–Off The Record Research. He calls his process *market checks* and it operates like this: One member of the team is assigned to constantly scout the external competition and internal company departments. This person determines what activities these areas are performing, what changes these actions may cause that may affect the mission, what these activities indicate is seen in the immediate future of the marketplace that the team leader may not see, and what actions the other groups are planning to deal with the perceived changes. If the manager arranges for information concerning similar issues to be brought into the group and constantly updated, the chances are slim that his or her team will fail in its mission. The elimination of mission failure will ensure that the leader retains the confidence of the team.

PERFORMANCE FAILURE

There are times when the mission is attainable and the vision is proper for the team, but the group still fails to achieve them. In this situation, the leader should thoroughly investigate the circumstances surrounding the failure. This investigation begins with the leader's asking the following questions:

- Was the project properly planned?
- Was the project beyond the expertise and capability of the team?
- Did the team possess the proper training to accomplish the task?
- Did the environment change, and did the change go unanswered?
- Were there proper amounts of the required resources available to the team?

If the leader answers no to any of these questions, therein lies the reason for the failure. Failure that starts out with simple mistakes only increases internal resistance to the mission. If the team perceives the possibility of failure, its members are far less likely to support the mission (no one wants to work aggressively on a project knowing that it will fail). It is the rare individual who is willing to work when the proper resources, training, time, and safety measures are not provided, especially if the person feels that he or she will be held responsible for any failure.

When failure in performance is encountered, the professional leader looks long and hard for the reasons. If the leader has acted responsibly when setting up the team, has provided it with professional support, proper resources, and training, and has made sure that the team operates in safe conditions, and still the team fails to execute, perhaps there is reason to believe that the team may have caused the failure. Even in these circumstances, however, the leader is never really free of some of the responsibility for failure.

LEADERSHIP FAILURE

To the failures of leadership that were covered earlier, two more sins can be added:

1. *Simple-mindedness:* Sometimes referred to as *obtuseness* or even as harshly as *stupidity,* this sin is committed by those leaders who do not recognize the need for change. Leadership is situational, and when situations change, leaders must change and make those changes clear to their teams. If leaders do not do this, they have failed utterly. They may still occupy the position, but they will no longer be leading.

   Think of leading a team as heading a school of fish swimming in the ocean and it is easy to understand the effect obtuseness can have. When the lead fish zigs, the school zigs. When the lead fish zags, the school zags. But when the lead fish stops paying attention to the environment and does nothing, mistakes occur. The lead fish, unaware of changes in the environment, can swim right into the mouth of a larger fish, and when this happens, the school has to scramble for its life. The school will find a new lead fish that knows how and when to zig and zag properly.

Leadership is like being the head fish; those who allow themselves to become unaware of the environment, staff needs, or the actual circumstances surrounding the team will always lead the group into peril. This type of behavior should cost the leader the right to lead.

2. *Arrogance:* Another sin is arrogance. Leadership is all about the willingness to embrace responsibility. This means that leaders must act in a responsible manner at all times. It is unwise for leaders to display a self-serving attitude and an ego swelled with power, because there is always someone around who is willing to challenge authority or, worse yet, to undermine it.

Superior leaders do not put much stock in the titles or trappings normally associated with their positions. Instead, they put the needs of their teams before their own and concentrate on maintaining good relationships with the individual team members.

It Is the Manager's Responsibility to Lead

The archives of business are full of stories about people in managerial positions who, when insubordination occurs in the team, assume that the responsibility for the existing negativity belongs to the team rather than to its leadership. Leaders who make this assumption have taken the first step toward obscurity. In fact, those managers who continually look for someone to blame are extremely poor leaders. The attempt of leaders to shift the responsibility for failure to others will cause increased resistance within their teams. This action is universally considered poor leadership and has no place in a dynamic nursing environment.

One of the basic responsibilities in leading a team is to demonstrate the willingness to listen to what the team is saying—not just the superficial dialogue that passes between leader and team members but the interpretation of the communication as well. For example, when the group tells the leader that things are going well, the interpretation could be, "Provide more leadership." When the group begins to question the authority of the leader, what is really being said is, "Accept the responsibilities you have been given." And when a group openly challenges the leader, it is expressing a desire that the person in charge listen and find a better way to elicit cooperation. The human animal is not, by nature, reluctant to follow. As a matter of fact, the vast majority of humanity consists of followers, so when a group of people rebel against leadership, it is a safe bet that the action has been taken solely because other methods of seeking assistance have been tried and failed.

Good leaders continually ask themselves, Am I exercising leadership? Am I responsible? Am I eliciting the cooperation of the team, or am I commanding? Am I asking questions and listening to the answers I am being given? Am I placing the needs of the team ahead of my own needs and my ego?

Leading a team involves the expenditure of energy and the completion of work. It is not enough to embrace the responsibility of team leadership. To be a superior team leader, the nurse manager must eliminate barriers to the unit's success. However, there are times when those barriers are total fabrications of an individual's mind. Human beings are continually drawing lines in the sand: "I'll go this far, and after that, it is someone else's responsibility." If the leader does this, the leader is not totally embracing the responsibility of leadership, and his or her team will see and know it.

It Is the Team Leader's Job to Embrace Responsibility

Many would-be leaders fail to embrace responsibility because they continually provide themselves with conscious and unconscious reasons to avoid it. "I want the team to grow into its capabilities" and "I can't do everything" are statements that demonstrate a lack of willingness to embrace responsibility.

Embracing responsibility means that, even if the leader has delegated responsibility to another, the leader never really lets go of his or her own responsibility. Instead, the leader acts as a sort of backup, someone who will provide a helping hand or a listening ear. The leader is there, checking on progress, asking questions, providing resources, helping to meet changes in the environment, but carefully staying out of the light just enough so that good follow-up doesn't become micromanagement. In truth, a good leader shares responsibility with the team, rather than delegating it. This means that, although the team may have the operational responsibility, the leader maintains active support by offering guidance and helping the team stay out of trouble and, at the same time, safeguarding his or her position of ultimate responsibility.

If group members feel that their leader has left them completely alone, they may react by feeling that the leader is no longer needed or that the leader doesn't care enough about them.

It Is the Team Leader's Responsibility to Elicit Cooperation

Few people can simply ask a group for support and receive 100% of its capabilities. This challenge is acknowledged in the actions taken by the leader to elicit cooperation. Rare is the individual who is so admired by the team that the group is willing to perform without first witnessing effort by the leader.

Eliciting the cooperation of the group means gaining everyone's cooperation, not just that of the dedicated and hardworking. The greater the proportion of team members who actively support the leader's point of view, the greater the opportunity for success. Why? Because individual team members reinforce each other's viewpoints.

There is also the proverbial "rotten apple" syndrome to consider when eliciting cooperation. If a nurse manager is not able to obtain cooperation from the entire team, he or she runs the risk of leaving an individual who has opposing views in the middle of the group. One negative individual can easily counter the support of an entire group. It is a fact, albeit a bewildering one, that the negative displaces the positive faster than the positive erases the negative.

Nurse managers obtain support for their ideas by providing their groups with as much information as possible. The old saying about keeping the troops in the dark and on a steady diet of manure (commonly known as the "mushroom approach") is far more than a nasty joke. What really makes this expression deplorable is that this is a common practice. Many, many leaders use this approach until it backfires on them—and that only happens once. Every team has a right to be kept informed, and the leader should take great pains always to respect that right.

Really good leaders never keep their teams in doubt. They establish a regular process of communication, whether through team meetings, informal conferences, or a team newsletter—the mode doesn't really matter. Dynamic leaders share all of the information they can, and when asked about information that, for whatever reason, should not or cannot be shared, they never lie to their teams. Instead, they simply tell the team members that they haven't been authorized to discuss that issue and that when they are able, an answer will be forthcoming. It is better to be considered left out of the loop than to be thought of as a liar.

Communication is a two-way street. The team and the leader both have a right to information, and each has a right to quick responses from the other. A leader who delays in providing information because he or she fears the impact is not helping the team. If the team delays in transmitting a message to the leader that a problem exists, the leader's ability to alleviate it may be limited. If the leader delays in providing additional information that will help the team work through a challenge, a failure may result.

Finally, eliciting cooperation is something that continually travels in full circles. When the team members see the leader providing information and support, they will be more willing to give their support, and when the leader sees the team being more supportive, the leader is almost always willing to provide more information. The leader has the responsibility to start this cycle and keep it going. If the leader approaches this process half-heartedly, the results are often worse than if nothing is done. The leader must understand that, when action is required, only with the full cooperation of the team will success be achieved.

It Is Everyone's Responsibility to Tell the Truth

Few people lie outright, but most people don't tell the truth, the whole truth, and nothing but the truth. Many people in the healthcare industry, and in much of society for that matter, place value on evasion and partial disclosure. People constantly work in environments in which it is both acceptable and preferable to behave so. However, the individual developing a team must make every attempt to eliminate this practice. Failure to make full disclosure and to live with the consequences of this disclosure often brings organizations and the people who operate them to the brink of scandal and turns minor infractions into major embarrassments. An example can be seen in the Monica Lewinsky scandal. If President Clinton had owned up to his relationship with Ms. Lewinsky, he would have received a certain amount of ridicule, but the matter would never have been sufficient to warrant impeachment proceedings. Instead, he was accused of perjury for lying to a grand jury, an act that could have caused him the presidency.

So why do people lie? Are there really such things as "white" lies? Can lying ever be permissible? Most societies say that lying is permissible if telling the truth would cause people pain. But in the stress-filled environment that is the nursing unit, something that one person can handle may well cause another person pain, and many nurses use lies to spare themselves more than to spare other people.

Establishing truth as the foundation of teamwork is fundamental to team success. Truth, however, begins at home. Members of the nursing unit team, and especially the leader, must be honest with themselves before others can appreciate them for being so. The probability of truth is established in a team by requiring each member to convey information accurately. In itself, this is a form of the truth. Team members learn to trust one another by knowing that they can rely upon what they are told. Truth is critical to the success of a team. A team, and most certainly a team leader, should never condone the presence of liars or individuals who deliberately misrepresent information. These people and their habits, regardless of their intentions, will ruin the team.

SUMMARY

- There is no concrete approach one can take to develop a team, no single method of building a relationship of trust, communication, and directed energy. Leaders can only give their best efforts to this purpose.
- Team building is far easier if leaders remember the following three key concepts of leadership:
  1. Elicit cooperation; don't demand it.
  2. Listen carefully.
  3. Place the needs of the team above one's own.
- Organizations that are team oriented traditionally outperform command-based organizations.
- It is highly recommended that the team concept be applied whenever possible to help the nursing unit and nursing leader create the opportunity for success.

FINAL THOUGHTS

Preparing the nursing unit and each member of its staff to perform as a dynamic team is the one true responsibility of the nurse manager. If the staff members can be molded into a smoothly running, cohesive team, the success of the unit and the nurse manager is guaranteed. When the members of an exceptional team pull together to perform even the most mundane of tasks, the quality of patient care is always enhanced.

Nurse managers should make it their top priority to develop and reward team performance. It is the one sure way to guarantee an exceptional nursing unit.

THE NURSE MANAGER SPEAKS

For many years, the nursing profession has lagged behind the general business world in promoting teamwork and leadership as the number one priority. Although there are many excellent reasons for this, the development of both qualities must now be increased in today's demanding and ever-changing nursing environment.

Teamwork is the essence of performance, because a well-developed team will always outperform a group of outstanding individuals. Being a high-quality individual performer is no longer enough to be considered exceptional. Today, the exceptional performer is the individual who builds quality into the team and, as a result, into the nursing unit.

SUGGESTED READINGS

Ackoff RL: *The democratic corporation: a radical prescription for re-creating corporate American and rediscovering success,* Oxford, UK, 1999, Oxford University Press.

Adams S: *Don't step in the leadership: a Dilbert book,* Kansas City, Mo, 1999, Andrews McMeel.

Ailes R, Krausher J: *You are the message: getting what you want by being who you are,* New York, 1989, Doubleday.

Alessandra A: *The platinum rule,* New York, 1998, Warner Books.

Allee V: *The knowledge evolution: expanding organizational intelligence,* Newton, Mass, 1997, Butterworth-Heinemann.

Baskin K: *Corporate DNA: learning from life,* Newton, Mass, 1998, Butterworth-Heinemann.

Bennis W: *The corporate culture survival guide,* San Francisco, 1999, Jossey-Bass.

Bennis W, Nanus B: *Leaders: the strategies for taking charge,* ed 1, New York, 1985, Harper and Row.

Blanchard K: *The heart of a leader: insights on the art of influence,* Colorado Springs, Colo, 2004, Honor Books/ Cook Communications.

Boylan M: *The power to get in,* New York, 1998, St. Martin's Press.

Bridges W: *The character of organizations: using jungian type in organizational development,* Upper Saddle River, NJ, 1993, Prentice-Hall.

Brown JS: *Seeing differently: insights on innovation,* Cambridge, Mass, 1997, Harvard Business School Press.

Bruce A, Pepitone J: *Motivating employees,* New York, 1999, McGraw-Hill.

Cameron KS: *Diagnosing and changing organizational culture: based on the competing values framework,* Reading, Mass, 1998, Addison-Wesley.

Carlson R: *Don't sweat the small stuff at work,* New York, 1999, Simon and Schuster.

Connor D: *Managing at the speed of change,* New York, 1993, Villard Books.

Covey S: *The seven habits of highly effective people: powerful lessons in personal change,* New York, 1990, Fireside.

Detmer JW: *Breaking the constraints to world-class performance,* Milwaukee, 1998, ASQ Quality Press.

Donnithorne LR: *The West Point way of leadership,* New York, 1993, Doubleday.

Elfers J: *The forty-eight powers of law,* New York, 1998, Viking Press.

Goleman PM: *Working with emotional intelligence,* New York, 1998, Bantam Books.

Greenberg J: *Behavior in organizations,* Upper Saddle River, NJ, 1999, Prentice Hall.

Harbour J: *The basics of performance management*, Shelton, Conn, 1997, Productivity.

Helgesen S: *Web of inclusion: a new architecture for building great institutions*, New York, 1995, Doubleday.

Hersey P: *Management of organizational behavior*, Upper Saddle River, NJ, 1998, Prentice Hall.

Hill N: *Napoleon Hill's keys to success*, New York, 1997, Plume.

Hill N, Stone C: *Success through a positive mental attitude*, New York, 1992, Simon and Schuster.

Hirschhorn K: *The workplace within: psychodynamics of organizational life*, Cambridge, Mass, 1990, MIT Press.

Jenson W: *Simplicity: the competitive advantage in a world of more, better, faster*, New York, 2000, Perseus.

Johnson S: *"Yes" or "no": a guide to better decisions*, New York, 1993, HarperBusiness.

Kirschner R: *Dealing with people you can't stand*, New York, 1997, McGraw-Hill.

Kriegel R, Brandt D: *Sacred cows make the best burgers*, New York, 1997, Warner Books.

Lissick M, Roos J: *The next common sense*, London, 1999, Nicholas Brealey.

Lloyd K: *Jerks at work*, Franklin Lakes, NJ, 1999, Career Press.

Mackay H: *Swim with the sharks*, New York, 1988, Ivy Books.

Mackay H: *Pushing the envelope*, New York, 1999, Ballantine Books.

Maister D: *True professionalism: the courage to care about your people, your clients and your career*, New York, 1997, Free Press.

McCormack M: *What they don't teach you at the Harvard Business School: notes from a street-smart executive*, New York, 1988, Bantam Doubleday.

Melohn T: *The new partnership*, New York, 1996, Wiley.

Muihead BK: *High-velocity leadership: faster, cheaper, better*, New York, 1999, HarperBusiness.

Musashi M, Harris V: *The book of five rings*, New York, 1992, Bantam Books.

Randall K: *The twelve truths about surviving and succeeding at the office: and some that aren't very nice*, New York, 1997, Berkley Trade/Penguin.

Reiman J: *Thinking for a living: creating ideas that revitalize your business, career, and life*, Athens, Ga, 2001, Longstreet Press.

Roberts W: *Leadership secrets of Attila the Hun*, New York, 1994, Time Warner.

Schon D: *The reflective practitioner: how professionals think in action*, New York, 1984, Basic Books.

Scott C: *Organizational vision, values, and mission*, Menlo Park, Calif, 1994, Crisp.

Sennett R: *The corrosion of character*, New York, 1998, Norton.

Senge DP: *The fifth discipline: the art and practice of the learning organization*, New York, 1994, Doubleday.

Stone D: *Difficult conversations: how to discuss what matters most*, New York, 1999, Bantam Books.

Wheatley M: *A simpler way*, San Francisco, 1996, Berrett-Koehler.

Managing Training and Education in Health Care

OUTLINE

LEARNING SYNOPSIS

Upon successful completion of this chapter, readers will possess a fundamental understanding of the role played by training and education in the operation of a healthcare facility and nursing unit, and their importance to the patient's attitude, perception, and treatment.

OBJECTIVES

1. Describe the critical aspects of the modern training model
2. Explain what a training needs assessment is and how it is developed
3. Describe how the organization's training activities are planned and implemented after the training needs assessment is completed
4. Identify the learning principles that guide the development of training activities
5. Discuss the major aspects of social learning theory and explain how this theory applies to the nursing unit
6. Identify the aspects of adult educational theory that apply to the nursing unit
7. Discuss why the evaluation of training is important and why it is one of the most controversial aspects of training programs
8. Discuss the importance of patient training and describe the methods that can be used to provide it

Every individual associated with the healthcare industry is unique and possesses a different level of formal education, professional training, individual skills, and personal ability. Nevertheless, a few common threads can be observed in every nursing unit. For example, staff nurses will have attended a formal nursing school at an accredited university, and new unit clerks will have graduated from high school and attended either a trade school or a college. However, the completion of formal education, no matter to what level, does not necessarily make an employee proficient in his or her specific job. Many employees start work without having developed all of the skills and knowledge necessary to perform their jobs at the level expected. This situation is exacerbated by the fact that the healthcare industry is dynamic and requires the continual development and/or enhancement of performance skills. As practices and technology change and improve, the complexity of performance increases, so that there is a continuing need for specialized training. One of the nurse manager's major responsibilities is to assist his or her subordinates in developing the specific job skills necessary to perform well in the unit. This activity is usually referred to as *training.*

Most early educational theories were based on the belief that the fundamental purpose of the educational process was to transmit the totality of human knowledge from one generation to the next, in a sort of educational continuum. This was a workable assumption only as long as the quantity of knowledge was small enough to be managed collectively by the educational system and the rate of change in that knowledge remained relatively insignificant. In today's highly technical world, however, these conditions simply do not apply. Instead, the nursing profession operates during a period of explosive expansion of knowledge and continual technologic change. Nursing is an environment in which cultural and technologic change is the only constant. This means that it is no longer possible to pass the totality of human knowledge from one generation to the next. In fact, it is extremely hard to keep pace with the changes on a minute-by-minute basis. The effects of this dynamic environment on education are twofold:

1. *Formal education is no longer primarily or exclusively directed toward children:* Over the past three decades, the focus of formal education has shifted greatly to encompass more and more opportunities for adults. In fact, many of the educational tools being developed are specifically formulated to fit the working and living patterns of adults.

2. *An educational partnership has been created:* The dynamic nursing environment has forced the healthcare industry to foster a partnership between the educator and the working professional so that learning occurs every day in and outside of the working environment using both structured and unstructured methods.

Today, the process of intellectual and performance enhancement (education) is considered to be something that occurs constantly during conscious human activity and can be continued even in dormant periods of rest. Therefore, people who wish to lead others or who endeavor to guide the direction and quality of performance in the healthcare industry must be aware of several issues pertaining to education:

- How people learn
- What they need to learn
- What learning processes can be used
- How to teach

Most people, in fact, will need to be taught how to learn or, at a minimum, how to enhance their learning skills so that they can learn efficiently enough to keep pace with the changing environment that surrounds them and to absorb new information as it becomes available and affects them.

Every organization in the healthcare industry has its own specific goals and is affected by the evolution of the goals of the industry at large. The attainment of these goals requires the organization to involve itself aggressively in the training of its staff, because, without trained personnel, the organization will fail. For this reason, most hospitals employ specialized training personnel. These trainers are either independent training contractors or hospital employees who are assigned directly to the nursing service or serve in special training and education departments.

Internal training departments are generally responsible for administering ongoing employee training and developing specialized programs; however, nurse managers are often extensively involved in the training process. For example, a new employee must be taught performance standards, specific performance requirements, and specialized tasks as well as receive instruction in new nursing or medical practices applicable to the unit.

Trained personnel are the key to the successful operation of a nursing unit and of the hospital overall. Proper employee training almost always leads to higher individual productivity, fewer accidents or mistakes, lower patient risk, high morale, greater pride in performance, and, ultimately, enhanced patient care.

Regardless of whether educational activities are planned for the unit's staff or the organization's customers, the basic model of the training function and the basic procedure remain the same. Fig. 21-1 illustrates the training process. Note that this process strongly resembles the healthcare process because it includes the following:

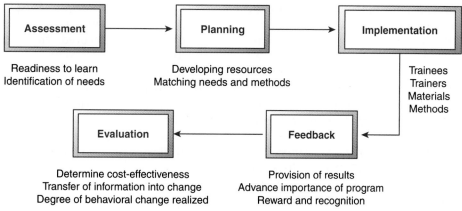

Fig. 21-1 ■ The modern training process.

Assessment: the procedure that provides information about an individual's willingness and readiness to learn and specific learning needs (i.e., skill level, ability, attitudes, and knowledge); often referred to as a needs analysis

Planning: the process of obtaining and/or developing training resources to present to the trainee and coordinating training needs with organizational capabilities, required time lines, and educational methods

Implementation: the gathering together of the individuals who will provide the training (trainers), the individuals who will receive the training (trainees), and all of the materials and equipment needed to carry out the training program

Feedback: the process of providing the participant, supervisor, and organizational management with the results obtained and with opportunities to advance the educational process or affect the degree of behavioral change produced by the training program

Evaluation: an investigation to determine whether the training was effective, to what degree the objectives were achieved, and whether the information presented in the program was actually applied on the job

TRAINING

Needs Assessment

The first step in the development of a training program or the establishment of an educational process is to determine that a need for it actually exists. An organization should not commit its resources to a training activity unless, in the best judgment of its responsible management (including nurse managers), the training is necessary to achieve some organizational goal such as better patient care, reduced operating cost, or more efficient or satisfied personnel, and no other method is available to produce the necessary behavioral change.

In the healthcare industry, training is not an end; it is a means that can be used to achieve a goal. Training is considered an end in itself only by those organizations that are in business to provide it, such as a center for education or a training development company.

Because of the importance of approaching training conservatively and using it as a resource, one of the decisions that management must make regarding training is where the training budget should be spent. This decision must be based on the best available data and is often made through an organization-wide planning process that centers on a SWOT analysis. A SWOT analysis takes a hard look at the organization, both internally and externally, to provide management with information in the following four major areas (which give the method its name):

1. *Strengths (S):* What are the things that the organization does as well as or better than its competition? What is it known for? Why do patients come to this organization instead of another? These factors can be anything from location to high-quality performance.
2. *Weaknesses (W):* What are the things that the organization does not do well but that are necessary? What are the things that place the organization at risk because of marginal or subcompetitive performance? Weaknesses, too, can be anything from location to low-quality performance.
3. *Opportunities (O):* What are the possibilities that are available to the organization? Where can it grow and what can it become? What is available in the community that can support enhancement? Opportunities can be anything from the

arrival of the latest technologic marvel to the creation of a new oncology department.

4. *Threats (T):* What can affect the organization's future negatively? What challenges are perceived as important? What in the environment can harm the organization if it is not neutralized? Threats can be anything from acute short staffing to the loss of the local university's school of nursing.

The results of the SWOT analysis are used to establish the major broad objectives that drive the organization. For example, a hospital might create five such objectives that will cover all of the areas in the organization, as follows:

- Improve the net income from 10% to 12%
- Decrease the overhead cost per patient-day from 28% to 25%
- Provide triage service
- Develop oncology research
- Increase the physician residency program by 25%

Using the data developed during the SWOT analysis, the organization can easily identify the things that must be done to ensure that it reaches each of the objectives it creates, at least one of which invariably involves supplemental training for members of the staff. Management looks at the way things are currently being done and then at the way things will have to be done if the goals are to be met. The difference is the amount of physical or behavioral change that must be brought about if the organization is to succeed. For example, consider the third organizational objective listed earlier, "Provide triage service." Management may find that training must be provided to emergency department nurses so that they will be prepared to handle critically injured patients on a timely basis; or a triage center that contains a dedicated operating theater may have to be built. Regardless of the details, what is needed to move the organization away from the way things are to the way things need to be is the physical or behavioral change needed to achieve the goal.

In an educational institution, the process of achieving behavioral change is fairly simple: determine what behaviors are needed to produce the result desired and then teach them (a statement that is greatly simplified but extremely accurate as a bottom line). The extent to which the training produces real behavioral change determines the degree of success achieved by the educational curriculum.

In the typical healthcare institution, however, the challenge of bringing about behavioral change is far more complex. This is so because of the different types of training that must occur, which include the following:

Specialized training for specific activities: The activities that can be made more effective through training

that changes behavior must be identified, and appropriate training programs must be either designed or procured. There is a continual need for this type of training, and a portion of the organization's training resources must be allocated to improving the performance of specific activities that will increase the organization's effectiveness.

Maintenance training: A great deal of training dedicated to enhancing or simply maintaining the level of performance is always being carried out in every organization. This is the type of training that is used to instruct both new employees and existing workers whose job skill requirements are changing (because of promotion, change of specialty, assumption of a new role, etc.). This maintenance or enrichment training demands a healthy portion of the organization's overall training resources and is not something the organization can do without.

Sadly, observation of the healthcare industry indicates that too many organizations continue to initiate training programs simply because these programs have been well advertised and marketed or because other businesses have found them useful. The dynamics of knowledge management dictate that such practices must give way to better utilization of the funds available for intellectual and performance enhancement. The problem is that there has never been a direct correlation between intellectual and technologic investments and improvements in business performance. Confirming this point, Dr. Erik Brynjolfsson, Schussel Professor of Management at the Massachusetts Institute of Technology's Sloan School of Management, noted, "The same dollar spent on the same system may give a competitive advantage to one company but become only an expensive paperweight in another."[1] This fact demands that the prudent organization not adopt an expensive training effort simply because a sister business may be doing so. The old, tired, and faddish practices must be reduced by systematically determining exactly what the organization's specific training needs are and using these needs as a basis for developing very specific training content. If carried out effectively, this approach will ensure that the funds spent for training programs will go only to the people and areas that specifically need them.

Planning and Implementation

After the organization's needs have been determined, the next logical step in the training process is planning, the goal of which is to match the previously identified needs with the resources available. Nurse managers usually participate in this planning, because it determines how training will affect their staffs and patients; however, the planning process is something that can be delegated. Many managers routinely delegate this task to their exceptional subordinates or to a specific staff nurse who may be designated as the unit's preceptor (a staff member who supervises the training of another).

The actual training program that is developed through this planning process can take advantage of the organization's closed-circuit television system, can be provided by training specialists employed by either the nursing service or a training and education department, or can be part of a comprehensive learning program such as the one in which you are currently enrolled. Today, technology provides nurse managers with a wide variety of resources to use in training their staffs.

In studies conducted in the early 1980s, researchers K. N. Wexley and G. P. Latham suggested that three main questions need to be considered in the assessment and planning of training programs, as follows[2]:

1. Is the individual trainable? (not all people are)
2. How should the training program be arranged to facilitate learning?
3. What can be done to ensure that what is learned during training will be transferred to actual performance?

Unfortunately, no well-developed and thoroughly tested theories of learning are available to help managers answer these questions, so they must rely on some simple learning principles and basic knowledge about training methods to develop their training interventions. Managers can also draw on theories of motivation to help ensure that trainees have the desire to learn and to apply any skills or concepts that are taught.

There is one well-known truth, however: *Change cannot occur solely as a result of a training program.* Training programs inform; by themselves, they do not produce behavioral change. Change occurs because the instruction presents high-quality information *and* the participant accepts it *and*, on his or her own, the participant makes an internal change that allows that person to perform in a different manner. Alternatively, and far more likely, someone who has control over the participant's future career tells the individual that the individual must change his or her behavior to bring it in line with the information presented in the training program *or else.* In short, someone whom the participant respects and/or who has direct influence over the participant's career creates the biggest reason that the change recommended in the training program is accepted and ultimately implemented.

Management—and in nursing units this means the nurse managers—is the only group in any organization that can effect behavioral change. This is true because management is the only group that has a direct influence on or exercises direct control over employees' future success in the organization.

Learning Principles

Four basic principles guide the development of training activities and create the success of educational programs. Two principles facilitate learning; the others determine the degree of transfer from the training context to performance on the job.

READINESS TO LEARN

Before any performer can benefit from formal training, he or she must be ready (willing) to learn. Readiness refers to the maturity level and experience that comprise the learner's background and is a critical factor in determining the individual's willingness to accept something new. Consider the simple process of learning mathematics. Students are not taught algebra, for instance, until they have developed an understanding of basic math, and after algebra they take geometry, trigonometry, and calculus, in that order. The logic in this progression is based on the fact that readiness to learn, at any stage of development, depends primarily on the learning that has occurred through the student's previous experience.

A training program will fail to achieve its objectives unless the skills and knowledge necessary to prepare the student to learn are considered in its development. It is extremely difficult to learn a new sequence of behaviors if the component actions on which it is based have not been learned previously. Maturational factors also influence readiness to learn. There are limits to the amount of information a person can acquire and retain at any one time.

MOTIVATION TO LEARN

Motivation affects performance by serving an energizing function. In simple terms, an individual who is motivated will work harder to achieve a given result. The following two factors are aspects of motivation:

1. *Process:* how behavior is inspired, controlled, maintained, and diminished
2. *Content:* which specific things motivate different people

Motivation plays an important part in the training process in several key areas, as follows:

Attendance: Participants must be motivated to go to the training presentation and to attend to the training content.

Reinforcement: Anticipation of benefits can provide motivation, reinforcing the desired behavioral change and encouraging practical application of the information presented in the training program. If learners are informed in advance about the benefits that will result from learning the content and adopting the modeled behavior, their motivation is strengthened. Furthermore, anticipation of benefits can strengthen retention of what has been learned observationally by motivating people to encode and rehearse modeled behavior that they value.

Attention: Motivation is, of course, one of the things that guides attention. It is difficult *not* to hear compelling sounds or to look at captivating visual displays.

Acceptance of change: Attendance at a training course and even completion of the training material does not guarantee that anything will be learned from the experience or that any portion of the desired behavioral changes will be realized. Participants must be motivated to accept what is being presented. A small percentage (approximately 5%) are completely self-motivated and about an equal percentage will never be motivated, but the 90% who can *become* motivated will do so only if someone they respect or someone who has authority over their future success tells them they must (Fig. 21-2).

CONDITIONS FOR PRACTICE

Years of research into adult learning have shown that, when a complex task is to be learned, the task should be divided into its major parts and each part should be presented separately. Learning can begin with the least complex element and continue through to the most complex, or the parts can be learned in their actual sequence in task performance. By arranging the training program in this format, participants will grasp the material faster and relate it more easily to the performance of an actual task. The process of learning through incremental presentation, however, should not be completely divorced from learning the whole.

Repetitive demonstration of the whole helps participants understand what the goal is and where individual training sessions will ultimately take them.

When a training program is developed, the content should be broken down into its major behavioral parts so that it can be learned in a systematic progression. The material should be presented until the participant can recall it with acceptable accuracy. The sequence of the presentation should be organized so that, when all of the parts have been covered, the trainee will be able to put them all together and practice the whole behavior.

Practice is more effective when it is spaced out over a period of time rather than providing it all at once, especially when any type of motor skill is involved. The reason is rather simple: if the trainee has to focus on one thing for long periods of time without some diversion or interruption, the quality of learning and degree of retention will suffer. This situation can be compared with a college student's cramming for an examination. The test scores that are achieved are usually high, but the amount of information absorbed from the effort is relatively low. Adults learn differently than do students in an academic environment. They are unable to focus on the training material for long periods of time because they have other pressures and obligations, such as regular job performance, family, and home life. Consequently, when the learning is spaced out over time and reinforced by practical application, long-term retention of the information presented is much higher and the transfer of the learned information to the work environment is much more effective.

TRANSFER OF TRAINING

The ultimate goal of any educational program is the conversion of the information presented into actual learning in the mind of the student and then into practice on the job. Learning is not the same thing as training. *Training* is the process of presenting information; *learning* is the process of converting the information received into behavioral change. Researcher H. C. Ellis suggested that the transfer of training to the

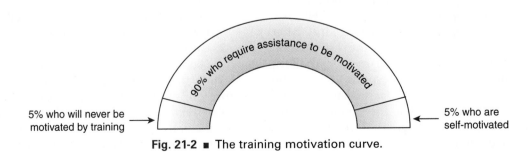

Fig. 21-2 ■ The training motivation curve.

work environment can be maximized if the following two conditions are met[3]:

1. *Similarity:* The more closely that training conditions resemble the participant's actual working conditions, the more successful the assimilation process will be. The vast majority of performers have very great difficulty in transferring training from one field to the next. For example, if nurse managers participate in a course on leadership requirements that was originally developed for the general business community, they will have greater difficulty assimilating and applying its content than they would if the program addressed the leadership requirements of the nursing profession—even if those requirements are exactly the same.

2. *Practice:* If the training program provides the participant with the opportunity to practice the performance being recommended, the amount of information retained will be greater than if no practice is permitted.

One of the authors of this book, educational consultant Dr. James Hawkins, suggested that the amount of behavioral change actually seen in the workplace will be directly proportional to the amount of importance management places on the training program.[4] If managers participate in the program by exerting direct influence, the amount of information that will be applied in the working unit will be significantly higher than if managers leave the training to the education department to oversee. If significant behavioral change is to occur, participants must know that they are expected to alter their performance as a result of the training. If the management team that has direct influence over the future success of the participants communicates the necessity for change by a process of reward and recognition of excellence throughout the training process, then participants will consider the training important and the change necessary.

The new behaviors introduced by the training program will not become part of participants' work performance until these behaviors have become part of long-term memory. If the information in the training course is to become incorporated into participants' long-term memory, it must be reinforced though practical application. This practical application can start in the training classroom in the form of practice lessons and performance workshops, but the most effective method of ensuring that the information is transformed into actual behavior (i.e., is put into long-term memory) is to make sure that the information is applied in the work unit. Until participants actually use the information to change the way in which they perform the requirements of their jobs,

the amount of change produced by the training program will remain small, regardless of the quality of that program.

Memory

The ability of an individual to retain what he or she has learned is not as relevant to the effectiveness of a training program as it is to the ability of the participant to put the information learned into actual practice on the job. Although the ability to retain is influenced to some degree by the individual's intellectual aptitude (i.e., the better the memory, the more effective the learning), the most critical factor in retention is how quickly the training can be reinforced through practical application.

The difficulty of participants in recalling from memory the information presented in a training program begins with the fact that human beings have two types of memory: short term and long term.

Short-term memory (or working memory) is the mental system that temporarily stores the information to which attention is currently directed and allows processing and use of this stored information. The short-term memory capacity of the average individual is very limited and is directly affected by the environment. Under the best conditions (when no influences are present in the environment to reduce retention) only a few storage or processing activities can be carried out simultaneously by even the most intelligent humans. The greater the environmental influences reducing the individual's ability to focus on the information contained in short-term memory, the shorter the time that the information will be retained.

Long-term memory represents the parts of an individual's experience that have been processed through short-term memory and stored for long-term use. Items in long-term memory range from individual letter or word codes to more general things such as strategies for processing and maintaining information. In fact, it has long been believed that the average human stores memories of every experience in life and can recall those memories at will if given the proper retrieval cues.

There are a variety of ways to facilitate the transfer of the information presented in a training program into long-term memory. Practice is perhaps the simplest strategy that can be used. Practice, or rehearsal, is generally an interactive process, and because it repeatedly brings the information into short-term memory, it increases the likelihood that the information will move into long-term storage. Adult learners generally have the capacity to rehearse several different items at the same time and can therefore absorb most of the information presented in any training program. In fact, the more rehearsal an adult performs, the easier it is for the person to recall the actions or information learned.

If the items to be learned are grouped into specific behavioral changes desired, retention is increased. If the training program is organized so that participants can deal with one behavior at a time, long-term retention of the material presented is enhanced. If the material is presented verbally, as in a lecture-based seminar, the amount of information presented must be reduced dramatically. The more content that is presented, the less that is transferred into long-term memory. If the verbal presentation is enhanced with graphic displays, the amount of information presented can be increased without significant loss of retention. If the verbal material is augmented with graphics and, in addition, the opportunity for practice is given, then long-term retention is greatly enhanced.

The organization of the training material can also enhance retention. For example, if the training material is presented in a logical, sequential pattern so that one part builds on another, then a higher proportion of the information will be learned (i.e., will pass into long-term memory). Such an organization of the material does not necessarily need to be imposed by the training course, because the human mind has the capability to organize information on its own. The more mature the individual participant, the greater the ability to organize the information presented and the more likely that the information will be retained.

Social Learning Theory

Social learning theory describes how people learn through imitation and observation. According to this theory, people can observe their own behavior and that of others and use these observations as a basis for future behavior. The theory also suggests that future behavior is a result of the consequences of behavior in the past and that how a person behaves over time influences what that person becomes. People think about when to employ various behaviors and try to use certain behaviors to increase the likelihood of producing positive consequences. If the action taken causes the anticipated positive consequences to occur, then the likelihood is greater that the action will be repeated (Fig. 21-3).

Social learning theory is based on behavioral theory, and it builds on many of the principles of reinforcement and the assumptions made regarding its operation. As researcher A. Bandura explained in his 1977 work *Social Learning Theory*,[5] except for rudimentary reflexes, people are not equipped with a large repertoire of instinctual behaviors. Instead, average humans expand their capabilities through a process of direct experience and observation.

The results of performance influence an individual's willingness to repeat certain behaviors. As stated earlier, when a behavior is rewarded or receives a positive response, the likelihood that the behavior will be repeated is high. Those behaviors or actions that result in negative consequences are less likely to be repeated. The process whereby successful behaviors are retained and behaviors that leads to no positive consequences or to negative consequence are dis-

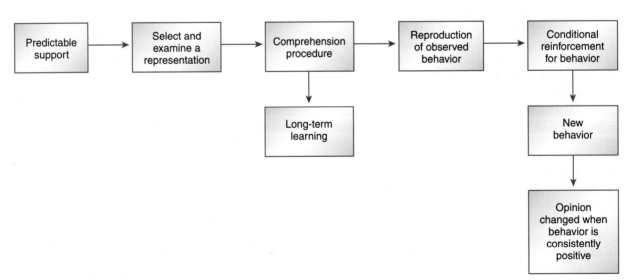

Fig. 21-3 ■ The process of social learning. (From Hawkins JA: *American business management,* Honolulu, 1998, The Directions Corporation.)

carded is referred to as *differential reinforcement*. Not all learning is accomplished in this manner, however. Differential reinforcement cannot explain the speed with which a human can learn, the learning that occurs without evidence of behavioral change (no-trial learning), and the survival of the human species.

According to the social learning theory of behavior, information about oneself and the nature of the environment is developed and verified through the following four different processes:

Direct experience: People derive much of their knowledge from the direct experience that occurs as a result of their actions.

Vicarious experience: Information about the environment is frequently extracted from substituted experience; that is, observation of the effects produced by someone else's actions.

Judgment of others: When direct and vicarious experience is limited, people can develop and evaluate their speculations about the environment from the judgments voiced by others.

Logical determination: After people acquire rules of inference from active, vicarious, or social experience, they can use these rules to evaluate the soundness of their reasoning through logical processes, either inductive or deductive.

Social learning theory also implies that anticipation of reinforcement is one of several factors that influence what is observed and what gets performed. If an individual knows or has reasonable expectation that his or her behavior will produce a positive outcome or at least avoid a negative one, his or her attentiveness to the actions will be greater. This suggests that learning that occurs through a process of observation will be more effective when the observer knows in advance about the benefits of adopting the behavior.

Simply attending to another's behavior is insufficient to cause learning and retention, however; several additional processes must occur. According to social learning theory, behavior is learned through symbolic coding, cognitive organization, and symbolic rehearsal before it is actually performed. Only after these cognitive processes have been completed will the individual attempt the actual behavior. If the first attempt leads to positive consequences, the behavior will be used again in the future. This is the motivational process that maintains the new behavior and ensures that it will be retained for future use. Through observation, the individual understands how and in what sequence response components must be combined to produce a positive new behavior. Most people guide their actions far more by paying attention to learned or observed processes than by relying on the outcomes of their personal behavior. This is a major

reason why it is so vital to maintain a positive working environment.

Modeling conveys information to observers regarding potential new responses and the way in which responses can be combined to form new behaviors. This information can be transmitted through physical demonstration, graphic imitation, or verbal narration. A large proportion of social learning actually occurs as a result of the casual observation of the behavior performed by others. People also learn to perform desired behaviors by reading about how to behave and by exposure to a wide variety of different media sources, especially television.

Relapse Prevention

In his work *Relapse: Conceptual Research and Clinical Perspectives*, D. C. Daley[6] presented a model for increasing the long-term retention of newly trained behaviors. The method he recommended is built around the development of several self-control and coping strategies.

According to Daley, the first step that should be taken to increase retention of trained material is to make the individual participants in the training program aware of the relapse process itself. In most circumstances, training programs represent themselves as being very successful in developing long-term retention; however, in actuality most are not. Most programs make no attempt to provide information on what might make presented material vulnerable to memory loss; therefore, participants are not prepared to avoid situations in which the trained behavior will be unsuccessful.

If the training program presents information that will help participants pinpoint situations that are likely to sabotage their retention, long-term retention will be enhanced. Trainees should be taught the following:

- To anticipate high-risk situations
- To identify coping strategies for avoiding high-risk situations
- To recognize that slight slips or relapses are predictable after any training program, but that these momentary lapses do not have to become long-term relapses

The importance of providing this information, according to Daley, is that if training participants are exposed to situations where failure can occur, such instruction will prepare them to compensate for the situation well in advance of encountering it. This advance mental preparation for demanding situations will help to prevent small relapses from leading to absolute failure due to what Daley called the "abstinence violation effect." This effect occurs when feelings of guilt caused by a small violation of the training content lead a training participant to deny the possible effectiveness of the trained behavior. Such denial almost guarantees that a small slip will end up with the participant's total rejection of the training content and the behavioral change for which it asks. To minimize the likelihood of such rejection, the training program should encourage the participants to discuss possible failure situations and help them develop effective means of coping with them. Success is greatly increased when the training program provides an opportunity for the participants to work through these potential situations by encouraging practice in the nonthreatening environment of the training classroom. When participants become comfortable working with the situation in practice sessions, they are preparing themselves to effectively manage the situation if it should occur in the normal working environment. Participants who are not given this opportunity or who are not provided with information regarding the potential for these lapses are far more likely to let a small lapse cause them to totally reject the information presented by the training course.

Adult Education Theory

For most of the first half of the twentieth century, the only educational concepts and techniques available were those that had been developed to educate children in a formal setting. It was generally assumed that anyone who was trained in basic educational theory and practice and was reasonably good at managing the development and logistics of educational programs could be a good trainer of adults. One of the primary discoveries of research conducted in the 1970s, however, was that adults learn far differently than do children. Based on this research, a variety of techniques for helping adults to learn were developed. The primary architect of this revolutionary thinking, M. S. Knowles,[7] suggested that the significant differences occur mostly as a result of the differing environments for adult and child learning. According to Knowles, the differences in adult and child education relate to the following four basic elements:

1. *Individual self-concept:* Children generally view themselves as being dependent on others, but as they move toward adulthood, they become increasingly aware of themselves and their own decision-making capability, and they become very capable of self-direction. This change in attitude toward oneself from dependency to autonomy characterizes the maturation process. Adults tend to resent being in situations where they are shown a lack of respect, talked down to, judged, or otherwise treated like children. Therefore, people who teach adults should present themselves as facilitators rather than as authoritative lecturers, and whenever possible, the adult learner should have some input into what is taught.

2. *Experience:* Adults have accumulated a vast quantity of knowledge through their life experiences, whereas children have not. The possession of this experience often causes adults to make choices regarding information they are taught and the format in which it is received. In adult education, this experience base should be valued, because the instructor can use theory to integrate and formalize it (i.e., the educator knows the theory, but the trainees have the experience).

   In contrast to children's education, which is oriented toward one-way communication, assigned readings, and audiovisual presentations, education of adults should include experiential learning, two-way and multidirectional communication such as group discussions, role playing, teamwork exercises, and skill practice sessions. This way, the experiences of all participants can be brought to bear on the problem being discussed.

3. *Readiness to learn:* The main task of primary education is to sequence learning activities for children in a manner that fits their developmental characteristics. Adults, however, have already completed their basic education in reading, writing, mathematics, speech, and so on, and their developmental tasks increasingly relate to the social roles that form their immediate concerns, such as working, living, family, and recreational activities. In primary education, the teacher decides both what will be learned and how and in what sequence learning will take place. In adult education, greater success is realized when the participants themselves help to identify what they wish to learn and the sequence in which the material will be presented. The adult trainer acts less as a teacher presenting compulsory material and more as a facilitator helping participants form groups to diagnose their learning needs.

4. *Time perspective:* Primary education has always been considered as preparing for the future rather than promoting readiness for the present. This means that the principal thrust of primary education is to ensure that students store up information for use on some future date. To facilitate this type of learning, teachers present

neatly packaged information that is designed for future use by subjects. In adult education, however, learning is problem centered rather than subject centered and focuses the energy of the participants on defining and solving problems that may be faced in the present.

Staff Development

The educational programs presented in hospitals generally include information for patients, families, staff, and members of the general community. In fact, most of the presentations that are given can be categorized into two main areas: (1) staff development and (2) patient education.

Staff development, sometimes known as *in-service education*, refers to the continuing education presented by the organization aimed at improving staff members' general knowledge or ability to perform job-related tasks. Staff development also includes management training and other areas of staff enrichment such as leadership training and training in assertiveness, counseling skills, and group process skills.

ORIENTATION

When an individual becomes an employee of an organization, he or she must get started properly. One of the best ways to ensure that this happens is through an educational process commonly referred to as orientation. Among other things, a well-planned orientation reduces the anxiety that new employees feel when beginning a new job. In addition, socialization into the workplace contributes to unit effectiveness by reducing dissatisfaction, absenteeism, and turnover.

The proper orientation of new employees is the joint responsibility of the organization's training staff and the nurse manager. In most institutions, during orientation the new employee attends a formal presentation conducted by the hospital's human relations department. This formal presentation is followed by an on-site orientation to the working environment, which should be conducted by a nurse manager. Most organizations have a well-designed plan for orientation that clearly defines the responsibilities of each participant in the program so that nothing is omitted from the new employee's experience. Fundamentally, the human resources staff provide information involving organizational matters that are relevant to all new employees, such as information regarding the cafeteria, benefits, parking, and work hours. Nurse managers concentrate their orientational efforts on those things unique to the employee's specific job and the nursing unit to which he or she will be assigned.

! CRITICAL POINT

Although the schedule of the typical nurse manager typically puts the manager at or near the limits of endurance, the orientation of a new employee should always be considered as a primary function of the job. Although it is certainly within the realm of tasks that can be delegated, this textbook does not recommend that the nurse manager ever do so. Orientation of a new employee should include going over the unit's mission, goals, objectives, and performance standards once again. Even if these were covered during the employment interview, things are very different on the first day of employment. No one in the nursing unit can convey the importance of these issues like the nurse manager. In addition, this is the perfect time to establish a relationship of cooperation with the new employee by working with the individual to establish goals and objectives for the first 90 days of employment.

Employees first entering the workforce often have unrealistic expectations about the amount of challenge and responsibility they will encounter in their first job, and when they find themselves performing menial and undemanding entry-level tasks, they often become discouraged and disillusioned. The result is dissatisfaction with the job, low productivity, and possible resignation from the job. Therefore, one function of orientation is to correct unrealistic expectations. Nurse managers need to outline what is expected of new employees very specifically and, at the same time, assure them that they will eventually be able to progress to more challenging tasks. Such job previews should cover the informal or nonconcrete aspects of the job, because employees could possibly have more unrealistic expectations about these aspects than about such concrete areas as pay scale or hours.

Most people, regardless of how well they have been oriented, begin a new job with a high level of anxiety. This uneasiness often makes it very difficult for new employees to function as productive members of the unit. The difficulty stems from the fact that even the most professional new employees either simply do not hear all of the information they are given or spend a lot of energy attempting to integrate and interpret the information, which means that they end up missing some critical points. Employees who are allowed the time to assimilate into the pace of the unit gradually and whose peers and supervisors are sensitive to the demands of assimilation actually perform better and are much happier than those who are immersed in the unit's activities immediately after walking through the door. Slower immersion has been documented to increase the learning rate of the new employees, increase productivity, and lower absenteeism and tardiness.[7]

Because nurse managers play an extremely important role in the orientation process, everything that they expect of new employees should be discussed openly and specifically. New employees will adapt far more rapidly and become far more productive if they understand what is expected right from the beginning of their employment. Everything, including standards of performance, attendance requirements, the way to treat patients, and feedback to expect in a performance appraisal, should be discussed.

PRECEPTOR PROGRAMS

The preceptor process, in which a new employee is partnered with an outstanding member of the existing staff, provides a means for the orientation and social adaptation of the new nurse as well as a mechanism for recognition of exceptionally competent staff members.[8] Members of the staff are selected to serve as preceptors based on their clinical competence, organizational skills, ability to guide and direct others, and concern for the effective orientation of new employees. Although the vast majority of preceptors in a nursing unit will be staff nurses, an exceptionally qualified unit clerk might serve as a preceptor for all nonnursing employees joining the unit. The primary goal is for the preceptor to assist the new employee in acquiring the knowledge and skills necessary to function effectively in the unit.

Selection as a preceptor gives the outstanding staff member an opportunity to sharpen and demonstrate his or her leadership skills and increase personal and professional satisfaction, while at the same time offering the new employee the advantage of an on-the-job training program tailored specifically to his or her needs.

In most preceptor programs, the new nurse works closely with the preceptor through the first 3 weeks of employment or until the preceptor feels that the new employee can function effectively with reduced supervision. The duration of the relationship varies based on the new employee's individual learning needs and/or hospital policy.

The preceptor's role is that of welcoming mentor, teacher, resource, counselor, role model, and evaluator.[9] By discharging these duties carefully and professionally, preceptors lend an air of exceptional welcome and professionalism to the unit for new employees. To ensure that assimilation is complete, preceptors concern themselves with proper socialization of the new employees within the group just as much as with familiarizing them with unit functions. Preceptors teach any procedures that are unfamiliar and help new employees develop any skills that will be needed but have not yet been learned. In addition, preceptors act as resource personnel for new employees on matters concerning organizational functions as well as policies and procedures.

New employees also find it convenient to use their preceptors as counselors to help them make their transition to the unit. If, for example, new employees notice discrepancies between their educational preparation or their expectations and the actual work in the unit, their preceptors are valuable allies in helping them adjust to the realities of employment.

Preceptors also serve as role models as they introduce the new employees to work-related tasks and show them how to set priorities, solve problems, make decisions, manage time, delegate tasks, and interact with others. In addition, preceptors evaluate new employee performance and provide both verbal and written feedback to encourage development.

Individual organizations establish programs whereby deserving staff members are trained as preceptors. Large organizations generally do this through the internal education department, and smaller ones through the human resources division. Whichever department actually conducts the training will ensure that each designee receives training in what role the preceptor should play, what the principles of adult education are, how to provide skills training, how to plan and evaluate instruction, how to write learning objectives, and how to provide both formal and informal feedback.

STAFF DEVELOPMENT METHODS

Staff development is usually considered to occur on two levels:

1. *Internal:* training efforts conducted in the nursing unit. These efforts usually include on-the-job training, workshops for unit nurses, and inservice programs.
2. *External:* training efforts conducted away from the nursing unit. These efforts typically include, but are not limited to, formal workshops presented by a human resources or training and education department in the hospital and all training activities conducted outside the hospital, including college courses, conferences, and continuing education workshops.

The different training programs available in healthcare facilities are too numerous to describe in this chapter; however, the model against which these various training programs should be evaluated is worth discussing. If a training program is to be effective for adult education, it must include at a minimum the following three elements:

1. Presentation
2. Practice
3. Feedback

Effective skill training should provide an opportunity for the participants to practice the desired terminal behaviors taught by the course and to receive feedback about their performance. It is not good enough simply to present the material and leave the participants to practice the behaviors on their own. Nor is it good enough to demonstrate a procedure, allow the employees to practice it, and not provide feedback on their efforts. To be effective, adult training programs must incorporate all three steps.

The most widely used training method in the nursing profession is called *on-the-job training (OJT)*. Such training is often accomplished by assigning the trainee to an experienced nurse, preceptor, or even the nurse manager. The trainee is familiarized with the given procedure, practice, or skill and then is expected to learn by observing the experienced employee and by performing the actual task under direct supervision. Training is generally repeated until the trainee can perform the assignment within acceptable limits. This method has many positive features, including the following:

Cost-effectiveness: Trainees learn effectively while providing some of the necessary nursing services. Moreover, the need for outside training facilities and reliance on professional trainers is reduced.

Avoidance of transfer-of-training problems: Transfer of training to a new environment is usually not an issue because training occurs while the participant is actually performing the job.

Care should be taken when using any form of OJT. Although OJT has been a source of continual benefit to almost every organization that uses it, this does not mean that it can always be relied on to produce positive results. OJT often fails because it is not a formalized process, and many trainees and their instructors simply do not take it seriously. In addition, very few designated OJT instructors actually know how to apply learning theory, and as a result of their ignorance, the concept of providing presentation, practice, and feedback is often neglected.

The following suggestions are worth considering during the implementation of an OJT program[2]:

- Those employees who function as OJT trainers must be assured that providing training to new employees does not jeopardize, but in fact enhances, their own job security, pay level, seniority, and/or status.
- Individuals who are assigned the collateral duty of OJT trainer should be informed that this additional responsibility will be considered when rewards are allocated.
- When possible, OJT trainers and trainees should be paired carefully to minimize any differences in background, language, personality, attitudes, or age that might inhibit communication and understanding.
- OJT trainers should be selected based on their proficiency, professionalism, ability, desire to teach, and willingness to assume additional responsibility.
- Personnel chosen to be OJT trainers should be carefully trained in the proper methods of instruction.
- Assignment as an OJT trainer should not be viewed as authority to fail to perform the requirements of the trainer's primary job. OJT training should not be viewed as a vacation from primary duties.
- Trainees should be rotated among different OJT trainers to ensure that all trainees have the advantage of working with the very best trainers and to expose each trainee to the specific backgrounds and knowledge of a variety of skilled personnel.
- OJT trainers and nurse managers must understand that the overall efficiency of their units may be negatively affected when OJT occurs.
- OJT trainers and nurse managers must ensure that close supervision is provided to each trainee to prevent any major mistakes and the learning of incorrect procedures. The importance of supervision cannot be overstated.
- OJT should be used in conjunction with, and not as a substitute for, other training approaches. The training received on the job should include theoretical as well as practical knowledge; for example, knowledge of fluid and electrolyte balance is essential to nurses who administer intravenous fluids.

Box 21-1 lists the key actions that should be taken when preparing for and conducting OJT. Note that the list contains the three fundamental steps described

---

BOX 21-1

Key Behaviors for On-the-Job Training

1. Write down each task to be taught, including all individual steps.
2. Explain the objective(s) of the task to the employee.
3. Demonstrate the task.
4. Explain the major points of the objective and give a copy of the objectives to the employee.
5. Demonstrate the task a second and perhaps a third time, if necessary.
6. Assist the employee in performing the task.
7. Constructively critique the employee's performance and have the employee repeat the task.
8. Have the employee perform the task until he or she is comfortable.
9. Provide meaningful feedback, phrased in positive terms.
10. Continue to have the employee perform the task as often as possible.
11. Continually provide constructive criticism and praise.
12. Do not attempt to do the work for the employee.

earlier which, if done correctly, should provide a quality learning session: (1) present the material, (2) allow the employee to practice the skill, and (3) provide positively expressed feedback about the practice performance. These actions also incorporate most of the elements of learning theory discussed earlier in this chapter. Fig. 21-4 provides a sample form that can be used by OJT trainers to write down the actual steps and key elements of the task to be trained before they provide any information to the employee in the training process.

AUDIOVISUAL TECHNIQUES

Because of the continual growth in the healthcare industry, the constant changes in technology, and the increasing number of people requiring training, there has been a continuous call to make the training process efficient enough to accelerate the learning process. To meet this increased demand for training, many organizations have begun to use advanced training techniques such as distance training programs, films, closed-circuit television, audiotapes, videotapes, computer-assisted instruction, and interactive computer

Job Performance Development Sheet

Department: _____

Unit: _____

Job to be trained: _____

Job breakdown developed by: _____

Date breakdown developed: _____

Important Steps to Be Performed Logical Sequence of Operation	Recommended Procedure How the Task Should Be Done

Fig. 21-4 ■ Sample job performance development sheet.

training. These methods allow an instructor's message to be delivered in a uniform manner at multiple locations simultaneously. When used in conjunction with a traditional lecture presentation, these procedures can add depth to the instruction, provide remedial training processes, and create an opportunity for participants to perform real-to-life procedures without the risk of endangering a patient. One of the most significant advances made is reduction in the cost of training programs. Today, using distance learning techniques, nurse managers can instruct their entire staffs on virtually any procedure without missing a single minute of patient care time.

Audiovisual materials can be used in almost every training and development situation, in both simple and complex programs. However, it is important to remember that audiovisual resources are teaching aids, not educational programs. These devices support the educational process, but practice and feedback are also required for the training to be effective. Audiovisual methods are not designed to substitute for a well-developed training program and will not supply the necessary learning elements to ensure that behavioral change will occur. These methods are best used when the following conditions exist:

- There is a need to graphically demonstrate certain procedures that will be explained to the trainee, with practice and feedback provided.
- Events that are not easily demonstrated in the classroom must be shown to the trainee.
- Training is being presented in multiple locations or even on an organization-wide basis, and it is not economically feasible for the trainer to travel from place to place and not possible to assemble all concerned employees in one location. Note that in this situation, a videotape by itself will not be an effective training procedure unless it is connected to a distance learning program that supplies the other two requirements—practice and feedback.
- It is supplemented with live lecture, discussion, and/or practice.
- It is part of a well-developed distance learning program.

Even the best audiovisual materials need some introduction when they are incorporated into the training program. Viewers need to be instructed on what the purpose of the material is, what exactly they will be seeing, and what the training program wants each trainee to look for in the presentation. After the audiovisual presentation is complete, it must be critiqued for the trainees and each important point of the material restated so that it is reinforced well enough to be remembered. This reinforcement is best accomplished by either real-time or distance-based practice and feedback.

As noted earlier, audiovisual presentations should not be considered as stand-alone training events. Misusing them in this manner is often counterproductive to the desired learning process and potentially risky for the organization. They should be carefully selected, adequately introduced, and followed up with adequate discussion, practice, and feedback.[2,10]

EVALUATION

One of the most controversial issues in the training field is evaluation. Most professional trainers agree that a participant's progress should be evaluated to determine the amount of learning that has taken place, but few agree on the best method to be used.

The problem with evaluation starts with the organization itself. After purchasing a program or developing its own, the organization will use the program over and over again until someone in a position of authority decides that it is no longer useful or no longer meets the organization's needs, or, most common of all, attendance decreases. In many cases, the organization does an effective job of getting evaluations from the trainees after they have completed the program, but these evaluations generally center around how much the participants liked the program and seldom focus on how effective they thought it was. When the evaluations focus on the training program in this way, the vast majority are extremely subjective, based on the solicitation of opinions and personal judgments. Rarely are training programs evaluated in a way that is objective enough to determine whether they have caused a change in the intended behavior or organizational variable.

Most evaluation is accomplished at the end of the program using participant questionnaires, which traditionally provide very little information on whether the trainees learned anything in the program that they will carry through to the job. In short, there is a need for effective and objective evaluation for every training program, and such evaluation should never be omitted. To consider the matter from a purely budgetary point of view, think about the following: If the manager is going to spend the organization's money and the manager's valuable time developing or presenting a training program, then the manager should insist that the program include an evaluation that can determine whether or not it actually accomplished what it was intended to do. Training programs are used by organizations to bring about behavioral change, not to provide information.

If the current program or a program being considered cannot show how much actual change it can create, it should not be used.

Evaluating behavioral change is not an easy process. In fact, it is so difficult that the vast majority of training development companies don't even address the subject when they market their programs. Change is extremely hard to effect, primarily for the following two reasons:

1. Training programs present information; by themselves, they do not create behavioral change.
2. People don't like to change.

Therefore, to measure how much change actually occurs requires a process that goes beyond the presentation of information and creates a reason for accepting the change that is recommended by the training program. Generally, such acceptance can be accomplished only in one of the following two ways:

1. *Self-acceptance of the necessity for change:* The top performers in an organization (usually not more than 5%) tend to evaluate the quality of the suggested change and make the change internally without further provocation.
2. *Provision of a reason to accept change:* The vast majority of performers require a reason to accept the change being recommended. This reason can be personal (it will improve the person's performance, potential, or self), but most often it is motivational (the change must be accepted or else).

If it is so difficult to evaluate the results of training, then why do it? Obviously, there are many reasons, and a professional nurse manager considers as many as possible before choosing a program for the staff. Among the most critical are the following:

The justification of expended funds: It is far easier to explain how money was spent when one can talk in terms of what the expenditure accomplished. The best justification for tomorrow's training budget is the effective use of today's resources.

If objective data are gathered that show what a training program actually accomplishes to improve the day-to-day operation of the unit, rarely will money be cut from the training program budget. With good evaluation of cost-effective training, programs will continue to be funded.

Improve the program: Elements of the program that need improvement can be identified. The fact that a program once met the goals and objectives of the organization does not mean that it will continue to do so. In addition, as things change in the nursing environment, so should the content of the training program. If careful evaluation of the program is not conducted, erroneous, out-of-date, and incorrect information can be passed to participants.

With the advent of advanced technology, a proper evaluation process need not be an absent ingredient. Today, most of the traditional difficulty and cost of designing sound evaluation tools can be mitigated if nurse managers choose carefully. Most trainers, including the vast majority of professional training consultants, have little interest in evaluating their products. They want to sell the program, train the trainers, and move on to the next customer. They have no vested interest in staying committed to the success of their product in a specific organization. Nurse managers responsible for the expenditure of training dollars, however, should insist on the inclusion of an evaluation process in every program they use. Nurse managers must keep their organizations committed to finding out whether their training programs are effective by insisting on good evaluation. It is the responsibility of all nurse managers to ensure that the training programs they use are, in fact, effective, and if a program cannot prove its effectiveness, it shouldn't be used.

The effectiveness of the typical training program in the following four major areas can be evaluated:

1. *Trainee reaction:* Information about trainee reaction is usually gathered by means of a questionnaire completed at the end of a program by each trainee. The questionnaire generally contains questions concerning the program's content, quality of the instructor, objectives of the course, instructional methods used, physical facilities, meals provided, and other miscellaneous aspects. The specific things that the organization wants to know about the program, training session, and performance of the instructor are determined before the training is presented and are addressed in any questionnaire.

   However—and this is a critical point— favorable trainee reaction to a program does not guarantee that learning has taken place or that behavior has changed as a result of the program. Nevertheless, trainee reactions are important for the following reasons:
   - Reports of positive employee reactions help ensure organizational support for a program.
   - Trainee reactions can be used to assess the quality of the training and to determine whether the presentation actually met the goals of the program.
   - Reaction data provide information regarding the training experience (facilities, environment, instructor quality, etc.).
2. *Learning:* Learning is the knowledge imparted by the training program (i.e., facts, figures, infor-

mation presented) that can be recalled by the trainee after a reasonable time has elapsed. Knowledge is typically measured by paper-and-pencil tests, which can include true-false, multiple-choice, fill-in-the-blank, matching, and/or essay questions. High-quality training programs conduct the testing portion of the process after the elapse of a certain period (usually not less than 24 hours) between the time the trainee received the information and the time the test is completed.

3. *Behavioral change:* Verifying the acquisition of knowledge is not enough to confirm that a training program actually satisfied the purpose for which it was implemented in the first place. To do that, one must determine that the knowledge imparted was converted into behavioral change; that is, trainees must be able to do things differently after they have been trained than they did before they attended the training.

The conversion of knowledge into behavioral change is the single biggest challenge in training. In fact, the information presented during training rarely transfers in large measure from the classroom to the job. There are several different schools of thought regarding this failure, but mostly the explanation comes down to the following:

- *The information presented does not relate to the performance demanded:* Too much of the training experience focuses on the presentation of the theory and principles of the subject being taught, little of which actually translates into the performance behavior required on the job. There is a big difference between theory and practice. Many training programs test recall for factual material presented by lecture. A person attending such a training program may intellectually remember the information that was presented yet not have acquired any new behavior to use on the job. If a written examination is given at the end of such a program, it may well prove that the training did, in fact, cause learning; however, if behavior is not measured before and after the program, it is impossible to know whether or not behavior has been affected. This means that the behavior the participant used before attending the training must be known, because this forms the baseline for measuring change. Then the behavior used after the training must be evaluated using exactly the same tools used to measure the pretraining behavior. After the posttraining behavior is measured, it must be compared with the pretraining behavior before

any conclusion can be reached regarding a change in behavior. The transfer of learning from the classroom to the job is critical, and the use of behavioral criteria is therefore very important in the business of teaching new skills.

- *Insufficient reason exists to accept the recommended change:* In the typical organization, senior management spends a great deal of time and effort selecting training programs to elevate the quality of performance in the organization. In almost every case, however, as soon as the training program has been selected, most of these senior managers are never heard from again. This disappearing act does not happen because management doesn't care about training; in fact, nothing could be further from the truth. The fact is that management-level people struggle under tremendous workloads, short time frames, and high levels of stress. To ask these individuals to aggressively lead a training session is not possible. Therefore, what happens is that management designates someone to oversee the training effort in the organization (e.g., the education manager or training supervisor). This individual is tasked with ensuring that the purchased training program produces the behavioral change management desired when the program was bought.

The problem with this approach is that the education manager or training supervisor does not have influence over the future success of the people who receive the training. This means that a nurse from the cardiac unit can take a class on vascular tissue treatment that advocates a revolutionary method of treatment but, because of pressures to perform on the unit, never has the time to turn the knowledge gained into behavioral change in actual practice. The education manager or training supervisor, because he or she doesn't work in the cardiac unit, will never know if the new treatment was used because his or her influence over the cardiac nurse ends immediately at the end of the class.

What must be done is to involve the member of management who has immediate control over the future success of the trainee. The person who writes the annual performance review for the cardiac nurse needs to witness the use of the new procedure and hold the nurse accountable for performing it. When the new procedure is not used, the supervisor needs to ask why not, and when it is employed, the supervisor needs to recognize and reward its use. Additional members of the management team, up to and including the senior member of the management committee, can become involved by participating in a program of recognition. Assume, for example, that a specific cardiac nurse performed exceptionally well in the training class. The instructor could give the nurse's name to the education manager and the education manager could pass it along to the hospital administrator, who could call the nurse and congratulate the nurse on his or her success. It doesn't matter what senior managers do to promote the importance of the training; what is important is that they do *something*. Even the busiest executive can find time for a telephone call to congratulate a member of the staff, especially if that telephone call can promote performance excellence; if not, the executive needs to be replaced.

In reality, there is every reason to expect that the information presented in the training classroom will be converted into performance change in the nursing unit. The problem has been that there just hasn't been enough time to get the right people involved. Today, however, the technologic advances made in the training process can involve every member of management without interfering with their existing work schedules. What it takes is imagination and the desire to ask management to participate. Any nurse manager who is not willing to aggressively participate in his or her staff's training development should not be a manager. And the same goes for every other layer of management in the organization. Supporting the advancement of the staff is the fundamental job of management, and every member of the team must view it as a primary responsibility.

Another method that can be used to enhance the likelihood of behavioral change is to tie the objectives of the training program to an end result for the organization. Things such as reduced turnover, fewer grievances, reduced absenteeism, higher quality of care, and fewer accidents are normally expressed in quantitative data and can be easily tied to dollars. What a training program must do to cause behavioral change in the performance unit is to link this change to things that are understood by and important to the performer.

4. *Organizational impact:* It is often difficult to determine whether changes in given areas can be unequivocally attributed to a training program or are influenced by other variables in the organization, such as changes in competitiveness, changes in management, increased pay, new equipment, or better selection. When a training evaluation is performed, particular care must be taken in deciding on the length of time for data collection, the unit of analysis, the method of randomization, and other aspects of experimental design so that the effect of outside variables can be ruled out. The most important criteria for measuring results are those that are related closely to the key training behaviors. Despite all of the difficulties involved in assembling and analyzing cost-related data, the trainer should attempt to collect such information, because it provides evidence to management that training efforts do influence organizational effectiveness.

Fig. 21-5 is a form for assessing the cost-effectiveness of a proposed training program. This form can be used to determine the probable dollar benefit to an organization when it is conducting a training program. It is recommended that nurse managers review other methods for evaluating training programs by calculating human resource outcomes in terms of dollars.[11]

Another important thing to consider when determining the cost-effectiveness of a training program is direct meeting costs, especially for programs that are conducted off site. Off-site meetings and training events are among the most costly methods of training personnel and among the least effective in developing behavioral change. The form shown in Fig. 21-5 can also be used to evaluate the cost-effectiveness of these types of programs.[2,10] This form can be used to determine how time should be spent during the training days and whether increasing or deceasing the number of training hours will change the overall cost of the training program.

PATIENT EDUCATION

Over the past four decades, a number of trends have combined to bring into prominence the need for continual education in the healthcare field. The increasing effort to promote good health rather than simply to treat disease has significantly increased the amount of knowledge nursing personnel must have to perform effectively. This new focus and the resulting enhanced professionalism of healthcare personnel have led to a major change in the attitudes about and perceptions of health and healthcare systems. Today,

Training Program Cost-Effectiveness Evaluation

1. Name of training program evaluated: _____

_____

_____

2. Description of training program: _____

_____

_____

3. Is this program a legal requirement? ☐ Yes ☐ No
   If so, what is the legal basis for the requirement? _____

_____

_____

4. Difficulty of implementation: _____

_____

_____

5. Special implementation requirements: _____

_____

_____

6. Anticipated economic benefits derived from program: _____

_____

_____

7. Identifiable benefits:

	Potential Revenue Impact	X	Probability of Occurrence (0-1.0)	=	Probable Gross Benefit
A.	_____	X	_____	=	_____
B.	_____	X	_____	=	_____
C.	_____	X	_____	=	_____
D.	_____	X	_____	=	_____
E.	_____	X	_____	=	_____

8. Total identifiable costs:

	Potential Revenue Impact	X	Probability of Occurrence (0-1.0)	=	Probable Cost ($)
A. Trainer time	_____	X	_____	=	_____
B. Training time	_____	X	_____	=	_____
C. Training facilities	_____	X	_____	=	_____
D. Meals/coffee/snacks	_____	X	_____	=	_____
E. Cost of lost performance	_____	X	_____	=	_____
F. Cost of overtime	_____	X	_____	=	_____

Fig. 21-5 ■ Sample form for evaluating the cost-effectiveness of a training program.

Continued

9. Intangible costs and benefits: _____

_____

_____

10. Potential risks involved: _____

_____

_____

11. Risks involved in not acting: _____

_____

_____

12. Other considerations/assumptions: _____

_____

_____

Fig. 21-5—cont'd ■ Sample form for evaluating the cost-effectiveness of a training program.

the shorter hospital stays and early ambulation require that patients be well prepared before being sent home to convalesce. During this same period there has also been a marked increase in the incidence of long-term illness and disability, which requires that both patients and their families receive additional information to prepare them for adjustment to daily life. Finally, the significant increase in malpractice suits alleging that hospitals and medical staff did not fully inform patients about what they were consenting to and the size of the settlements these liability actions have generated have led insurance companies to demand increased emphasis on patient education.

As a result of these changes and the increased liability of healthcare organizations, the Joint Commission on Accreditation of Healthcare Organizations (JCAHO) has increased pressure on healthcare organizations in the area of patient education. That urgency has been supported by policy statements from the American Medical Association (AMA), the American Nurses Association (ANA), and the American Hospital Association (AHA) that have outlined responsibilities for educating patients.

A hospital has a responsibility to provide patient education services as an integral part of high-quality, cost-effective care. Patient education services should enable patients, their families and friends, when appropriate, to make informed decisions about their health; to manage their illness; and to implement follow-up care at home. Effective and efficient patient education services require planning and coordination, and respon-

sibility for such planning and coordination should be assigned. The hospital should also provide the necessary staff and financial resources.

Nurse managers fulfill several responsibilities in conjunction with the delivery of patient education, including the following:

Prepare and assess staff: Nurse managers are responsible for ensuring that their staff members are prepared to provide training to patients and their families. To discharge this responsibility, nurse managers must document what their staff members accomplish and continually assess the quality of their teaching, regardless of whether the instruction is conducted orally or through written text. Nurse managers have primary responsibility for ensuring that their staff members have patient teaching skills and that they are given the educational opportunities to develop these vital skills.

Maintain awareness of organizational effort: Nurse managers must be aware of the training programs used hospital-wide so that they will not waste valuable time in duplication of effort.

Serve on committees: Nurse managers' input to committees involved in patient education is critical to the success of any program, especially those in their areas of clinical specialty.

Assist with planning: Nurse managers must serve as subject matter experts in the development of effective training plans for the unit and the organization, especially when those plans are focused on the needs of their specific patients.

Manage the educational effort in the unit: Nurse managers must identify both the specific and general training needs in their units, coordinate the patient education activities therein, effectively delegate appropriate responsibility, and follow up to ensure compliance and progress.

Nurse managers may elect to perform patient instruction themselves or delegate that responsibility to the more outstanding staff nurses in their units. They can ask their organizations' education departments to assist in developing staff members' teaching skills or use group classes or videotape presentations being held on a hospital-wide basis. Nurse managers may select from a wide variety of different methods of delivering patient training, such as one-to-one sessions and more formalized group presentations. In addition, almost every organization maintains an extensive library of educational material to assist patients in learning the information necessary to meet their needs.

The professionalism of typical staff nurses is such that, almost to a person, they place high value on carefully instructing their patients; however, many of them feel personally unprepared to teach effectively. The most common cause of this feeling of inadequacy is a belief that they lack sufficient content knowledge, teaching experience, and mastery of instructional technique, or that they have insufficient time to do the best job possible. Nurse managers must work diligently to correct these perceived deficiencies and develop confidence in the nursing staff. One suggested method of accomplishing this is to encourage staff members to read and keep up with changes in their profession and particular specialty.

Patient education is a continuous process. Nurse managers must stress its importance and develop in nursing staff the willingness and desire to assume the responsibilities inherent in the provision of education. Training is something that can occur just about anywhere—while the nurse is caring for the patient at the bedside, during laboratory testing, in the hallway, and through television watching. Training can be accomplished by just about anyone in the hospital who has been given proper instruction, including nurses, managers, administrators, doctors, patient educators, specialized trainers, and, yes, especially nurse managers.

Challenges Faced in Teaching Patients

Even when patient teaching programs are professionally developed and conducted and incorporate all of the activities required for an effective learning process, they may not always be successful. Many different factors can limit their effectiveness, and professional nurse managers must plan to minimize these challenges. The following is a list of the major challenges that will be found in nearly every nursing unit:

Low priority: Many organizations, and many nurse managers for that matter, make the mistake of not giving training a sufficiently high priority in the daily work schedule. Experience indicates that if patient teaching is not given high priority by management, it either will not take place or will be done poorly—even if more than sufficient opportunity for effective instruction is present. To ensure that their nursing units continually set a high priority on patient instruction, nurse managers should see that the specific ingredients essential in establishing patient education are reinforced. These include the following:

- Maintenance of a positive attitude regarding the need for patient education by both the organization and the nursing staff
- Commitment from the hospital administration to support patient education by allocating time, money, and staff
- Inclusion of patient instruction responsibilities as a component of performance evaluation
- Operation of an effective reward program for those who perform quality patient training and, to acceptable limits, specific sanctions for those who do not support it
- Reinforcement and recognition for teaching efforts and accomplishments

Lack of time: Too little time is probably the most commonly raised defense for not teaching patients, but it is no more than a simple excuse. Many nurses are quick to cite a lack of time because of the demands of their heavy workloads or allude to inadequate staffing as the reason for inadequate patient teaching; however, professional nurse managers make sure that their staffs understand that patient teaching is an expected part of the normal workload, not an extra that is accomplished only if there is time. Training does require time, but most of it can be done as part of the job. It is not necessary to set aside a block of time specifically designated for teaching patients. Questions can be answered and information given at any time a nurse is providing patient care. In fact, any nurse who does not understand this point needs instruction in basic professionalism.

Lack of communication: Every staff member involved in patient care needs to know about the individual patient's learning needs. This information can be communicated throughout the nursing unit from shift to shift by documentation in the patient's chart. What training has been given and what needs to be performed should be charted. Charting patient instruction should be just as common and just as important as charting other patient needs and treatment.

Lack of knowledge: Nurses who lack proper training or believe themselves to be insufficiently prepared rarely will provide instruction to patients. The only truly effective method of dealing with ignorance is to teach what needs to be known and then work with the staff to develop confidence. Ignorance by itself is a problem that can easily be fixed. It does not become a concern unless it is ignored.

Lack of confidence: Lack of confidence is an offshoot of ignorance or the feeling of inadequacy that is fostered by lack of experience. Teaching patients is something that all nurses are prepared for and, by virtue of their position, are capable of providing. However, most feel that they somehow lack the qualities required to be effective. Nurse managers should continually remind their subordinates that theirs is a profession respected almost universally by the people they serve. Patients look to nurses for answers and instruction and only feel neglected when these are not provided. Every nurse can teach; those who say they can't simply don't try hard enough. Nurse managers can eliminate this excuse by providing a plan of education for the staff through inservice programs or attendance at training sessions, workshops, and other continuing education programs.

Lack of teaching skill: Nurses need to understand the principles of teaching to reach their full capability as patient educators. The more they comprehend teaching principles, the more likely they will be to teach. The ability to teach involves specific skills, including interpersonal sensitivity, the ability to communicate, the ability to develop trust and rapport, and the desire to recognize and anticipate needs.[12]

Lack of family involvement: Often, it is critical to get the patient's family involved in the instruction being presented. Nurse managers should ensure that members of the patient's family actively participate in any training session given, especially if they are to be involved in the patient's recovery.

Lack of continuity: Because many different people interact with the patient and family during the hospital stay, it is easy for the patient and family to become confused by the different interpretations of facts and material. To avoid this, it is helpful to maintain a detailed teaching record for each patient.

Poor patient motivation: Poor patient motivation can result from low self-esteem, a crowded schedule, lack of trust in and rapport with the staff, and just plain fear. Nurse managers should encourage every member of their staffs to work with each patient to develop rapport, trust, and confidence. People rarely follow those who *tell* them to do something; they almost always gravitate to those who *encourage* them to do something.

Patient's physical condition: Patients often cannot attend to the learning because they are weak or in pain. The elimination of this obstacle comes through good observational skills and timing. The training should be provided when the patient is ready to accept it, not when the nurse is ready to give it.

Patient's psychosocial adaptation to illness: The patient's adaptation to illness may affect his or her motivation to learn. Readiness to learn differs at the various stages of the adaptation process.

An effective way to promote patient teaching is to assemble a patient education planning group in the nursing unit to accomplish the following objectives:

1. Help counteract physician resistance, if physicians are included in the planning group
2. Help develop in the unit the attitude that patient education is important
3. Define staff expectations regarding patient teaching
4. Build staff nurses' knowledge of the learning process and teaching skills, with attention to elements such as role clarification, development of nurse-patient rapport, content review, appraisal of learning needs, assessment of readiness to learn, teaching strategies, and documentation

Education and Training Development in the Organization

Within the hospital, an excellent resource for patient education is the education and training department, whose services can be used to improve the nursing staff's teaching skills and competencies. This department typically offers courses, workshops, inservice training, and other patient education programs to improve the quality of patient teaching and promote consistency in the information disseminated to patients. Often the patient education coordinator position is located in this department.

Having a hospital-wide coordinator of patient education has been a national trend for more than two decades. Hospital patient education units have proven their importance by ensuring that the need for cost-effective programs is met. They have had a tremendous effect in organizations, reducing or even eliminating the duplication of efforts in program development and implementation that long taxed the budgets of hospitals. But the most effective contribution of these units is the centralization of planning, direction, and evaluation of patient education programs. The nurse manager should continually seek out the patient education coordinator for information, support, and assistance regarding any patient education needs or problems in the nursing unit. Instructors in this department are also educational resources for the nurse manager.

Record Keeping and Evaluation

All hospitals and health education programs must keep records of patient education, because these records can have a direct impact in any liability litigation initiated by or on behalf of a patient. Liability is a major concern of every healthcare provider, and judgments are almost always based on negligence. To ensure that the organization can prove that it has, in fact, made legitimate efforts to assist a patient and that those efforts conform to the requirements of the profession and the law, the patient's records must be maintained to provide a written account of what happened to the patient while he or she was in the hospital. These records are considered official documents and, as such, are admissible in court and can be subpoenaed; therefore they should be complete and accurate. Entries should be made when teaching occurs, and each entry should be dated and signed. Erasures should never be allowed, even to correct an erroneous entry, because, in a courtroom, erasures can look like attempted concealment. If these basic procedures are followed, liability can be dramatically reduced.

A variety of patient education records can be kept, including the following:

- Referral forms used when patients are billed specifically for an educational program
- Standing orders for educational programs
- A nursing assessment that includes information about a patient's educational needs

It is important to document what has been taught to the patient and family. Whether or not the patient has demonstrated comprehension or competency should be recorded; this can be ascertained by observing the patient, asking direct questions, and discussing specifics with the patient. However, the ability to verbalize an understanding of a concept is not definitive and does not necessarily indicate that a person has developed a certain skill. The nurse manager should make certain that adequate steps have been taken to ensure patient comprehension and that these steps are documented in the patient's records.

SUMMARY

- There is always a need for staff and patient education. This education should be based on adult learning principles.
- Most hospitals have specialized training personnel, but nurse managers also have a role in both staff and patient education.
- The basic training process parallels that of nursing: assessment of training needs, planning, implementation, feedback, and evaluation.
- Three questions need to be answered during assessment: (1) Can the trainee do what is required? (2) If not, is it due to lack of skill or lack of motivation? (3) If it is lack of skill, is training a current employee a more cost-effective approach than hiring a person who already has the skill?
- There are many aspects of learning that must be considered any training program: (1) Is the trainee ready to learn? (2) Is the trainee motivated to learn? (3) Are practice opportunities properly provided? (4) Is transfer of training facilitated? (5) Is too much material given to learn at one time? (6) Is feedback provided? (7) Is the program formulated for adults?
- Staff development includes orientation, formalized education, and on-the-job instruction.
- Although evaluation is done infrequently, it should be carried out after training intervention to confirm the success of the intervention. Elements evaluated include trainee reaction to the program, learning demonstrated, behavioral change achieved, and organizational impact.
- Patient education has increased because of the emphasis on maintaining health; reduction in hospital stays; and declared policies of the AMA, JCAHO, ANA, and AHA.
- Barriers to teaching include low priority for patient education, lack of time, lack of communication between care givers, lack of knowledge, lack of teaching skill, lack of involvement of the patient's family, and poor patient motivation.
- Educational records include billing records, standing orders for patient education, staff educational records, and documentation of results.

FINAL THOUGHTS

Nurse managers play a key role in the development of their staffs and the creation of a professional and amicable work environment. They must continually be supportive and strive to develop each member of the team to his or her highest potential. This development process should include all types and levels of training: in-house programs, consultant-provided training, formal education, and specialized instruction.

There is always a need for staff and specialized education. The basic elements of training parallel those of nursing and include the following:

1. Assessment of training needs
2. Planning
3. Implementation
4. Evaluation

Educational records include billing records, standing orders, staff educational records, and documentation of results. Patient training helps mitigate the risk inherent in health care.

THE NURSE MANAGER SPEAKS

Every individual within the healthcare industry represents a unique profile, varying in formal education, professional training, individual skills, and personal ability; however, most who are properly motivated to excel will work harder to achieve a goal or consequence than one who is not.

Not withstanding the typical professional quality of staff nurses, only the highest quality staff member should be selected for training and assignment as a preceptor.

Training the staff should be thought of as a primary duty and not something that others should do or have the responsibility for. It is nurse managers who bear the responsibility for enhancing the performance of their units, and one of the best methods of fulfilling that responsibility is to ensure that all of the staff continually train toward superior performance.

The manager bears the responsibility for ensuring that the information gained during a training session is put into practice in the work center. No one should be sent to training without the nurse manager's following up to see that the knowledge gained is turned into actual performance within the unit.

REFERENCES

1. Wicks GT: The cost of technology, *Information Week,* p 17, Sept 9, 1996.
2. Wexley KN, Latham GP: *Developing and training human resources in organizations,* Glenview, Ill, 1981, Scott, Foresman.
3. Ellis HC: *The transfer of learning,* ed 3, New York, 1992, Macmillan.
4. Hawkins JA: *American business management,* Honolulu, 1999, Directions Training Development Corporation.
5. Bandura A: *Social learning theory,* Englewood Cliffs, NJ, 1977, Prentice-Hall.
6. Daley DC: *Relapse: conceptual research and clinical perspectives,* New York, 1989, Haworth Press.
7. Knowles MS: *The modern process of adult education,* New York, 1970, Association Press.
8. May L: Clinical preceptors for new nurses, *Am J Nurs* 80(10):1824, 1980.
9. Murphy ML, Hammerstad SM: Preparing a staff nurse for precepting, *Nurs Educ* 6(5):17, 1981.
10. Breckon DJ: *Hospital health education,* Rockville, Md, 1982, Aspen.
11. Cascio WF: *Costing human resources: the financial impact of behavior in organizations,* Boston, 1982, Kent.
12. Corkadel L, McGlashan: A practical approach to patient teaching, *J Contin Educ Nurs* 14:9, 1983.

SUGGESTED READINGS

Craig RL: *Training and development handbook,* ed 4, New York, 1998, McGraw-Hill.

Crate MA: Nursing functions in adaptation to chronic illness, *Am J Nurs* 65(10):72, 1965.

Decker PJ, Nathan B: *Behavior modeling training: theory and application,* ed 2, New York, 2001, Praeger Scientific Publishing.

Douglas LM: *The effective nurse leader and manager,* ed 5, St Louis, 1999, Mosby.

Ellis JR, Hartley CL: *Managing and coordinating nursing care,* ed 2, Philadelphia, 1995, Lippincott.

Goldstein LL: *Training: program development and evaluation,* ed 2, Monterey, Calif, 1991, Brooks/Cole.

Hall DT: *Careers in organizations,* Santa Monica, Calif, 1976, Goodyear.

Loveridge CE, Cummings SH: *Nursing management in the new paradigm,* Gaithersburg, Md, 1996, Aspen.

Marquis BL, Huston CJ: *Management decision making for nurses,* Philadelphia, 1998, Lippincott.

Minor MA: Ten- and six-hour nursing shifts solve staffing problems, *Hosp Prog* 52:62, 1971.

Redman BK: *The process of patient teaching in nursing,* St Louis, 1980, Mosby.

Shaw ME, Corsini RJ, Blake RR, and others: *Role playing,* New York, 1980, Wiley.

Managing the Performance Appraisal Process

OUTLINE

LEARNING SYNOPSIS

Upon successful completion of this chapter, readers will possess a fundamental understanding of the importance of the performance appraisal process to the organization, the nursing unit, the nurse manager, and the individual healthcare employee.

OBJECTIVES

1. Identify the six fundamental assumptions of the performance appraisal process
2. Describe the basic and critical uses of the performance appraisal
3. Discuss how employment law affects the performance appraisal process and how performance appraisal can support the organization against legal challenge

4. Identify the major performance measurement issues that arise in the performance appraisal process
5. Describe specific methods that can be used in the performance appraisal process
6. Understand why the performance appraisal process is important, who within the organization usually bears the major responsibility for its effectiveness, and what challenges can occur to hinder the appraisal process
7. Identify and discuss methods that can be used to improve the performance appraisal process
8. Describe ways a nurse manager can document employee performance to facilitate the development of performance appraisals
9. Identify procedures that can be used to enhance the performance appraisal interview
10. Describe methods and processes the nurse manager can use to coach the staff toward success

The performance appraisal process used by organizations in the healthcare industry typically includes the following four elements:

1. Day-by-day interaction between management and employees during activities such as job performance, coaching, counseling, and disciplining
2. Written documentation such as commendations, critical incident reporting, and the completion of the performance review form
3. The formal performance appraisal interview
4. Follow-up to the formal performance appraisal that involves actions such as recognition, reward, coaching, and/or discipline as required

The primary goal of this chapter is to provide nurse managers with an improved understanding of the elements that contribute to the creation of the performance appraisal and that affect the entire process of performance review, which is one of the most critical responsibilities of managers at every level.

If a group of nurse managers were asked to list the things they liked least about their job, performance appraisals would probably be at or near the tops of all of their lists. It is the part of the job that most managers dislike most. If the same group of nurse managers were asked why they dislike writing and conducting performance reviews, most would be able to provide a long list of reasons such as the following:

- It is impossible to properly evaluate nursing performance.
- The form used to create the evaluation is not adequate to properly assess whether the employee has met the demanding performance requirements.
- Professionals don't need to be evaluated, and performance evaluation of a professional nurse is an inadequate measure of the dedication and professionalism required in the job.
- Low ratings may create marginal performance and severely limit opportunity.
- There is no proper way to gather enough information to rate accurately.

For these and a great many other reasons and excuses, those nurse managers charged with generating performance appraisals typically do not consider this task to be as important as other aspects of their jobs and consequently spend very little time developing such appraisals properly. The result is usually that the average ratings given are higher than are actually earned.

What about the staff nurse's perspective on performance appraisal? Take a moment to reflect back to your own most recent performance review and think about the process in the context of the following three questions:

1. How prepared was your manager when he or she presented the appraisal?
2. How accurately did the feedback you were given portray your actual performance during the reviewed period?
3. Did the evaluation process help you improve your performance?

If your answers to these questions are, "Not as prepared as necessary," "Not very accurately," and "No, it did not help me improve," then your response is typical of the way most people would respond if asked similar questions about their own performance appraisals.

None of this negative feeling regarding performance appraisals should be construed as a recommendation to do away with the performance appraisal process, however. To the contrary, this chapter advocates keeping the performance appraisal because it is critical to the overall effectiveness of the healthcare organization and the continued professionalism of every nurse in it. The problem with performance appraisals is not the fact that they are necessary but the manner in which they are prepared and presented. This chapter provides information that, if followed, will prepare nurse managers to do a better job of performing this critical task. Before the specifics of creating and presenting appraisals are dealt with, however, let's take a minute to describe the many and varied factors that affect the way appraisals are done.

ASSUMPTIONS

The discussion in this chapter is based on the following six fundamental assumptions:

1. *Performance reviews should be future oriented.* One of the most fundamental reasons for providing performance reviews is to assist employees in improving their future performance.
2. *Appraisers can improve their evaluation performance.* Managers can become more accurate in the development of their ratings and more professional in providing constructive feedback to the individual being appraised. Although the performance appraisal process is a difficult part of the nurse manager's job, there is little reason that managers cannot become more skilled at it. Often, the difference between the development of an excellent performance review and a marginal one has little to do with the performance of the individual being evaluated and everything to do with the attitude of the nurse manager toward the requirement to write the review.
3. *The form is never the issue.* Very few nurse managers actually like the performance appraisal form they are required to use; however, citing the poor quality of the form as an excuse for not fulfilling one's responsibility for developing quality performance reviews is unprofessional. Remarks like "The form takes too long to complete," "The form is contradictory," "The form requires me to make judgments that I lack the data to make," and so on, reflect managerial weakness and should be avoided, especially within hearing of subordinates.
4. *Excellent year-end reviews start with observation and documentation.* A good performance review does not simply happen when the nurse manager sits down to write it. Instead, a high-quality formal year-end review begins with the nurse manager's carefully observing the day-to-day performance of the person who is to be evaluated

and then appropriately recording the observed behaviors, both good and bad, so that they will not be forgotten as the year progresses.
5. *Supervisors always evaluate their employees' performance.* It is a fundamental responsibility of management to observe and evaluate the performance of subordinate personnel against the standards and requirements of their job descriptions and the organization. In fact, the only question is whether the evaluation is conducted informally through verbal exchange with the employee or takes the more formal structure of a written performance review; both require specific feedback to occur between the nurse manager and the employee.
6. *Quality review practices will not always be effective.* The recommendations in this chapter will not work with every employee on the staff. In fact, it is a generally accepted belief with the managers interviewed during research for this book that at least 5% of all employees will not benefit from a performance review, no matter how professionally developed and delivered. However, even if one assumes that this is true (and many, many argue fervently that it is not), this does not relieve nurse managers of the responsibility to professionally develop and deliver performance reviews to all employees within their charge.

THE MANY USES OF PERFORMANCE APPRAISAL

Many progressive organizations use the performance appraisal process as the cornerstone for making a number of key administrative decisions in areas of critical concern to employees, such as salary increases, promotion decisions, transfers, demotions, and even terminations of employment. If this marriage between administrative requirements and performance analysis is accomplished properly, the accurate performance appraisal process that results will allow the organization to gain better performance and align collateral programs such as reward and recognition systems. In addition, the performance appraisal process can be an effective method of ensuring that ongoing programs focused on employee development are an active part of the employment process. This might be realized by having the manager work with each employee early in the review cycle (immediately after the last review is the best time to start) to develop an action plan designed to improve the employee's overall performance. The manager and his or her employee can collaborate to design a program incorporating a variety of developmental activities such as formal training, academic course work, simple on-the-job coaching, or a some combination of these. Then, when the manager sits down to write the next performance review for the employee, the manager can use the action plan as an objective tool for evaluating the employee's progress.

Another critical reason for having an effective performance review process is the absolute necessity for every organization to comply with the federally mandated Equal Employment Opportunity Act (Title VII of the U.S. Code). If employment practices such as promotion, salary increases, job assignments, and even termination of employment are based on performance appraisals, it is far less likely that the organization can be called into question regarding its compliance with state and federal law. This is a critical point, because the implementation of an effective performance review process can do much to limit an organization's liability when employment lawsuits are brought. The history of the healthcare industry is littered with the stories of employees who have successfully brought legal action against organizations over employment decisions and won in open court. Having and rigidly adhering to an effective policy of using performance appraisals as a major factor in employment decisions has proven to be a strong deterrent against unwarranted allegations.

Regardless of what logic an organization might employ when it comes to the use of performance appraisals, no use will be effective if the appraisals do not accurately reflect employees' job performance. If an individual manager, when assigning an employee his or her performance rating, does so in an inaccurate, unfair, or inappropriate manner, a mediocre employee may get a promotion that might better be filled by another individual, additional employees may not receive the training they need to maximize their performance, or the organization might not be able to effectively tie the performance evaluation to motivational and performance programs such as recognition and rewards. Any of these situations reduces overall performance in the organization and acts to decrease the individual employee's motivation. What is most important, however, is that they can result in the hospital's involvement in a costly and embarrassing lawsuit. There is no room for mediocrity in the performance evaluation process; managers must be able to write and support accurate performance evaluations.

THE LAW AND ITS EFFECTS ON PERFORMANCE APPRAISAL

Since the U.S. Congress passed Title VII, the legal system has seen an overwhelming number of litigations centered on employment decisions. A majority of these cases have concerned promotions, terminations of employment, and compensation decisions in which performance appraisals have played an important role.[1] In many of these legal actions, the court system has not been kind to the healthcare industry, ruling that the employment decision being litigated was illegal because the organization's performance appraisal system was in some way impaired. Although it is almost impossible to guarantee that any organization's performance appraisal system will always be legally defensible, there are things organizations can do to help ensure that their procedures will at least be nondiscriminatory. Some of these (e.g., the type of performance appraisal form used) may not lie within the sphere of control of the individual manager. However, managers can attend to the following basic guidelines that can help to decrease the potential for a finding of discrimination or other poor outcome in litigation:

Frequency and form: Every performance appraisal should be conducted at least annually and should be made in writing.

Common information: The information contained in the performance appraisal should be shared, in its entirety, with the evaluated employee, and the employee should be compelled to sign the performance review form acknowledging that he or she has seen it.

Written response: The employee should be provided with sufficient time and opportunity to respond to the content of the performance review in writing.

Appeal: The organization should have available a simple, easily understood mechanism by which an employee can appeal the results of his or her performance appraisal.

Sufficient observation: The manager drafting the performance appraisal should have an adequate opportunity to observe the employee's actual job performance. If adequate time has not been available for proper observation, such as when the manager works days and the employee is on the night shift, the information required to draft the appraisal should be gathered from other sources, and those sources should be named in the report and should sign the report indicating their participation.

All managers must understand that the observation period begins on minute 1, day 1, following the previous performance review. Too many supervisors tend to wait to gather information until just before they write the performance review. This practice is not only incredibly unfair to the employee, it is highly unprofessional and has even been judged unlawful. Employees do things, good and bad, every day of the year. Managers should not miss the opportunity to collect data that can help in developing an excellent review by realizing only at the last moment that information gathering is important to their success.[2]

Documentation: Notes recording both critical incidents and casual observations should be kept to document each employee's performance over the entire evaluation period. These notes should be shared with the employee during the course of the evaluation interval. It is very important that managers not rely on their memories, no matter how good they might be. Memory, by and large, has very poor credibility in a court of law.

Training: No manager who writes performance reviews should be allowed to do so until he or she has completed a comprehensive training program on how to do it correctly. The manager should be trained, at a minimum, how to perform the following four tasks:

1. Carry out the performance appraisal process
2. Determine exactly what reasonable job performance is
3. Complete the evaluation form
4. Conduct the feedback interview

Objectivity and performance orientation: To the highest degree possible, the performance appraisal should be based on the employee's actual behavior (what the employee did compared with what he or she was expected to do). This observed behavior should be assessed against goals and objectives that are measurable and objective. The evaluation should not be based on subjective judgments of elements such as personality traits (e.g., initiative, attitude, congeniality).

Managers absolutely must not place themselves in situations that come down to "I think" or "she said, he said." When it comes to a manager's word against an employee's, the court system has tended to lean heavily in favor of the employee, even to the point of allowing personal lawsuits against the errant manager.

PERFORMANCE MEASUREMENT ISSUES

Whether or not a manager has had the opportunity to supply formal input as to the type of performance appraisal instrument used by his or her organization is not important. This has absolutely no bearing on whether the manager can write a high-quality performance review. In fact, those managers who complain about such a situation are simply using it as an excuse to cover up some other challenge, such as a poor attitude or unprofessional conduct. What is

important is that the manager have a thorough understanding of the essential issues in the performance review process so that he or she can deal effectively with the many constraints that affect how appraisals are actually developed. Specifically, the manager must know more than the simple mechanics of writing a performance review; for example, the manager must also understand the underlying approach (absolute or comparative judgments) used by the performance appraisal system and the effect that is to be achieved by it.

Basic Approach

To begin, managers need to determine whether the evaluations they will make are to be absolute or comparative.

ABSOLUTE

Well-developed evaluation systems are based on absolute judgment; that is, the individual's performance is evaluated against a standard that is well known to both the manager and the employee undergoing review. This standard reflects what the manager perceives as being reasonable and acceptable performance for a staff nurse and what has been discussed in detail with the employee at the very beginning of the review period. When evaluations are absolute, the employee's performance can be judged as exceeding or failing to meet the standard for acceptable performance. If the standard was discussed with the employee at the beginning of the review period and was known by the employee to represent expected behavior, then if the employee fails to measure up, a poor review rating should not come as a surprise to the employee.

Under an absolute rating system, evaluations are based largely on the judgment of the manager; however, the subjective element should be minimized by ensuring that the standard against which the manager judges the employee's performance aligns with the organization's performance standards and with the highest goals of professionalism and conduct for the nursing profession.

COMPARATIVE

When evaluations are based on comparative judgments, the manager rates subordinates by comparing each employee with others performing the same or a very similar job. This means that a specific nurse's performance evaluation will be based on the level of performance of his or her peers. A good analogy is the university professor who grades on a curve. When this system is used, the evaluation received by each person in a particular job category is based on the manager's comparative judgment of the relative standing of the person being reviewed among his or her peers.

Because evaluations based on this system require the manager to comparatively rate all of the employees with a particular job description, not all of the employees being reviewed will receive a high rating. Some ratings will be low, some will be in the middle, and only a few will be high. This approach is contradictory to the way in which most managers prefer to rate their employees; that is, the tendency of unit managers is to rate others, especially others with skills similar to their own, as high performers. Given the basic premise of comparative evaluation, it is no surprise that most nurse managers develop their ratings using absolute judgments. Rating scales based on the two kinds of judgment are presented in Fig. 22-1.

Focus of Evaluation

In today's healthcare organization, every nurse must perform in a variety of demanding professional and supportive activities. To ensure that the multidimensional nature of the staff nurse's job is accurately taken into account, the typical form used for the

---

Absolute and Comparative Judgment

Comparative Judgment

Rate each staff nurse you supervise by comparing his or her performance against all others you supervise

	Bottom 10%	Next 20%	Middle 40%	Next 20%	Top 10%
1. Initiative/enthusiasm	☐	☐	☐	☐	☐

All staff nurses supervised

	Bottom 10%	Next 20%	Middle 40%	Next 20%	Top 10%
2. Dependability	☐	☐	☐	☐	☐

All staff nurses supervised

	Bottom 10%	Next 20%	Middle 40%	Next 20%	Top 10%
3. Job knowledge	☐	☐	☐	☐	☐

All staff nurses supervised

	Bottom 10%	Next 20%	Middle 40%	Next 20%	Top 10%
4. Policies/regulations compliance	☐	☐	☐	☐	☐

All staff nurses supervised

Absolute Judgment

Rate each staff member on how well he or she meets the standards for satisfactory performance

	Does not meet	Meets few	Meets	Exceeds	Far exceeds
1. Initiative/enthusiasm	☐	☐	☐	☐	☐
2. Dependability	☐	☐	☐	☐	☐
3. Job knowledge	☐	☐	☐	☐	☐
4. Policies/regulations compliance	☐	☐	☐	☐	☐

Fig. 22-1 ■ Differentiation between absolute judgment and comparative judgment in performance appraisal.

performance appraisal requires that the manager rate the staff nurse along a variety of different performance dimensions, such as creativity, initiative, job knowledge, and human relations (the ability to work well with others). In developing the form used to document an employee's performance (the performance appraisal form), the typical organization also focuses on general performance characteristics such as results obtained and behaviors exhibited.[1] The style and focus of the appraisal form created by the organization's management will affect the entire review process. The importance of the form cannot be overemphasized, and it is every manager's responsibility to provide constructive feedback to organizational administrators so that the form can evolve to fit the changing needs of the nursing unit.

TRAITS AND PERSONAL CHARACTERISTICS

Most older performance appraisal systems focused attention on documenting the personal traits and characteristics of the individual receiving the evaluation (e.g., emotional stability, ability to perform in demanding circumstances, performance under stress).[2] Different traits and characteristics were included on the form, and nurse managers were required to rate their staff nurses independently in each area. These ratings were typically heavily subjective, and nurse managers performed them following the organizational requirement to use either absolute or comparative judgment. In most cases, these performance appraisal systems based on personal traits and characteristics were used primarily because the cost to develop them was relatively low and they could be used for a variety of different job positions.

The past decade has seen a significant shift away from the old-style trait-oriented systems, however, largely because of their inability to support the organization's position during litigation. Too many instances have occurred in which these subjective trait rating systems have yielded lower scores for minorities and women than for men, and in every such case discovered, the organization has experienced huge financial repercussions. Today, both federal and state law require organizations to demonstrate the validity (job-relatedness) of the appraisal ratings given to every employee. When an organization that has failed to comply with these laws has become involved in a legal challenge, the organization has almost always been found to be guilty of illegal discrimination.

Another reason that organizations have moved away from trait rating is the lack of applicability of this form of appraisal to employee growth and development. Today, the underlying reason for the performance appraisal is to assist in the employee's development. Because trait ratings are almost entirely subjective in nature and ambiguous in content (initiative, for instance, can have a hundred different definitions or interpretations), trait-oriented systems have proven to be of little use in helping an employee enhance his or her performance.

RESULTS

Today's business environment is exceptionally demanding, and all organizations, even those holding Internal Revenue Code section 501(c)(3) status as not-for-profit institutions, must focus on maintaining positive cash flow and bottom-line performance. Today, if a hospital has a 75% occupancy rate, a 15% staff absenteeism rate, and several pending malpractice suits, its future is bleak, no matter what its past success has been. Today, it is absolutely necessary for a hospital to keep its bottom line positive, and to do so, senior administrators have turned to performance appraisal as a means of motivating employees.

Little argument exists that results-oriented performance appraisal systems are, at least theoretically, vastly superior to the old-style trait-oriented systems, because employees know in advance what results they are supposed to accomplish and their objectives are quantifiable, objective, and easily measured. The most significant problem faced by a healthcare institution that is contemplating a shift to a results-oriented appraisal system is that, in practice, it is not easy to come up with readily measured, concrete objectives for many healthcare jobs. For example, one important aspect of a staff nurse's job—providing a high quality of patient care—is not easily quantified; other aspects, such as the average number of minutes that elapse before the nurse answers a patient's call button, may be easily quantified but may not be worth the cost of measurement. In addition, use of a results-oriented system does not guarantee that the staff's future performance will be enhanced, because simply telling someone that he or she failed to accomplish a goal does not, by itself, teach that person how to accomplish it in the future. Therefore, although extremely good reasons exist to implement a results-oriented appraisal system in an organization, it does not make good business sense to rely totally on such a system.[3,4]

BEHAVIORS

The weaknesses of both appraisal systems discussed previously have led many healthcare institutions to adopt a behavior-oriented performance appraisal system rather than endure the challenges and pitfalls of the older versions. Unlike the earlier trait- and results-oriented appraisal systems, the behavior-oriented system focuses on what employees actually do—not what is expected, or what it would be nice for them to do. An example of such an appraisal is shown in Fig. 22-2. Because the behavior-oriented system provides all employees with specific information on how they are expected to behave, it is less likely to lead to legal problems and its behavioral focus is far more conducive to employee development. In spite of these obvious advantages, however, use of a behavior-based appraisal system is not without drawbacks. Probably the most compelling disadvantage is the fact that a behavior-oriented appraisal system is often extremely time consuming and expensive to develop and is generally applicable to a narrow range of jobs at most and possibly to as few as one. This shortcoming can be observed in Fig. 22-2, which lists a series of behaviors that were identified by interviewing a number of staff nurses and their immediate supervisors. Unlike the more general trait dimensions seen in Fig. 22-1, these behaviors would be applicable only to staff nurses and not to other performers working in the same unit.

COMBINATION OF ELEMENTS

The events of the last three decades have forced healthcare institutions to become more concerned with employee productivity, and, as a result, many have developed appraisal systems that combine all of the types of evaluation just discussed. This type of review process has, as its core, evaluation of performance against specific assigned goals and objectives. For example, a nurse manager and a staff nurse together will develop a series of goals that are performance related, trait sensitive, and behavior based. Together they agree that these goals will form the

basis for the majority of the employee's performance evaluation, but the employee also understands that his or her review will consider general personal characteristics and specific behaviors, in addition to these goals.

SPECIFIC EVALUATION METHODS

Traditional Rating Scales

Traditionally, the most commonly used performance appraisal format has been the conventional rating scale, which typically focuses on personal characteristics and traits. Research conducted by H. G. Heneman, D. P. Schwab, J. A. Fossum, and others in the mid-1980s provided much-needed clarification regarding traditional rating scales. They found such scales to have the following four characteristics[5]:

1. *Several performance dimensions typically are examined in the review process.* These dimensions (e.g., "dependability") are not normally based on an extensive job analysis but are almost always arbitrary.
2. *Performance dimensions are general.* This generalness allows them to be applied to a wide variety of jobs. In fact, it is not uncommon for an organization to use the same rating scales for all of the employees in the organization.
3. *Performance dimensions are equally weighted.* An overall performance appraisal score is derived based on this equal weighting. No dimension is viewed as more important than any other dimension.

Behavior-Based Performance Appraisal

Rate each staff nurse based on what you consider to be the actual performance exhibited against known tasks required of the job being reviewed

	Unacceptable	Needs improvement	Average	Above average	Excellent	Outstanding
1. Records medication as required	☐	☐	☐	☐	☐	☐
2. Communicates information received from physician's rounds to nursing personnel	☐	☐	☐	☐	☐	☐
3. Keeps nurse manager or charge nurse informed of changes in patient's condition	☐	☐	☐	☐	☐	☐
4. Reports faulty equipment and safety hazards and follows up to ensure action has been taken	☐	☐	☐	☐	☐	☐

Fig. 22-2 ■ Example of a behavior-based performance appraisal.

4. *Subjective standards (absolute judgment) form the basis for the ratings made.* Because of this subjectivity and differences in opinion from one supervisor to the next, identical behavior on the part of two separate individuals may result in completely divergent ratings simply because different supervisors have varying perceptions of what constitutes satisfactory performance.

When a performance review is completed using a traditional rating scale, nurse managers (appraisers) must accomplish the following two tasks:

1. Make their ratings reflect the employee's performance over the entire evaluation period
2. Rate the individual against an internal standard of performance

A common complaint of both those undergoing these performance reviews and those executing them is that a performance dimension which forms part of the evaluation (e.g., leadership) is irrelevant to the job in question or the supervisor does not know exactly what the dimension means. Such complaints arise because the organization uses a single appraisal form for a variety of different jobs and because the performance dimensions are not always associated with rigid and well-defined behaviors.

Essay Evaluation

The essay evaluation is, without a doubt, one of the most difficult approaches used to assess an employee's performance. When this format is used, the nurse manager is expected to describe an employee's performance over the entire evaluation period by writing a narrative that details the performance strengths and weaknesses of the individual being appraised. This method is almost always used as part of an overall review process that incorporates several other approaches. When it is done correctly and objectively, the essay provides valuable data that can be used in the appraisal interview. If the method is used without the support of other techniques, however, its effectiveness is limited for a number of reasons.

One of the most obvious of these reasons is the fact that the development of an essay evaluation can be extremely time consuming. This is because the format requires managers to express themselves in writing, which is something that many experience extreme difficulty in doing. In addition, the essay format has proven to be very hard to defend in court because many of the written comments are difficult to tie closely to actual job performance. A large percentage of evaluators weaken their positions even more by filling the essay with subjective statements and innuendo. Therefore, essay evaluations are far more effective and carry far less risk when they are used in combination with other evaluation formats and when the information they contain can be tracked back to notes that were taken by the originator of the report and that cover the entire evaluation period.

Writing effectively is an extremely difficult task, and one that many clinicians and technicians do poorly. If managers must write a narrative or essay describing the performance of their employees, they should exercise restraint and include nothing that cannot be validated by other records. The possible need to perform this type of evaluation is a good reason why every manager should take a course or two in creative writing at the university level. Once an individual rises to the management level, technical skill becomes only one of the abilities required to perform effectively; writing well is certainly another.

Forced Distribution Evaluation

The forced distribution evaluation approach to performance appraisal is similar to that used by a college professor when grading on a curve. Nurse managers who use this approach rate their employees in a predetermined and very rigid manner (see the comparative judgment items in Fig. 22-1). For example, if the scale used for rating the employees is divided into five different categories, managers may be required by hospital policy to spread their employee ratings equally across all five categories. Obviously, this is not a popular form of evaluation among nurse managers because, in both premise and practice, it severely constrains the ratings that can be given. It is not uncommon to hear high-quality nurse managers give voice to complaints like, "I have two exceptional employees, but this evaluation system only allows me to place one of them in the category they both deserve" or "I don't have any employees who deserve to be rated in the lowest category."

Because of this general dislike of the forced distribution evaluation system and the fact that it is extremely difficult to support in the legal system, this system is not commonly used today. When an organization does employ such a difficult form of evaluation, it is almost always because nurse managers have previously given all of their employees high ratings. Even then, it is normally used in conjunction with other forms of evaluation.

Behavior-Oriented Evaluation

Behavior-oriented evaluation, as noted earlier, focuses on specific and preestablished behavior in appraising individual performance. Because of this, it has tremendous advantages for the organization. For example, (1) new employees immediately have specific information on how they should behave, what exactly is expected, and how they will be reviewed; and (2) the reliability of this method is widely accepted by the court.

A number of different types of behavior-oriented rating systems exist, but the most frequently used share similar approaches, have a number of characteristics in common, and typically are developed as follows:

Identification of critical incidents: In developing the grading system, groups of workers—which generally include individuals who actually perform the job and their immediate supervisors, all of whom are very familiar with the job's requirements—provide written examples of critical incidents or of what exactly constitute exceptional and unsatisfactory job behaviors.

Creation of performance dimensions: The critical incidents identified by these groups of workers and supervisors are classified by theme to create behavioral groupings called performance dimensions. Examples of performance dimensions are "direct patient care" and "nurse-physician interaction."

Use of complex statistical procedures: To arrive at a clearer definition of the required behavior, a subset of the original pool of critical incidents is developed. This procedure is used to eliminate items that do not clearly reflect the performance dimension into which they were grouped, that overlap with other critical incidents, or that were inadequately described.

From the earlier discussion of how behavior-oriented rating scales are developed, it is easy to see why this type of review applies to a single job description and can be extremely time consuming and expensive to develop. For these reasons, behavior-oriented systems are generally developed in organizations where a large number of individuals hold the same position, such as staff nurse.

The biggest advantage of behavior-oriented rating systems is the fact that actual jobholders and supervisors develop them. This professional collaboration makes these systems more acceptable to highly educated performers because they tend to trust the professional effort that went into creating them. In addition, because of the credibility thus created, the reviewers typically have faith in the system and are motivated to use it.

Management by Objectives

Whereas the other approaches to performance evaluation center on an employee's personal characteristics or behavior, management by objectives (MBO) focuses on the results the employee accomplishes. Although there are many variations on this technique, basically MBO involves the following three steps:

1. *Establishment of performance objectives:* To initiate the MBO program, management develops a number of performance objectives that will be accomplished by an employee or group of employees during a prescribed time period. These objectives can be established at a variety of different levels: (a) by senior management if the program will be organization wide; (b) by a department head, such as the vice president of nursing, if the program will be departmental; (c) by a nurse manager if the program will affect only the nursing unit he or she directs; or (d) by a nursing supervisor for a single or small group of employees. The objectives can be formulated by the management representative or by a committee that includes both management and staff.

   The individual performance objectives should have the following characteristics:
   - Each should be defined in specific, quantifiable terms.
   - Each should include a specific performance time frame; usually this is accomplished by including a deadline date. Each objective can include its own specific time frame, even if it applies to a single individual.
   - Each objective should be written in such a manner that it both challenges the employee or employee group and, at the same time, makes each performer feel that the objective is attainable.

2. *Evaluation of employee performance:* The second part of any well-developed MBO program is the actual evaluation of the employee's performance. Typically, the evaluation is accomplished by the manager responsible for the MBO program and the individual employee or group of employees tasked with completing the objectives specified. The focus of the discussion is how well the employee(s) satisfied the requirements of the objectives. The management representative must make this meeting positive, upbeat, and growth oriented. The purpose of the meeting may be to discuss the accomplishment of the original objectives, but the meeting should also focus on developing in the employee(s) the confidence to want to accomplish the next set of objectives.

3. *Evaluation of the MBO program:* Every time an objective is established and actions are taken toward its accomplishment, something should be learned from the exercise by both management and the employee performer. An MBO program

is an excellent means for the nurse manager to learn more about what it takes to motivate an employee, how to structure the next objective more effectively, and how to implement and manage change in the unit. It is absolutely essential that every MBO program be carefully analyzed so that it can be developed into a learning situation for all personnel involved and for the organization as a whole.

MBO systems have not found much success in the healthcare field because of the difficulty in establishing challenging, clear, quantifiable goals for many of the healthcare jobs that are built around variable patient needs. However, this does not mean that a well-developed MBO program cannot work in the nursing unit. What it takes is an environment in which cooperation, professionalism, and teamwork are the hallmark and in which working together for the good of the unit and the customers of that unit (patients and other units) is the life's work of every member of the team. In short, a good MBO program can work anywhere if enough care is put into its development and management. As with any other motivational performance program, the key to a successful MBO program is leadership.

PERFORMING THE EVALUATION

Although the individual organization certainly has the right to determine who will perform employee evaluations, the employee's immediate superior is almost always charged with this responsibility. This assignment is not only logical but also provides the best opportunity for reducing the risk to the organization that the evaluation process can create. The immediate supervisor is the one person in management who is most familiar with a specific subordinate's performance, and therefore is the one person in the best position to evaluate it. There are always exceptions to this basic assumption, however. In some work environments the immediate supervisor may not have sufficient knowledge of a specific employee's performance to accurately evaluate it, yet may be compelled to complete the performance evaluation form anyway. In this situation, it is the professional duty of that supervisor to develop information regarding the individual's performance and document its source(s) so that he or she can write the performance review without making vague and/or inaccurate observations.

Nurse managers must remember that each time they write a performance review, they are shaping the future of the employee and the organization. Writing performance reviews is one of the most important responsibilities of management and should never be taken lightly. A poorly developed review can dramatically damage a good employee's future, make it possible for a marginal employee to advance to a position of responsibility, or create a significant liability for the organization. If these three reasons are not enough to ensure that every nurse manager takes this responsibility seriously, then consider the fact that both federal and state courts have repeatedly found the originator of a performance review to be as liable as the organization when the performance review has been judged to harm an employee.

As members of the management team, nurse managers should realize that writing a performance evaluation is a cornerstone event in their performance. Effective evaluation is one of the major tools managers have at their disposal to influence the quality of the performance environment, and therefore evaluation is always a critical job function. Nurse managers need to develop an objective approach to writing reviews for their employees and take steps to eliminate subjectivity. At no time should nurse managers allow personal preferences, opinions, friendship, or any other such influence to affect the review process. Nurse managers do not have to like a subordinate, approve of the subordinate's personal life, or establish a friendship with the subordinate to obtain good performance from that person. Ambiguity, opinions, and emotions have no place in an objective review. How well performance meets the standards, rules and regulations, job description, and mutually developed objectives should be the only criterion. In other words, every performer should receive the performance review he or she earns. If nurse managers remember their responsibility, they will take the review process seriously and take the steps necessary to ensure that their evaluation work represents their employees, themselves, and the organization in a professional manner.

Things such as whether the nurse manager likes the form that is used, approves of the format that has been prescribed, or likes the performer are not important. Performance reviews are serious business and should always be treated as an important part of the nurse manager's job responsibilities.

POTENTIAL PROBLEMS

Regardless of the type of appraisal used in the organization or the type of appraisal device employed, there is always the potential for challenge to the accuracy of the performance evaluation system. If and when these challenges and problems arise, they can have a dramatic effect on the usefulness of the performance review. If a performance rating can be shown to be inaccurate for any reason, it can do more harm to the organization that simply making it culpable in a lawsuit.

Leniency Error

It is very common for managers of highly technical or highly educated staff to overrate individual performance; that is, to rate performance at a higher level than has actually been demonstrated. This management failing is often referred to as *leniency error*. This shortcoming can be witnessed when a nurse manager rates all of his or her staff nurses as "above average" or better, when it is obvious that not everyone is an exceptional performer. Although most nurse managers can provide a litany of "reasons" for this practice, such conduct by a member of management is totally unacceptable. In fact, most of the reasons cited aren't really reasons at all but are excuses, such as the following:

- I want my nurses to respect me.
- It's difficult to justify giving someone a low rating.
- I have to depend on this person.

Leniency error is a serious problem when viewed on an organizational level and a serious professional failing if scrutinized on the individual level. The willingness of a manager to award undeserved or inflated performance ratings can create severe problems for the manager, the staff in general, the working environment, and the healthcare organization as a whole. Take a minute to carefully evaluate the following scenario: Nurse Manager Paula Jones gives Staff Nurse Betty Brown a mark of "above average" in medication inventory control when her performance was actually below average. Consider the following potential problems that can be created[6]:

- Nurse Brown may think that Nurse Manager Jones is not in touch with the nursing unit and the quality of the day-to-day performance of her nurses. "If she were," reasons Ms. Brown, "I never would have gotten that mark."
- Nurse Brown might be satisfied with a mark of "above average" and may not work to improve her performance.
- Other higher performing nurses who are aware of Nurse Brown's failings may learn of the mark and, instead of talking with Ms. Jones to understand it, may become resentful because they feel the mark is undeserved. Resentment can lead to (a) lower performance by the normally higher performing nurse, (b) lack of trust and confidence in Nurse Manager Jones, and (c) tension and stress in the nursing unit, all of which can create an environment in which performance is no longer considered important.

- Nurse Manager Jones, because of the unjustified mark, may be unable to initiate disciplinary action against Ms. Brown if the latter's performance does not improve, and, if she attempts to do so, may potentially expose the institution to legal action.
- Nurse Manager Jones may lose the respect and trust of her senior managers if they become aware of continued problems with Ms. Brown and are unable to rectify the situation without risk of legal action. Suppose that Ms. Brown's poor performance causes a patient to receive the wrong medication or too much medication. Suppose that the mistake was severe enough that Ms. Brown was fired, and Ms. Brown decides that the termination was unjustified because, after all, she was an "above average" performer. If the case goes to a state or federal labor mediation board, there is every reason to believe that Ms. Brown will be right back in the unit in her old job with a large chunk of the hospital's money in her pocket as compensation for the trouble to which she was put.

Giving a mediocre performer lenient ratings almost always backfires in the end, and nurse managers can pay a tremendous price for their unprofessional conduct. At the very least, a lenient rating will make it difficult to initiate corrective action such as disciplining or demoting the person.

The greatest damage that can be done by a habit of leniency appraisals, however, is the demoralizing effect it can have on the unit's best and highest quality performers. It is these hard-working professionals who deserve to be set ahead of the nonperformers. These high performers keep the nursing unit operating efficiently and safely, and if the nurse manager fails to recognize their excellence by making a clear distinction between their marks and those given marginal performers, the overall performance of the unit will soon suffer. In truth, leniency error by the nurse manager will always be viewed as a positive attribute by the lower performing nurse and as a severe failing by the more professional performer.

Recency Error

Another factor that makes it difficult to develop quality performance reviews is the length of time covered by the average review. The vast majority of businesses, including healthcare organizations, require that performance reviews be accomplished on an annual basis. Evaluating even a single employee's performance over such an extended period is an extremely difficult cognitive task, and the greater the number of employees the manager supervises, the more demanding it becomes. To this is added the fact that the typical manager, when he or she sits down to compose an evaluation, tends to recall only the performance that occurred within recent memory and forgets most of the more distant events, even if they were more representative of the actual overall performance level. Given this tendency, the typical performance rating usually reflects what has been contributed lately rather than what was demonstrated over the entire evaluation period. This challenge is referred to as *recency error,* and it can create a host of ills, including legal and motivational problems, as follows:

Legal challenge: If the question of a performance review is ever taken to litigation and it can be proven that a single evaluation that was supposed to have reflected 12 months of performance actually is descriptive of only the 2 to 3 months immediately prior to the writing, the validity of the organization's entire appraisal process can be brought into doubt.

Motivation: The manager committing recency error demonstrates to all employees that they must perform at a high level only near the time of their performance review. This attitude leads to a level of performance and quality of service that is inconsistent and generally unsatisfactory to the patient. Managers who are guilty of recency error do a significant injustice to their teams, their individual employees, and everyone their unit serves.

As does leniency error, recency error benefits the poorly performing team member and is always detrimental to the overall operation of the unit. When employees who perform in a superior manner throughout the entire year see known mediocre personnel receiving ratings similar to theirs, overall unit performance suffers. The result of recency error is always lower performance from the consistently superior performer and unchanged or even reduced performance from the mediocre employee. Fortunately, there is a simple fix for recency error: managers must keep copious notes documenting each employee's performance throughout the year, from review to review, and use these notes to develop the individual's performance review.

Halo Error

Sometimes an appraiser fails to differentiate among the various performance dimensions (e.g., job knowledge, communication skills) when evaluating an employee and assigns ratings on the basis of an overall impression, positive or negative. When this occurs, some employees will receive a high rating, others an average rating, and a few a below average rating in all dimensions, regardless of their specific skills in individual areas. This is referred to as *halo error.*

Halo error can be deceiving, because it can actually appear that the evaluation has been written accurately. For example, if an employee is performing in an excellent manner, or at an average level, or even below expectations, he or she has *earned* the right to receive the marks that reflect his or her performance; this is not halo error but an actual reflection of the employee's performance. Halo error is apparent when the employee receiving the review is rated exactly the same in all categories, because as a general rule, most people perform at different levels in accomplishing the various tasks assigned to them. In some areas performance is excellent, in some average, and perhaps in some needs additional work to meet expectations. A truly objective performance review will reflect these different performance levels as well as individual strengths and weaknesses.

Ambiguous Standards

Many organizations and even some individual evaluators get themselves into trouble in the evaluation process because they use words that are not specific or that do not precisely describe behavior. These organizations and individuals weaken their positions by using words such as the following:

- Outstanding
- Excellent
- Above average
- Average
- Below average
- Unsatisfactory

The challenge results because different evaluators have different interpretations of exactly what these words mean. This ambiguity is often viewed as a problem in evaluation standards and can lead to significant weakening of an organization's position in the event that a disagreement over a performance review ends up in court.

Today, many organizations have eliminated this potentially risky situation by insisting that evaluative reviews judge employee performance against individualized goals and objectives. If words such as those listed earlier continue to be used, these organizations provide clear definitions specifying exactly what each word means in the organization, such as the following:

Outstanding: Clearly exceptional. Performance level rarely achieved and not expected to be achieved by more than 5% of the top performers in the group.

Excellent: Superior performance. Performance level exceeds all standards for this evaluation point.

Above average: Performs slightly better than required by performance standards

Average: Meets all performance standards.

Below average: Meets some but not all performance standards.

Unsatisfactory: Fails to meet any performance standards.

The best means available to a healthcare organization for eliminating this type of risk is to convene teams of professionals to determine exactly what these terms will mean in specific circumstances. For example, managers can meet to determine what might constitute an "outstanding" mark in patient care. Once the group has reached a decision, the standard is set, and all nurses providing patient care must meet that standard to achieve that specific rating.

Unsubstantiated Written Comments

Very few evaluation forms fail to provide places for the evaluator to write comments that support the marks given or that shed additional light on the overall performance of the individual being evaluated. Intelligent and capable nurse managers will use this opportunity to provide justification for the ratings they have given and to comment on the individual's potential for advancement, record objectives for the reviewed employee for the next marking period, or identify specifically what they mean by individual words and/or marks.

It is extremely important that managers not include in these comment blocks any unsubstantiated remarks or evaluative comments that are not supported by hard, previously established standards of performance. Personal opinion, innuendo, and other unverifiable comments can only weaken the position of the organization and evaluator and can increase potential liability in a civil action. Negative and vague comments should not be put in this section. However, these sections also should never be left blank.

Writing comments is far easier if managers detail employee performance as the year progresses by keeping notes and other documentation that will help them remember exactly how each individual performed and why. The problem is that all too many managers leave the preparation of the performance review until the very last minute, which makes writing an effective and professionally developed review extremely difficult.

Managers must remember that the performance evaluations they write will be reviewed by their immediate supervisors and quite possibly by a member of senior management. These senior managers will form opinions of every nurse manager's capability from the quality they see demonstrated in these evaluations. Consider the following remarks by a manager:

> As the vice president of a major division in a large metropolitan hospital, I personally evaluate all of the performance reviews written by the various managers who report to me or to one of my subordinate managers.
>
> When I find evaluations that are vague, negative, and/or poorly constructed, I make a very strict evaluation of the individual manager who wrote it. I hold that any professional manager who cannot write an objective, supportive review of a subordinate does not have the qualities I look for in an exceptional performer. My primary thinking is that the non-performing manager does not have the best interests of the individual, unit, or hospital in mind. No outstanding or excellent manager would risk the loss of support of a single performer, risk the pecuniary investment made by the hospital in the performer, or willingly place the institution in a potentially grave legal position. Therefore, none of these managers receives any grade higher than "average" on their personal reviews.

IMPROVING THE ACCURACY OF THE PERFORMANCE REVIEW

If the performance appraisal is to fulfill its primary functions, it must encompass all facets of the job performance expected of the individual being evaluated and must be free of error. These seemingly simple tasks have historically proven to be very difficult to accomplish. Today, however, many means are available to the average reviewer to help improve the quality of the product generated.

Skill of the Appraiser

If evaluators are to accurately describe and evaluate the specific performance of an individual, they must do the following:

1. *Understand the behavior:* Evaluators must know and understand precisely what the evaluation is asking for (i.e., what the performance must be to achieve a specific grade).
2. *Observe:* Evaluators must observe the actual performance to be evaluated over the entire marking period and must be able to recall it accurately.
3. *Understand the appraisal form:* Evaluators must know how the organization intends the eval-

uation form to be used and precisely what each dimension being evaluated means (e.g., What does "initiative" mean? What is meant by "acceptable conduct"?).

To the degree that any of these elements is lacking, the performance review is degraded. To put it more simply, if the appraiser does not understand how to perform the evaluation, how can the organization expect a quality review to be conducted? Therefore, the organization has the responsibility to ensure that every individual tasked with writing evaluations be trained effectively. It should never be assumed that an individual knows how to write a performance review simply because he or she has many years of experience.

Every nurse manager's ability to write effective performance reviews can be enhanced. The organization can develop detailed job descriptions that clearly identify the expectations of a specific job, can provide clear definitions of terms to be used in evaluations, and can even encourage nurse managers to take writing classes so that they will understand the potential impact of their written statements. The organization can overlap managerial assignments so that other supervisors can contribute comments to an individual's performance review if they had occasion to witness any of that person's performance. In fact, organizations that employ shift labor should ensure that supervisors and nurse managers collaborate in developing performance reviews. Just how important it is for the organization to provide descriptive definitions of terms used in evaluations can be seen from the following comments by a Navy chief of nursing:

> As a serving naval officer, I was tasked with developing annual performance reviews for the nurses who were subordinate to me in my assignment as chief of nursing. The U.S. Navy is not a benevolent institution, but rather a highly competitive and demanding one. In this extremely competitive environment, the only real means the Navy has to evaluate a nurse's potential for advancement is the annual performance review. The Navy takes these reviews as holy writ and once written, they become the chief means of identifying officers who are worthy of promotion.
>
> To ensure that every nurse is evaluated fairly, objectively, and against expressed performance standards, the Navy issues lengthy and specific guidelines for writing performance reviews. In these documents, it clearly defines what is meant by words, and what words are appropriate in what circumstances. For instance, the word *good* is defined in naval rules as meaning "average." If a reviewing officer's written comments use the word *good* to describe the performance of a clearly superior nurse, a career has just

been ruined. One mark of "average" in the competitive promotional environment in which we work means there will be no promotion, and if a nurse is passed over twice, he or she is compelled to leave the service.

> We take words very seriously.

Nurse managers are encouraged to actively keep a running record of the performance of every nurse whom they supervise. These notes should include comments describing both acceptable and unacceptable behavior. All too often, nurse managers who keep notes on their staffs document only the negative occurrences they witness. A year is a very long time to hold observations in one's head. Nurse managers routinely demonstrate their human failings by forgetting all of the good things that a person does and remembering only a few isolated negative events. Or, worse yet, they only write down occurrences that they witness a few weeks before the review is due.

Motivation

It is foolish to assume that just because an individual is appointed to a management position he or she will automatically become motivated to appraise all subordinates accurately.

In fact, nurse managers have a wide range of very important tasks to perform in discharging their duties. Many of the matters to which they must attend are considered critical, urgent, and even life threatening. Under these conditions, it is easy to see how even the most professional nurse manager can come to view a performance review as something that can be accomplished "later." What is not understandable, however, is the persistent feeling of many managers that performance reviews are not particularly important. Performance review is a fundamental responsibility of management. It has a strong impact on morale, motivation, performance excellence, and risk management in the organization. Carrying out this responsibility to anything less than the utmost of one's ability is unprofessional, and such behavior indicates that the individual should not be a manager of others or hold a position of responsibility in the organization.

Of course, there are some who hold that a nurse manager should be rewarded for performing the appraisal process well. Although recognizing excellence is certainly important and any well-founded effort to do so should be applauded, the discharge of one's fundamental duty does not fall into the category of the exceptional. Writing a performance review should always be a minimum expectation of someone holding the position of nurse manager. It is a responsibility and should never be treated as less, nor should a nurse manager expect to be rewarded for accomplishing it. In fact, nurse managers who do not perform this function to the best of their ability should be reassigned to a nonmanagement position with less important responsibilities.

DOCUMENTING PERFORMANCE

When managers undertake to evaluate others' performance, they are embarking on one of the most difficult tasks in their area of responsibility. To begin with, the time period involved in the typical appraisal is lengthy (usually 1 year). This means that professional nurse managers are tasked with conducting the appraisal interview every day for 365 days, not 1 day once per year. This demanding process is made even more difficult by the fact that the typical nurse manager has several individuals to evaluate. The pressures of a demanding profession, the stress of an ever-changing environment, and the incredible urgency of life-and death decision-making create a situation in which faces can run together and one person's performance can blend with another's. One way to deal with this situation is to write critical incident reports, or reports of behavior and events that stand out from the ordinary, either positively or negatively.

Positive Behavior

Positive behavior is probably the most frequently ignored or poorly documented. Why? Because the expectation in many people's minds is that a nurse should perform positively, and his or her doing so does not necessary make the situation noteworthy. But the truth is that excellence not only characterizes single incidents but also is seen in consistency. Therefore, even seemingly insignificant things, when gathered together, can separate good from excellent and exceptional from incredible.

When annotating a positive action (behavior), nurse managers are free to use any system they desire (few organizations mandate use of a specific form). Regardless of the format used, however, the following four things should always be recorded:

1. Name of the employee: Who did it?
2. Date of the incident: When was it done?
3. Brief description of the incident: What happened?
4. Action taken: What did the nurse manager do or say at the time of the incident?

If nurse managers do nothing but record incidents of positive performance, they are bound to enhance their ability as performance evaluators and make the task far less agonizing.

Why don't more nurse managers engage in this type of reporting? Probably because many feel it to be an unnecessary task, or at least one of extremely low priority. Timing is also a problem. The best time to record an incident is immediately after it happens, but too many times the small things are overshadowed by the urgencies of the nursing unit; time slips away and the incident is forgotten.

Keeping a few 3 × 5 inch cards in one's pocket can easily eliminate this slow slide to nondocumentation. Fig. 22-3 shows how to prepare these cards so that they can be available for quick completion.

The nurse manager can fill out the card right in front of the performer as the manager is critiquing or acknowledging the positive action. The fact that staff members know that positive performance is recog-

---

Critical Incident Report

Employee name: _____

Date of incident: _____

Description of occurrence: _____
_____
_____
_____

Action taken and comments: _____
_____
_____
_____

Fig. 22-3 ■ Example of a card for critical incident reporting.

nized, commented on, and then recorded is usually enough to boost performance in the unit and acts almost immediately to reduce such critical problems as turnover and absenteeism.

After the end of the shift, each card filled out is placed in the appropriate team member's personnel file. Then the cards are pulled out at review time.

The fact is that staff members do far more good and positive things over the course of a reviewing period than they do negative things. The typical ratio measures in the hundreds to one. It is a shame that what most nurse managers remember are the few negative occurrences or only those positive things that happened within the last few weeks leading up to the review.

Negative Behavior

When a member of the staff does do something that is not positive, there is typically less reluctance on the part of the nurse manager to document it. Many organizations even mandate that these negative incidents be recorded and train nurse managers how to do so.

Documenting these incidents can be extremely uncomfortable for both nurse managers and noncompliant nurses. Nurse managers must be careful to exercise sensitivity when writing negative reports, and the reports should not be completed within sight or earshot of other staff members. Nevertheless, such reports must be compiled.

Without doubt, documenting moments of failing can be stressful for nurse managers. Many think of themselves as lurking about the unit waiting for something negative to happen; in fact, many actually do. But professional nurse managers know that the difficulty of documenting negative incidents can easily be offset if they also document the positive occurrences in the unit.

Critical Incident Reporting

Because most nurse managers are extremely busy, many feel that completing these critical incident forms is not a good use of their time. The truth, however, is that these reports are actually labor-saving and time-conserving actions. Think of it this way: spending a little time recording a behavior is far better than spending a great deal of time laboring through a performance review. The average critical incident can be written up in less than a minute, but writing a performance review without sufficient documentation can take days to accomplish.

One of the most important aspects of critical incident reporting is how it is demonstrated to the staff. If managers use this method only to record

negative actions, then chances are great that the staff will come to despise the process and every manager who employs it. The view of the staff then will be that management is "spying" and "lurking;" waiting for negative things to happen. If managers record both good and bad events, however, and make a bigger fuss over good things than over bad ones, staff members will tend to support the process. Also, if staff members understand that the purpose of the reports is to ensure that employees ultimately receive a higher quality performance review, many will even endorse it.

One other truth about critical incident reporting can be noted. It has a remarkable effect on performance in the unit, and long before the first performance review is written. When employees know that what they do gets written down, they tend to do better, especially if they know that the nurse manager records the positive things they do. Believe it or not, the typical performer will be less afraid of this process than eager to be a part of it. People want to be remembered for the good things they do, and if that is how the nurse manager presents this process, almost all members of the staff will improve their performance so that they can have their actions recorded.

Managers must observe the following principles when engaging in critical incident reporting:

Stick to the facts: The manager should record what actually happened, not what makes people feel good or what the manager thinks might have occurred.

Write objectively: The manager should not dramatize or color the incident in any way. The manager should simply write down the facts. This is an excellent example of a case in which the KISS principle (*keep it short and simple*) is applicable.

Speak plainly: Don't use jargon or acronyms. Use simple, clear words that express the meaning clearly.

Make the note specific and behavior oriented: Words like *careless* or descriptions like *difficult to supervise* should be avoided. Instead the manager should state what was done or why the employee was "difficult" and exactly what "difficult" means.

Inform the staff member: When the manager records the behavior, the manager should inform the staff member that he or she has done so. Positive actions can and perhaps even should be recorded publicly, but negative incidents should be documented only in private.

Record both the good and the bad: The manager should let it be known that both types of incidents will be recorded but should emphasize the positive aspect as much as possible.

Managers should keep in mind that the only true purpose of critical incident reporting is to enhance the performance review process. If the process is conducted in a positive and forthcoming manner, however, nurse managers can generate considerable support and enhance performance in the unit long before the first review needs to be written. On the other hand, if the process is handled poorly, managers can decimate a productive nursing unit. Morale and performance are unpredictable and fragile, and professional nurse managers deal with them very carefully.

What kind of reaction can a manager anticipate? The fact is that good performers like to have their actions documented, and poor performers usually do not. Therefore, a manager will observe different types of reaction. What is important is not to respond to either type. The manager should simply be objective; record good, marginal, and poor behavior; and give more emphasis to the positive than to the negative. The unit will respond favorably, and as for those individuals who don't, well, let them leave. Either way, the manager will be improving the unit's overall performance.

CONDUCTING THE APPRAISAL INTERVIEW

The appraisal process starts with and centers around the development of an accurate and well-supported appraisal; however, nurse managers must not think that their work is complete once the appraisal has been prepared, because nothing could be further from the truth.

If one of the primary reasons for developing the review is to promote improved performance by the unit and the individual, then it follows that even the most professionally prepared review must be delivered in a proficient and motivational manner. This is accomplished primarily through the performance appraisal interview.[7]

Preparing for the Interview

Preparing for the interview requires more than just gathering up the report, arranging for a quiet place, and ensuring that no interruptions will occur. In fact, much of the preparation concerns not specific activities but rather mental preparation that reminds the nurse manager exactly what goal he or she is trying to achieve by conducting a professional interview; namely, to build a favorable perception on the part of the employee so that the appraisal process is viewed as a positive occurrence and the source of recognition and future opportunity. To ensure that this perception is reinforced, the organization and the individual nurse manager should make a concerted effort to link performance reward systems to the appraisal process.

Part of the nurse manager's mental preparation must be to realize that not all of his or her employees are going to share the manager's viewpoint and that a percentage will openly disagree with the manager's assessment. In fact, only a few performers (usually the very best in the unit) will not have some disagreements. Most professionals, and this certainly includes nurses, have a very clear view of themselves as above-average performers. For nurses, this opinion is rooted in the fact that, to become a nurse, one must successfully complete a demanding and difficult course of education—one that continually drives home the point that service as a nurse marks the performer as a cut above the average. Reality, however, is not quite so supportive. Although it is certainly true that nurses and nurse managers perform in a demanding and highly professional career field, this by itself does not make the individual an above-average performer in that field. If one compared the field of nursing with other professional fields of endeavor, one would have little doubt that the average nurse must meet far more demanding criteria and performs in far more demanding circumstances than do many other career professionals. The appraisal process does not compare across a variety of career fields, however. It looks at one career field, nursing, a field in which every professional performs under similarly demanding circumstances and in critical situations. The appraisal system compares nurses against nurses, and even in the smallest unit, some are going to be exceptional and some are going to be marginal. It is the job of the nurse manager to make sure that every nurse under his or her charge understands this basic fact.

One of the best ways for nurse managers to prepare themselves to face the challenges of the appraisal interview is to clearly understand that they are only presenting an evaluation that has been earned. If nurse managers are doing their jobs correctly as their employees move through the appraisal period, employees should know before entering the appraisal interview what type of review will be received and what marks it will contain.

Preparation for an appraisal interview begins the moment the previous one finishes. Nurse managers have the responsibility continually to inform, facilitate, guide, encourage, and motivate employees throughout the appraisal period. If they do this, they will find the actual appraisal interview to be easy to conduct. At the very least, neither the manager nor the recipient of the appraisal will receive any surprises.

Certainly, nurse managers should ensure that the appraisal interview is conducted in a setting that is nonthreatening, private, and free from interruptions. But this type of preparation is the professional icing on the cake. It will help the interview go smoothly, professionally, and quickly, but it will not guarantee that the evaluation is better received. To ensure that an appraisal is accepted in the same professional manner that it is created, competent nurse managers develop and present it every day of every week in the appraisal period.

While conducting an appraisal interview, nurse managers should be sure to bring up specific examples of the behavior that has caused the given ratings. This is particularly important when the appraisal contains lower marks and is absolutely essential if any rating is "below average" or worse.

It goes without saying that the performance appraisal is a document whose circulation is limited to senior management of the organization, the nurse manager, and the individual receiving it. Nurse managers should not discuss the appraisal with anyone outside the chain of authority. If assistance is required in the development of the appraisal, it is highly recommended that nurse managers limit their choice of sources to their immediate supervisors and their human resources departments. If senior management assistance is necessary to prepare the appraisal, it should be obtained only through the nurse manager's supervisor. It is not professional to discuss an employee's performance appraisal with other managers unless it is done in the abstract, with names and specifics left out.

Carrying Out the Interview

Nurse managers can usually anticipate that interviews will progress smoothly if they have prepared their employees through a program of counseling and guidance throughout the appraisal period. Only extremely rarely does an employee resist accepting his or her marks if the employee has been continually informed as to what they will be. If there has been little or no guidance or discussion regarding performance during the appraisal period, however, or if the ratings are substantially different from what the employee has been led to believe they will be, the nurse manager can and should expect resistance.

The first step in conducting the interview is to ensure that the room being used provides a non-threatening environment. This means that the nurse manager's office is not a good choice for presenting the appraisal. It is far easier to get an individual to relax in a neutral environment than in one where the trappings of authority are conspicuously displayed. In addition, selecting a neutral environment usually ensures that interruptions will be less likely.

Once the employee has joined the nurse manager in the interview location, a certain amount of time should be given to establishing rapport and letting the employee relax. Quiet, professional small talk or a brief conversation regarding a mutual interest can accomplish this. Care should be taken, however, that this time is limited and does not consume the time set aside for the interview.

The nurse manager should set the proper tone for the interview with the employee. One of the key elements to establish is that the appraisal interview is a place to work together to create a means to improve the nurse's opportunity in the upcoming appraisal period. If such a mutually productive environment is to be created, the nurse manager must understand that every employee has a different tolerance level for criticism. Once this level is exceeded, the only thing that will be elicited in the employee is defensiveness. Although shortcomings certainly must be discussed, they should not be the focus of the interview. To the contrary, the focus should be upbeat, positive, and constructive. Instead of "This is what you haven't done," the conversation should be more like, "What can *we* do differently to achieve improvement?" An individual can tolerate far more criticism if it is interspersed liberally with positive comments aimed at improvement.

The importance of remaining positive and not exceeding the criticism limit becomes even more acute if the employee is receiving a marginal appraisal. Typically, the nurse manager will present an extensive list of the negative factors that have led to the assignment of poor marks. This is done to "provide justification." However, if the nurse manager has prepared the employee properly for the interview throughout the appraisal period, there is little need to present the defense's case for the marks, no matter how bad they might be, because the employee will already know what the reasons are.

The way the interview is conducted, the climate of the interview, and, in most cases, the attitude of the employee, all depend on the behavior of the nurse manager. It is the manager's responsibility to develop the evaluation system, perform the interview every day of the appraisal period, and create a positive, upbeat environment to discuss what is contained in the appraisal. It is also the nurse manager's responsibility to ensure that the employee leaves the interview room ready and willing to perform professionally and positively. The nurse manager bears the responsibility for performance in the nursing unit, and every action that he or she takes in the interview should be orchestrated to ensure that the overall performance of the unit will be enhanced because of the interview. If the nurse manager spends time ensuring that the interview is conducted properly, he or she will spend far less time on damage control. As the old maxim says, "It is far easier to prevent a fire before it starts than after the house burns down."

The nurse manager should follow these key steps during an interview to enhance the way the employee perceives it:

Put the employee at ease: As was stated earlier, many employees, even the most professional, are uneasy about the appraisal process. This is especially true for new employees and for those who suspect they will be receiving a marginal appraisal. To ensure that the appraisal is a two-way communication process, the nurse manager must find ways to get the employee to relax. Some use small talk, such as conversation about the weather or the unit in general. Others begin by providing an overview of the process that is about to take place. No one method has consistently proven successful, because there is no guaranteed method of reducing tension. Once again, the best way to accomplish this is to adequately prepare the employee throughout the performance period.

State the purpose of the interview: The purpose should always be to identify and initiate a process of helping the employee to perform at an improved level during the next appraisal period. This is applicable regardless of whether the employee is currently a substandard performer or is the very best of the best.

Identify the rating system: The nurse manager should go over the different marks that are available on the appraisal form and provide specific examples of what type of behavior is necessary to earn each mark.

Go over the employee's ratings: Carefully and thoroughly, the nurse manager should discuss each and every rating assigned on the employee's appraisal and provide specific examples of demonstrated behavior that led to that mark's being given. This must be done even if the ratings are "above average" or better. Traditionally, managers do a good job of describing those behaviors that generated less than acceptable ratings but frequently gloss over those things that the employee did well. By doing so, they are putting a negative light on the appraisal process. Positive comments are vital to the success of the overall process. It is important to discuss positive behaviors with every employee, and every employee will have exhibited many such behaviors during the evaluation period. The absolute belief that positive actions outweigh the negative can be seen in the following story:

> Upon assignment as a nurse manager, I was informed that one of my primary duties would be to evaluate the performance of my staff nurses. The vice president of nursing in our hospital, Ms. Margaret Tan, was a woman of vision who took the development of subordinate

personnel extremely seriously. "Before you can evaluate anyone," she often said, "you need to understand how people work."

Ms. Tan told me that people work on a behavioral basis; that is, they do one thing at a time, even when they think that they are juggling a variety of different things. She proved her theory, at least to her and me, by stating her belief that when an employee was observed, you could actually count the behaviors in every performance. For example, a nurse doesn't simply take blood pressure readings, he or she (1) talks to the patient to get the patient to relax, (2) places the pressure wrap on the upper arm and verifies that it will not bind or restrict, (3) places the stethoscope into her ears and against the vein, (4) pumps the pressure wrap, (5) monitors elapsed time, (6) records the blood pressure in the patient's chart and (7) talks to the patient again to provide reassurance.

Ms. Tan believed that the average nurse performed several thousand of these positive "behaviors" before he or she would commit any error that was worthy of discussion by a supervisor, and the wise nurse manager remembered that even the worst single performance is only a single event in the life of tens of thousands of positive ones. "Wise managers," she said, "remember to remind their nurses of all the positive things that they do even as they are providing disciplinary instructions regarding an error."

Solicit feedback from the employee: The prudent nurse manager is constantly eliciting the employee's reaction to what is being said by encouraging dialogue. If the employee seems reluctant to share, then the nurse manager needs to ask questions that compel more than a one-word answer. When confronted by an employee who disagrees with a point in the appraisal, the nurse manager must remain calm, positive, and open. Becoming defensive or falling back on one's authority is never productive, and the wise nurse manager refuses to use the type A management* response, "Because I said so." The manager must remain positive and maintain an atmosphere of mutual respect at all times.

When the employee opens up and begins to talk, the nurse manager must respect that person's viewpoint, even if it is totally the opposite of the manager's. Giving the employee respect and

---

*Type A management was first identified by G. Z. LaBorde in *Influencing with integrity* (Palo Alto, Calif, 1987, Syntony Publishing). It is management that is directing, controlling, and demanding, and is applied through the use of full authority.

credibility is not the same thing as being "easy" or submissive. The nurse manager shows respect when he or she paraphrases the employee's comments so that the employee knows the manager understands what has been said and then encourages the employee to provide reasons why he or she is in disagreement, citing specific behaviors. It is impossible to create a win-win situation in the appraisal interview if the nurse manager does not take the time to find out how the employee feels.

Shift the focus to the future: The nurse manager needs to move the conversation on to what the manager and the employee can do together to ensure that the future is positive and productive. How can the nurse manager help the employee? What does the employee need to do to ensure that the next period's marks are higher? Together, the nurse manager and employee should agree on specific ways in which performance can be enhanced and then write them down. Again, the professional nurse manager understands that, although guidance and objectives need to be developed for all pertinent behaviors, not all of them need to be discussed during the appraisal interview. As noted earlier, all employees have a limit as to how much criticism they can endure, and some of the discussion can occur after the interview is completed.

One of the best ways to facilitate the development of performance objectives is to ask the employee what he or she would do to improve performance. Once the employee has voiced his or her thoughts, the nurse manager can add his or her own, and together, as professionals, they can blend their ideas into specific behaviors that can be measured over specific time frames.

Provide unofficial follow-up: The fact that performance objectives have been developed does not mean that they will be accomplished. It is the role of the nurse manager to ensure that the employee gets started toward achieving the objectives and stays on track. The manager accomplishes this by using unscheduled unofficial reinforcement visits. A reinforcement visit is an unofficial stop conducted by the nurse manager as a normal part of his or her job: when the nurse manager encounters the employee during the normal discharge of his or her duties, the manager asks about the employee's progress on the objective and offers assistance. The manager provides no criticism and no new guidelines, just a friendly question and an offer of assistance. That is enough to let the employee know that the nurse manager has not forgotten the objective and considers it important enough to ask about it.

All these steps are for naught unless the nurse manager takes the time to express confidence in the employee, and there is no acceptable reason for not doing this—even if the employee is the worst performer in the unit.

Once the appraisal interview is concluded, the nurse manager should develop a plan for ensuring that all of the objectives agreed upon in the interview are actually accomplished. This plan should include formal meetings where progress against each an objective should be discussed. During these periods, progress is assessed and no deficiency is ignored. If progress is being made, the nurse manager should congratulate the employee and recognize the effort made. If the deficiency is not being improved, that too should be discussed. Ignoring deficiencies will not make them go away, and the prudent nurse manager knows it is his or her job to keep the employee on track.

COACHING FOR SUCCESS

"The performance appraisal is built on individual moments, not great leaps" (p. 67).[8] The success of the employee is based largely on the degree of motivational guidance and direction setting provided by the employee's manager. People—all people—want to do well and will make a concerted effort to emulate the actions of those for whom they work. This desire to excel is pointed up in the following anecdote:

> One of my jobs as a nurse manager was to provide training events for my staff in a wide variety of disciplines and technical specialties. The subject I most enjoyed teaching was leadership and teamwork. To prepare myself to deliver these training events, I often attended off-site seminars given by professionals in the business world. At one of these seminars, I heard a business consultant ask the group, "How many of you went to work yesterday with the intention of doing a bad job?" When not a single person in the audience raised a hand, the consultant said, "And neither did any of your employees."
>
> He then went on to share with us what he claimed was one of the biggest secrets in the business world. He said, "People do what gets recognized."

It's just that simple. People respond with what gets recognized, looked for, and rewarded. If the nurse manager is the type who looks for problems, then he or she will probably find them without much effort. However, if the manager is the type who looks for and recognizes excellence, then he or she just as likely to find that. People always attempt to fulfill expectations, no matter what their level of responsibility.

Truly effective coaching is not an event that is typically "planned," but it is one that requires preparation. No nurse manager should ever approach an employee to coach unless he or she has prepared beforehand.

This preparation need not be time consuming or involve volumes of research, but it does need to include the following two elements:

1. *Familiarization with the challenge to be addressed:* The nurse manager should make sure that he or she has the facts correct. The manager should know what the problem is, what progress has been made up to this point; what part, if any, of the challenge remains; and what the manager is prepared to do to facilitate continued improvement.
2. *Preparation for the employee's reaction:* The exceptional nurse manager will know each member of his or her staff well enough to be prepared without too much effort, but managers should spend some time scanning the employee's file to identify any peculiarities, potential challenges, and motivational opportunities.

Coaching is a challenging part of the nurse manager's job but can be one of the most beneficial. It is performed best when the challenge to be discussed is still in its initial stage (i.e., is not a big problem). For example, a nurse who did not give a patient her medicine at the prescribed time should be coached for improvement as rapidly as possible. The best time is as close to the first infraction as the nurse manager can arrange it. The more quickly performance issues are dealt with, the easier they are to remedy. If the challenge is not providing the medication on time, the manager should not wait until that error has occurred several times or a pattern of this behavior has emerged. "Can you help me understand why Ms. Jones's medication was not given on time this morning?" is a far easier question to deal with than, "Can you tell me why you are frequently late passing out medication to the patients?" The former is more objective, more identifiable, and far less likely to trigger the subordinate's defense mechanisms.

Coaching is a positive action. It is not a process in which "reactive management" should be exercised. Competent nurse managers know that a problem worth identifying has occurred, and they also know that, before they confront the errant subordinate, they need to have both a recommended solution to the problem and a method of ensuring that the unacceptable behavior is not repeated. Both of these must be presented in positive, constructive, and proactive terms. Consider the following two examples and judge for yourself which coaching effort will help improve performance:

NURSE MANAGER 1

Ms. Jones's medication wasn't given on time this morning. What's the matter with you? Don't you know the hospital could be sued? You could be fired.

NURSE MANAGER 2

Ms. Jones's medication wasn't given on time this morning. Please help me understand why that occurred. I know you realize that this problem can cause significant liability for the hospital and for yourself personally. Before it becomes an issue, is there something we can do to prevent it from happening in the future?

Carefully examine these two approaches to identify which of them best embodies the key coaching behaviors listed in Box 22-1.

Truly exceptional nurse managers understand that the vast majority of employees really want to

---

BOX 22-1

Key Coaching Behaviors— SFRISEF

1. *State the problem.* Phrase the challenge in specific behavioral terms.
2. *Focus on the problem.* Keep your conversation focused on the challenge that needs to be addressed. Avoid references that reflect on the person, especially negative ones.
3. *Reinforce the urgency.* Stress the potential impact of not resolving the problem. Make sure that a nonthreatening and positive tone is used. *Do not* gloss over the severity of the problem, but stick to the facts and phrase your discussion so that it does not communicate a threat.
4. *Identify the cause.* The purpose of coaching is to rectify the current situation and enhance future performance, so ask the employee why the deficient performance was allowed to occur. Again, keep the tone positive and nonaccusatory.
5. *Solicit solutions.* Ask the employee what can be done to eliminate future occurrences, and perhaps what you can do to help. Don't accept ambiguous responses such as, "I'll work on it." Make sure that a specific and understandable solution is reached.
6. *Establish the solution.* Make sure that the employee and you agree on the solution and that each understands his or her role in future prevention.
7. *Follow up.* Never leave future behavior to itself. Follow up within a reasonable time and verify that the solution has been implemented. Recognize the effort if it has and discipline the employee if it hasn't.

perform well. Trust and belief in the staff can go a long way toward ensuring that a positive, efficient, and high-performance environment exists in the unit. Therefore, the coaching session should give the employee the benefit of the doubt and should not be used to determine guilt or innocence. The goals of coaching are (1) to make the employee aware that management knows that a challenge exists, and (2) to avoid future occurrences of a problem. Type A management is not conducive to building trust or improving performance. Instead, the professional nurse manager understands that extenuating circumstances may exist that can cause even the best of performers to make a mistake.

Some mistakes occur, however, when outside factors such as personal problems have been brought to work. If this is the case, a coaching action can rapidly deteriorate into a counseling session. Every nurse manager must remember the limits of his or her ability in this area. Most nurses are not trained in marriage counseling, individual therapy, or drug or alcohol rehabilitation, and therefore care should be exercised. The nurse manager's role is that of manager, not physician or priest. Although every nurse manager should be able to recognize symptoms of depression, alcohol and drug abuse, and even spousal abuse, each should remember that the hospital employs professionals to help employees when they require assistance with such problems.

SUMMARY

- Developing performance appraisals is one of the most demanding and important aspects of a nurse manager's job.
- Accurate appraisals provide a solid foundation for administrative decision-making (salary increases, promotions, etc.) and employee development.
- Performance appraisals, if not accomplished properly, can expose the organization and the individual nurse manager to legal liability.
- There is no acceptable excuse for a nurse manager's failure to do a good job of developing the performance appraisal.
- Leniency is not an appreciated virtue in the working environment. Not only does a lenient appraisal not reflect the actual performance rendered, it weakens the organization's ability to pursue future disciplinary action.
- The nurse manager has the responsibility to improve his or her ability to rate accurately and to write a comprehensive, objective, and accurate performance review for every staff member in his or her unit.

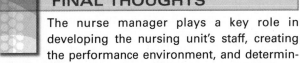

FINAL THOUGHTS

The nurse manager plays a key role in developing the nursing unit's staff, creating the performance environment, and determining the level of excellence each staff member is willing to achieve. One of the best ways this professional can contribute effectively to the creation of an exceptional unit is by providing objective, well-written performance appraisals. Performance appraisals are far more than a means of providing feedback to the individual performer. They also serve the follow functions:

- They are a way of recognizing excellence.
- They are a means to identify shortcomings and suggest constructive and positive actions that can be taken to enhance future performance.
- They are an effective team-building tool.
- They are a source of support for and verification of the individual's historical performance.
- They serve as a legal document that can be used to support the organization's position in litigation.

THE NURSE MANAGER SPEAKS

It is the responsibility of nurse managers to learn how to develop an effective performance appraisal. They ensure that each appraisal is devoid of emotion, personal opinion, and innuendo. They must objectively speak to the specific behaviors demonstrated during the evaluation period.

Performance reviews should be viewed as a fundamental part of every nurse manager's responsibility. Although they may not be as critical as emergency patient care, if they are done wrong, they can prove to be just as deadly. If challenged in court, a poorly developed appraisal can result in a huge financial loss for a healthcare facility.

Individual nurse managers are liable for the comments they make in performance appraisals. The only way to eliminate any potential of personal liability is to (1) be objective, and (2) reinforce statements with critical incident reports.

Good managers carefully build a reputation for excellence by making sure that all appraisals and coaching are done with future improvement as their goal.

REFERENCES

1. Latham GP, Wexley KN: *Increasing productivity through performance appraisal,* ed 2, Upper Saddle River, NJ, 1993, Prentice-Hall/Addison-Wesley.
2. Carroll SJ, Schneier CF: *Performance review and appraisal systems: the identification, measurement, and development of*

performance in organizations, Glenview, Ill, 1982, Scott, Foresman.

3. Rakich J, Longest BB, O'Donovan T: *Managing healthcare organizations*, Philadelphia, 1977, Saunders.

4. Rowland HS, Rowland BI: *Nursing administration handbook*, Germantown, Md, 1980, Aspen Systems Corporation.

5. Heneman HG, Schwab DP, Fossum JA, and others: *Personnel/human resource management*, ed 2, Homewood, Ill, 1995, Irwin.

6. Chapman EN: *The manager's survival guide*, ed 5, Chicago, 1998, Science Research Associates.

7. Moore T, Simendinger F: Evaluation is a two-way street, *Superv Nurse* 7(6):58, 1976.

8. Hawkins J: Coaching for success. In *Advanced business techniques*, Honolulu, 2001, Directions Corporation.

SUGGESTED READINGS

Ashton JT, Wilkerson J: Establishing a team-based coaching process, *Nurs Manage* 27(3):48N, 1966.

Beaulieu R, Shamian R, Donner J, and others: Empowerment and commitment of nurses in long-term care, *Nurs Econ* 15(1):32, 1997.

Beer M: Performance appraisal: dilemmas and possibilities, *Org Dyn* 9(3):24, 1981.

Belasco JA, Stayer RC: *Flight of the buffalo*, New York, 1994, Warner Books.

Benner P: *From novice to expert: excellence and power in clinical nursing practice*, Menlo Park, Calif, 1984, Addison-Wesley.

Bray D: Orientation critical pathway. In *Nine day pathway*, Colorado Springs, Colo, 1997, Memorial Hospital Emergency Department.

Bruce A, Pepitone JS: *Motivating employees*, New York, 1999, McGraw-Hill.

Kahn RL: *Occupational stress: studies in role conflict and ambiguity*, New York, 1964, Wiley.

Kanter RM: *Men and women of the corporation*, ed 2, New York, 1993, Basic Books.

Kidd P, Sturt P: Developing and evaluating an emergency nursing orientation pathway, *J Emerg Nurs* 21(6):521, 1995.

Kolb DA: *Learning style inventory*, Boston, 1985, McBer and Company.

LaBorde GZ: *Influencing with integrity*, Palo Alto, Calif, 1987, Syntony Publishing.

Yoder-Wise PS: *Leading and managing in nursing*, ed 3, St Louis, 2001, Mosby.

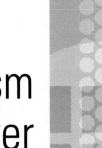

Managing Absenteeism and Turnover

OUTLINE

LEARNING SYNOPSIS

Upon successful completion of this chapter, readers will possess a fundamental understanding of how the challenges of absenteeism and turnover affect the nursing unit, the organization, and the healthcare industry; what the primary causes of these problems are; and what procedures can be followed to reduce their severity.

OBJECTIVES

1. Identify the fundamental reasons that absenteeism and turnover occur in the nursing unit
2. Describe the possible consequences of absenteeism and turnover, both adverse and desirable
3. Discuss proven methods for controlling absenteeism and turnover
4. Identify the real cause behind absenteeism and turnover in the nursing profession and describe what, specifically, nurse managers can do to combat these challenges in their areas of responsibility

Absenteeism and turnover historically have represented major challenges for the healthcare industry, but in today's demanding environment, the critical shortage of trained professional nurses makes these problems two of the foremost facing the industry. This chapter examines these two so-called withdrawal behaviors, provides nurse managers with an understanding of each problem, and furnishes some important suggestions on how nurse managers might reduce the challenges these problems present in their areas of authority. This discussion covers the following topics:

- Logical circumstances that create these costly behaviors
- Possible consequences of absenteeism and turnover, both adverse and desirable
- Proven methods that can be used to control the impact of both absenteeism and turnover

One of the keys to controlling these challenges is to develop an environment of trust and cooperation, and for that reason, individual leadership qualities and staff motivational suggestions are also discussed. Because absenteeism is quite different from turnover, however, the two withdrawal behaviors are examined separately. The purpose of this chapter is to offer nurse managers insight into what they can do to increase employee attendance and retention in their units. The intention is to provide the information necessary to deal proactively with these issues, and therefore an action-oriented emphasis is adopted. The chapter provides nurse managers with a variety of strategies for actively managing and even eliminating absenteeism and turnover in their nursing units—a management tactic far better than the traditional approach used in too many hospitals worldwide of merely living with the devastation wrought by these extremely serious behaviors.

ABSENTEEISM

One of the most basic challenges faced by nurse managers is that, for their nursing units to provide high-quality patient care, they must have properly trained personnel to perform the various tasks demanded—in the right skill mix, in the correct numbers, and at the proper time. It is a fact of life that when staff nurses are absent from their units, patient care suffers, both directly and indirectly. The problem is easy to understand: when the proper number of skilled personnel are not available, the shortage leads remaining staff to rush through patient care, take shortcuts, or overlook needs, and the result can only be a reduction in the quality of nursing care delivered. Another costly challenge occurs when the organization is compelled to pay nurses overtime rates when the relief nurses fail to show up for their shifts. The

additional expense of the double shift cannot usually be absorbed by the typical healthcare organization and so is ultimately passed on to the patient. Because hospitals operate on narrow profit margins, they simply do not have the financial resources available to cope with an extensive and expensive pattern of absenteeism and turnover. The best level of management at which to deal with these challenges effectively is the level closest to the absent staff nurses: that is, the nurse manager. Therefore, in nearly every healthcare organization, it is the nurse manager who must effectively address these significant problems.

Accurately determining the degree of decline in patient care caused by absenteeism or the cost, in hard dollars, directly attributable to absenteeism in the typical nursing unit is extremely difficult. However, the fact that absenteeism in healthcare institutions is both pervasive and expensive has been well documented. Annual surveys conducted by the Bureau of National Affairs since 1985 have consistently shown that healthcare employees have one of the highest absenteeism rates of any employee group in any industry.[*] When the data from the surveys conducted by the Bureau of National Affairs from 1980 through 1999 are combined, then the average absenteeism rate per healthcare employee is found to be approximately 6.5 days per year. If this is converted into hard dollars by adding just the cost of the absent nurse's salary and benefits and the cost of a fully competent replacement, then the estimated annual cost of a single nurse's absenteeism is conservatively estimated at slightly more than $3,200.[†] This figure, as staggering as it is, is not the highest estimate. In fact, it has been suggested that the cost of absenteeism may be as high as three times the amount that the absent employee would be paid during the time he or she is absent, or approximately $4,650. If these figures are used only as reference points, then the estimated annual cost of absenteeism per nurse can be considered to fall between $2,500 and $5,000 per year—a figure that, even at the low end, is far more than the average healthcare institution can afford.

---

[*]More information can be found on the website of the U.S. Bureau of National Affairs (http://www.bna.com).

[†]This amount was calculated using the average U.S. salary for a registered nurse of $45,000, a benefit average of 40% of the annual wage, an average number of days scheduled for work of 264, which yields an average per-day cost for a single registered nurse's salary and benefits of $238.64. Added to this figure is the cost of a replacement nurse's time-and-a-half salary without benefits—$255.68. Figures were obtained from the U.S. Bureau of National Affairs.

The costs of absenteeism, however, go far beyond its immediate effect on the quality of patient care and institutional dollar costs. The most dramatic impact of absenteeism is not on the purse strings of the institution but rather on the personal and professional lives of the staff nurses who must carry the additional workload it creates. A significant contributor to this burden is the fact that the staff nurse who shoulders the extra duty must do so in an environment in which there is overwhelming short-staffing even in the best of times. This already critical situation is further exacerbated because the nurses in residence are required to provide continually increasing quality of patient care despite the impact of their missing colleagues' absenteeism. Nursing is demanding work, and when individual staff nurses must carry out their responsibilities in an environment of continual personnel shortage, especially for extended periods of time, even the most professional can suffer both physical and mental strain. All too frequently, it is the norm to expect resident nurses to omit authorized breaks, hurry through or completely miss scheduled meals, work long and difficult hours, abbreviate their interactions with patients, pass up continuing education workshops, cancel scheduled nonwork activities, and even forsake their personal and family contacts. Absenteeism is not something that is remedied by the availability of a replacement nurse; even if a temporary replacement is called in, the work flow of the hospital unit will not be fully maintained. Instead, valuable and extremely scarce time will be consumed explaining standard hospital procedure and expectations to replacement or agency nurses. Moreover, even if the nursing unit is brought up to full head count by the use of replacement personnel, the professional capabilities needed to delivery quality health care will not necessarily be available. In fact, it is almost routine to assign the predictable duties to the replacement nurse (the administration and nursing staff do not have confidence in his or her ability) and spread the more difficult and demanding tasks among the regular staff. When this practice becomes the organizational norm, the acute workload and the greatest share of the pressure and stress remain on resident nurses. The delivery of quality nursing care is not a matter of numbers alone, but rather requires a combination of numbers, talent, experience, proven capability, trust, and confidence.

It is no surprise, then, that absenteeism receives a great deal of attention from senior administrators throughout the healthcare field. For the nurse manager, the immediate question may be, "What can I do to reduce the recurrent absenteeism problem in the individual nursing unit?" Although this is certainly a logical and necessary question, a satisfactory answer starts to emerge only after the manager clearly understands what causes someone to absent themselves from their responsibilities.

An Employee Attendance Model

Absenteeism is not a single challenge; instead, it actually comes in two different forms. Thus, any attempt to understand and define the phenomenon must include discussion of the following:

1. *Voluntary absence:* absence in which the employee intentionally fails to show up at the work assignment to attend to another aspect of his or her life, or an absence that is definitely within the control of the employee. For example, not coming to work to attend a family outing or social function, or to carry out another obligation.
2. *Involuntary absence:* absence that is not within the normal control of the employee, such as taking a sick day to recover from the flu, another virus infection, or some other legitimate illness.

These definitions would be reasonable if employees did not routinely abuse sick leave, but because the practice is rampant, and even encouraged, throughout the industry, it is often difficult for nurse managers to distinguish between these two categories of absenteeism in the nursing unit. Of course, there are some common indicators that can be used to assist in making the determination, such as the following:

- The absences regularly occur on Fridays and Mondays, weekends, and days adjacent to scheduled holidays.
- The absence is for a single day.
- The absence is repeated at regular intervals.
- No symptoms of the reported illness are apparent the day before or the day after the absence.

Some organizations have tried to distinguish between voluntary and involuntary absenteeism when they measure the phenomenon. Traditionally, most healthcare institutions have calculated absenteeism in terms of total time lost, that is, the total number of days of absence in a given period (usually 1 year), a practice that has proven somewhat insensitive to a single illness of long duration. Others base their absenteeism evaluations on the total number of distinct periods of absence regardless of their duration. In these cases, frequency of absence is used as an indirect estimate of voluntary absenteeism.

Distinguishing between the frequency of absence (number of absences) and the total time lost due to absenteeism generally makes sense to nurse managers. For example, a staff nurse who misses seven Mondays in a row would be credited with seven absence periods *and* seven total days absent. In contrast, an individual who misses seven consecutive days of work would have only one absence period with a total of seven days lost. At first glance, it is almost certain that the first staff nurse is much more prone to voluntary absenteeism than is the second. As a result, the first nurse would be expected to receive lower markings on his or her performance appraisal than would the second nurse. Research based on statistical analysis of absenteeism records[1] bears out this assumption, because it has been shown consistently that the performance appraisal ratings given by nurse managers concerning employees' attendance were much more closely related to absence frequency than to total days lost. This suggests that many nurse managers consider the pattern of the absences to be a more serious problem than the number of workdays actually lost.

Although many models are available that gauge attendance and absenteeism, the model developed almost three decades ago by R. Steers and S. Rhodes[2] remains particularly useful for the practicing manager even today. Their research was confirmed in additional work by M. E. Hardy and M. E. Conway in 1988,[3] and by C. Haddock in 1989.[4] (The discussion in this chapter is limited to the sections of these works that are particularly germane to the nurse manager.) According to the Steers and Rhodes model, an employee's attendance at work is largely a function of the following two variables:

1. The individual's ability to attend
2. The individual's motivation to attend

The research conducted by Steers and Rhodes[2] showed that an employee's ability to be at work at the proper time (attend) is affected by such factors as illness, accidents, family responsibilities, and transportation problems (Fig. 23-1). No matter what the specific reason for the absence, most nurse managers view the ability to attend as being linked very closely to what was defined earlier as involuntary absenteeism. Steers and Rhodes also considered the ability to attend to be influenced by a variety of personal

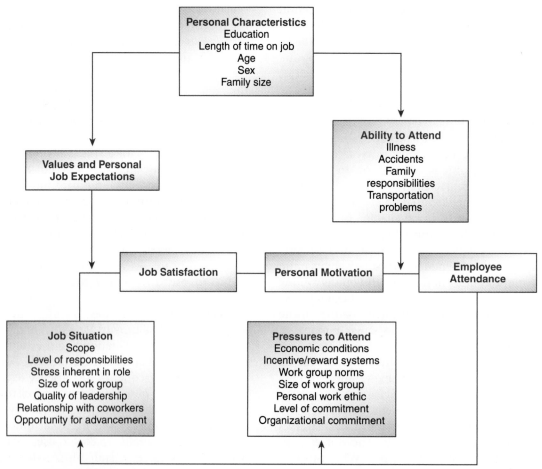

Fig. 23-1 ■ Factors influencing employee attendance. (Data from Steers R, Rhodes S: Major influences on employee attendance: a process model, *J Appl Psych* 63:391, 1978.)

characteristics, in addition to the general factors given earlier. For example, working women with young children, who traditionally accept most of the responsibility in the family for child rearing, may have more reasons not to attend than do others. This tendency is believed to get worse when the professional woman has a larger family, the theory being that as the number of children increases, so does the likelihood that family problems will occur that are sufficient to draw the mother away from her responsibilities in the workplace.[5]

Motivation to attend is somewhat different. It is generally influenced by a variety of factors, including the following:

Job satisfaction: This factor includes how adjusted and happy the employee is in carrying out the responsibilities of the job and how content he or she is with all the other aspects of the occupation and employment situation. An individual who is satisfied with the important features of his or her job is typically more motivated to meet the attendance requirements imposed by the job than are those who are not. The level of satisfaction is directly related to the degree to which the employee believes the characteristics of the job are compatible with his or her personal values and expectations.

There are very specific aspects of every job that have a significant influence on the average employee's satisfaction with the work, including the following:

- Leadership provided by the employee's supervisor
- Extent to which the employee believes the job is "enriching" (job scope)
- Level of stress involved
- Relationship with co-workers
- Opportunity for advancement

Values and personal job expectations: The importance attached to this influence can vary greatly from performer to performer. For example, many staff nurses desire a job situation that affords promotion opportunity, whereas others are not at all interested in leaving direct patient care. One nurse may be very sensitive to working for a type A (authoritarian) nurse manager, whereas others may not be negatively affected. These differences among nurses make it necessary for nurse managers to influence employee satisfaction on an individual basis; that is, they need to make an effort to establish symmetry between the characteristics of the job and the individual employee's values and expectations. Generally, nurse managers are limited in their ability to accomplish this fit because of constraints on their power to change the job situation (environment) and the type of individual who is hired.

Pressure to attend: Several outside pressures can influence an employee's motivation to attend work, whether or not the employee perceives the job as being attractive. The following are among them:

- Economic conditions: What is the job market like? Is there opportunity to change jobs relatively easily or is the market tight with few jobs available? The research of Steers and Rhodes[2] indicated that, during times of high unemployment, there is a direct correlation between job satisfaction and the work environment, which suggests increased pressure to maintain a good attendance record out of fear of losing one's job.
- Personal work ethic: To what degree does the employee view the performance of his or her job as a responsibility? Does the employee feel that by accepting a job he or she has obligated himself or herself to support the requirements of that job, or does the employee simply feel that he or she has been hired to perform a function and that is the extent of it?
- Work group ethic: What is typical of performance in the work group? Is absenteeism viewed as acceptable or is it frowned upon by both management and peer-level performers? Research conducted by G. Johns in the mid-1980s demonstrated the important influence of group norms, either pro- or anti-absenteeism, on attendance behavior.[6]
- Organizational commitment: To what degree is the organization committed to providing a working environment that is professional and conducive to the individual needs of the employee? For example, the organization might have an incentive system that rewards attendance or that imposes sanctions for failing to attend work.

The following are three important points regarding the Steers and Rhodes model (see Fig. 23-1):

1. *The model shows that both ability and motivation to attend must be present.* These conditions are essential if maximum employee attendance is to be achieved.
2. *The model has been validated.* A number of empirical studies support the basic elements of the model.
3. *The model provides a useful framework for understanding.* Nurse managers can use the model to attempt to understand why their unit's staff nurses are absent and what specifically they might do to improve attendance.

The Management of Absenteeism

The model based on the research of Steers and Rhodes is useful for understanding why absenteeism occurs and for developing managerial strategies for controlling it. This is true even if some of the influences that lead to absenteeism, such as transportation difficulties and child care problems, are typically beyond the influence of the nurse manager. The goals of the nurse manager should be to provide a positive work environment, to change policies that reward absenteeism, and to use performance appraisals as a motivational tool.

PROVIDE A POSITIVE WORK ENVIRONMENT

Providing a positive work environment not only is an area that is under the influence of nurse managers but is actually one of their primary responsibilities. The type of environment in which work is performed directly reflects the type of leadership provided by the unit manager. If the manager is fair, objective, approachable, willing to support the staff, trusting, and encouraging, the work environment will tend to be the same way. In *The New Partnership*, author and industrialist Tom Melohn demonstrated that the qualities of leadership can have a dramatic effect on the success of an organization.[7] He stated, "In the final analysis, it is the joy of management that provides true meaning in my life in business" (p. 103). What he meant by "the joy of management" is the feeling that a manager gets when he or she helps another and shares in the happiness and pride that result when together they achieve something special—something important to both of them. Melohn provided the secret to being an effective manager when he said, "By helping others, you help yourself. Each day brings a new challenge, to marshal diverse human resources toward common goals. When we help each other, we all achieve our personal objectives. That is the true joy of management" (p. 9).

What Melohn said largely comes down to the following when applied to the problem of absenteeism: If a unit has an absenteeism problem, it is very likely that the nurse manager is the major cause. It is not the desire to have an exceptional nursing unit, or a willingness to work hard, or the fact that the nurse manager is the most proficient and capable technician that makes for a quality work environment. Although these things certainly have value and are positive influences, none can guarantee that the unit will thrive. The following, however, are some values that will:

Honesty: The nurse manager must never lie or tell partial truths to his or her employees. Employees tend to see things in black and white, not in shades of gray. For example, if a nurse manager tells an employee that he or she has no knowledge of the necessity for overtime work and the employee later learns that the nurse manager actually did know that overtime was going to be required, the employee will consider that the nurse manager willfully lied, even if the nurse manager did so because he or she was instructed by a senior manager to not tell anyone (something that happens all too frequently).

Trust: The nurse manager should not demand trust from others but should take the personal risk and give it freely. It has been proven over and over again in every work situation that when a manager trusts another to do a good job, almost invariably the person will do it well. Trust does not mean blind faith. Good supervisors follow up on all job assignments, but it is the manner in which this follow-up is accomplished that is important. "Is there anything I can do to help you?" is much easier for the employee to deal with than "What is your status now?" Respect and sensitivity do not make one a "weak" manager. To the contrary, they strengthen bonds.

Equality: There should be equality not in authority but in respect for one another. Too many managers set themselves up as being superior to those who work for them. Nothing in a manager's job description grants superiority, and no one likes being treated as a lesser contributor. Everyone in the unit should be treated well, fairly, with respect, and in a way that promotes a feeling of self-worth.

Mutual respect: The manager should treat others as valued members of the team. Each individual, regardless of position, education, or capability, performs a vital function in the nursing unit. One of the biggest flaws nurse managers tend to exhibit is a feeling of superiority. Although it is true that the average nurse manager is generally better educated, has more experience, and is more clinically and technically proficient, those things do not make the manager superior. If the nurse manager finds value in his or her subordinates, the subordinates will enjoy working in the environment and show up more often.

Self-worth: Promoting self-worth is about making people feel good and instilling pride in accomplishment. Wise managers recognize excellence and let it be known when one of their subordinates excels. Managers should be proud of their teams and work consistently to generate pride in others.

Dignity: Everyone should be treated as an important asset. No one should ever be talked down to, ridiculed, belittled, or reprimanded in public. Tearing another person down does not make one superior.

Recognition: The nurse manager should never take credit for another's work; instead, the manager should take pride in an employee's accomplishments. If a member of the staff does his or her job well, the manager should mention it to the person, and do so in front of others. Although the subordinate might feign humility and appear not to want the recognition, only extremely rarely does the person not enjoy the recognition. Recognition should be something of value (it should not be overdone), but it should not be a scarce commodity.

Teamwork: Most organizations, even at the unit level, are quick to declare themselves a team or to claim that they believe in teamwork, but in reality almost none truly practice teamwork. On a real team, the players are tasked with playing and the coach is charged with ensuring that all of the conditions necessary for the team to play well are met. Choice assignments are given out to players, but, more importantly, so are difficult ones. For example, hiring a new employee is almost always the prerogative solely of the nurse manager, but if a nurse manager really believes in teamwork, he or she will aggressively solicit input and assistance in the hiring process from junior members of the team. Dr. Larry Price, former head football coach of the University of Hawaii, distinguished business school professor, and celebrated radio and television personality, had the following to say about teamwork while speaking to the executive management group of the Bank of America[8]:

> Teamwork is a shared event. Team members enjoy each other. I don't know why, but they do. They do more than work with each other; they are excited about helping one another. A real team player will stop at any time to help a fellow worker. If one member of the team has a problem, every member of the team has the same one; they share their problems.

Most people like and enjoy working with other people and do not enjoy working alone. Most people like teamwork, feel good working with others to achieve a common goal, and value a sense of belonging, purpose, and unity. The problem with teamwork is that far too many managers don't fully commit themselves to the team; they are more concerned with themselves. Subordinates can sense this, so when the uncommitted manager speaks about teamwork, the single most influential thing created is resentment. If nurse managers are going to create teams, they have to commit themselves to it.

Caring: Caring is probably the most important part of a positive environment and the strategy necessary to create one. Managers must care more about others than they do about themselves and must be willing to place the needs of others ahead of their own needs. When they do this consistently enough that others perceive them as caring, then those others will be willing to extend themselves on the manager's behalf.

WORK TO CHANGE POLICIES THAT REWARD ABSENTEEISM

The work environment needs to discourage the use of sick days. A sense of teamwork should be built that is so strong that a staff nurse will actually feel guilty about being legitimately ill, because he or she will know that another member of the team will have to pick up the slack caused by the illness. Although nurse managers should never discourage the legitimate use of sick leave (sick nurses should not come to work and expose patients and co-workers to illness), they should do everything in their power to ensure that every member of the unit understands how he or she supports the other members and the team as a whole, and exactly how that person's absence weakens the team's capability. People need to be taught to accept their responsibility for the professional quality of the nursing unit, because everyone shares in that responsibility. Everyone is an important part of success and should be encouraged to accept his or her role.

Although the Steers and Rhodes model clarifies several influences that can result in absenteeism problems, all managers must understand the key factors that create absenteeism in their particular units. As managers work to increase their knowledge, they may need to gather information from a variety of different sources, including the following:

- Subordinates
- Human resources department
- Other nurse managers and senior management

In the attempt to make sense of absenteeism, careful study of absence patterns can be particularly informative and can provide answers to questions such as the following:

- Is the absenteeism problem distributed equally across all staff nurses?
- Does the unit have a higher absenteeism rate than other nursing units?
- What is the average duration of the absences (1 day, 2 days, 3 days or more)?

■ Does absenteeism occur in a consistent pattern (e.g., predominantly on Mondays and Fridays, before holidays, or shortly before a person quits)?

Although the usefulness of answering these questions is fairly obvious, their importance will become even clearer as specific strategies for controlling absenteeism are discussed.

Many nurse managers, after reflecting on the factors that affect the ability of staff nurses to attend work, conclude that there is nothing they can do as individuals to reduce absenteeism. Nothing could be further from the truth. Although it is certainly an obligation of the healthcare institution to regulate absenteeism, the one person who can be most influential in solving the problem is the individual nurse manager. For example, the hospital could sponsor a day care center to relieve the child care concerns of working mothers, but if the nurse manager doesn't create a performance environment that is empathetic and supportive of nurses with these concerns, the typical staff nurse may not perceive the organization's efforts as an enhancement. Nurse managers absolutely should make an effort to encourage organizational management to consider offering some cures, but that is not the limit of their responsibility. Nurse managers are responsible for the performance of their nursing units, and they must work with their staffs to identify needs and develop systems to solve them. Some of those solutions may involve working in conjunction with fellow nurse managers to persuade the organization to offer brick-and-mortar solutions such as a child care center, but the vast majority of successful solutions are those that are developed collaboratively by the individual nurse manager and the members of his or her unit.

Not only must nurse managers make it known that attendance is considered critical to the success of the unit, they also must work with every member of their staffs to develop plans for reducing illness and solving child care problems. Nurse managers should use their innate creativity to expand the list of possible actions that can be taken in their units. Typically, the only limits on what nurse managers can do are their own inventiveness and their ability to sell the need for the solution to senior management.

Clearly, the easiest way for nurse managers to control absenteeism in their units is to improve the individual staff members' motivation to attend. To accomplish this, according to the Steers and Rhodes model, nurse managers must influence both employees' job satisfaction and the pressure to attend that employees feel. They can accomplish this by aggressively pursuing a process of continual improvement of the unit that includes the following objectives:

Increasing satisfaction: Very often, increasing satisfaction is a simple matter of enhancing the staff member's job by adding more responsibility and autonomy and more challenging tasks. Assignments to address these additional aspects of performance need to be positive. Simply loading up someone's wagon until it overflows is neither productive, helpful, nor a demonstration of leadership.

Reducing job stress: Nurse managers can also work to reduce job stress by providing timely and reliable information to employees.

Building group cohesiveness: Nurse managers should encourage socialization outside of work when possible to help build group cohesiveness. Creating reasons for employees to come together (e.g., unit picnics, social functions, and organized celebrations after work) is one way to do this. Consider the following example:

> After being assigned as the nurse manager of a large El Paso–based regional medical center, I soon began to realize that one of the major elements missing in our unit was a feeling among the staff nurses that they were appreciated for what they contributed. Everything was more or less an expectation of senior management, and when the expectation was not met to their liking, the boom was lowered, and hard. I knew that my staff needed to be shown that their efforts were appreciated.
>
> To show my appreciation, I called for a meeting to take place during the changeover from day shift to evening shift. I even asked the night crew to come in early for the meeting, which caused no small amount of grumbling. When the nurses got there, I left my assistant in charge of the desk along with one of the recent hires and led all of the rest toward the floor's conference room. When the first nurse started to enter, she stopped in her tracks. There on the wall was a simple sign that said, "Thanks! You're great!" The room was full of balloons, and there was a small buffet on the table. As each nurse entered the room, I placed a flower lei around his or her neck and told each one something special I valued about his or her contribution. (I rotated my assistant and her young nurse into the party as well.)
>
> We stayed and talked for nearly an hour, enjoying the camaraderie and banter that is shown by people who respect and admire each other. Afterwards, I stayed and cleaned up the room.
>
> The next day, the morning shift came in expecting me to place demands on their time as payment for the celebration. When none were made, one of the senior staff nurses approached

me and asked me why I had created the party and what I wanted.

Feigning shock at her questions, I said, "I don't want anything, and the only reason was that I thought it was time to say thank you."

Slowly, even somewhat warily, my unit pulled out of the strictly business atmosphere that my predecessor had demanded. You could hear occasional laughter coming from the nurse's lounge and even see the staff greeting each other warmly. Charts that never were kept up before suddenly were up to date *and accurate*. Patients stopped bending my ear with complaints and instead offered compliments on the kindness being shown.

We still have our "thank you" celebrations—once a month. But now, the staff and I take turns setting them up and supplying the food. Whether or not these little celebrations caused the turnaround or not, I can't definitely say. But I do know that working on 3 West is far more enjoyable today than it was before we had our first one.

Improving opportunity: Nurse managers should help improve opportunities for individual staff member advancement by working with each individual to improve his or her knowledge, skill, and team qualities. Managers should take the time to look into what types of training are needed by individual staff members and make arrangements for it to be obtained. Managers should work with each staff member to understand what he or she wants and what his or her goals are, and to show that they care. People respond to caring with an increased willingness to support the needs of the unit.

Improving employee relations: Nurse managers can also work to enhance the relationships between co-workers, at least by considering co-worker compatibility when scheduling work and creating work teams.

Preparing the staff for the unexpected: Almost all nurses enter their first job with unrealistic expectations of what it will be like. In the collegiate world of nursing school, a great deal of time and energy are spent in telling nursing students how special they are, how great it feels to be a nurse, and how much opportunity being a nurse offers. But when day 1 on the job is finished and all of the nurse's grandiose expectations have not been fulfilled, disappointment can set in. Creative nurse managers deal with this and other aspects of job satisfaction, and ultimately attendance motivation, by providing realistic job previews before hiring.

USE THE PERFORMANCE APPRAISAL AS A MOTIVATOR

One of the best tools available to nurse managers for focusing attention on the importance of good attendance is the employee performance appraisal. The simple fact that managers will be measuring attendance and discussing it with the employees tends to establish it as being important in the performance unit. During every performance appraisal interview, nurse managers should discuss the employee's attendance record and communicate the effect it has had on the appraisal and the unit's overall capability (e.g., impact on patient care, co-workers, and overall proficiency of the unit). If the organization links merit compensation to the performance appraisal, no small part of the evaluation should focus on attendance. The simple truth is that if an employee has a history of not being in the unit at the times he or she is scheduled to work, his or her performance cannot be worthy of a merit increase.

In fulfilling their leadership role, nurse managers must always remember that they are models for the behavior expected in their employees. Nothing will communicate the importance of attendance more than the manager's personal behavior. Attendance is one of those areas in which employees will definitely emulate the behavior they observe in their managers. Although it is not guaranteed that employees will all have good attendance records if their nurse manager does, it is absolutely certain that if the nurse manager has poor attendance, so will everyone else in the unit.

In addition to communicating the importance of attendance during the performance review and through their personal example, nurse managers continually need to reinforce the importance of good attendance to every member of their staffs. This can be accomplished in a group setting such as a staff meeting, in one-on-one informal coaching sessions, in other private one-on-one sessions, or even in informal, unscheduled conversations, as follows:

Group settings: Here nurse managers should emphasize the cost of absenteeism (e.g., expenditures of budget dollars, the cost to and impact on fellow employees). These are areas in which employees can receive the most help from managers in the group setting, because many are ignorant of the impact of their absences.

Private coaching sessions: When nurse managers conduct any form of coaching with an employee, critical areas of performance such as attendance are open for discussion. It never hurts to gently remind even the unit's most reliable and professional staff how important their attendance is.

Disciplinary coaching sessions: When coaching a poorly performing member of the staff, nurse managers may want to raise not only all of the other issues concerning attendance but also the potential for progressive discipline. This discussion can include such things as the impact of excessive absenteeism on interpersonal relationships with other members of the staff as well as its effects on merit pay, advancement opportunities, and even job retention.

Conversations with peers: Possibly the most effective means of controlling absenteeism is peer pressure. When peer pressure is brought to bear against absence-prone individuals, only rarely does the person fail to respond positively. Nurse managers should encourage open dialogue between the staff members, with the caveat that such dialogue be positive. For example, a respected co-worker's discussion of the hardships that have been caused by an employee's absence is often far more effective than the nurse manager's delivery of the same message.

Using a variety of communication strategies, nurse managers should create an official and unofficial communication process that continually points up the problems created by employee absenteeism for all concerned.

Absenteeism Policy

Not uncommonly, the established organizational policy of providing sick leave actually hinders managers' efforts to reduce absenteeism in their units. Although absenteeism policies differ slightly, in most healthcare institutions employees accrue paid sick days; for example, one paid sick day for every month employed. These "earned" sick days are usually accruable up to a specified maximum. This benefit, established as a reasonable allowance for those who are legitimately ill, in many cases actually rewards undesirable behavior. A prime example of this negative impact can be seen in the case of an individual who, through longevity, has reached the maximum allowable number of accrued days of sick leave. After this number has been reached, the employee loses all sick leave he or she earns if it is not used. The thought "Well, I'll lose it if I don't use it" soon establishes itself. This attitude is especially prevalent in a unit in which there is an absenteeism problem. Previously excellent, reliable employees who have not been an absentee problem can quickly become one when they begin to justify absences with "use it or lose it" thinking. Such a "use it or lose it" policy typically has a dramatic effect in promoting absenteeism when employees who know they will be leaving

the organization learn that they will be paid nothing for unused sick leave. These exiting employees tend to use up their allotment of paid sick days prior to leaving.

Over the past decade, many progressive healthcare institutions have taken a close look at their absenteeism policies with the idea of revamping them to promote the desired behavior (good attendance). In a few organizations, management has changed the policy to allow sick days to accumulate without the typically restrictive upper limit. Then, when an employee leaves the institution, he or she is paid for sick days that have not been used. Other organizations allow retiring employees to add unused sick days to the total amount of time they have actually worked, which enables them to retire earlier or with a higher retirement allowance. Research by S. Panyan and M. McGregor examined the effectiveness of a policy of paying a small but specific amount of money for each unused sick day. Absenteeism fell by more than 35% during the first year. Over the next 3 years, absenteeism averaged less than 50% of the rate before implementation of this new policy.[9]

Healthcare managers are typically exceptionally intelligent and well educated, and most have come to realize that employees use sick days for many things that do not approach the clear definition of illness, such as carrying out personal business. To combat this tendency, these administrators now provide another innovative approach for managing absenteeism: substitution of "personal days" or extra vacation days for unused sick days. If nothing more, this approach has helped employees respond in a more professional manner by eliminating the need for them to lie (i.e., to say they are sick when they are not). In addition, creating personal days has helped nurse managers provide adequate coverage because they have advance notice of when an employee is going to be absent. By substituting personal days for sick days, employees no longer feel compelled to tell their supervisors something that is not true, and nurse managers now have time to plan for a replacement—a win-win situation.

Not quite as common is the practice developed by a select few organizations of special incentive rewards for good attendance. These rewards consist mostly of cash bonuses but also include other equally desirable prizes. Some very creative organizations have gone so far as to create lotteries that are available only to employees with acceptable attendance records. Some such programs have resulted in documented declines in absenteeism of as much as 40%.[10]

In almost every instance, changing the hospital's paid sick leave policy is beyond the scope of authority of the typical nurse manager. However, when a group of respected professionals band together and make a concerted effort to move forward, they can be very effective in getting even the most conservative administration to initiate high-quality and innovative changes. Simply stated, it makes good sense to reward the behavior that is desired and to discourage through a process of well-orchestrated disciplinary action that is undesirable.

Although this text has not dealt much with the subject of discipline, the effective use of well-documented and progressively applied disciplinary actions (i.e., a well-grounded and legally compliant strategy) has a place as a deterrent to excessive absenteeism. Most of these disciplinary processes are quite simple: the organization puts together a formal policy that details exactly how much absenteeism is considered acceptable and circulates it to all employees. Once an employee reaches the limit, prescribed disciplinary steps are instituted. It is extremely important that nurse managers, in performing the role of supervisor, follow the discipline policy very precisely. However, managers must remember that discipline is a negative motivator, and its use as a strategy for reducing absenteeism is limited by the fact that its success rate is not generally high. To comply with federal and state employment laws, managers cannot initiate disciplinary action until the rate of absenteeism has exceeded acceptable levels. Those employees who are prone to creating absenteeism problems are, if nothing else, well informed. They know what the limits are and are usually very careful not to exceed them. The result is that nurse managers continue to have an absenteeism problem in the unit, but one that they cannot easily address through the use of progressive discipline.

A Systems Perspective

Although a variety of different approaches have been discussed that can, in the right circumstances, improve employee attendance, every nurse manager needs to understand that no universal remedies exist for dealing with this problem. In addition, every nurse manager must understand that one thing should be avoided at all costs, and that is a quick-fix approach. Placing a Band-Aid on a small cut is probably the correct medical approach, but absenteeism is no small cut. It is a torn artery in the fabric of the nursing unit. To treat such a potentially dangerous condition, the nurse manager must go beyond the obvious and superficial and take a systems approach; that is, the nurse manager (and the entire organization, for that matter) must examine absenteeism as part of an evaluation of the entire work environment. To develop this approach, the nurse manager must stand back and ask himself or herself the following questions:

Is there really an absenteeism problem? Just because employees are periodically absent from their assigned place of duty does not mean that the performance unit has an absenteeism problem. Previously, this chapter mentioned that it was foolhardy for nurse managers to insist on zero absence. Not only is this a demonstration of exceptionally bad leadership, it can ultimately cause the nursing staff to overreact and result in such things as physically ill nurses being present in the unit, where the harm their illnesses can cause to patients may outweigh the benefits their skills can provide..

If there is a problem, what can be done about it? If careful analysis and comparison with other units indicates that there is actually an absenteeism problem, then the nurse manager needs to acquire a clear understanding of why the absenteeism is occurring. Such an investigation can involve conversations with various parties (e.g., higher-level supervisors, absence-prone nurses) as well as an examination of absence patterns (e.g., does most absenteeism occur in the month before an employee quits?). The results of such an investigation should provide the nurse manager with a better understanding of how to attempt to manage the problem.

This textbook describes many different leadership and management skills that have a bearing on the control of absenteeism in the nursing unit. The process of control is best started before the applicant is actually hired, when the nurse manager presents a logical and realistic view of life in the nursing unit. The reason is that if people know what to expect from the beginning, they are less likely to be disappointed. Consider the following story:

> When I was a nurse manager in a large healthcare organization, one of my primary responsibilities was to hire replacement staff. My technique was, to say the least, very different from that of my colleagues and caused our human resources (HR) division more than a few headaches.
>
> When HR sent applicants for interview, I felt it was my job to tell each and every one of them what life in the unit was really like. I began by telling them of my expectations for performance (i.e., good was simply not good enough). I told them about the long hours, the existence of overtime, and the heavy patient load that we dealt with. In fact, I told them in the first few minutes every reason I knew why they should *not* accept a job in my unit.
>
> When the director of HR confronted me with her concerns regarding my interviewing techniques (she felt I caused her to expend more resources finding acceptable applicants than did other nurse managers), I responded by stating that (1) my unit actually spent

less of her time and resources than most of the other units, because I required her services far less than any other unit due to the fact that we enjoyed a very low turnover rate; and (2) it was my obligation to tell every applicant the truth. If that meant that HR spent more time looking for the right applicant, then so be it. I strongly believed then, and believe even now in my position as vice president of the nursing division, that it is far better to spend money looking for the right applicant and informing that person of exactly what to expect so that he or she can make a logical choice if offered a position (not all nurses accepted a job that I offered) than it is to hire people who don't really fit, train them to perform, deal with all of the headaches they cause while on the job (absenteeism and poor performance), and then ultimately have to find a replacement when they quit.

Spend money to find quality people, tell them the facts, support them with proper training and leadership, and the major problems of absenteeism and turnover will take care of themselves. That's my formula.

Leadership—whether it is manifested through telling the truth during the interview, creating a performance environment that promotes initiative and excellence, or providing a reward system centered around a performance appraisal that recognizes excellence—is the key to solving absenteeism. Merit pay and advancement are the instruments of a leadership-based environment that provide structure and tangibility to performance. Nurse managers must understand that they cannot motivate any employee to come to work unless they provide a reason to do so. Monetary reward for attendance is not a problem solver; it's a Band-Aid. The problem of absenteeism will be solved when nurse managers provide caring and nurturing environments in which performance is expected and in which the expectations are demonstrated daily by the people who create them. Absenteeism is a symptom, not the disease.

Most healthcare organizations are operated by an exceptionally well-qualified group of professional administrators. These people are focused on the cost-effective operation of an organization that is truly difficult to manage. The proof of excellence is always its cost savings to the organization. If nurse managers concentrate on developing professional, nurturing environments, their efforts will be noticed because they will be reflected in the organization's bottom line.

Turning a nursing unit into a center of lower cost per patient-day starts with inspiration and perspiration. The problem is that the development of a leadership-based organization takes longer than the development of one in which authority is used to provide direction. There are more obstacles to overcome and more challenges to face, and more creativity

is required; but the reward and opportunity that can be achieved far outweigh the effort that is demanded.

Providing a leadership-based nursing unit is not a sign of weakness. To the contrary, it is a sign of strength, capability, and perseverance. Being a leader does not mean being easy. In fact, a leader actually demands and receives far more in the way of performance and compliance than does the toughest autocrat. The difference lies in how the manager asks for these things. An autocrat, for example, might demand that a staff nurse not miss more than a certain number of days per year, or else. The leader might let it be known that absenteeism is a serious problem, solicit ways that the staff can work together to eliminate it, implement them (giving credit to the staff), reward the compliant employees, and then celebrate achievement when there is a genuine reason to do so.

In the past, short-term solutions to the problem of absenteeism have placed many healthcare organizations in conflict with public law. Some organizations have suggested that because such a strong correlation exists between the marital and parental status of the nurse and absenteeism, it would be wise not to hire women in these higher risk categories. Aside from the fact that there is absolutely no real proof that a married woman with children will be absent more than a single, childless woman, such a position is illegal everywhere in the United States. Under Title VII of the U.S. Code, it is illegal to discriminate on the basis of sex and marital status, and although the law doesn't specifically preclude discrimination based on parental status, there have been many instances in which policies based on the existence of children have been contested and in which organizations have been found not to be in compliance with the spirit of the law and therefore culpable.

In summary, absenteeism is a difficult and serious problem in the healthcare field. The demands and pressures typically associated with healthcare jobs and the tendency to run organizations short-staffed create an extremely difficult situation—one that calls for creativity, initiative, respect for others, a belief in the value of employees, and a willingness to place the needs of others before one's own. In short, absenteeism is a problem that can be solved *only* through leadership, example, and the objective evaluation of performance against well-developed standards.

TURNOVER

According to *Webster's Ninth Collegiate Dictionary*, *turnover* means "an upset, reversal, or shake-up," and the impact that turnover has on the nursing profession and the individual healthcare organization is just about summed up in this definition. In fact, nursing is considered to be the profession with the highest rate of turnover in the United States. Throughout the last decades of the twentieth century, the average annual turnover rate in healthcare organizations was between 18% and 25%.[11] Although this level of turnover is atypical of a professional-level career field, the fact that it was posted during a time of acute shortages of trained personnel and during a time of national economic downturn is nothing short of incredible. The impact of this level of turnover becomes clear when it is compared with the national average in all professional fields, which was a mere 6% to 9% during the same period, or about one-third of that in health care.

The importance of turnover can also be seen in what it costs the industry. If one accepts the assumption that is taken as holy writ in the business world—namely, that a new employee receives the equivalent of 1 year's salary in training before he or she is proficient in the job—then one can see how much turnover costs. Assuming that the average nurse's salary is between $25,000 and $30,000 in the first year on the job (it is usually more) and that the industry hires approximately 18,000 new nurses per year, then the healthcare industry spends $450 million to $540 million each year in training costs alone just to bring a graduate nurse to proficiency in the vocation. If 18% to 25% of those hired leave within the next year, the industry loses $225 million to $270 million a year through turnover of newly graduated nurses.*

Just as the costs of absenteeism are hard to measure, the total costs of turnover in the healthcare industry are extremely difficult to compute. However, if one adds together all of the myriad expenses associated with the hiring of a new nurse (e.g., recruitment, interviewing, selection, orientation, skill development training) and the temporary replacement of a nurse who quits or is fired (e.g., temporary replacement costs, in-house overtime expenses), the potential risk to quality patient care, and the legal exposure of the organization, the costs certainly must be considered significant. Note that these costs are all bottom-line dollars. This means that if they were not spent, they would be part of the organization's profit. This expenditure of what should be profit dollars (spendable income) is one of the most significant reasons why healthcare institutions feel they must run lean (employee fewer workers than might be considered optimum), why they don't offer higher

salaries, why more state-of-the-art equipment isn't available, why benefits are not better, and, finally, why there isn't more opportunity for rewards and special compensation packages. Think about the many things that the average nurse manager does not have that would help him or her operate an exceptional nursing unit, and it is a good bet that many would be available if the organization could just control turnover.

No matter how it is computed, turnover in the nursing field is an extraordinary expense that needs to be sensibly managed. The process of management starts with understanding exactly what turnover is. Turnover was defined by W. Mobley in the 1982 book *Employee Turnover: Causes, Consequences and Control*[12] as "the cessation of membership in an organization by an individual who previously received monetary compensation from that organization" (p. 72). Simply viewing the phenomenon as something bad is not enough. This antediluvian view of turnover is not going to help nurse managers deal effectively with this costly and pervasive phenomenon in their units. Instead, organizations need to help nurse managers by determining the reasons for the departure of an employee. Turnover can be categorized into the following types:

Voluntary turnover: The individual left of his or her own accord.

Involuntary turnover: The individual was asked to leave.

Dysfunctional turnover: The departing employee had a history of exceptional performance.

Functional turnover: The departing employee's performance was considered to be acceptable but not exceptional (i.e., mediocre).

Every healthcare organization must examine the departures of its employees to determine if their exits are, in fact, indicative of a turnover problem. This means that the organization must analyze the data trails left by the employees so that the real reasons for departure can be established and patterns defined. Then, and only then, will the organization truly know whether or not it has a turnover problem and, if so, what might be done to reduce or eliminate it.

This chapter focuses primarily on voluntary turnover. If a healthcare organization, through its analysis of employee departures, determines that a significant amount of involuntary turnover exists, the corrective action is to review the process it uses to recruit, interview, train, and motivate its employees.[13]

Measurement of Turnover

As was true for absenteeism, every nurse manager attempting to reduce turnover in his or her nursing unit must understand exactly what constitutes

---

*Figures are based on data received from the Bureau of National Affairs and the American Nurses Association. These figures have a 5% to 8% margin of error.

turnover. Understanding the problem begins with developing an appreciation of the complexity and variety of the issues involved.

When nurse managers study turnover, the first question they must ask is, "Was the turnover voluntary or involuntary?" On the surface, this question appears to be relatively easy to answer (did the employee quit?), but in truth, the real answer can go very deep and may not be obvious to anyone except the departing employee. For example, some employees may be given the opportunity to resign before they are fired, which can complicate the answer. Consider for a moment: if a nurse quits to keep his or her record clean and to avoid being fired, is the job termination voluntary or involuntary? In almost every instance, this type of separation is considered voluntary.

Not only is there the complex matter of determining whether turnover was voluntary or involuntary, but the following two other issues need to be considered:

1. The reason for turnover
2. The functionality of turnover

DETERMINING THE REASON FOR TURNOVER

The traditional approaches used by healthcare institutions to determine the reason(s) for voluntary turnover have included the exit interview and the personnel questionnaire.

Exit Interview. The exit interview is a brief discussion between the departing employee and either a member of the human resources department or the nurse manager. The purpose of the interview is to determine exactly what are the reasons for the departure. Although, at least on the surface, the exit interview appears to be a straightforward means of obtaining this information, many researchers question the validity of any data gathered in this manner. For example, research has shown that the reasons given by departing employees during exit interviews differ considerably from those given on questionnaires completed several months after the employees left their organizations.[14]

The single biggest cause of this difference in information is believed to be the fact that future employers often ask applicants for references from prior employers. The exiting employee, anticipating the need for a good reference, is more likely to give less critical or "safe" responses to questions during the exit interview. In fact, it is very rare when departing employees say anything negative about the organizations they are leaving or about their immediate supervisors. Obviously, the tendency for a departing employee to provide safe answers during an exit interview makes determining exactly what causes turnover a rather difficult chore.

Questionnaire. The data gathered during the exit interview can be clarified, at least to some degree, by sending questionnaires to former employees several months after job termination. The former employee must be given a realistic measure of assurance that his or her responses will be treated as confidential and will not be included in his or her former personnel file. The sole purpose of such questionnaires must be to establish the reasons for employee turnover.

Co-Worker Input. Some organizations validate exit interviews by discussing the situation with the former employee's co-workers. It is very common for co-workers to know exactly why an employee left, and under the right circumstances (e.g., their remarks will be confidential, they trust the personnel department representative), many of these co-workers will provide valuable input.

DETERMINING THE FUNCTIONALITY OF TURNOVER

One of the best methods available to nurse managers to evaluate the impact of an employee's departure is to categorize the turnover as being either functional or dysfunctional.[15] When different employees leave an organization, their impact is directly proportional to the type, quality, and quantity of work they performed. For example, the departure of a high-quality performer will be a greater loss to a nursing unit and the hospital than the exit of a mediocre employee. Another way to look at the situation is in terms of dollars and cents. If a nurse can be replaced with relative ease, the cost to the hospital and the unit will be far less than if his or her replacement is difficult to locate.

What all of this means is that the type of turnover that is most difficult to live with is dysfunctional turnover, or the departure of high-quality and difficult-to-replace employees. Functional turnover, on the other hand, is the type that involves the departure of easily replaced or poorly performing employees.

The type of turnover that should receive the most attention from nurse managers is dysfunctional turnover. In contrast, functional turnover may be a blessing in disguise. After losing a poor performer, the organization may, if the right effort is applied, actually acquire a much better employee.

One of the important impacts on the nursing unit is the hard dollar cost of turnover. When calculating the total cost of the loss of an employee, the nurse manager must consider how that loss effects the operating budget of the unit. Did the outgoing employee have a high salary and a significant benefits package? Can the replacement employee be hired for less money, or will it cost more in salary and benefits? The work of D. Dalton and W. Todor[16] points up the complexity of the distinction between functional and dysfunctional turnover. Using actual payroll records, they showed that, when the costs and benefits of voluntary turnover are assessed, one also needs to be sensitive to overall costs. For example, they demonstrated the importance of examining whether the departing employee had a vested pension as well as the dollar savings that might result because of the difference between the departing employee's salary and the replacement employee's starting salary.[16]

When nurse managers consider turnover, they must keep a sense of perspective to understand the costs and benefits of voluntary turnover in their units. The common belief that turnover is always a bad and disruptive process must be replaced with an appreciation of the various circumstances that cause it to be or not to be a problem that merits the nurse manager's attention.

The Effects of Turnover

When turnover is discussed, the conversation most often centers around what it costs the organization in terms of hiring expense, training costs, overtime, and salary. Although turnover definitely has dramatic effects on a healthcare organization and its ability to perform, a discussion of the effects of turnover that stops at this point is incomplete. Turnover not only has a negative effect on the organization itself, it can be detrimental to a wide variety of different activities that occur within its walls. Things like patient care, co-worker morale, unit discipline, and continuity of effort can be dramatically affected.

The flip side, however, is that many of the effects are not negative at all, or at least don't have to be. Voluntary turnover, as discussed previously, does not have to have a negative connotation and in fact can have dramatically positive results. Almost every working adult can remember a case in which someone left his or her work unit and the departure sparked a noticeable improvement in performance, attitude, teamwork, and camaraderie. This means, then, that anyone who analyzes the cost of turnover in a unit needs to consider that it can have both positive and negative impacts. In fact, what may be considered a negative impact by certain members of the nursing unit might be cause for celebration by others.

NEGATIVE IMPACTS

The perception of negative or positive impacts aside, turnover always has certain direct costs associated with it, especially when it involves a highly technical employee such as a staff nurse. Fig. 23-2 details some of the costs absorbed by an organization when a member of the staff departs. The replacement costs shown are composed of a variety of direct and indirect expenses typically incurred as a result of personnel turnover (e.g., procurement of the new hire, adjustment and training costs for the new hire, and separation costs for the departing employee).

Real dollar values need not be assigned to every factor listed in Fig. 23-2 in order to see the significant expense that turnover represents for the organization. Keep in mind also that every dollar spent to replace an exiting employee is a bottom-line dollar that, if not expended, could supply additional revenue to the stockholders, increased technology to the hospital, salary increases to deserving performers, and a wide range of patient care–related enhancements.

The sad fact is that turnover-related costs do not end with the dollar expenses incurred by the organization. Turnover can and often does have a severe impact on the remaining employees, especially those who had a direct working relationship with the exiting employee. In the book *Personnel Management,* researchers R. Steers and T. Stone[17] suggest that turnover is often interpreted by the employees who remain on the job as a rejection of themselves as co-workers and of the job itself; perhaps even more damaging is the recognition that better job opportunities actually do exist.

Problems that occur in the unit because of abnormally high turnover affect everyone who is associated with the troubled performance center. Temporary fixes can easily backfire and can themselves create more stress and decline in performance. Hiring a temporary employee, although certainly a viable and immediate answer to the loss of a staff nurse, can cause problems in the work flow because the temporary replacement is normally not as proficient as the departing staff nurse, is more ignorant of hospital routine and expectations, and typically lacks the special skills required in a specific unit.

The biggest loser of all in the turnover challenge, however, is the patient. The exceptionally high monetary expenses associated with turnover can affect the hospital's ability to provide services and specialty treatments and will almost certainly cause delay, postponement, and even cancellation of potentially profitable new ventures.

POSSIBLE POSITIVE IMPACTS

Virtually nothing occurs in the nursing unit that does not have the potential for positive consequences, and turnover is no exception. As was mentioned earlier, there are several major areas in which turnover can actually deliver positive results, including the following:

Performance enhancement: There is every reason to believe that if nurse managers properly and thoroughly select top-quality performers to replace departing staff increased performance will result;

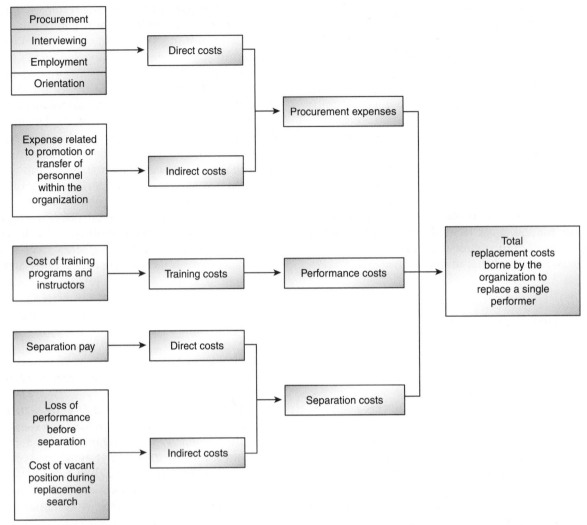

Fig. 23-2 ■ Costs the organization must absorb when a staff member leaves the organization. (Data from Cascio W: *Costing human resources,* Boston, 1982, Kent Publishing.)

that is, new employees will bring with them different skills, work ethics, and personal capabilities. The opportunity exists to improve the unit's performance if nurse managers properly carry out their responsibilities in hiring new staff. Consider the following story:

After assuming the position of nurse manager, I began to change things in the unit. I expected performance to meet hospital standards, personnel to be punctual, and employees to restrict personal pursuits to time spent away from the unit. Each individual was informed that performance appraisals would be based strictly on performance and that a program of continual observation would be instituted and good records would be kept so that actual performance throughout the year would be remembered.

Although I thought my requirements embodied the fundamental elements of leadership, they caused quite a stir among the unit's staff. We were staffed with a heavy percentage of older nurses who were used to not being compelled to attend meetings, to be at work at the proper time, or to comply fully with hospital dress and performance standards. To make a long story short, my unit's turnover rate skyrocketed with the transfer of nearly all of my senior staff nurses to other parts of the hospital.

We reacted to these losses as if they were a blessing, instead of a curse. I worked closely with the human resources manager and, together, we built a mental picture of the type of nurse replacements I felt would be best for the unit and the hospital. We set strict interview procedures, and many of the applicants interviewed did not meet our expectations.

Those whom we did accept brought with them higher performance capabilities, better individual skills, and far better overall attitudes than the departing nurses had had. As a result, and after a period of adjustment, my unit's performance started to move off the chart in a positive direction. Our absenteeism fell to almost zero, our professional performance became the hallmark of the hospital, and our teamwork and interpersonal relationships grew proficient and rewarding.

The next time I inherit a nursing unit, I hope I am lucky enough to have some significant turnover.

Improvement in interpersonal relations: The potential always exists for conflict among performers, especially in the higher-skill professions. Belief in one's ideas, capabilities, and skills runs deep in the average worker, and many times when these individual qualities conflict with those of other workers, disagreement and personality clashes result. Turnover can eliminate some challenges of this type because the departing employee usually takes the conflict with him or her.

Improved opportunity: Many times an employee departure will reduce the amount of competition for promotion and other advancement in the unit, as well as offering the opportunity to free up some budgetary resources for distribution to other performers in the form of salaries and reward programs. This is especially true when older, higher-salaried individuals leave.

Innovation and change: Many times, the existence of well-established employees who are used to things being done in a certain manner causes the nursing unit to be resistant to change and innovation. New hires almost never suffer from this malady, even if they are exceptionally qualified and experienced. Turnover can result in fresh ideas and acceptance of change by the nursing unit and by the individual nurses who remain after the departing ones have left.

Temporary pay increases due to availability of overtime: Although the need for overtime is most frequently thought of as a negative impact of turnover, overtime and its accompanying pay increase can actually help some employees. It is extremely common for many employees to want to work overtime. Perhaps the "get on and stay on" type of overtime is damaging, but well-developed and time-limited overtime can actually be a boon to performance. This area is one in which nurse managers can really shine in front of their staffs if they handle overtime requirements in a well-thought-out, professional, and unbiased manner.

Policy changes and enhancements: Not frequently but occasionally, a unit will lose a well-established and respected member of its team because of disagreements with unit or organizational policy. When this happens, there is often significant sentiment present to get the offending policy changed, which enhances the environment for those who remain. Although this is certainly an extremely high price to pay for change, such a situation does happen and should be considered a potential opportunity.

Decrease in the likelihood of staff reductions: Voluntary attrition can have a very positive impact on the frequency of layoffs. In poor economic times and in periods of increased government regulation, it often becomes necessary for healthcare organizations to reduce their staffing levels to remain profitable. If sufficient numbers of staff leave of their own accord, the need to force an employee to depart (lay an employee off) becomes less likely.

A Model of Employee Turnover

Since turnover has become an issue of concern in the healthcare field, a variety of different models have been developed to help clarify the turnover process. Each of the variants has its strengths and weaknesses, but none of them provides an absolute answer to the challenge of turnover. The model shown in Fig. 23-3 holds the most interest and potential for nurse managers as they struggle to deal with turnover in their units. This model, derived from one first developed by J. March and H. Simon,[18] is relatively straightforward and easy to understand, yet it does a credible job of

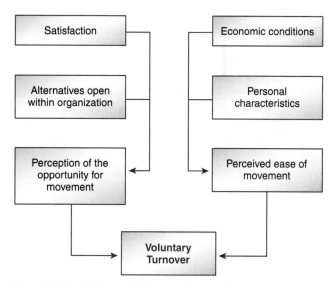

Fig. 23-3 ■ Primary influences on voluntary turnover. (Data from March J, Simon H: *Organizations,* ed 5, New York, 1974, Wiley.)

illustrating the primary influences that affect voluntary turnover. The following discussion places greater emphasis on those sections of the model that are most relevant for nurse managers.

The model depicts voluntary turnover as derived from perceptions; that is, how the typical employee views both the *opportunity* for and the *ease* of moving out of a currently held position. Perceived ease of movement depends on the nurse's personal characteristics (e.g., education, specialization, age, marital status, number of contacts at other healthcare institutions) and the current economic conditions in the marketplace (e.g., number of job openings in the nurse's area of expertise and interest at other healthcare organizations and at nonhealthcare institutions hiring nurses for open positions, even if not associated with nursing).

Perceptions of the opportunity for movement, like perceptions of ease of movement, can be affected by a variety of different factors, two of which are (1) the availability of alternatives in the same healthcare institution, and (2) the level of personal satisfaction with the current job. Generally speaking, the more employees believe that transfers within the organization are possible and the more satisfied they are with their jobs, the more content they will be with the institution and the less likely they will be to leave. Employees find comfort in the fact that they can move from one unit to another, perhaps to relieve themselves of shift work, reduce overtime, or escape a personal difference with a co-worker. Perceived opportunity for movement is an area in which a competent and professional nurse manager can exercise tremendous influence in reducing voluntary turnover.

Job satisfaction has a tremendous effect on perceived desirability of movement. The higher the individual employee's satisfaction level in his or her current job, the less likely he or she is to quit. Job satisfaction is influenced by a wide variety of factors, including the professionalism, leadership ability, and capability of management; relationships with associates in the unit; the quality of patient interactions and relations with physicians; and, probably the most discussed, the shift to which the person is assigned.

In dealing with turnover, nurse managers must be aware of the following three important factors:

1. *Variety of influences:* A variety of factors act to create a situation in which turnover increases or decreases, and even the best manager cannot influence all of them.
2. *Need for assessment:* The nurse manager should assess why each employee leaves the unit. This is best accomplished by working closely with the human resources department.
3. *Need for planning:* Every nurse manager must realize that any action he or she takes to reduce turnover in the unit may have consequences that are less than desired and may even be negative. Because of this, the nurse manager absolutely must thoroughly consider and plan any strategies for dealing with turnover long before such strategies are implemented.

Strategies for Controlling Turnover

The turnover model shown in Fig. 23-3 provides an effective framework for developing methods of managing turnover in the nursing unit. The nurse manager's goal should be to positively influence those factors within his or her control that can help to reduce dysfunctional voluntary turnover. Little or no time should be spent on functional turnover, because most of it actually benefits the nursing unit. Direct control measures are those that can be implemented by the nurse manager himself or herself; indirect measures include collaboration with other management and human resources personnel when they are actively engaged in improving the institutional policies or procedures that affect turnover.

As can be seen easily from Fig. 23-3, when nurse managers wish to decrease voluntary turnover, they will achieve the best results when they focus on reducing staff members' perception of how desirable it might be to change positions. Because nurse managers typically can do little to change the economic conditions that influence the healthcare environment, they should not spend large amounts of time attempting to do so.

Once again, because the average nurse manager's ability to positively influence the perceived ease of movement is rather constrained, he or she should focus efforts on influencing the desirability of movement, where a profound impact can be made. For example, it is usually within the nurse manager's authority to facilitate or restrict movement of personnel within the same healthcare institution. If the manager notices that one of the staff is becoming burnt out from working in a specific area of specialization, the manager might be able to keep the employee in the organization by encouraging him or her to transfer to another unit. Unfortunately, not many nurse managers will take this proactive view. To the contrary, most will aggressively take steps to prevent such a transfer, especially if the employee is a top performer. The feeling is almost always that the manager does not want to lose a top-performing employee. This viewpoint is extremely shortsighted, however, and does not adequately consider the needs of the organization. If the efforts of the employee to transfer to another unit are blocked, he or she will often retaliate by leaving the organization altogether. Nurse managers must understand that they have a dual responsibility. They must look out for the welfare of their units *and* they must look out for the welfare of the organization. In most instances, the best way to solve this dilemma is to act in the best interests of the employee. It is not professional to take the short-sighted view and work selfishly to maintain personnel within one's own unit. If an employee wishes to leave, the unit will best be served by allowing the transfer.

The best way to prevent internal transfers or to reduce the desire in an employee to leave the unit is not to restrict transfers, which is almost always detrimental, but instead to build up the unit and one's personal leadership ability so that the employee cannot find as desirable a situation elsewhere in the organization and fears that it might not be available outside of the hospital. People work where they feel good, where they are respected, and where they feel they can contribute their very best. If nurse managers work to create an environment in the unit that provides these fundamentals as its foundation, there will be very few, if any, transfers.

A Systems Perspective

Absenteeism and turnover share a common thread: both are employee withdrawal behaviors; that is, both provide an avenue of escape for the employee, one temporarily and one permanently. In almost every case, the desire to withdraw from a place of occupation stems from personal dissatisfaction. Given this almost universal cause, it is not surprising that many of the effective strategies for reducing absenteeism discussed earlier can also have a positive and sometimes dramatic effect on turnover.

One of the cardinal rules when dealing with turnover, just as when dealing with absenteeism, is to avoid attempting a quick fix. Band-Aids won't work here either. The reduction of turnover is achieved only when sound management and leadership practices are in place and the professional working environment is built on respect, loyalty, and recognition of effort.

In addition, nurse managers must realize that any efforts they make are generally followed by nay-saying by different members of the staff. Even when an honest effort is made to assist a top performer, someone in the staff is likely to feel slighted. Nurse managers must understand that individual acts of support will never reduce turnover or increase job satisfaction; instead, what is required is a comprehensive demonstration of leadership that encompasses every employee, fairly and objectively. Nurse man-

agers must anticipate challenges and prevent them from occurring. Every day, they need to demonstrate professionalism, caring, and concern for the welfare of the staff—all of the staff, without exception. Reducing turnover comes down to following the three principles of leadership emphasized throughout this text:

1. *Elicit support:* Nurse managers should not demand performance, they should encourage it. They should not make people feel obligated, but make them feel excited. They should not make staff feel used, but make them feel like contributors. When nurse managers do this, every member of the staff will be excited to work in the unit, and very few, if any, will want to leave.

2. *Listen:* The staff can teach nurse managers just about as much as they are willing to learn. When staff members feel that their ideas and concerns are being heard and paid attention to, then they will not want to leave. When they feel that they have a voice that contributes to the success of the organization and are not considered to be the cause of its problems, then they will want to stay. To accomplish this, nurse managers need to listen to every word that is being said as well as to every word that is *not* being said. Listening means being able to comprehend what is going on around one. It is more than hearing words, it is recognizing the feelings, listening to the body language, and understanding the unspoken words being screamed when an employee shows a poor attitude and disobedience.

3. *Place the needs of others ahead of one's own:* If nurse managers want staff members to stay, then they must make staff members feel that they are important. Nothing should ever be done for personal gain, it should be done for the enhancement of the unit and the staff. Nurse managers should not expect from others, but give to them, and all that they desire will be returned. Employees are not petulant children; they are reasoning, comprehending, and capable, thinking adults. They can see when managers do things for themselves and their own personal benefit, and they can tell the difference between what results from those actions and what occurs when their managers look out for their welfare—just as you could when you were not in management. When managers give out work assignments, they should keep the dirty jobs and give out some of the career-enhancing ones. In other words, they should delegate, not dump. They should let their staffs have their successes and celebrate with them.

In summary, it must be stressed that the nurse manager does not have to be satisfied with a unit in which a high turnover rate exists. Contrary to popular belief, keeping people in a given location comes down to the quality of the environment that exists there, and because the working environment and its quality are the responsibility of the nurse manager, he or she has control over most of the turnover that the unit will experience. Employees have proven over and over again that they will remain in a position for extended periods of time as long as they feel that they are recognized for their contributions, respected for their professionalism, and made to feel as if they are part of the solution and not part of the problem.

Certainly, every nursing unit will experience some turnover, and some of it will be significant because it will involve the unit's best people. High-quality people will leave to take senior positions elsewhere in the hospital or transfer to another organization for a more responsible position, and that is good. When such an exit occurs, the smart nurse manager makes a big deal of it. The manager lets everyone know that one of his or her best people is leaving for a promotion or for enhanced opportunity, and why. The "why" is because the departing employee learned how to excel from the nurse manager who let him or her do so. After this happens several times, the nursing unit will develop a reputation for opportunity and advancement: "Hey, people get promoted after they work there." Let the grapevine work wonders for the unit. Once it does, there will be no shortage of highly qualified replacements lining up for a chance to work in a nurturing, positive, and promotion-enhancing environment. The best way to control turnover is to be a good leader and to provide an environment that encourages initiative, applauds success, and views mistakes as opportunities for learning. Good people will find out quickly, and the unit will never have a significant turnover problem—or an absenteeism problem, either, for that matter.

There will also be those nonperformers who want to leave. Once they find themselves in a high-activity unit where performance is the letter of the day and where they will go nowhere but out if they don't perform well, they will want to leave, and quickly. But who cares? Their departure is an opportunity for the unit. Replace them with quality performers, treat those performers exceptionally well, and encourage staff members to reach for their very best every day and the unit will conquer both absenteeism and turnover.

Managing turnover and absenteeism is about leadership and the quality of the nurse managers responsible for providing it. High-quality nurse managers work hard every day to reduce these potential challenges, and they head them off by performing the unexpected, by doing more than is necessary, and by caring about each and every employee. The reward for this is obviously an exceptional nursing unit but, even more, almost unlimited opportunity for the nurse manager who can deliver it.

SUMMARY

- Historically, healthcare institutions have had serious problems with excessive employee absenteeism and turnover. Fortunately, there is much the nurse manager can do to control their effect on the nursing unit.
- Annual costs of absenteeism are a significant reason why desired salary increases and equipment, technology, and other patient care enhancements are not always available.
- The Steers and Rhodes model of attendance behavior is particularly useful for the nurse manager. It suggests that absenteeism is directly related to an individual's ability and motivation to attend. This places absenteeism within the control of the nurse manager, who is the person in the organization who has the greatest opportunity to influence it positively.
- Nurse managers can influence turnover through the use of effective leadership, which involves: (1) eliciting the support of others, (2) listening, and (3) placing the needs of others ahead of their own. Leadership techniques such as coaching, building self-worth in the employee, recognizing effort, rewarding exceptional performance, and setting a personal example help create the best possible working environment.
- In attempting to deal with an absenteeism problem, nurse managers must adopt a systems perspective, investigate why the absenteeism is occurring, communicate to both staff nurses and the personnel department the problems absenteeism creates, and work diligently to build a working environment that reduces it.
- Turnover averages between 18% and 25% in the healthcare industry. This means that 18% to 25% of the people who are working on January 1 of any given year will have left the organization before December 31 of that year.
- The consequences of turnover are many: lost productivity, especially if high performers leave; increased training expenses; the cost of temporary replacements and/or overtime for remaining nurses; and reduced quality of patient care.
- It is important to determine if turnover is functional or dysfunctional and if it constitutes a problem or an opportunity for the unit.
- To manage turnover effectively, nurse managers must understand the underlying causes and build a work environment that meets those challenges and

provides a quality of working life that is hard to find in other places.

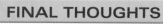

FINAL THOUGHTS

One of the greatest pleasures nurse managers receive from the job is the ability to work with other people. As with many things, however, one of the greatest strengths often presents the majority of the challenges. Problems such as absenteeism and turnover are only two of the challenges that will be faced by nurse managers, but together or separately they have the potential to be the most significant. If nurse managers want to be successful, these challenges must be dealt with in a manner that minimizes their effects on patient care and staff morale. Solid leadership skills, personal example, and documentation of accomplishment and performance without prejudice and with objectivity are critical to any successful effort.

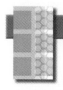

THE NURSE MANAGER SPEAKS

When attempting to control absenteeism and turnover in the nursing unit, the nurse manager must use initiative, foresight, and quality leadership.

All employees respond better when they work in an environment that has high expectations tempered with equal parts of concern and respect. Today's employee needs to be led well, given responsibility, and trusted to perform.

Being a good leader and creating a work environment that promotes attendance and low turnover does not mean that the nurse manager has to be easy or soft. Neither is it necessary to set the performance requirements low to ensure that they can be achieved. To the contrary, a nurse manager can have very high expectations and demand quality performance as long as he or she gives back respect and trust, and as long as he or she encourages excellence and does not tolerate poor performance.

Leadership is the cure for absenteeism and turnover, and it is never about being lax, soft, or easy.

REFERENCES

1. Breaugh J: Predicting absenteeism from prior absenteeism and work attitudes, *J Appl Psych* 66:555, 1981.
2. Steers R, Rhodes S: Major influences on employee attendance: a process model, *J Appl Psych* 63:391, 1978.
3. Hardy ME, Conway ME: *Role theory: perspectives for health professionals,* ed 2, Norwalk, Conn, 1988, Appleton and Lange.
4. Haddock C: Transformation leadership and the employee discipline process, *Hosp Health Serv Adm* 34(2):185, 1989.
5. Muchinsky P: Employee absenteeism: a review of the literature, *J Vocat Behav* 10:316, 1977.
6. Johns G: Unresolved issues in the study and management of absenteeism from work. In Goodman P, Atkin R, editors: *Absenteeism,* San Francisco, 1984, Jossey-Bass.
7. Melohn T: *The new partnership,* New York, 1996, Wiley.
8. Price L: Speech at a training seminar given to the Bank of America, 1995.
9. Panyan S, McGregor M: How to implement a proactive incentive plan: a field study, *Pers J* 55:460, 1976.
10. Stephens T, Burroughs W: An application of operant conditioning to absenteeism in a hospital setting, *J Appl Psych* 63:518, 1978.
11. Bureau of National Affairs: *Bulletin to management,* Washington, DC, March 2001, The Bureau.
12. Mobley W: *Employee turnover: causes, consequences, and control,* ed 3, Reading, Mass, 1994, Addison-Wesley.
13. Heneman H, Schwab D, Fossum J, and others: *Personnel/ human resource management handbook,* ed 4, Homewood, Ill, 1989, Irwin.
14. Hinrichs J: Measurement of reasons for resignations of professionals: questionnaire versus company and consultant interviews, *J Appl Psych* 60:530, 1975.
15. Dalton D, Krackhardt D, Porter L: Functional turnover, *J Appl Psych* 66:716, 1981.
16. Dalton D, Todor W: Turnover: a lucrative hard dollar criterion, *Acad Manage Rev* 7:212, 1982.
17. Steers R, Stone T: Organizational exit. In Rowland K, Ferris G, editors: *Personnel management,* Boston, 1982, Allyn and Bacon.
18. March J, Simon H: *Organizations,* ed 4, New York, 1991, Wiley.

SUGGESTED READINGS

Cabot SJ: Easing the pain of separation, *Provider* 21(4):57, 1995.

Decker P, Moore RC, Sullivan E: How hospitals can solve the nursing shortage, *Hosp Health Serv Adm* 27(6):12, 1982.

Hersey P, Blanchard K, Johnson DE: *Management of organized behavior: utilizing human resources,* Englewood Cliffs, NJ, 1996, Prentice-Hall.

Irvine DM, Evans MG: Job satisfaction and turnover among nurses, *Nurs Res* 44(4):246, 1995.

Latham G, Napier N: Practical ways to increase employee attendance. In Goodman P, Atkin R, editors: *Absenteeism,* San Francisco, 1984, Jossey-Bass.

Taunton RL, Perkins S, Oetker-Black S, and others: Predictors of absenteeism among hospital staff nurses, *Nurs Econ* 13(4):217, 1995.

Managing the Collective Bargaining Environment

LEARNING SYNOPSIS

Upon successful completion of this chapter, readers will possess a fundamental understanding of how collective bargaining and the presence of union representation influences management of the nursing effort in the unit.

OBJECTIVES

1. Describe how healthcare labor relations are affected by U.S. labor law and how healthcare union representation is organized
2. Cite the reasons that healthcare professionals join labor organizations
3. Discuss the effects of unions and professional organizations on nursing and the administration of health care
4. Describe methods of recognizing when organizing efforts are underway
5. Discuss the various aspects of the nurse manager's role in labor relations

For most of the last half of the twentieth century, the U.S. economy struggled through the demands of shifting from an industry-based to a service-based economy. Those organizations intent on unionizing the American workforce noted this trend and worked hard to organize vast numbers of service employees. The collective bargaining effort began slowly in the United States during the turbulent management-labor wars of the 1920s but did not reach a point of significance until the mid-1970s.

The healthcare industry, at least at first, was not well represented in legislation passed by the U.S. Congress before World War II. In fact, national labor laws initially excluded the vast majority of healthcare employees. The Wagner Act (also known as the National Labor Relations Act) (http://encarta.msn.com/encyclopedia_761573039/National_Labor_Relations_Act.html), which passed into law during 1935 and is now the prevailing document establishing most of U.S. labor law, originally excluded all public employees. This meant that any healthcare facility that was operated by either the state or the federal government was not required to comply with its provisions. The Wagner Act did not specifically exclude private and nonprofit organizations, however; in fact, the National Labor Relations Board (NLRB), the enforcement body created by the act, initially established jurisdiction over these types of organizations.

The Wagner Act was modified in 1947 with the passage of the Taft-Hartley Act (29 U.S.C. §§ 141-187 [2000]), which did exempt private and nonprofit healthcare facilities from federal collective bargaining laws. In fact, not until 1967 did the NLRB actually claim jurisdiction over healthcare organizations that were classified as proprietary (i.e., privately owned and for profit). This "jurisdiction" was not exercised effectively until 1974, however, when the U.S. Congress once again modified the Wagner Act with new legislation (Public Law 93-360) that lifted the Taft-Hartley exclusion and compelled private and nonprofit hospitals, nursing homes, health maintenance organizations, health clinics, and all other healthcare institutions to comply with the provisions of federal labor law.

The modifications brought about by the 1974 legislation were more than a little overdue. The healthcare industry had grown into a behemoth that at the time employed more than 5 million people. During the years since the passage of the first legislation that had exempted health care from compliance, explosive growth had occurred in both the size and cost of health care in America. As the industry grew, many of its primary organizations became extremely large and complex, with annual increases in expenditures that far exceeded the inflation rate. This growth was further accelerated by the fact that in health care, unlike in many other service industries, labor requirements were not reduced by the development of new technology. In fact, even today, work in the typical healthcare organization remains extremely labor intensive, and healthcare organizations are beset by a host of employee relations problems. These problems have been made more acute by the fact that health care is predominately a professional-level industry; that is, most of its decision-making members are highly educated and technically oriented. When these highly skilled individuals work in close proximity to one another, the ensuing conflicts are far more than simple interprofessional tensions and rivalries. One of the most serious of these problems is that the salaries of most healthcare employees have lagged significantly behind those of comparably educated groups in other service sectors, with the vast majority of the salary dollars going to only one of the many contributing professions.

Another major factor contributing to the problems that now permeate the healthcare industry is the dramatic change in its basic structure in recent years. The previously widespread provision of charity-based services in hospitals has declined significantly and has been replaced by third-party benefit systems and health maintenance organizations. Insurance companies, which in the early part of the twentieth century were minor contributors in the industry, have become a major, even dominant influence in the last four decades. One big change is the way in which federally funded and regulated insurance programs like Medicare and Medicaid have become institutionalized. These significant changes and the extremely high cost of health care today have combined to mark the industry, at least in the minds of lawmakers in the U.S. Congress, as an industry out of control. Long-held beliefs such as the view that private and nonprofit healthcare facilities should be immune from collective bargaining because of the danger that wage increases may be passed on to sick patients no longer hold credence. In fact, it was this new environment and the concern over runaway costs that caused the U.S. Congress to enact the 1974 amendments to the Wagner Act forcing healthcare employers to comply with U.S. labor law.

HEALTHCARE LABOR RELATIONS

Today, all private and nonprofit healthcare organizations are required to comply with U.S. labor law. If healthcare organizations were as easily classified as those in many other industries, this might not be a significant problem. In the healthcare industry, however, a major question is what, exactly, constitutes a private healthcare institution and what makes it different from a public organization. For example, it is common for a hospital to be operated by a private, for-profit organization but for its assets to be owned by a public agency. This dichotomy between ownership and management has led to bitter arguments over the classification of such institutions, and no end to the conflict appears to be in sight.

Recent NLRB rulings, however, have repeatedly driven home its belief that when the organization that employs and directs the institution's management is different from the entity that owns the physical assets of the facility, it is the status of the former that determines whether or not the healthcare facility falls under NLRB's jurisdiction. What this basically means is that if a healthcare facility is operated on a day-by-day basis by a private organization, it is subject to U.S. labor law.

Although there are literally hundreds of organizations representing the employees of the healthcare industry, the major collective bargaining agents are the Service Employees International Union, the National Union of Hospital and Health Care Employees, and the American Nurses Association and its constituent state nurses associations. Today, a number of nurses working in the United States are covered by some kind of labor contract. This trend started in the early 1970s and has continued to grow steadily ever since, with peak years showing increases as high as 14%.[1] Many people are now predicting that unionization will continue to grow, both in the actual number of hospital employees represented and in the number of different occupational groups represented.[2] This trend continues as the new millennium advances, even though the overall number of unionized workers in America is declining.

As stated previously, the major U.S. laws that govern collective bargaining are the Wagner Act and the Taft-Hartley Act. Although these two pieces of legislation were enacted more than a decade apart and represent distinctly different viewpoints (the Wagner Act was written as a prolabor document and the Taft-Hartley Act has a promanagement slant), they were combined to form much of the Labor-Management Relations Act of 1947. As noted earlier, the Wagner Act, as amended, established the NLRB, the major administrative body. The NLRB has five members, who are appointed by the President and confirmed by the Senate.

Section 7 is the heart of the original Wagner Act and when translated into lay terms essentially means[3]:

> Employees shall have the right to self organization, to form, to join, or to assist labor organizations, to bargain collectively through representatives of their own choosing, and to engage in other concerted activities for the purpose of collective bargaining or other mutual aid or protection, and shall also have the right to refrain from any or all of such activities except to the extent that such right may be affected by an agreement requiring membership in a labor organization as a condition of employment as authorized in Section 8(a)(3).

This portion of the law clearly states that all employees covered by the act have the right to choose whether or not to join a union unless the organization in which they are employed is covered by a closed-shop agreement. In a closed shop, union membership is considered a condition of employment.

The Wagner Act, as amended, also outlines specific actions that, if taken by either employers or unions, are considered unfair labor practices. For employers, the prohibitions are the following:

An employer may not assist or dominate any labor organization. A company may not form any part of the union's administration or its organizational structure. A company may not cause a union to be swayed by the presence of company employees within its ranks. Management may not contribute financial or other support or otherwise dominate or interfere with the development or administration of a labor union.

An employer may not discriminate in its hiring, assignments, or other terms of employment on the basis of union membership. A company cannot institute hiring and employment procedures that restrict the operation of a union, the hiring of a union sympathizer, or the continued employment of an individual who attempts to organize his or her fellow workers.

An employer may not penalize or discriminate against any employee who charges an employer with violation of the act. An employer may not take retaliatory action against any employee who initiates legal action against it for labor violations, either real or imagined.

An employer may not refuse to bargain in good faith with any union over issues of wages, hours, and conditions of employment. Good faith is generally defined as "acting in a manner that promotes a mutual solution or that works in a direction to obtain that solution." Therefore the employing company must be willing to negotiate with the intention of seeking compromise on or resolution of demands made by the union, its members, or its representatives.

For unions, provisions regarding unfair labor practice include the following:

Unions may not coerce employees in the exercise of their section 7 rights. A union may not use undue influence in soliciting the right to represent any employee, group of employees, or companies as a whole.

Unions cannot demand or require that an employer violate anything in the act. The union cannot cause an employer to break the law, either knowingly or out of ignorance.

Unions cannot engage in or encourage individuals to engage in strike or refusal to handle some type of product when the object is to accomplish any of the following: (1) to cease handling nonunion products, (2) to force an employer to bargain with any uncertified labor organization, (3) to require excessive initiation fees, (4) to force an employer to pay for services not rendered, or (5) to picket to force recognition.

Unions must bargain in good faith in all actions covering wages, hours, and conditions of employment. Numerous NLRB rulings have provided an excellent definition of "good faith." Basically, it means that if one party proposes, the other counterproposes.[4]

Specific Bargaining Issues and Concerns

Amendments to the U.S. Labor Law passed in 1974 speak specifically to significant issues faced by healthcare organizations and have provided a certain degree of latitude in the implementation of the law in the industry to minimize the prospect of work interruptions that might cause impairment of the services provided to patients. These sections were written so that a healthcare organization faced with a labor slowdown or strike is provided with sufficient time to make temporary provisions for the care of patients or residents. The special circumstances in this industry are reflected in the restrictions placed on union organizations and union organizers with regard to access to healthcare employees. Although in most labor situations it is relatively easy for internal union organizers to gain access to employees, such is not the case in a healthcare organization.

NO SOLICITATION

In 1976 an NLRB decision held that the no-solicitation rule prohibiting union organizers from operating in any area of a healthcare institution where patient contract was possible was ambiguous and not in keeping with the spirit and intent of the public labor laws. On appeal, however, the NLRB decision was overturned by the Tenth U.S. Court of Appeals, which held that the needs of patients far exceeded the organizing rights of employees, no matter how well intended. This decision remains in effect, and today all union organizing activities are prohibited in any area of a healthcare institution to which patients or residents have access. However, this ban does not mean that all union activi-

ties are barred from these areas. For example, passive organization can and does frequently occur when employees wear union pins or buttons that call for organization.

The 1974 amendments also created a different set of rules for negotiations in which healthcare facilities are involved. Instead of conducting good faith negotiation, in a healthcare organization, the party that desires to change the existing terms of a contract is required to inform the other party in writing within 90 days and not less than 60 days before the expiration date of the current contract. Both parties are enjoined from striking or locking employees out during this 90-day period or until the actual date of expiration of the existing contract, whichever date is later. These provisions give the healthcare organization more than sufficient time to make alternative arrangements for patient care in the advent of a strike by organized labor.

STRUCTURE OF BARGAINING UNITS

Before 1984, the NLRB required that all healthcare bargaining units be organized according to specific functional occupations. The frequent attempts that were made to place registered nurses in mixed bargaining units invariably ended with the nurses' remaining as a separate bargaining unit in the organization. Other major bargaining units were (a) technical employees, such as licensed practical nurses, x-ray technicians, and laboratory technicians; (b) maintenance and service employees; (c) administrative and clerical employees; and (d) physicians, when organized.

Most of these line-style bargaining units changed when the NLRB ruled in 1984 that maintenance employees at St. Francis Hospital in Memphis, Tennessee, could not organize into their own distinct bargaining unit. This decision ran counter to the pre-1984 NLRB interpretations, which had used a traditional "community of interest" test for determining acceptable bargaining units. Previously, up to seven distinct bargaining units had been allowed to exist in a hospital, one of which was designated for registered nurses. The St. Francis decision, in a significant change from previous policy, eliminated the seven distinct units allowed previously and reconstituted them into only two—professional and nonprofessional.

In March 1987, however, the U.S. Court of Appeals for the District of Columbia reversed the NLRB's decision in the St. Francis case and remanded the case back to the NLRB for further consideration. The NLRB then designated the following eight separate bargaining units for most healthcare organizations:

1. Employed physicians
2. Registered nurses
3. Professionals not otherwise grouped

4. Technical employees
5. Skilled maintenance employees
6. Administrative employees (business office and clerical)
7. Security employees
8. Other nonprofessional employees

Nursing homes, psychiatric hospitals, and rehabilitation facilities were exempted from this 1987 decision, and the NLRB's rules for organization were bitterly contested by those institutions large enough to mount a challenge. Finally, in 1991, the U.S. Supreme Court upheld the NLRB ruling regarding the St. Francis case and opened the market for the minimally organized healthcare industry to union representation.

MULTIPLE-GROUP BARGAINING

In many of the states that have healthcare bargaining laws, a history of multiemployer bargaining exists in the healthcare industry. For example, it is quite common to find a state government entity or a regional healthcare association acting as the bargaining agent for large numbers of organizational employers.

The reverse situation is also found in which a union bargaining agent represents workers in several different healthcare organizations (e.g., one agent represents all of the registered nurses in an entire city's municipal hospitals). To date, the NLRB has not disallowed or moved to modify this multiple-group bargaining process.

Effect of Unionization in Health Care

Over the years, many different opinions have been expressed to provide answers to why employees unionize. Although opinions vary, it is believed to come down to this simple statement: *employees join unions to increase their power in negotiations.* Research conducted by the authors showed that when employees of a nonunionized organization have turned to a union, they have done so because management has created a situation that is intolerable to the employees.

This statement was discussed with several labor union leaders during the research conducted for this book, and not a single one found any fault with it. The union leaders we talked with actually admitted that if management would provide an environment that provided employees with the security, income, and negotiating ability that the employees felt respected their commitment to the success of an organization, there would be no reason for unionization.

It's not all about money, however. In fact, it appears from research conducted for this book that better salaries appear about sixth from the top in the list of priorities for most employees. Among the issues of concern to employees are the following:

- Poor quality of immediate supervisors
- Arbitrary treatment by management
- Lack of promotional opportunities
- Poor working conditions
- Poor communication
- Job inequities
- Inadequate benefits

The simple fact is that employees, when faced with problems such as the foregoing, form a union to represent their needs instead of quitting their jobs.

Numerous studies have attempted to measure the effects of healthcare unionism on wages, employment, and, ultimately, costs.[5,6] Most research on wage levels has turned up significant reasons for organizing unions. For example, one study[7] that examined the salaries of professional employees found that, among the 15,000 registered nurses interviewed, the annual salary was an average of 4% to 7% higher for nurses who were represented by a bargaining agent than for those who were not. Research conducted for this book verifies this figure, as the values the authors determined nearly matched the 7% level. These findings, however, are not anything close to an accurate representation of the salary differential between unionized and nonunionized employees across the nation. In fact, unionization, which tends to be geographically specific, has had little effect on the wages received in the northeastern United States and in California, although unions in this areas have been extremely effective in organizing professional nurses. Nevertheless, when the total compensation of professional staff is considered nationwide, the union to nonunion differential is about 8% in favor of unionized employees.

Given the relatively small gains in wages and benefits realized through unionization, another question must be asked: Has unionization caused employers to reduce the number of employees under contract? The answer is that historically unionization has indeed caused a slight decrease in the actual number of employees retained under contract in specific organizations, but the reduction has tended to be relatively small. This lack of significant reduction in the size of the workforce was not caused by the employers' benevolence or liking for unions. Rather, it was due to the fact that, as wages were bargained upward by the unions, the increasing cost of doing business was simply passed on to the patients (or third-party payers) by the employers. Today, however, the tendency is for hospitals to respond to further salary demands by unions by reducing the total number of employees in the workforce. Because employers receive fixed fees for services under a payment system based on diagnosis-related groups, it is impossible to imagine that they are not managing their costs by reducing staff.

A fact of business is that a for-profit organization must meet its responsibility to return the investment of its stockholders. When faced with fixed levels of income and increased demands for better salaries and benefits, the healthcare organization is in a quandary. The past practice of simply passing on the expense to patients (and third-party payers) has hit a hard ceiling and has led to a major decrease in support from the communities that the healthcare organizations are licensed to serve. Although it is still realistic to believe that a certain amount of the cost of unionization is passed on to patients, a larger amount is made up by the retention of fewer higher-wage employees and by the increase in employee efficiency achieved by certain work rules demanded in union contracts (e.g., regulation of the length of work breaks). Ultimately, the costs and benefits of collective bargaining today probably balance each other out.

WHY PROFESSIONALS JOIN UNIONS

As noted earlier, there is much speculation about the question of why professionals join unions. Over the years, the reasons given for this have not been altruistic, because membership in unions continues to increase even in times of prosperity. This means that employees' desires for unionization become stronger as employees recognize the availability of money. In short, professionals unionize because they realize that they have greater negotiating power as a group than as individuals, and this power is critical as they attempt to get what they believe is their fair share of the organization's income. These same studies show a dramatic decrease in unionization in periods of recession and depression. This pattern has been seen since the very early days of American trade unions.

As was also noted earlier, however, money is not the only reason for unionization. Today's employees, especially well-educated and professional employees, expect more from the job than compensation. The number one reason cited to the authors by healthcare professionals for unionization was the poor quality of first-line supervision available to them. The problems caused by poorly trained and irresponsible nurse managers are the major factors contributing to employee unhappiness today.

The environment in a typical healthcare organization is not a great deal different from that in many other business organizations. It is a labor-intensive environment within a large, impersonal, capital-intensive organization. This combination creates a dependency relationship because the worker must rely on the organization for both a job and a reasonable wage. To control this relationship, the organization establishes a system of authority in the workplace that provides the employer with control over the employee's job security, tenure, and wages. The employee then counters this authority relationship through unionization. Organization by the workers therefore presents a credible threat to the employer, because it tends to equalize the economic relationship and rationalize the employment relationship.

Employers always view organization by workers as a threatening situation because collective rather than individual bargaining increases the strength of the workforce. A back-and-forth relationship is established as workers attempt to control the labor market by restricting the organization from purchasing labor without paying a predetermined minimum wage or asking the union to supply that labor, or both. The union wants to guarantee job security and income while negotiating rules and procedures that protect employees against arbitrary employer actions.

The truth is that most professionals join unions because of the low quality of the managers for whom they work. In fact, if the quality of first-line managers were to improve significantly, there would be far less reason for unionization of the professional workforce, and there would be far less strife between management and labor in the individual organization.

NURSES, UNIONS, AND PROFESSIONAL ASSOCIATIONS

Collective bargaining is not, by any stretch of the imagination, a new movement in the occupational field of nursing. In fact, nurses have been concerned with their economic and general welfare for more than a century. The first organization was established by nursing leaders in 1893. This primitive collective bargaining organization was called the American Society of Superintendents of Training Schools for Nurses, and its express purpose was to promote the general welfare of nurses through education.[8] This initial foray into the field was quickly followed by the establishment of the Nurses Associated Alumnae of the United States and Canada a mere 4 years later. This organization became an international association for all nurses rather than just those interested in education. In 1911, this association became the American Nurses Association (ANA).

In these early years, working conditions for nurses were extremely poor and salaries were even worse. The nation, in the middle of a general economic depression, was fighting for its very life. The healthcare industry was not left untouched by the Depression and dramatically reflected the poverty, poor working conditions, and lack of growth found in virtually every other sector of the American economy. In fact, the conditions under which the average nurse worked were miserable beyond belief, characterized by excessively long hours, absolutely no fringe benefits, and substandard wages even for that period. Just before the total collapse of the world economy in 1929, many nurses began to realize that if conditions were ever going to improve, they would have to band together and organize. In 1928, just a year before the collapse of Wall Street, the ANA, through its legislative policy, began to demand specific improvements in the general welfare, health, and education of nurses.

Throughout the war years, conditions for nurses steadily improved. In 1945 the executive director of the California Nurses Association, Shirley Titus, chaired a committee for the ANA to study employment conditions. As a direct result of the work of the Titus committee, the ANA adopted what was later called the Economic Security Program. This reform program, however, had virtually no success in improving conditions for the nursing professional. The program failed largely because the ANA adopted a no-strike policy shortly after its enactment. Although this no-strike policy was later rescinded, its effects, together with the passage in 1947 of the Taft-Hartley Act, which excluded nonprofit hospitals from any legal obligation to bargain with their employees, left nurses with virtually no power to bring about change in their working conditions or salaries. Under these circumstances, the nursing profession was left with few options except work stoppages, mass resignations, and informational picketing. None of these activities, however, was very effective in improving the day-to-day plight of the nurse.

The amendments to the Taft-Hartley Act passed in 1974 and later referred to as the Nonprofit Health Care Amendments (Public Law 93-360) allowed nurses to take legal actions to ensure that collective bargaining included the conditions of employment. These amendments resulted in the following changes:

- Unions representing healthcare interests are required to provide a 10-day prestrike notice.
- Strikes and lockouts are not permitted during the notice period.
- Unions must provide advance notice in writing of the intent to modify contracts and to terminate contracts. Notice must be given to employers, federal mediation services, and a recognized conciliation service.
- A board of inquiry was established to resolve disputes.

- Employees are allowed to be exempt from mandatory financial support and membership in a union on bona fide religious grounds.
- Mediation procedures must provide for the involvement of federal mediators and recognized conciliation service organizations.

The amendments largely gave the NLRB the right to determine the composition and size of bargaining units; however, all decisions made by the NLRB are now subject to review by the 12 U.S. circuit courts of appeals (each of the 12 federal judicial districts has a single court of appeals).

In the decades following the passage of these amendments, many state nurses associations qualified themselves as legal bargaining agents for nurses. In addition, in 1982, the ANA modified its organization to become a federation of state nurses associations. This change provided individual states with greater and more direct representation for their member nurses. Over the last 30 years, a myriad of union organizations, including some exceptional outside unions such as the teamsters union, the meat packers union, and the American Federation of Teachers, have sought permission to organize nurses in the workplace. In 1980, Barbara Nichols, then ANA president, stated that the ANA "currently represents more registered nurses for collective bargaining purposes than all the other labor organizations combined."[9]

The dramatic changes in the healthcare environment, which have been driven largely by profit and insurance considerations, have created a situation in which collective bargaining looks increasingly attractive to nurses. These changes have severely restricted average nurses from practicing their craft as they believe it should be practiced and from influencing their working conditions. Today, there is a very real belief that collective bargaining can be a viable means of improving salaries, personnel policies, and benefits.

Almost from the beginning, the participation of state nursing associations as bargaining agents has created a wide division in the ranks of nursing. Some nurses believe that a professional organization should not serve as a labor organization. These nurses feel that such an arrangement represents a conflict of interest with regard to professional purposes and standards. Others, however, believe that there is no conflict and that the promotion of nurses' economic security and general welfare is a major responsibility of the organization. Even as the new millennium advances, this conflict continues to be a significant source of division among ANA members.

A major difficulty with the representation of nurses by state nurses associations, and one that will sooner or later be tested through legal action, is the conflict that is created by allowing nurses serving in supervisory positions to have membership in the association. How, it is argued, can supervising nurses (including both nurse managers and supervisors) whose job requires them to administer union contracts belong to the same organization that serves as the bargaining agent for nurses? The almost universal belief among those who oppose representation by state nurses associations is that this situation creates at best divided loyalty and at worst conflict of interest.

Those who support the role of state nurses associations as collective bargaining agents counter that collective bargaining is only one responsibility of the organization and that no legitimate reason exists for preventing supervisory personnel from enjoying the benefits of membership. These proponents emphatically believe that nurses in administrative positions *can* belong to the same organization that represents the profession in general. Opponents, of course, argue otherwise. Some administrative nurses have taken the question to heart and resigned from their professional associations, either because they disapprove of the associations' acting as bargaining agents or because of the effect the associations' decisions have on them as administrators.

Legal action has been taken against specific state nurses associations charging them with violating federal labor laws because association board members have held hospital administrative positions. Nevertheless, the NLRB has consistently ruled that associations are *not* violating labor law if board members are not actively participating in labor relation activities. When board members have been found to be so engaged, however, and in fact do control the finances of an organization or give local units collective bargaining advice, federal appeals courts have ruled that the associations *are* in violation.[10] Furthermore, where it has been proved that a definite conflict of interest exists, the NLRB has moved to revoke the specific nursing association's certification as sole bargaining agent.[11] These dual governmental and professional association requirements create a quandary for state nurses associations, because following the NLRB stipulations may cause them to be in violation of ANA membership rules if their bylaws are changed to exclude nurses in administrative positions from holding office in the organization.

HOW TO IDENTIFY THE BEGINNINGS OF ORGANIZATION

How do nurse managers detect the beginnings of union organization in their units or in the healthcare organization? What can they do about it?

The second question is easier to answer than the first, and the answer is that nurse managers cannot restrict the organization efforts of a union unless those efforts put organizers into contact with patients. Managers may prohibit union organizing activities on the nursing floor where patients are present, but they cannot demand that their staff nurses not attend a union organizing event after hours.

Nurse managers should suspect that union organizing activities are occurring or that the staff are in the organizing phase of unionization if they can answer yes to any of the following 10 questions:

1. Have union authorization cards or pamphlets been found on the organization's premises?
2. Are employees conducting or attending union-sponsored meetings outside of the organization?
3. Are clandestine meetings being held at the homes of staff nurses?
4. Has there been a sharp increase in the number of peer-level social gatherings?
5. Are strangers and former employees repeatedly mingling with employees outside of the organization as the employees come to and from work?
6. Has there been an increase in the number of incidents in which a gathering of employees stop their conversation and walk away when a supervisor approaches or the employees stop talking when managers are within earshot?
7. Has the number of complaints about salary or employment conditions been increasing?
8. Has the number of complaints about scheduling, staffing, content or frequency of inservice training programs, or unclear or overlapping job classifications been rising?
9. Has the rate of turnover changed?
10. Are there other factors that seem to be separating the workers from the administrators?

THE NURSE MANAGER'S ROLE

Nurse managers working in a healthcare organization in which the nurses are covered by a union contract participate actively in administering the contract in a variety of ways, depending on what exactly is contained in the contract. For example, a union contract will almost always specify broad items such as salaries, work hours, and working conditions, but it may also include indirectly related items such as deduction of dues from paychecks and grievance procedures. Although the human resources office will administer most provisions of the union contract, nurse managers will invariably assist in the administration of the grievance process. In addition to issues relating to discipline, nurse managers' responsibilities usually will entail the first and second steps of the grievance procedure.

Grievances

Grievances are complaints filed by union members with the union that report alleged violations of the contract. They are usually classified as follows:

Misunderstanding: The violation occurred because of ignorance or a simple mistake with no prejudice intended. The action leading to this type of grievance is usually a result of (a) the circumstances surrounding the grievance, (b) a lack of familiarity with the contract, or (c) an inadequate labor agreement. In almost every instance, the person filing the grievance is motivated by self-interest in that he or she is acting to protect a perceived contractual right. This type of grievance is common and almost inevitable—even when a mature and efficient labor-management team administers the contract.

Intentional contract violation: A portion or portions of the union employment contract was deliberately violated. Violations of this sort usually are caused by an effort to capitalize on ambiguous contract language or historical practice.

Symptomatic problem outside the scope of the labor agreement: The action taken, by itself, was not a direct violation of the contract, but the results of the action caused one. This form of violation has historically proven to be the most difficult to identify and prevent. In almost every instance, however, the employee filing this type of grievance is simply trying express dissatisfaction or frustration. Generally, these grievances occur because of (a) a personal problem between the individual filing the grievance and something or somebody in the organization, (b) union politics, or (c) unfavorable contract language. Most of these grievances are highly emotional because they grow out of dissatisfaction.

All grievance procedures are negotiated by collective bargaining and are clearly described in the labor agreement. In most cases, the procedures to be used involve a series of progressive steps and time limits for submission and resolution of grievances.

The Grievance Process

The steps described here are representative of the procedures that might be used to resolve a grievance. Nurse managers must understand that the specific steps used in a given organization and for specific types of employees may differ. Managers must also be aware of the contractual requirements that cover each classification of worker they supervise and conduct themselves accordingly.

Probably the only part of the grievance process that is universal is the very first element, which is the requirement that the aggrieved employee talk informally with his or her immediate supervisor as soon as possible after the incident in question occurs. The union worker has the right to have a representative of the bargaining agency present during this informal discussion.

The following four steps are usually preceded by informal discussion, but, as noted earlier, these steps may or may not occur depending on the provisions of the union contract:

Step 1—Written request: If the grievance cannot be resolved during the informal discussion, a written request to move to the next step must be presented to the aggrieved employee's immediate supervisor within a specified number of days (usually 10 workdays). The supervisor is usually mandated to provide a written response to this request within a specified number of days (usually no more than 5 working days). If the response generates any further request for informal discussion, the employee, his or her supervisor, and the contract agent (union) must be present at this meeting.

Step 2—Written appeal: If the aggrieved employee deems the written response provided by the immediate supervisor unsatisfactory, he or she may submit a written appeal to the next level of management requesting a meeting of all parties within a specified period of time (usually 10 working days). This meeting can include a variety of different people, but the employee, a union representative, the organizational grievance chairperson (if one is appointed), and the manager to whom the appeal was addressed must be present. The meeting does not have to include the immediate supervisor. Once again, a written response must be generated within a specified period of time.

! CRITICAL POINT

In most bargaining units, the positions of representative agent and grievance chairperson are filled by different people. The grievance chairperson is usually an officer in the bargaining unit.

Step 3—Formal meeting: If the written response from senior management does not resolve the issue, a formal meeting is called that includes the senior manager, the aggrieved employee, the union representative, and the organization's director of personnel. The purpose of the meeting is to talk through the grievance with the intent of establishing agreement and resolving the grievance. The normal response periods are applied in this step as they were in steps 1 and 2.

Step 4—Final arbitration: The final step is usually some form of mandatory arbitration. This process is normally not invoked unless the issue is very serious or no solution can be reached through lesser means. Arbitration meetings may include all of the parties to the grievance, including the immediate supervisor, and a neutral third party will always be present. The contract will require submission of the grievance to arbitration within a specified time after step 3 is completed.

! *CRITICAL POINT*

In specifying the grievance procedure, contracts usually include a statement in each mandated resolution step stating that if the contractual time limits are not observed by one party, the grievance may be considered resolved in favor of the other party and further action will not be allowed. In addition, each individual contract specifies how an arbitrator is to be selected.

STRATEGIES TO RESOLVE GRIEVANCES

The suggestions provided in the following sections can be applied in nearly every contractual situation to assist in the resolution of grievances.

Observe Common Courtesies and Demonstrate Respect. The objective of any grievance procedure is to achieve resolution, not to conquer or achieve for oneself. Professional nurse managers understand that they must return to work with the aggrieved employee after the grievance is resolved; therefore, they make a point of treating all parties to the grievance with courtesy and respect.

Don't Use Position to Intimidate. It is never a good management practice to threaten or deceive a member of the staff; professional nurse managers know this axiom of management and seldom try to do so. This is not an uncommon tactic, however—and this is a sad commentary on the level of professionalism shown by the typical nurse manager. In fact, there are nurse managers who employ these unsavory tactics as general rules of management. Any employee intent on pursuing a grievance through to resolution will almost always uncover such a ruse, and if this happens, the manager using it will pay a significant price for the effort.

Share Information. The manager should not withhold information that might have a bearing on the grievance. Not only is willful withholding of pertinent information totally unprofessional, it may also be grounds for job termination. The basic rule is to bargain in good faith. Nurse managers represent the organization, and their actions reflect on themselves, their supervisors, and the administration as a whole. Many senior members of management will not tolerate this form of behavior in a subordinate manager—and none should.

Demonstrate Unity. Nurse managers must never openly demonstrate their personal feelings or opinions regarding internal disagreements or disputes among management. As members of the management team, they must understand the importance of presenting a unified position. It is absolutely certain that the bargaining unit will do so.

Never Willfully Delay the Proceedings. Speed and attention are essential. In fact, almost every union contract insists upon it. Nurse managers who use delaying tactics only exacerbate the emotional aspects of the grievance procedure. Keep in mind that managers must work with the aggrieved party after the grievance has been resolved. If they delay the proceedings, they may further impair that working relationship. On the other hand, no manager should rush to respond. Nurse managers should take the time necessary to research the issue and respond effectively. They should make sure that the organization is being properly represented by considering all of the facts.

Don't Focus on Fixing Blame. Union-management relations are adversarial. Nurse managers must recognize this. If managers make mistakes, they can expect those on the other side to take full advantage of them—that is their job. Managers should look at such occurrences as learning experiences; they should learn from the exposure and not repeat their mistakes a second time. There is a big difference between making a mistake out of ignorance and failing to learn from previous experience. Ignorance, by definition, is a temporary condition remedied by knowledge. Mistakes made after objective lessons have been learned are a demonstration not of ignorance but of idiocy, which is usually a permanent failing.

Remain Objective. Managers should keep control of their feelings and not allow themselves to become emotionally involved. Keeping your perspective about the issue, the process, and even the outcome will encourage a positive result for all parties. Remember, after the grievance process is over, the manager must return to work with the employee , and both will need to be in a fame of mind that promotes acceptance of, and respect for, each other.

Anticipate Positions and Responses. There is an old saying that a true professional never asks a question to which he or she doesn't already have an answer. The same holds true for involvement in a grievance procedure. The truly professional nurse manager will anticipate the other party's position and carefully evaluate it before responding to a grievance. In fact, the implementation of decisions or the filing of grievances is almost always a negotiation process requiring a well-planned strategy.

Don't Be Limited. Managers should make sure that they support their positions completely. Grievance proceedings are not the time to hold back. Nurse managers must represent the position of the organization with the utmost skill, and that always means using all of the resources available. One of these resources, and possibly the most effective, is guidance from managers higher up in the chain of authority. There is seldom a "new" problem. Senior managers are generally experienced professionals who have seen a good many grievances during their working histories. They will always have advice and can be an excellent source of constructive criticism. When seeking the advice of seniors, however, nurse managers should remain aware of the fact that not all of them are going to be capable people. One should never solicit the advice of a fool.

Be Available. Refusing to meet with the aggrieved employee or his or her representatives is just not good management. To begin with, how can anyone represent the best interests of the organization if he or she hides from this responsibility? Nurse managers should never refuse to meet with the aggrieved employee or his or her representative(s). The right to be heard and to be represented is a fundamental advantage of being affiliated with a collective bargaining unit, and when union representatives are shunned, any future action they undertake usually assumes the cast of zealotry.

Remember That the Bargaining Unit Representative Is Not a God. Although the union representative occupies a unique position, he or she is never immune from reprimand or discipline. These people are employees of the same organization as the nurse manager, and many may be far less capable, educated, or experienced. At all times, these people are responsible for their conduct. In fact, when they are not actively playing their union roles, they are just as bound by the rules and regulations of the institution as is the nurse manager. When the parties to the grievance return to the unit, after the grievance is completed or during the procedures, the nurse manager has every right to a full day's work and an acceptable level of performance. In the process of handling grievances, however, the representative (agent) is not to be considered an employee and most certainly should not be viewed as a subordinate. He or she must be given the respect accorded to any outside representative or advocate of the employee who filed the grievance. The key here is to be respectful, professional, and wary.

Don't Lose Control. Grievance resolution can, by nature, become extremely heated. It is very difficult to maintain composure when being personally attacked, which sadly is the tactic taken by many aggrieved employees. When emotions start to run away, the nurse manager should stop the proceedings, take a break, or reschedule, but keep his or her cool. The nurse manager should not let the emotional outburst create a hole the manager can't dig out of. Neither party to a grievance has to tolerate personal abuse. The manager should never let the proceedings get to that point. The meeting should be adjourned and rescheduled at a time when discussion can continue on a more objective level.

Understand That Being Right Doesn't Eliminate Others' Right to Appeal. Regardless of the nurse manager's status, he or she is not obligated to accept the validity of the grievance. In many cases, nurse managers, when first confronted with a grievance, deny its allegations based on nothing more than a feeling that none of the cited violations has occurred. But no matter what position the nurse manager takes or how correct he or she might be, the aggrieved employee still has the right to pursue the grievance and move on to the next step in the procedure.

Don't Worry About What Is Fair. Emotional claims that something is not fair have no bearing on the employee's grievance and are not something to which the nurse manager needs to respond. What is "fair" is for the contract to determine. If necessary, a neutral third party can be engaged to determine fairness by interpreting the contract. A cardinal rule of management is that what one person considers fair may be totally unfair in the eyes of another. Fairness is an arbitrary concept and therefore not part of management. Instead, intelligent nurse managers rely on objectivity and compliance with standards.

Be Open Minded and Accepting. Nurse managers should make sure not to close off their minds to other opinions. In fact, it is the hallmark of excellence to be prepared to make reasonable compromises and accept alternative solutions within the framework of the contract, no matter who might originate them.

Understand the Issue. Nurse managers should be sure to understand the real issue. Truly professional nurse managers make it their business to be aware of both the strengths and weaknesses of the grievance—from both points of view.

Think Toward the Future. Solutions to a grievance may have wide-reaching ramifications. Before the nurse manager agrees to anything, he or she should think through the compromise completely from a variety of different viewpoints and then have it analyzed by another member of management. The nurse manager should not commit to something that can alter the position of the company or infringe on another part of the contract. It is a fact that solutions are often the beginning of change; therefore, the professional nurse manager always thinks ahead.

Don't Settle for a Quick Fix. Band-Aids don't stop arterial bleeding and they don't settle grievances or solve problems. Taking the easy solution is never fixing the problem. Accepting a quick fix may go completely against the principles of sound judgment and flexibility that are absolutely necessary for effective grievance resolution.

Know When to Say No. Nurse managers must understand just how far they can go to resolve a grievance; that is, where exactly their limits of authority lie. Professional managers are never afraid to say that something is beyond their ability to control. They know that this is a fundamental part of management and rarely exceed their bottom line in searching for a compromise.

Observe Established Time Requirements. Time limits are established contractually. If the nurse manager does not comply, the loser will be the organization. Managers should make sure that they do not lose future bargaining ability by ignoring an established deadline. It is far better to pass the baton on to the next level than to lose one's rights by failing to comply in a timely manner.

Be Careful. Intelligent nurse managers are always aware that a grievance can set off a series of chain reactions that can result in some truly bizarre solutions. Managers should mitigate this risk as much as possible by being extremely careful how they respond to anything in writing.

Make Sure Communication Is Understood. Managers should not make the mistake of assuming that just because they make a statement their audience understands an issue the same way they do. Effective communication is a truly fine art, and good nurse managers understand that when dealing with something as important as a grievance, sharing knowledge in a clear, concise manner is very important. Communication, especially in a difficult situation, can easily be tainted by one's temperament so that the message received is even more likely to be misconstrued. Managers must never assume that they or their messages are understood. Instead, they should follow up with well-developed and sensitive questions that will help them know that their messages have been properly interpreted.

Remain Humble. Although it may be human nature to let one's pride in a victory swell one's ego just a little, winning in a grievance is only complete if both parties return to work satisfied that they have come away with something. Gloating over a win, although it may be a typical human failing, is just that—a failing. The objective of management is to produce a win-win situation in everything that is done. If nurse managers keep their attitude positive and their feelings humble, they will truly end up winners.

Investigate the Facts Thoroughly. A grievance is a delicate situation, and one that is best handled in an objective and informed manner. The best way to deal with emotion is to remain calm and keep to the facts. This takes a bit of investigation on the nurse manager's part—dispassionate investigation. The nurse manager should keep his or her mind on the facts and not succumb to the emotional aspects of a grievance. The manager should get all the facts and information, witnesses' testimony, and documentation and study them well, then go into the arbitration well armed with accurate information. This will help the manager overcome the emotions that surround the grievance better than any other single item in his or her favor. During the investigation, the manager should not forget to look for similar previous occurrences or circumstances and ascertain their outcomes.

THE GRIEVANCE HEARING

Nurse managers should keep in mind that although the grievance hearing is actually conducted in an informal manner, it is anything but an informal situation. All nurse managers must take these circumstances extremely seriously. Managers should approach a hearing in a positive yet cautious manner and keep their opinions and personal feelings to themselves. Objectivity is the goal of management, and that can be achieved only by not taking things personally. Managers must keep their heads and remember the hints provided in the following sections.

Keep the Meeting Low Key. The nurse manager should start by putting the aggrieved party at ease. The nurse manager must be a model of discretion and professionalism during the meeting. Good management skills and good personal manners, such as not interrupting or openly disagreeing with the aggrieved party, should always prevail. Instead, the nurse manager should let the employee state his or her opinion and position freely. The manager should watch his or her body language; shaking one's head can be just as aggravating as open disagreement.

Listen Aggressively. The nurse manager should listen dispassionately. If the manager lets his or her emotions start to take over, the manager will not hear what is being said. Instead, the manager should ask the aggrieved party's permission to take notes and then do so. Eye contact should be maintained, and the manager should remain active in the discussion by nodding his or her head occasionally. Notes should remain fixed on the statements being made; doodling is to be avoided. The manager should not read into what is being said; rather, thoughts should be kept on the subject at hand.

Maintain Composure. One of the cardinal rules of management is never to lose control of oneself. In the grievance meeting, the manager is very likely to hear comments that are personal and offensive, but the manager must not respond in a like manner. Instead, the manager must discuss the problem with the aggrieved party calmly and with an open mind. The manager should never let himself or herself get into an argument and should never deliberately antagonize the employee. The best sessions are those that the nurse manager views as a negotiation, not an opportunity to win. Winning is not important; returning the employee to work in a positive and constructive frame of mind is. Although nurse managers must—we repeat, *must*—represent management's position positively and aggressively, that does not mean that managers must do so at the expense of the employee or themselves. They should keep themselves under control at all times. Things said in anger often come back to hurt in the most damaging ways. Consider the following story:

> I once worked with a nurse manager who was extremely aggressive in her pursuit of what she felt was right and wrong in her unit. Although she was an extremely competent professional with years of nursing experience, looking back, Mrs. Hudson was anything but a good manager. She often managed her unit through the use of intimidation and subjectivity and was very prone to playing favorites among the staff. Senior management tolerated her behavior because we felt that her clinical skills made up for her management inadequacies and we did not want to risk losing those qualities by removing her from a management position. That was the worst mistake I have ever made as a nursing director.
>
> One day, Mrs. Hudson hired an extremely capable and very experienced staff nurse and assigned her as a supervisor in the unit. The supervisor (we'll call her Jane) was a woman who spoke her mind and often came into conflict with Mrs. Hudson's management style. During one of these disagreements, Jane filed a grievance that was supported by the nurses union.
>
> During the initial grievance meeting, Mrs. Hudson openly criticized Jane and made threats regarding future employment if she did not drop her claim. When Jane asked her why she was so hostile, Mrs. Hudson yelled, "Because I don't like you and never have." The union representative who had come with Jane to the meeting stopped the conversation immediately. Further discussions between management and the union broke down.
>
> Feeling that she had been personally injured, Jane quit and filed suit against Mrs. Hudson and the

hospital. The ensuing court action was settled by terminating Mrs. Hudson's employment and paying Jane $1.8 million in damages.

Deal with the Facts. The nurse manager should make sure that the aggrieved party stays with the facts of the issue, and as the employee speaks, should make notes regarding the employee's side of the story. This is best done by asking dispassionate, logical, open-ended questions that help to clarify unclear or dubious points. Although the nurse manager need not question what is said or take exception to it, it is important to distinguish between fact and opinion.

Never Assume That You Are Correct. The nurse manager's position as part of management in no way guarantees that he or she is right. The nurse manager's job is to consider the facts surrounding the issue, and this cannot be done properly if the manager does not carefully consider the aggrieved employee's viewpoint. The manager should never assume that the employee is wrong. The nurse manager's job is to look for solutions, not to form opinions of right or wrong. Objectivity is the key to solving most grievances. The manager should be positive, be upbeat, be thorough, and remain neutral.

Do Not Act as the Judge. Different people can look at the same situation and come away with different opinions. A nurse manager's job is to investigate the allegations thoroughly, look at them objectively, and carefully weigh any decision. The manager must never make snap decisions. The manager should think things through, talk with others that the manager respects and that are in a position to assist, and avoid opinionated judgments at all times. The manager must remain objective and remember that the grievance procedure has specified time limits, for the benefit of management as well as the employee. These time limits should be used and time taken to prepare a decision. The manager should avoid admitting mistakes, because such an admission may weaken management's position in later settlements, even if no mistake was actually made.

Make a Fair Decision. After the nurse manager has carefully weighed the facts and has made sure that he or she is not reacting to the situation but instead is being objective and analytical, and when it is within the manager's jurisdiction, the manager should make the correct decision. It is recommended that a decision never be made without consulting another manager, preferably a more senior and experienced one. Once the decision has been made, however, it should be communicated to the aggrieved party promptly and within the specified time frame. Delaying in hope that the situation will improve or go away is not professional and is most often foolhardy.

Decisions, especially ones that may put a nurse manager in a negative light, are often difficult to make. Although consultation with senior management is always encouraged, if the decision is within the manager's area of responsibility and the manager has considered the facts properly, then the manager should make the decision. Management is a tough job; making unpopular decisions is the toughest single part of that tough job—but it is also the most critical.

Indecision is something that can run through a performance team and kill its willingness to perform. Nurse managers should never allow themselves to be indecisive.

SUMMARY

- The 1974 healthcare amendments to the Wagner Act forced most healthcare organizations into compliance with U.S. labor law. Publicly owned hospitals administered by private firms are also included.
- Many unions and state nursing associations represent nurses' interests by serving as collective bargaining agents under federal labor law.
- The Wagner Act defines the rights of individuals in collective bargaining, outlines unfair labor practices of unions and organizations, establishes the NLRB, and provides for remedies.
- The process of collective bargaining is different in health care than in other fields of endeavor to ensure that patients are not harmed. Most bargaining units are structured along occupational lines.
- The effects of unionization on healthcare costs have been negligible. There is little research showing effects on nurses and nursing practice.
- Nursing unions often act like craft unions in that state nurses associations frequently serve as the direct representatives for nurses in collective bargaining. This sometimes creates concern, because many feel that this duality of purpose creates a conflict of interest between labor and management.
- The nurse manager's major responsibility in collective bargaining is to represent the interests of management and administer the contract.

FINAL THOUGHTS

Nurse managers should evaluate their management skills and take continuing education courses to improve them. Motivational techniques are particularly important for those who direct the work of others, because they must work through their subordinates to accomplish the mission they are assigned. They must be able to listen carefully to staff concerns and represent the staff's wishes to senior management with objectivity. Labor relations is one of the most important areas about which a professional nurse manager must be knowledgeable.

The nurse manager should not serve as the organization's chief negotiator in collective bargaining sessions. That role should be left up to the organization's legal representation. Once the contract has been finalized, however, the nurse manager must become informed of its content and keep a copy within easy reach.

THE NURSE MANAGER SPEAKS

There are advantages and disadvantages to collective bargaining. The process tends to equalize the power between administrators and staff because the staff gains power through organization. If collective bargaining is handled properly, the professionalism of both management and staff can be enhanced through the process, as follows:

- Nurses gain control of their practice.
- Grievance procedures become viable and important methods of promoting teamwork.
- Systematic and equitable divisions of labor can be established.
- The quality of service to the patient can be enhanced.
- Economic security can be improved.

If, however, the situation is allowed to become adversarial, long-term damage can be done. The following are a few examples of such harmful effects:

- Unionization can come to be considered unprofessional.
- Unions can interfere with the management of the organization.
- Leadership for unions may become difficult to obtain.
- Nurses may lose their objectivity and view their work as a job instead of a career.

Everyone is best served when both management and union conduct themselves as professionals—not as people on a mission.

REFERENCES

1. Dilts DA, Deitsch CR, Rassuli A: *Labor relations law in state and local government*, New York, 1992, Quorum Books.
2. Evans M: Laboring for union nurses. With CAN's first win outside California competition is heating up to organize registered nurse: some say that's good for providers, *Modern Health Care* 23(21):6-7, 1, 2005.
3. Wagner Act, 198, U.S.C. 238 (1935), codified as amended at 29 U.S.C. §§ 151-169 (2000).
4. Allen RE, Keavenly TJ: *Contemporary labor relations*, Reading, Mass, 1983, Addison-Wesley. (This source provides excellent information for a discussion of good-faith bargaining and labor law issues.)

5. Fossum JA: *Labor relations,* ed 4, Dallas, 2002, Business Publishers.

6. Davey BW, Bognanno MF, Estenson DL: *Contemporary collective bargaining,* ed 6, Englewood Cliffs, NJ, 2001, Prentice Hall.

7. Link CR, Landon JH: Monopoly and union power in the market for nurses, *South Econ J* 41(4):644, 1975.

8. Miller RU: Collective bargaining: a nurse dilemma, *AORN J* 31(7):1195, 1980.

9. Nichols B: Belonging to your professional organization: a commitment to personal growth and professional development, *Imprint* 27(4):18, 1980.

10. Lorenz FJ: Nursing administration and undivided loyalty, *Nurs Adm Q* 6(2):67, 1982.

11. NLRB v. North Shore University Hospital, 724 F.2nd, 269 (2nd Cir. 1983), 259 NLRB 852.

SUGGESTED READINGS

Allen RE, Keavenly TJ: *Contemporary labor relations,* ed 4, Reading, Mass, 1997, Addison-Wesley.

Autry JA, Mitchell S: *Real power: business lessons from the Tao te ching,* New York, 1998, Riverhead Books.

Betts VT: Nursing agenda for healthcare reform: policy, politics and power through professional leadership, *Nurs Adm Q* 20(3):1, 1996.

Cummings S: Attila the Hun versus the hen: gender socialization of the American nurse, *Nurs Adm Q* 19(2):19, 1995.

Ellis JR, Hartley CL: *Managing and coordinating nursing care,* Philadelphia, 1995, Lippincott.

Huber D: *Leadership and nursing care management,* ed 3, St Louis, 2005, Mosby.

Hunt JW: *Employer's guide to labor relations,* ed 11, Washington, DC, 1999, Bureau of National Affairs.

Miller RU: *The impact of collective bargaining on hospitals,* ed 4, New York, 1991, Praeger.

Pfeffer J: *Managing with power,* Cambridge, Mass, 1992, Harvard Business School Press.

Tappen RM: *Nursing leadership and management: concepts and practices,* Philadelphia, 1995, FA Davis.

Vestal KW: *Nursing management: concepts and issues,* Philadelphia, 1995, Lippincott.

Whetten DA, Caeron KS: *Developing management skills,* Reading, Mass, 1998, Addison-Wesley.

Wywialowski EF: *Managing client care,* ed 3, St Louis, 2004, Mosby.

Yoder-Wise PS: *Leading and managing in nursing,* ed 3, St Louis, 2003, Mosby.

Motivating the Professional Staff

OUTLINE

LEARNING SYNOPSIS

Upon successful completion of this chapter, readers will possess a fundamental understanding of how motivation is created in the nursing unit, what processes might be used to increase motivation, and how work might be designed to obtain the maximum performance from employees.

OBJECTIVES

1. Identify factors that motivate individual performers
2. Describe different content theories of motivation
3. Describe different process theories of motivation
4. Identify methods and processes that can potentially be used to increase staff motivation

The word *motivation* is derived from the Latin *movere,* meaning "to move." All human behavior is motivated by something, and very few behaviors in what are considered "normal" human beings are completely random. Some human behaviors are genetically determined and therefore arise because of instinctive processes, but the vast majority occur through the establishment of a system of goals and the satisfactory attainment of these goals. Generally, most people do what they do for specific reasons and to obtain desired results. The reasons may not always appear to be logical or rational, but most often they are systematic or predictable. It is this latter characteristic that makes the study of human motivation both possible and practical, particularly from an organizational point of view. Although the concepts discussed in this chapter are relevant to human behavior in general, the chapter focuses primarily on how they apply to the healthcare industry and, in particular, to the motivational problems frequently encountered by nurse managers as they direct the efforts of their staffs.

IS IT NECESSARY TO PROVIDE MOTIVATION?

Proper motivation is unquestionably an important aspect of performance in the healthcare environment. The healthcare institution, like any other business organization, requires people who can function effectively if it is to provide adequate service (in this case, patient care) to its customers. This fact implies that, as an organization, the healthcare institution must both motivate qualified personnel to seek employment in the institution and then supply enough motivation to retain them on the job. Continuous personnel turnover is one of the most severe challenges facing any business today. It means higher-than-normal training costs, lower overall performance, inefficiency, and continual disruption to normal staff functions. In addition, the process of continual recruiting is expensive in terms of time, money, and other assets. To keep turnover under control, it is imperative that once employees are on the job, proper motivation be supplied by their managers so that employees become and remain capable of performing work of the required quantity and quality.

Managers must develop an understanding of motivational processes not only so they can motivate employees to meet daily performance requirements, however, but also so they will have a better awareness of the effects of other factors such as leadership, job design, and incentive systems on overall employee performance and satisfaction. Almost all other leadership qualities are developed to enhance the ability to influence employee motivation, on both an individual and a group level. The primary concern of managers is

how to use motivational tools most effectively to ensure good performance.

WHAT MOTIVATES THE INDIVIDUAL PERFORMER?

Most theories of motivation share the following three concerns:

1. What engages and stimulates human behavior
2. How to direct specific behaviors toward the accomplishment of some preestablished objective
3. What methods can sustain the desired behavior over a specified period of time

In a variety of ways, all of the motivation theories considered in this chapter attempt to address these fundamental points. The degree of success or failure of any of these views of motivation depends on three things:

1. The ability to define motivation adequately
2. The ability to forecast with a certain amount of accuracy how people will react to specific stimuli
3. The ability to provide practical ways of influencing people to accomplish organizational objectives

The major theories of motivation have some fundamental differences that allow them to be classified into at least the following two different groups:

1. *Content theories:* those theories that emphasize individual needs or the rewards that may satisfy those needs
2. *Process theories:* those theories that emphasize how the motivation process works so that an individual's efforts can be directed into performance

CONTENT THEORIES OF MOTIVATION

Content theories of motivation traditionally have been divided into (1) *instinct* theories and (2) *need* theories.

Instinct Theories

Instinct theories are much older than need theories and date back to the mid-1890s. According to these theories, "instincts" or natural actions can be separated into different categories such as the following:

- Purposeful and goal-directed action
- Blind, mechanical action

Regardless of exactly how instincts were viewed, all researchers of the time characterized instincts as inherited or innate tendencies that predisposed individuals to behave in specific ways. One version of the instinct theory originated with Dr. Sigmund Freud, who noted that individuals are not always consciously aware of their desires and needs. This fundamental belief formed the basis for part of his treatment, and

Freud tended to focus on the notion of unconscious motivation when discussing instinct.[1]

As long ago as the early 1920s, however, instinct theories came under increasing criticism on a variety of different grounds. The difficulties raised included the following:

Large number of instincts: By the mid-1920s, the list of instincts had swelled to include well over 6,000 individually identified tendencies, which made it extremely difficult to determine specific reasons for a particular behavior by invoking one or a small combination of instincts.

Uncertain relationship to behavior: Although every individual was assumed to have a complete set of instincts, continuing research made the medical community ever more aware that an increasingly large proportion of instincts did not seem to be strongly related to specific behaviors.

Difficulty of distinguishing between instinctive and learned behavior: As research advanced, many psychologists began to question whether Freud's unconscious motives were really instincts or were, in fact, learned behaviors. This criticism led, in part, to the development of a second category of content theories focusing on the concept of learned needs.

Need Theories

Although there are a large number of need theories, the most popular are those developed by Abraham Maslow,[2] Clayton Alderfer,[3] and Frederick Herzberg.[4]

NEED HIERARCHY THEORY

Maslow attempted to bring a high degree of order to the concept of needs by categorizing all needs into five broad groups and organizing these groups into a hierarchy. This hierarchical organization reflects Maslow's view that the needs he identified operate in a specific order. The lowest-level needs primarily control an individual's behavior until these needs are satisfied; then needs at the next highest level energize and direct behavior until they are satisfied; and so on up the hierarchy.

Fig. 25-1 and the following list present the five levels of needs identified by Maslow, from lowest to highest[2,5]:

1. *Physiologic needs:* These are the most fundamental of all human needs and include such things as the need for food, water, and shelter.
2. *Safety needs:* After the fundamental necessities are met, humans set out to satisfy the need for personal safety, such as bodily safety.
3. *Social needs:* Sometimes referred to as *belongingness* needs, this level of need includes such things as the need for friendship, affection, and love.

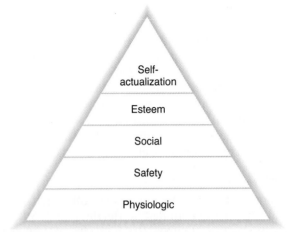

Fig. 25-1 ■ Maslow's hierarchy of needs. (Data from Maslow AH: A theory of human motivation, *Psychol Rev* 50:370, 1943.)

4. *Esteem needs:* This level of need involves the striving for things such as recognition, appreciation, and self-respect.
5. *Self-actualization needs:* This level of need includes the desire to develop one's potential.

Maslow's need theory, although not new, is still frequently used in the nursing profession to provide a fundamental understanding of human behavior. Nurses are instructed to view the patient's needs in this hierarchical order and to direct nursing care toward meeting the more critical lower-level needs before providing assistance to the patient in meeting the more lofty ones. Over time, however, Maslow's theory, although it provides a basic and totally acceptable explanation of human needs, has proven to be less useful in management, in which the focus is on predicting behavior and directing appropriate change.

EXISTENCE-RELATEDNESS GROWTH THEORY

Over the years, Maslow's hierarchical theory of motivation has been modified by a variety of researchers, one of whom was Alderfer. In his existence-relatedness growth (ERG) theory, Alderfer suggested that there are three, rather than five, need levels, as follows:

1. *Existence needs:* This level includes Maslow's physiologic and safety needs.
2. *Relatedness needs:* These include Maslow's safety and social needs.
3. *Growth needs:* These include Maslow's needs for self-esteem and self-actualization.

Alderfer's ERG theory is similar to Maslow's in that it assumes that the desire to satisfy the needs of a given level is not activated until all of the needs at the levels below it have been met. However, ERG theory suggests that if an individual becomes frustrated in trying to solve higher-level needs, a regression to and reemphasis on the needs of the next lowest level in the hierarchy can occur.[3,6]

Alderfer's model also suggests that more than one level of need may be operating at any given time. This makes it somewhat less rigid than Maslow's inflexible hierarchy. In essence, Alderfer presents nothing really new or substantially different from Maslow, and the criticisms of Maslow's theory in terms of its relevance to management are applicable to Alderfer's modified need hierarchy theory as well.

TWO-FACTOR THEORY

The concept that motivation is identical to job satisfaction was first expounded by Herzberg in 1959.[4] In his collaborative writing, Herzberg stated that job satisfaction and job dissatisfaction are not two ends of the same continuum; rather, these seeming opposites in fact fall on two different continua. This view was based on research conducted by Herzberg and his associates which showed that the factors leading to job satisfaction are very different from those leading to job dissatisfaction and that the behaviors resulting from these two states are also quite different.

Herzberg believed that the circumstances that prevent job dissatisfaction are related to external, non-performance factors, such as the following:

- Satisfactory pay
- Adequate technical supervision
- Up-to-date and pertinent company policies
- High-quality administration
- Satisfactory working conditions
- Job security

Herzberg suggested that employees need these so-called extrinsic factors to avoid experiencing dissatisfaction with their jobs. This is a very real concern to a short-staffed healthcare industry, because dissatisfied employees are more likely to be absent, file grievances, perform poorly, or look outside the organization for fulfillment.

It is important to note, however, that the presence of all of these extrinsic factors will not guarantee that any specific employee will receive satisfaction from the job or will be motivated to perform well. Satisfaction and motivation are not achieved by providing these types of benefits. Instead, they result from intrinsic on-the-job factors such as the following (which are listed in no special order):

- Recognition and praise
- Responsibility for one's own or another's work
- Advancement or changing status through promotion
- Sense of achievement for performing a task successfully

The more visible these intrinsic factors in the work environment, the greater the potential for an employee to experience job satisfaction and the greater the opportunity for the organization to develop the individual's motivation to perform the assigned job in a high-quality manner.

The results obtained by Herzberg, however, appear to be quite specific to the research methodology he used. Even though Herzberg's hygiene factors (generally lower-order needs) and satisfiers (generally higher-order needs) have enjoyed a popularity among managers second only to Maslow's needs hierarchy, the preponderance of the evidence produced by subsequent research indicates that his theory, too, is inadequate for creating an environment in which work is engaging and fulfilling.

PROCESS THEORIES OF MOTIVATION

In spite of their popularity, the content theories fall short of truly being able to diagnose exactly why an individual behaves in a particular manner. To develop effective means of accomplishing this, content theories have been augmented by what have become known as process theories. These new theories differ from content theories in that they do much more than simply *explain* behavior; they actually offer a means of *understanding* it. Understanding is critical to a manager's performance because it supplies a means to predict what an employee will do on the job under a specific set of circumstances. That capability, of course, implies the ability to control or influence the individual employee's behavior.

Reinforcement Theory

One specific process approach that has been used to study motivation is reinforcement theory, which basically views motivation as a learning process.[7] According to this theory, behavior is something that is learned through a process called *operant conditioning*, in which a specific behavior becomes associated with a particular consequence. This response-consequence relationship becomes stronger as time passes, or, in more simple terms, the response-consequence relationship is *learned* by the individual. The resulting behavior is referred to as *operant* because the individual is perceived as *operating* on his or her environment to obtain a desired consequence.

To produce a desired behavior using operant conditioning, one must control or manipulate the consequences of the behavior. Consider the following example:

A nursing student correctly administers an intramuscular injection and the patient remarks that "it didn't hurt at all." The patient's praise is immediately followed by acknowledgment of the successful act by the nursing instructor, who says, "Well done!"

In this instance, the praise of both patient and instructor are desired consequences (obtained by the student nurse) that occur only when the behavior (giving the injection) is performed properly. Each time this behavior-consequence sequence occurs, the desired behavior is strengthened and the learning process is enhanced.

The focus on desirable consequences (e.g., praise, money, favored task assignments) is nothing more than the process of supplying *positive reinforcement*. Positive reinforcement is a stimulus that, when introduced into a situation, has the effect of strengthening the probability that a certain operant response will occur. If one follows this line of thought just a little further, it is easy to see how a behavior that leads to positive consequences tends to be repeated, whereas a behavior that leads to negative consequences tends not to be repeated. Obviously, both processes are important in an organization.

There are times when managers need to have employees do things that they are not currently doing and there are times when a manager wishes that employees would not do things that inhibit effective performance. The principle that behavior is related to the consequence of that behavior was once referred to as the greatest business secret in the world, because although it is well known, it is rarely applied in most of the professional and business environments today.[8]

Reinforcement increases the frequency or magnitude of a behavior. This relationship is depicted in the left column of Fig. 25-2, which indicates that the frequency or magnitude of a behavior can be increased by either positive or negative reinforcement. In the former, some positive consequence or stimulus (e.g., praise) is applied for the express purpose of increasing a desired behavior. However, behavior may also be increased by removing something undesired from the environment, as shown in the lower left quadrant of the figure. This is known as *negative reinforcement* and is sometimes categorized as either escape or avoidance learning. If the individual's behavior can terminate the offensive stimulus, the process is called *escape* learning. If a behavior can prevent the onset of an offensive stimulus, the procedure is called *avoidance* learning.

The following examples should make the difference between positive and negative reinforcement quite clear:

> A staff nurse does a thorough job of charting and has her performance reinforced by the nurse manager through the provision of praise. This is *positive* reinforcement.

A nurse who has continually been reprimanded for being tardy arrives for work on time and therefore is not criticized for being late. In this case, the staff member has engaged in avoidance learning by increasing effective or desired behavior to prevent a reprimand from the nurse manager. This is an example of *negative* reinforcement.

As shown in the right-hand column of Fig. 25-2, there are also two different ways to decrease the frequency or magnitude of a behavior. In the second example given previously, the nurse manager wishes to stop a behavior that is incompatible with effective job performance (i.e., tardiness). When the manager delivers a undesired consequence to reduce the occurrence of an undesirable behavior, the procedure is commonly known as *punishment*. When a desirable consequence is removed to decrease behavior, the procedure is known as *extinction*. Punishment is considered to be an active process, whereas something like ignoring the behavior (i.e., providing no reinforcement for it) is considered passive. A passive approach on the part of a manager is rarely an effective form of motivation.

It is highly recommended that nurse managers emphasize positive reinforcement when seeking to alter the performance of a subordinate, because repeated studies have demonstrated that it is the most effective way to change behavior. This statement should not be construed as meaning that other reinforcement procedures are inappropriate or ineffective, however. Certainly punishment, especially if severe enough, will produce an immediate and drastic change in behavior, which is why it is used so frequently. Termination of undesirable behavior achieved

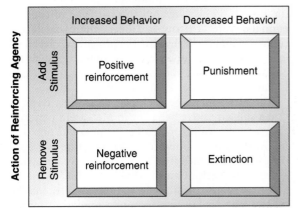

Desired Behavioral Response

Fig. 25-2 ■ Relationship between reinforcement (stimulus) and the frequency or magnitude of a behavioral response. Delivery of reinforcement increases the frequency or magnitude of a behavior.

through punishment is generally not permanent. Typically, the performer will only suppress the undesirable behavior for as long as the reinforcing agent (the person imposing the punishment) is monitoring the situation and the threat of further punishment is present. Punishment is a negative management response and may cause an employee not only to avoid exhibiting a given behavior but to evade the reinforcing agent and the job as well. In short, a manager who relies on punishment as a primary means of changing behavior is likely to create an environment in which lower job satisfaction, greater absenteeism, and eventually greater turnover will outweigh any gains in performance.

! CRITICAL POINT

It is the manager's responsibility to develop an environment in which the employees produce at maximum capability. Quality performance, whether it takes the form of delivering a specialized service or providing general patient care, is rarely achieved in a working environment managed through threat and intimidation. Although punishment is an effective management tool, great care should be used in implementing it, and it should be regarded as a final recourse for dealing with undesirable behavior. A manager's job is to motivate and excite the performer into achieving the desired level of performance, and this can only be accomplished in an environment in which positive reinforcement is the primary motivator.

Extinction, as shown in Fig. 25-2, occurs when no positive consequence exists for a behavior. When the extinction process is implemented, the belief is that the undesired behavior will eventually cease if nothing is done about it (i.e., no reinforcement is provided). This is a relatively inefficient way to change an employee's behavior, however, because it may take a great deal of time. The best combination of actions is to carefully address the undesired behavior in as positive a manner as possible (i.e., extinguish) *and* simultaneously positively reinforce the desired behavior when it occurs. For example, positively address recurring lateness and significantly praise punctuality. This is a behavior-consequence relationship that is far easier for the employee to understand than simple extinction and is much more effective from a managerial point of view. After all, only very rarely is it desirable for an employee to do nothing; rather, the manager's job is to encourage employees to do something different. Whatever that something is, it must be appropriate and constructive in terms of job performance.

One of the most significant problems with operant conditioning in the minds of many managers is that it does not provide a means to elicit the desired behavior from employees so that this behavior can be reinforced. Instead, managers must wait for employees to perform in the desired manner before positive reinforcement (a desirable consequence) can be administered. The obvious solution to this dilemma is to simply *tell* employees what they should be doing and what they should not be doing. In most situations involving highly educated professionals, this should be sufficient to elicit the desired behavior, which then should be positively reinforced. However, telling people what to do is a process that must be handled delicately.

WARNING !

Another significant drawback to operant conditioning is that ignoring undesirable behavior can cause a backlash from those employees who conscientiously perform the desirable behaviors. Employees are always aware of the negative performance of their peers and will continually observe to see how the manager deals with it. If they perceive that the negative behavior is not going to be remedied, the good performers are likely to turn against the manager (worst-case scenario) or engage in the negative behavior themselves (unsatisfactory scenario).

Sometimes, positive reinforcement is simply not sufficient to rectify undesirable behavior. For example, consider the situation in the following story:

Margaret, a nursing assistant, rarely came to work less than 20 minutes late. Her uniform was perpetually wrinkled and often soiled; her personal hygiene routinely left something to be desired; and her general attitude was unpleasant. Margaret's nurse manager decided that a procedure called *shaping* would be the most appropriate method for dealing with the errant assistant. Shaping involves selectively reinforcing behaviors that are successively closer approximations to the desired behavior. Margaret was not ignorant of the expectations of her job and the type of conduct expected from her; she had been reprimanded and counseled innumerable times on appropriate job behavior. Therefore, her problem could not be considered to be caused by a lack of knowledge; rather, it appeared to have its roots in a simple lack of motivation.

The nurse manager attempted for over a week to find a single positive behavior in Margaret's performance and demeanor to reinforce but could not. The following week, however, she identified several occasions on which she could positively recognize Margaret's performance. One day, for example, Margaret came to work only 10 minutes late, and the relative punctuality was promptly reinforced by the nurse manager. Similarly, as Margaret seemed to have made at least an attempt to comb her hair, she was positively reinforced for her improved appearance. On every occasion, however, the nurse manager was met only with a grunt and an occasional icy glare from Margaret, who continued about her own business. After a few weeks, however, she seemed to respond more favorably to the positive recognition and increased interest (rewards) being provided by the nurse manager. With increasing frequency, Margaret's comb appeared to have wandered through her hair (on some days even more than once), and although her uniform was still somewhat wrinkled, it was now clean each day.

Within a period of approximately 2 months, Margaret's performance, although not perfect, had improved enough to meet minimum standards, and she was no longer an embarrassment to her colleagues and the hospital. Moreover, her disposition improved, and she actually began to develop some friendships with other members of the staff. Over the period of monitoring, Margaret's appearance and hygiene improved for the most part and became acceptable overall, and her punctuality, although by no means perfect, did start to show small glimmers of improvement. Although she was clearly no superstar, Margaret came to be regarded as a valuable and necessary member of the staff.

The main point of this story is that behavior modification can be achieved using the principles of positive reinforcement if they are implemented carefully. That is, each successively closer approximation to the desired behavior must be reinforced and well established before the desired behavior can begin to materialize. When people become clearly aware that rewards are contingent on a specific behavior, their behavior will change eventually. Nurse managers must ensure, however, that the change to acceptable behavior progresses rapidly enough to meet the available time frame. An employee should not be given forever to make a change. Instead, as part of a positively orchestrated consultation process, the employee should be told exactly what the expectations are and given a definite time period in which to achieve them. During that period, every time an improvement is noted, the employee should be recognized for the achievement. On the other hand, failure to comply with minimum standards or a refusal to attempt to bring individual conduct in line with expectations should never be tolerated. Nurse managers must provide a positive environment for all of their employees, not just for the ones who fail to perform.

Behavior modification works quite well when the following conditions can be met:

- Rewards can be found that are viewed as positive reinforcement by employees.
- Rewards can be controlled or made contingent upon performance by supervisory personnel.
- Recognition and rewards provided do not impair continued improvement.
- Recognition and rewards provided do not impair the performance of others.

One should note that not all rewards work equally well for all individuals, and the same rewards, or a system of rewards in general, may not continue to generate improvement effectively over a long period of time. If a nurse manager praises a subordinate several times a day every day for the same accomplishment, or in the same manner for different accomplishments, the praise will soon begin to lose its value (i.e., it will cease to be a positive reinforcement). As with most other motivational processes, care must be taken not to overdo what can be a good management tool. In other words, a *continuous schedule* of reinforcement—that is, delivery of the reinforcer every time a desired behavior occurs—may cause that reinforcer to lose its effectiveness (Table 25-1).

The use of *partial schedules* of reinforcement (e.g., reinforcement of the desired behavior after every second or third occurrence or after a specific time period) may prove helpful. When a *fixed-ratio schedule* of reinforcement is used, for example, the individual receives reinforcement after performing the desired behavior a specific number of times. This method requires very close monitoring by management to ensure that the errant employee is reinforced according to the set plan (every so many occurrences of the behavior) and for rather obvious reasons is not very practical. However, if the nurse manager reinforces the desired behavior on a fairly regular or frequent but varying basis (a *variable-ratio schedule;* see Table 25-1), a planned course of reinforcement might prove to be quite feasible. Using this method, the nurse manager would provide reinforcement on an average of every second or every third demonstration of the desired response, for example. A *fixed-interval schedule* of reinforcement is quite common in many organizations. An example of this form of positive reinforcement is the distribution of weekly or monthly paychecks.

Over the past few decades, many applications of continuous and partial schedules of reinforcement have produced extraordinary results. For example, it is well known that the continuous schedule of reinforcement is the fastest method of establishing a new behavior, whereas the use of a partial schedule of reinforcement achieves the desired results at a generally slower rate. On the other hand, a behavior established on a continuous schedule extinguishes very quickly as soon as the reinforcement stops, whereas a behavior that has been established on a partial schedule of reinforcement continues for a much longer period of time following the cessation of reinforcement. In addition, research has shown that the use of money as a form of continuous reinforcement

Effects of Different Reinforcement Schedules

Reinforcement Contingency	Schedule of Reinforcement	Effect on Behavior When Applied	Effect on Behavior When Removed
	Continuous reinforcement	Fastest method to establish a new behavior	Fastest method to extinguish a new behavior
	Partial reinforcement	Slowest method to establish a new behavior	Slowest method to extinguish a new behavior
	Variable partial reinforcement	More consistent response frequencies	Slower extinction rate
	Fixed partial reinforcement	Less consistent response frequencies	Slower extinction rate
Positive reinforcement Avoidance learning		Increased frequency over preconditioning level	Return to preconditioning level
Punishment		Decreased frequency over preconditioning level	Return to preconditioning level
Extinction		Decreased frequency over conditioned level	Return to conditioning level

Data from Behling O, Schreisheim C, Toliver J: Present theories and new directions, *Ext Suppl Abstract Serv* [APA Journal Supplement Abstract Service], 1979.

achieves more rapid and often measurably higher results than the use of other reinforcing agents such as praise and recognition. However, it is also well documented that as soon as the money stops, so does the behavior—almost immediately. Overall, research has shown that money is a poor motivator over the long term.

Although the ability of positive reinforcement to change behavior has been well documented, little research has been done on what specific agents are reinforcing to particular individuals and why preferences occur. Basically, a certain consequence of behavior truly becomes reinforcing only when the mind of the individual receiving the reinforcement accepts it as such. Not all rewards—or all punishments, for that matter—are effective behavior-modifying agents for all people. In fact, a seemingly infinite number of different things can motivate people. It is important to note that basic reinforcement theory makes no attempt to explain individual preferences regarding reinforcing agents and punishment variants.

Expectancy Theory

Expectancy theory was first introduced by Victor Vroom in 1964 as an explanation for specific work motivations.[9] Expectancy theory approaches behavior from a different direction than does reinforcement theory (which focuses strictly on observable behaviors). Vroom's approach suggests that people's thoughts regarding the environment and their personal evaluation of the events that affect it (i.e., their expectations) are important in determining future behavior.

The major difference between expectancy theory and reinforcement theory (behavior modification) lies in their views on how people react to their environment: expectancy theory holds that people react consciously and actively to the occurrences in their environment, whereas reinforcement theory suggests that people passively react to forces (reinforcement contingencies) that are present in their environment. Expectancy theory examines conscious choice behavior, whereas reinforcement theory focuses on the learned stimulus-response bonds that are formed as a result of positive reinforcement. There is one area in which the two theories agree, however: both of them place a strong emphasis on the role of rewards and their relationship to the performance of desired behaviors.

Expectancy theory contends that an individual is motivated by his or her expectancies or beliefs about future outcomes (i.e., the consequences of behavior) and by the value the individual places on those outcomes.[9,10] The following three factors are important in determining exactly when and where a given individual will work to his or her full capabilities or deliver maximum effort:

1. *Expectancy:* the belief that certain effort (an action or behavior) will lead to specific performance
2. *Instrumentality:* the belief that performance will lead to a certain outcome (i.e., either a reward or a punishment)
3. *Valence:* the value or desirability of an outcome

These three factors combine to indicate the level of effort an individual is willing to expend to fulfill a specific performance requirement.

To achieve maximum performance from their staffs, nurse managers must determine whether each individual believes that his or her efforts will result in achievement (expectancy), whether the individual believes that this achievement will yield rewards (instrumentality), and how these rewards are valued (valence) (Fig. 25-3). These three factors are multiplied together to determine the amount of effort an individual will exert: effort = (expectancy × instrumentality × valence). When effort is expressed in this manner, it is easy to see how a reduction in any specific area will affect overall motivation (effort). For example, if a person does not believe that he or she is capable of performing a task (expectancy), *or* the individual believes that there will be little chance of reward for the work (instrumentality), *or* the value of the outcome (valence) is low, the amount of motivation that person will feel to perform the requirement is reduced. In fact, because these factors are multiplied together, a zero value for any one of them results in zero motivation.

Expectancy theory also takes into account multiple outcomes. For example, consider the promotion of a particular staff nurse to the position of nurse manager. Although the staff nurse offered the position believes that such a promotion is a positive reward for the competence and performance she has displayed in her present duties, she also understands that there are some potential negative outcomes that accompany such a promotion, namely, working longer hours, losing the close camaraderie enjoyed with other staff members, and no longer being the person to whom everyone (staff, administrators, patients, and physicians) relays complaints.

Thus, to achieve maximum employee performance (motivation), the nurse manager should always ask the following three questions when considering potential rewards for a staff member:

1. What does this staff member believe about her or his ability to do the work (expectancy)?
2. What is the probability that the work will lead to positive outcomes (instrumentality)?
3. What is the desirability of those outcomes (valence)?

Equity Theory

Equity theory suggests that the amount of effort expended by an individual to accomplish a job and the amount of satisfaction that person receives from the job depend on the perceived equity of the work situation.[11] In this context, perceived *equity* simply refers to a person's belief that her or his contribution to a specific assignment is rewarded, proportionately speaking, in exactly the same way as another's contribution. This does not mean that the reward received is identical to that received by another contributor; the exact contributions of each person may differ, and therefore the rewards received by each must also be allowed to differ. A given person's contribution is a combination of a variety of tangible and intangible elements such as ability, education, experience, and effort. Rewards include such things as pay, prestige, and fringe benefits. Given the potential variations in these different factors for different individuals, equity theory is actually concerned with the conditions under which employees perceive their contributions to the job and the rewards obtained as being fair and equitable. To fully appreciate this approach, managers must understand the distinction made earlier between a situation that is *equitable* and a situation that is *identical*. Equity in no way implies that every individual should receive the same thing in the same amount or at the same frequency. Instead, the concept of equity suggests that those employees who bring more to the job, who perform a more arduous task, or who work harder to achieve results deserve more in the way of rewards.

According to equity theory, as long as the individual perceives the *ratio* between his or her outcomes and inputs to be approximately equal to that of other individuals in similar or comparatively similar circumstances, a state of equity exists. For example, there are very few employees who don't understand that registered nurses and nursing assistants have unequal salaries, and most understand that these two different types of employees bring different and unequal education and experience to the job. Therefore, their task assignments and the salaries each group receives

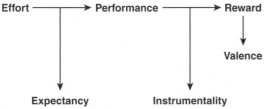

Fig. 25-3 ■ Representation of expectancy theory.

for performing those tasks are usually perceived as equitable. In this case, the difference in inputs (education and experience) offsets the difference in outputs (rewards). Inequity occurs when an employee's outcome/input ratio is perceived to be noticeably different from that of a person with whom comparison is relevant. The person with whom the employee draws a comparison may be a co-worker, a person performing a similar job for a different employer, or an "ideal worker," or it may even be the employee himself or herself at some other time or in some other job situation. When a person perceives an imbalance between inputs and rewards, then and only then will a difficulty arise.

It is not equity but inequity that motivates a change in behavior, and once this change is achieved, it may either increase or decrease actual effort and job performance. Equity, by itself, simply motivates a change in the status quo. From a practical viewpoint, nurses who see the nursing assistants' salaries increased without a corresponding increase in nurses' salaries may be motivated to attempt some sort of behavioral change. On the other hand, no change in salary or an equal percentage salary change for both groups will generally motivate everyone to continue at the current level of performance. Again, the nurse manager must be aware of the difference between behavior and performance. Reducing inequity may or may not change performance.

It is very difficult to predict exactly what specific individuals will do or how they will react when they perceive a lack of equity. However, the following basic principles may help:

- It is logical to assume that most people will try to maximize rewards and minimize contributions.
- Almost all people are more resistant to changing their ideas about their own rewards and contributions than they are to distorting their perceptions of the contributions and rewards of those with whom they compare themselves.
- Contributions and rewards that are perceived to be central to an individual's self-esteem and self-concept will be more difficult to change than those that are not viewed as important. For example, if registered nurses perceive that a salary increase given to nursing assistants implies a loss of their own status, they will be more inclined to attempt some type of change.
- Changing a person's reaction to a perceived inequity will be more difficult once the individual's comparison of self to others has stabilized. In other words, the manager must act when the salary increase is announced, or a change will be unlikely to occur.

- Leaving the situation is the least likely thing an individual will do. Usually this occurs only after all other attempts to restore perceived equity have failed and the individual comes to the realization that the perceived inequity will remain—regardless of whether this belief is justified.

People may follow a number of different avenues to restore what they believe to be equity, including the following:

1. *Increase or decrease the actual contribution:* Individual effort is especially likely to be changed. For example, nurses may attempt to increase their status by assuming an increased number of patient care assignments, spending more time charting, or exhibiting other behaviors that reflect a higher level of effort.
2. *Attempt to persuade a comparison group to increase or decrease input:* For example, a registered nurse who perceives a salary inequity as described in earlier examples might attempt to persuade the nursing assistants to perform their work at a slower pace.
3. *Persuade the organization to change rewards:* Individuals may attempt to persuade the organization to change either their own rewards or those received by the comparison group (e.g., make salary changes).
4. *Distort individual effort:* An individual may psychologically distort the importance and value of his or her own contributions and rewards ("How could they run this unit without me?").
5. *Distort the comparison group's contribution:* The individual may distort the importance and value of the comparison group's contributions or rewards ("What can you expect from assistants?").
6. *Select a different comparison group:* The person perceiving the inequity might select another group for comparison; for example, a nurse perceiving an inequity between herself and an assistant might compare her contributions and rewards with those of her nurse manager.
7. *Leave the organization:* As noted earlier, this is the last form of escape from the inequity. It is used only when the individual perceives that the desired change will not occur.

The approaches listed as numbers 4 and 5 are the easiest ways in which perceived equity can be restored without actually changing performance levels.

Without doubt, the most extensively researched aspect of equity theory is the use of compensation as a reward. The focus on this element has been so great for one primary reason: pay is perceived as a valuable reward by most people (albeit not the most important reward). Its use has a variety of potential impacts, including predictability.

If one assumes, for example, that changing the level of job performance is more expedient than other reactions to inequity, certain predictions can be made regarding pay inequity. For example, employee efforts vary according to perceived underpayment or overpayment. Although most research has focused on overpayment inequity (probably because it is more controversial), it is just as easy to understand why individuals might change their behavior if they feel they are being cheated or underpaid, even if it seems less likely that they would increase their performance.

What is true is that the perception of inequity, regardless of what prompts it, will motivate changes in behavior. Therefore, the concept of equity may be seen as one of several potential social norms that operate within groups, particularly when the distribution of rewards is considered. Table 25-2 presents two different distribution rules for the allocation of rewards in small groups.[12] Which distribution rule (equity or equality) is appropriate depends on the goal of reward allocation, among other things. For example, when the goal is to maximize individual

productivity in a group, all rewards should be distributed equitably—that is, they should be allocated based on individual expertise and contributions. If, however, the manager's goal is to maximize harmony and, at the same time, minimize potential conflict within the group, then rewards should be distributed equally to all participants regardless of their contributions.

The degree of cooperation required for the performance of a task is another important factor to be considered when distributing rewards. If tasks are essentially individual (i.e., staff members carry them out on their own with no need for a high degree of cooperation), then equity should be the rule for allocating organizational rewards. On the other hand, if a high degree of cooperation and coordination is required for effective task performance (i.e., group or team tasks), then rewards should be distributed equally among group members.

It is critical that nurse managers differentiate between rewarding individual performance and rewarding group performance. If the goal is to get individual staff members to perform specific tasks (e.g., patient care, record keeping) in a competent and productive way, then any reward established to

---

TABLE 25-2

Rules for Allocation of Rewards

Distribution Rule	Circumstances in Which Rule Is Likely to Be Used	Factors Affecting Use of Rule
Equity (outcomes match contributions)	1. Goal is to maximize group productivity. 2. A low degree of cooperation is required for task performance.	1. What receiver is expected to do 2. What others receive 3. Outcomes and contributions of person allocating reward 4. Task difficulty and perceived ability 5. Personal characteristics of person allocating rewards and person performing
Equality (same outcomes to all participants)	1. Goal is to maximize harmony, minimize conflict within group. 2. Judging performer's needs or contribution is difficult. 3. Person allocating rewards has a low cognitive capacity. 4. A high degree of cooperation is required for task performance. 5. Person allocating rewards anticipates future interaction with low-input members.	1. Sex of person allocating rewards (e.g., women are more likely than men to allocate rewards equally) 2. Nature of task

Data from Leventhal GS: Fairness in social relationships. In Thibaut J, Spence J, Carson R, editors: *Contemporary topics in social psychology,* Morristown, NJ, 1976, General Learning Press.

provide motivation should be individualized. However, if the goal is to provide motivation on a group task (e.g., for a surgical nursing team), then performance will be maximized when staff members are rewarded for group rather than individual performance or, in cases in which the reward must be delivered on an individual basis, when rewards are allocated with the full agreement of the group.

The critical point here is that perceived fairness in the distribution of rewards can have a dramatic affect on the way individuals view their jobs and their organizations and can affect the amount of effort they are willing to expend toward task accomplishment. In many instances, inequitable rewards, especially underpayment inequity, lead to increased psychologic tension and lower job satisfaction in the individual performer and ultimately have an adverse impact on job performance.

In times of economic austerity, if no one receives a salary increase then employees may perceive the situation as being equitable if they believed the situation to be equitable before the economic downturn. In this specific circumstance, job satisfaction is rarely affected adversely.

Another key point that is similar to the point Herzberg made regarding extrinsic factors is simply that pay equity is important to keep a good motivational situation from going sour, but distributing rewards equitably will not necessarily improve an otherwise poor motivational environment.

Goal-Setting Theory

There are three basic propositions in goal-setting theory[13]:

1. Specific goals, like "Handle the medical needs of five critical patients," lead to higher performance than do vague goals such as "Do your best."
2. Specific goals that are difficult to accomplish lead to higher performance than do specific goals that are easy to accomplish, provided the goals are accepted by those asked to accomplish them.
3. Incentives such as money, knowledge of results, praise and reproof, participation, competition, and time restrictions affect behavior only if they cause individuals to change their goals or to accept the goals that have been assigned.

Thus, goal-setting theory, unlike expectancy theory and equity theory, suggests that it is not the reward or outcome of task performance per se that leads to the expenditure of effort but rather the goal itself. The only functions rewards play in this process are (1) to ensure the acceptance of an assigned task or goal, and (2) to induce individual performers to set more exact and difficult goals for themselves. It is the specificity

and difficulty of the goal that mobilizes energy and directs behavior toward goal accomplishment.

A number of studies provide compelling arguments for the establishment of specific goals by showing that they produce significantly higher levels of performance than is achieved with general goals or no goals.[14] As a matter of fact, these studies seem to indicate that the higher the goal that is established, the higher the level of performance that will be achieved. This is supported by the fact that the difficulty of the goal typically predicts 50% to 75% of the differences in individual performance levels.

WARNING!

The establishment of goals is critical to achieving the level of performance desired from employees. Although it is true that a higher level of performance will be achieved when a loftier goal is established, it is equally true that if the goal is too high and is perceived to be unattainable by the employee, performance will decline sharply. People are not motivated by goals they believe they cannot reach.

In reality, employees performing their normally assigned responsibilities rarely totally reject established performance goals. This is true because employees rarely dispute the right of their managers to impose goals, and in the case of nurse managers, the legitimacy of their relationship with staff nurses is one that is readily accepted by most nurses. As long as the goals and duties are perceived as being both reasonable and attainable, then setting specific, difficult goals will very likely produce higher performance—provided the higher level of performance is equitably rewarded *and* the individual is held accountable for task accomplishment.

Many executives believe that managers should be present to oversee performance. It has been well documented that the continual or at least frequent and unscheduled presence of supervisory personnel helps to ensure goal acceptance. Those supervisors who frequently absent themselves from the working environment or who are not available for long periods during the working day are likely to have employees who exhibit substantially lower productivity than the employees of supervisors who remain on the job with their subordinates. In short, good managers understand that nothing can be managed well from their offices.

It is also a fact that establishing specific, difficult goals will generally lead to higher levels of job performance regardless of whether the nursing staff participates in every decision regarding the setting of performance standards. In some organizations and for some managers, participation is a natural and encouraged form of management; in other establishments and for other supervisors, emphasis on participative management is lower. Although either approach is likely to be appropriate and productive provided managers are supportive of their employees, good long-term performance is best realized when performers are actively involved in establishing the goals and objectives they will be asked to achieve. Managers must understand, however, that how a goal is developed is not the most important determinant of its attainment. Supportiveness and encouragement, particularly when the tasks are difficult or undesirable, carry that distinction. These two qualities can go a long way toward obtaining acceptance of high-performance goals by the individual employee and ultimately may result in the achievement of significantly higher levels of performance.

SUMMARY OF MOTIVATION THEORIES

When motivational theory is discussed, one thing becomes very obvious, and that is that the use of a single approach to motivating staff members will most likely fail to maximize performance and satisfaction, especially over prolonged periods of time. Some methods will work better than others for certain people or in certain settings, and some methods won't work well at all. However, all of the various perspectives discussed previously on what motivates individuals in work settings can contribute something to managers' understanding of employee motivation and, ultimately, to their ability to influence it.

All the motivation theories described so far can be integrated to some extent by recognizing that all of them, including the process theories, are based on needs. For example, reinforcement theory does not specify what a reinforcing stimulus is or why it works. However, it seems reasonable to assume that such reinforcers actually change behaviors because they lead to the fulfillment of some underlying need. Similarly, expectancy theory says nothing about why an outcome has a strong positive or negative valence. We simply measure valences and assume that some outcomes are indeed motivational.

It may well be that the need for self-competency or self-efficacy (the need to cope successfully with the environment) can be used to integrate the various motivational perspectives.[15-17] Viewed in this way, all of the theories, both content and process, can be viewed as being linked by this common human need. Although it may be most helpful to specify particular needs or processes (e.g., reinforcement, equity, expectancy) to more precisely describe human motivational behavior, recognizing a common basis such as the need for self-competency points up the fact that utility can be gained from a variety of theoretical approaches.

In actual practice, it is this utility that is particularly important for nurse managers. It starts with the premise recognized by all content theories that people do have particular needs and that to varying degrees these needs must be fulfilled. A very simple example is the need for money, or at least the things that money can buy. Other needs are of a higher order and can be met only through proper job design and assignment of tasks (e.g., professionalism, altruism). Content theories acknowledge these needs but really do not say very much about how to satisfy them. In contrast, the process theories focus specifically on techniques and methods to improve performance and satisfaction, although these are not described in terms of need fulfillment. Nevertheless, to the degree that all motivation theories are based on underlying needs such as the need for self-competency, the techniques and methods presented by the process theories actually represent useful means for providing need fulfillment.

INCREASING STAFF MOTIVATION

Although this chapter has presented a large amount of information, one question remains unanswered: How does the nurse manager motivate staff? Fig. 25-4 provides a simple demonstration of how the various motivation theories are related to facilitate their application. First, though, the task to be accomplished must be defined. If this task is expressed in terms of a specific and difficult goal that is accepted by the staff member, then it is realistic to expect a reasonably high level of performance in most situations.

But how can the manager be sure that a given member of the staff will deliver a high level of performance? In theory, goals, professed ability, and apparent situational constraints combine to yield the perceived likelihood that a specific effort will lead to a given level of performance (goal accomplishment). This expectancy, when combined with the promise of valued rewards after goal attainment, leads to effort or motivation. Therefore, goal-setting and expectancy theories suggest that not only will the staff member know exactly what he or she should be doing but that the individual will also perceive that all potential rewards are contingent on performing properly so as to fulfill those requirements.

A staff member's ability and the situational constraints under which he or she operates combine with individual effort to produce the actual performance level. The nurse manager, when assigning tasks that

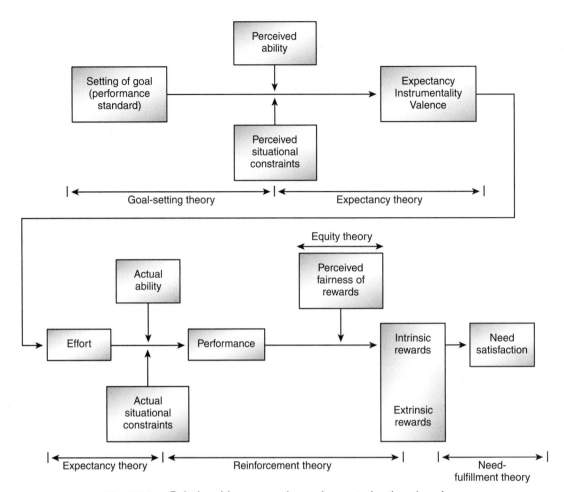

Fig. 25-4 ■ Relationship among the various motivation theories.

are commensurate with a staff nurse's education and experience, may take into account known ability levels. Performance may also be improved by removing as many situational constraints as possible (e.g., rotating shifts) or, at a minimum, providing assistance in overcoming them (e.g., assigning to the same shift for several consecutive days). When the nurse manager carefully manages these types of factors, the staff member's effort or motivation will actually be translated into effective job performance.

Expectancy theory also focuses on anticipated rewards. If the work is produced and the anticipated rewards are not received, then subsequent performance may be reduced. In reality, if employees are told that performance will in fact lead to valued rewards, and those rewards are perceived as being fair and equitable by staff members, then with very few exceptions improved performance should be realized.

Extrinsic rewards or reinforcements help to satisfy lower-order needs, whereas intrinsic rewards or reinforcements are likely to satisfy those of a higher order.

For example, money helps to satisfy the fundamental needs for food, clothing, and shelter, whereas recognition satisfies the higher-level need for self-esteem.

Rewards that are made contingent on performance and are perceived as being equitable will do a great deal to increase individual and team motivation and accomplishment. By themselves, however, rewards will do little to sustain motivation and performance over an extended period of time. To accomplish long-term performance enhancement, managers must rely on a combination of approaches, taking into careful consideration the individual needs of the staff members. This type of multilevel approach will be far more likely than any single method or technique to produce effective job performance. But beyond all that, the real key to effective motivation is the attitude demonstrated by management (i.e., that the things desired *can* be accomplished). Supplying motivation to the staff is not always easy, but it is certainly one of the most important parts of any manager's job. With practice and a little ingenuity, most managers will find that far more can be done than initially believed possible to motivate their staffs to higher levels of performance.

Motivation and Organizational Change

One of the questions that continually baffles management in every industry is why some employees resist change whereas others seem to welcome it. A very simple answer, but one that applies to most situations in which job changes are being contemplated, is that, in general, people are very reluctant to move out of their comfort zone, and that is precisely what change forces them to do (i.e., it moves people away from what they know, understand, and are generally good at). The work that an individual accomplishes forms a very important part of that person's life. Not only is considerable time spent on the job, but one's social standing and prestige as well as one's sense of self are very frequently related to the nature of one's work, one's job title, and, to some extent, the organization in which one is employed. This is especially true of individuals in the medical profession (physicians, registered nurses, physical therapists, etc.).

WARNING !

Today, many professional business consultants feel strongly about the provision of motivation and about exactly who in the organization is responsible for supplying it. The consensus over the last decade has shifted from the view that the responsibility is solely the managers' to the view that it is shared by managers and employees. Many of the more traditional consultants continue to feel that it is impossible for one person to motivate another effectively over the long term, whereas the liberal opposition at the other end of the spectrum continues to cling to the belief that it is solely a managerial responsibility.

The most thoroughly documented evidence available today, however, supports the view that managers are responsible for creating an environment that encourages individual employees to motivate themselves. If the environment encourages self-expression, opens channels of discourse between the manager and employees (feedback), and provides a system of goals and objectives and a well-understood set of expectations, the chances are excellent that it will also be an environment in which employees are highly motivated and professional in conduct.*

*LeBouef ML: Motivation in the 2000 workplace, Cambridge, Mass, 2001, Massachusetts Institute of Technology. The gist of this study is that it is not totally the manager's responsibility to motivate. The best and longest lasting motivation is that which comes from within the individual performer and is well received and encouraged by management.

Change, especially change that is not well understood or is perceived as being unnecessary, at best will move a performer out of his or her comfort zone and at worst will threaten the individual's sense of well-being and ability to cope with the environment. Given these potential effects, it is easy to see why change can be viewed as a frightening experience, especially when one is unsure of precisely why the change is being made and what will be expected once it has been implemented.

From the viewpoint of expectancy theory, when change is instituted, the likelihood that individual or group effort will lead to high performance is small unless high performance is specifically defined in the change. The reason is that if employees demonstrate high performance, they may not be sure whether their actions will generate valued rewards or negative social pressure from peers. Performance is inhibited in periods of change because the ability of employees to make good choices is limited by the fact that they don't always know what choices they actually have open to them. The resulting hesitancy to make a choice often results in minimal performance. Small wonder, then, that change can have such a devastating impact on both performance and employee satisfaction.

Change does not have to have a negative effect on the workforce, however. As a matter of fact, when it is properly managed, it can be one of management's best tools for influencing employee performance and job satisfaction. Change can be a productive performance enhancer if managers adhere to the key principles presented in the following sections when they introduce change.

IMPLEMENT CHANGE ONLY WHEN THERE IS A REASON FOR IT

Change for change's sake is most often perceived as being arbitrary, unnecessary, and an unreasonable use of power and influence. For example, consider those managers who, immediately on assuming a new position, begin by making changes to the procedures established by their predecessors. They may find a short time later that staff members are already actively resisting their leadership. They may also feel that staff resent them and anything they attempt to accomplish that is different from "the way things use to be." Their initial efforts, no matter how well intended, can create significant backlash and usually generate a predictable result: things will not go in the intended direction but will generally work themselves into a slowdown in performance and other negative responses from the staff (increased sick time, higher turnover, etc.). Such a situation is extremely difficult to correct; therefore, it is imperative that all who are responsible for change or have the power to effect it do so only when it is necessary to promote good order and performance in the unit. Even then, change should be attempted only after essential information regarding its need is shared with the staff.

Why, in the situation described earlier, would a professional staff actively resist a new manager's initial leadership efforts? Obviously, there could be an infinite number of reasons, but one of the most common is that staff members know the rules of the "old" game and don't like the fact that the "new guy" has attempted to change them. They resist change because it moves them out of their comfort zone (they knew the things they had to do to please the previous manager and the things they could reasonably get away with). The standards and expectations set by the new manager change the playing field, and the staff members still want to play the old game. The lesson to be learned from this scenario is that making arbitrary change just because one can is an excellent way for a manager to invite the active resistance and resentment of staff members, which is something that no manager can afford to let happen.

What, then, is a "good" reason for implementing change? The following three reasons are applicable in a wide variety of situations:

1. *To solve a problem:* Eliminating or reducing the effect of problems, either real or perceived, is an excellent reason to implement change and one that is nearly universally accepted by employees.
2. *To make work procedures more efficient:* Change may be instituted to eliminate the time wasted on relatively unimportant tasks. This effort should be accomplished in conjunction with the staff to increase their commitment to the change and reduce overall resistance.
3. *To reduce unnecessary workload:* Rare is the individual who wants to do more work than he or she has to in order to accomplish a job.

If managers focus on the changes prompted by one of these "good" reasons, then they can go a long way toward decreasing resistance and increasing acceptance of those changes they choose to implement.

INTRODUCE CHANGE GRADUALLY

A second fundamental rule regarding change is to introduce it gradually. Good managers never try to change everything all at once, even if a situation or environment desperately calls out for it. Too much change can be overwhelming for most performers. As a matter of fact, if there is anything worse than the feeling of ambiguity and powerlessness created by a single change in only one area, it is the total confusion that can be created when an individual must deal with changes in a large number of different areas at once. Intelligent managers introduce change slowly. Changes should be kept to one or two areas at first,

and then a tangible effort should be made to build on the success of those efforts. If managers move slowly and then celebrate their successes with their staffs, they will go a long way toward developing the trust and cooperation they will need to successfully introduce future changes. This recommendation, however, should not be construed as advocating that managers drag their feet to get something accomplished. Rather, what is being suggested is that change be an orderly and well-planned process undertaken in manageable increments.

PLAN THE CHANGE

Change should be thoroughly planned before it is attempted. Any change that is devised without sufficient planning or that is implemented on the spur of the moment is likely to result in a host of unexpected problems. Proper and careful planning of the change and the strategy that will be used when introducing it will greatly enhance the likelihood that it will be accepted and will significantly increase the opportunity for successful implementation.

The same principles apply when change is introduced to an entire group of employees. First of all, a need must be established by involving the staff in the recognition of a problem or in a discussion of ways to increase efficiency and reduce unnecessary work. When actively engaged by group participation, staff members are far more likely to become involved in producing solutions (creating change) than in resisting change. This procedure is made easier if the manager concentrates the group's discussion and effort on a single problem or change and on the specific actions to be taken by each member of the group. After initial successes are achieved, the group can move on to dealing with other problems. It is the manager's job to keep the group focused on the solution of the particular problem being discussed and way from what else can be achieved. In short, problem resolution (change) should be taken one step at a time.

Undesirable Jobs

Every organization has work that is considered less than desirable but that must be accomplished by someone from time to time. Traditionally, these "bad" jobs have been assigned to the best employees simply because that practice increases the likelihood that the jobs will be done properly. This approach is often counterproductive to good order and performance, however, because it may give the high-performing employee the impression that the reward for high performance is assignment to disagreeable tasks. Although, in the short run, most staff members will accept assignment to disagreeable tasks as being a necessary part of the job, over the long run, continual assignment to such tasks may have the effect of lowering motivation and increasing dissatisfaction with the job. Instead, task assignments should be made on an equal basis using fair and nonprejudicial methods. In short, the entire staff should share in the good and the not-so-good jobs in the unit.

It is not recommended that assignment to these "bad" jobs be used as a form of punishment for lower-than-expected performance. Marginal performers who believe that they are trying to meet expectations and who are continually saddled with bad assignments may feel that they have no opportunity to improve. It cannot be stressed enough that job assignments should be made fairly and with the best interests of all staff members in mind.

If every member of the staff is executing at approximately the same level of performance above an established standard (not a typical situation), equity and positive reinforcement become critical issues. If the undesirable jobs are regularly rotated so that no one is unduly penalized by having to repeatedly perform them, the perception of equity in assignments can be achieved. Another suggestion is to provide an incentive for completion of undesirable tasks in a timely and professional manner. This can be something as simple as allowing the staff member to choose from a list of preferred tasks when the undesirable job has been satisfactorily completed.

Individual preferences in assignment are important to the average performer and cannot always be anticipated by managers. In fact, what is considered desirable or undesirable to one member of the staff may be viewed quite differently by another. Managers who take the time to learn the individual preferences of their staff members and use them as incentives for performance have a powerful tool for motivating employees and fostering job satisfaction. Task assignment is only one of many potential incentives or reinforcements, but it can be a very powerful incentive when used properly.[18]

Job Design

The very early history of job design was one of job specialization and fragmentation. In early industry—well before the Industrial Revolution, in fact—general craftsmanship was very often plagued by inefficiency. To overcome these challenges and the deleterious effect they had on production, job specialization was developed. Early efforts caused significant increases in labor costs, however, and completion of products was often delayed as result of the specialization, in part because of the increased need for coordination among the specialists. With the Industrial Revolution and the advent of mass production, efficiency was increased by further fragmenting the work into highly specialized movements that were repeated over and over during the course of the working day. This had a staggeringly negative effect on production, however, because the monotony it produced significantly increased absenteeism. The typical managerial reaction to these early problems was an increased emphasis on discipline.

Continued efforts did change the scope of many jobs, however, and the process has improved steadily through advances in the way that the specialization and fragmentation of the total work effort are implemented. In the early days of nursing, for example, each nurse assumed all of the duties involved in caring for patients, including cleaning the patient's room. Today, however, nursing is increasingly divided into highly specialized areas or somewhat fragmented job duties, so that now a hospital may employ specialists in such areas as intravenous nursing and intensive care unit nursing.

One problem with the specialization of professionals is that the highly specific training required does not allow one to change emphasis or specialty easily during a career. The high degree of specialization in the nursing profession has often left many highly talented nurses bored with the monotony of doing the same thing over and over or dealing with the same types of patients day after day. The problem in the industry has been made more difficult by the fact that the types of work required have remained largely unchanged; therefore, the only solution has been job redesign. Today, in the healthcare industry, there is a definite trend back toward more general rather than highly specialized professional jobs. Consider the concept of holistic medicine and the concern for the psychologic as well as the physical needs of the patient, both of which have become increasingly important in the past decade. Another indication is the shift being seen from team to primary nursing. These examples show that the general movement in the profession is away from job simplification and toward job expansion.

Job expansion and job enrichment are two of the many different attempts that have been made to reduce the negative effects of specialization. *Job expansion* can be defined as the addition of performance tasks to increase the variety of skills and talents that staff members must use in the performance of their jobs. This type of job enlargement not only increases variety in the job but also provides the performing nurse with a sense of completion by allowing the individual to carry out a larger and thus more identifiable piece of the entire task. The problem with job enlargement, however, is that it is frequently viewed as "more work" rather than "better work" or work that entails greater responsibility and a higher level or different kind of professional skill. Intrinsic (higher-order) needs are particularly strong among nursing professionals, and simply assigning them more work as opposed to better work does little to satisfy those needs or to stimulate outstanding job performance.

In contrast to job expansion, *job enrichment* focuses on closing the gap between the doing and controlling aspects of the job. In job enrichment, employees are given greater latitude in selecting work methods, evaluating their work, and participating in decisions affecting either their jobs or the organization as a whole. Therefore, job enrichment is most often viewed by the staff nurse as the assumption of greater responsibility and control over the job, as opposed to a simple increase in the number of mundane tasks to be accomplished.

The purpose of job redesign is to create jobs that provide a higher level of internal work motivation, better quality of work performance, and greater satisfaction with the work, as well as lower absenteeism and turnover.[19] These desired results are more likely to occur in individuals who (a) experience a greater meaningfulness in their work, (b) feel a sense of responsibility for the results of their work, and (c) have feedback regarding the effectiveness of their work. This is illustrated in Fig. 25-5.

One might assume that professional employees such as nurses would experience these rewarding psychologic states as a result of their work. However, the nursing profession is staffed by human beings who are subject to the same ills inherent in every other profession. Lack of motivation, absenteeism, and turnover are problems that are serious enough to warrant discussion and certainly serious enough to merit particular attention by the nurse manager. Because the nursing profession is subject to these negative influences, motivational systems must be developed and implemented to retain highly talented and productive nurses in jobs in which their services are particularly needed. Job redesign tries to increase the degree to which an individual experiences meaningfulness, a sense of responsibility, and effective feedback, which lead to high performance and high job satisfaction. When the specific set of core job dimensions that research has shown to be related to these psychologic states is managed effectively, higher levels of job satisfaction almost always result.

Core Job Dimensions

According to job redesign theory, there are five core job dimensions that produce the critical psychologic states mentioned earlier. The first two are generally associated with job enlargement:

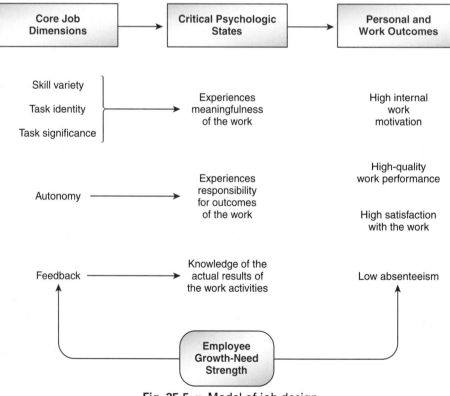

Fig. 25-5 ■ Model of job design.

1. *Skill variety:* the degree to which a job provides activities that involve the use of different skills and abilities
2. *Task identity:* the degree to which a job requires completion of a whole and identifiable piece of work; this entails doing a complete task from beginning to end

Job enrichment adds the following three additional core job dimensions that are important for creating the desired psychologic states:

3. *Task significance:* the degree to which a job has importance for the lives and work of other people both inside and outside the organization
4. *Autonomy:* the degree to which a job provides freedom, independence, and discretion to the staff member in scheduling the work to be accomplished and in choosing the procedures to be used in carrying it out
5. *Feedback:* the degree to which individuals are able to obtain clear information regarding the effectiveness of their performance; this may be apparent from the task itself or may be available from other individuals—particularly patients, other nurses, and the nurse manager

The following principles can guide the redesign of jobs to enhance these five core job dimensions:

Principle 1: The first principle is to form natural work units incorporating tasks that logically fit together. This helps employees to see the significance of their tasks and to feel a greater sense of responsibility for the outcome of what they do.

Principle 2: A related principle is that of combining tasks, which helps to increase perceptions of skill variety and task identity. By carefully combining tasks, a natural work unit can be formed, and both principles can be drawn upon to motivate and satisfy staff members.

Principle 3: The third principle is to establish client relationships. This principle is already followed in the nursing profession, where establishment of the nurse-patient relationship is a prerequisite to providing care. Patients provide direct feedback to the nurse on their perception of the nurse's work. In addition, the patient relationship tends to enhance skill variety because the nurse must practice the interpersonal skills necessary for effective communication with different patients. Finally, patient relationships affect autonomy in that the nurse must decide how to manage the relationships with patients and co-workers in the unit.

Principle 4: This principle calls for giving the individual added control over his or her work. Again, allowing staff nurses to participate in making decisions, selecting work methods, and evaluat-ing their own work increases the amount of autonomy experienced in the job.

Principle 5: This principle deals with opening feedback channels. This involves essentially two things: (1) the feedback from the nurse manager regarding job performance, and (2) feedback coming from the job itself (including feedback from patients). The latter form of feedback is more important because it is both immediate and specific. For example, staff nurses may be made responsible for evaluating their own performance, such as by noting patient response to their ministrations. Such nurses are continually reminded of performance quality without the intervention of the supervisor.

Proponents of primary nursing have argued that staff who work in units using this nursing method experience greater job satisfaction because the foregoing principles are applied.

Barriers to Job Redesign

Nurse managers should be aware of some of the common problems encountered during the redesign of jobs, such as role changes, value conflicts, reluctance to participate, a lack of desire for growth, and a frequent absence of predetermined goals.

CHANGE IN ROLE

The first problem that may be encountered in job redesign may also be the most important: namely, the nurse manager's role may change from that of leader and director of unit staff to that of coordinator of staff activities. Somehow, the notion of coordinator seems inconsistent with the cultural stereotypes of leadership. We tend to think of a leader as the person in charge or "the boss." This stereotype of leadership tends to include the unilateral and unquestioned use of power, with objectives, strategies, and evaluation defined strictly from the leader's perspective. Many managers treat this issue as a matter of "leadership style" and tend to regard it as a personality characteristic. This particular barrier, however, is one over which the nurse manager can exercise direct and explicit control.

In reality, a number of elements are involved in effective leadership other than the power afforded by virtue of job title and reporting relationships. Effective leadership is accepted leadership, and there are many ways in which to foster acceptance of the nurse manager's legitimate organizational power. The strategies and techniques described in this chapter, however, are tools meant to help nurse managers achieve individual and unit effectiveness. If achieving effectiveness means being the coordinator instead of the boss, then these strategies and techniques are what nurse managers should use.

VALUE CONFLICT

Another barrier to job redesign is that the values implicit in it may be at odds with those of the hospital administration. The notion of providing autonomy, feedback, and greater responsibility and self-direction in the performance of jobs may not be in tune with the philosophy and historical practice of the hospital hierarchy. However, matters that do not fall under management typically afford different degrees of responsibility, and there may be a good deal of flexibility within the limits of the rules. Job design is just another tool to use within the limits of the situation at hand.

RELUCTANCE TO PARTICIPATE

In some cases, staff members may be reluctant to participate in job redesign or other motivational efforts because they fear that increased productivity may have implications for their job security. That is, they fear that if productivity increases sufficiently, people may lose their jobs because they may no longer be needed to accomplish the work in the unit. In nursing, however, this seldom poses a significant problem because most nursing units are woefully understaffed. In this situation, increased productivity will not only ease the daily workload but, if properly managed (e.g., rewarded), is likely to result in greater satisfaction and organizational commitment and less absenteeism and turnover.

In addition, there is a tendency to focus on quantity and to ignore quality. Effective motivation of staff members involves both of these dimensions, but job enrichment most consistently increases job satisfaction and work quality rather than the quantity of work produced.

LACK OF DESIRE FOR GROWTH

Some people prefer to have their work very clearly prescribed, unvarying in its content or procedure, and highly predictable from day to day. For these people, job redesign is appropriate only when their jobs are not structured enough to suit their needs.

ABSENCE OF PREDETERMINED GOALS

Exact specification of what is to be accomplished by redesigning an individual's job is often lacking. Expectancy theory suggests that people know exactly what they should do to ensure that their level of performance is as high as possible. Therefore, development of clear goals and objectives, planning to define how the goals can and should be attained, and periodic monitoring of progress to identify needed

change in strategies or objectives are essential when implementing any job redesign measures. Job design may seem somewhat complex, but it is simply another technique that encompasses a variety of motivational strategies with an eye toward overall nursing effectiveness.

Climate and Morale

The job climate is defined as the accumulation of employee perceptions of the events, practices, and procedure of an organization or one of its subunits. When taken together, these perceptions are useful in characterizing the organization or subunit. Normally, a wide variety of climates exist in an organization. Examples of climates in the typical healthcare organization include the productivity climate, the safety climate, and the patient care climate.

One must be careful to specify the exact climate to which one is referring. For example, a nursing unit may be characterized as having a climate of high productivity when the work is usually completed at the end of each shift and patient satisfaction is generally good. When such a climate exists, nurse managers may be reasonably sure that their managerial efforts have been effective in motivating staff to high standards of performance.

Just as *climate* refers to group rather than individual perceptions, *morale* refers to the combined attitudes of all work group members rather than individual job satisfaction. Morale is essentially a matter of group spirit or cohesiveness and is almost tangible in the work environment. It is a critical element in the unit because it reflects what attracts the individual staff members to the group and indicates the degree to which group values and expectations (norms) are adopted by members as their own. Group norms are common expectations held by the members of a work unit with regard to such things as decision-making and productivity, and they become increasingly important as group cohesiveness is enhanced.

Group norms are productive to the extent that they are congruent with or support organizational goals. High morale can aid in pursuing productivity or effectiveness goals, and the nurse manager should never underestimate its potential impact. In contrast, low or negative morale may lead to or be associated with active resistance on the part of group members to leadership and motivational efforts. For example, there may be a norm to restrict productivity, a low standard for a "fair day's work" that is enforced by subtle group pressures. Low morale may be caused by a variety of different factors, but the largest contributing factor is poor management. If the unit is plagued by poor morale, the first place to look for the cause is the performance and practices of the nurse manager.

The phenomenon of "groupthink" (failure to explore alternative approaches or ways of thinking because most group members think in a certain way) represents a nonproductive group norm. Examples of the effects of groupthink are the failure to prepare for the attack on Pearl Harbor and the decision to undertake the Bay of Pigs invasion. Groupthink occurs frequently in organizations in circumstances such as the following:

- When the group is invulnerable to outside pressure
- When the group believes itself to be morally right, which inclines members to ignore the ethical and moral consequences of their decisions
- When the group rationalizes warnings and other forms of negative feedback
- When the group applies direct pressure on any individual who expresses doubts about the group's shared illusions or who questions the validity of arguments supporting an alternative favored by the majority
- When the group applies self-censorship (i.e., pressures individuals to conform to the group consensus)
- When the group provides a shared illusion of unanimity in the group

Under these conditions, the group typically limits its discussion to a few alternative courses of action. It can also fail to reexamine the course of action initially preferred even after learning of risks and drawback not previously considered and often makes little or no attempt to obtain information from experts. Group members are interested in facts and opinions that support their preferred policy but ignore those that do not. The group may also fail to develop contingency plans to cope with foreseeable setbacks that could influence or endanger the overall success of their chosen course. Given all of these potential hazards, it is easy to see how groupthink can be not only a counterproductive but a potentially dangerous practice.

Under more favorable conditions, however, high morale can be used as a positive motivating factor for increasing productivity. Again, the feeling of togetherness or group cooperation is the strongest determinant. Other motivating factors include the following:

- Agreement on goals
- Attainment of progress toward these goals
- Definition of specific and meaningful tasks necessary for goal achievement

Although not all of these are absolutely essential to bring about group cohesiveness and commitment to organizational objectives, they all can be developed through a process of careful planning, inclusion of staff members in diagnosing problems and developing action plans for their solution, and careful management of performance based on the principles and techniques outlined in this chapter. In short, morale can be a significant factor in either helping or hindering the nurse manager's efforts to motivate staff members.

SUMMARY

- Content theories of motivation define motivation primarily in terms of need satisfaction.
- Process motivation theories describe how motivational processes operate and prescribe specific actions for implementation by the nurse manager. Therefore, content and process theories provide different perspectives on what mobilizes, directs, and sustains efforts (motivation).
- Reinforcement theory views motivation as a process of learning which specific behaviors lead to rewards and which behaviors are either unrewarded or punished. Positive reinforcement (reward) is more effective in changing behavior (motivation) than punishment.
- Expectancy theory regards conscious choice as the determinant of motivation, both in what the nurse will do and in how much effort he or she will exert on a given task. Three factors are important: (1) the perception of the nurse that he or she can actually perform the task (expectancy), (2) the perception that task performance will result in certain outcomes (instrumentality), and (3) the perceived value or desirability of the outcomes (valence; i.e., reward or punishment).
- Equity theory considers the perceived fairness of the outcomes/inputs ratio for a given employee compared with the outcomes/inputs ratio for another employee in a comparable job or situation. Inequity may be perceived with either underpayment or overpayment (outcomes) and motivates the individual to do something to restore perceived equity.
- Goal-setting theory holds that establishing specific, difficult goals lead to higher performance levels than establishing either general goals or specific, easy goals.
- No motivation theory provides a complete description of the motivational process; each theory brings a different perspective and contribution to understanding and influencing motivation. Effective staff motivation is best accomplished by combining elements of the various theories and techniques to achieve complementary effects.
- In implementing change, the nurse manager should (a) introduce change only for a good reason,

(b) implement change gradually, and (c) plan change strategies carefully.

- Job design includes job enlargement and job enrichment, both of which may be used by the nurse manager to increase employee motivation.
- Barriers to job redesign include stereotyped perceptions of the nurse manager as the boss rather than as leader of a professional staff; organizational policies and values; reluctance to change; fears about job security; personal characteristics; and a lack of predetermined goals.
- Group cohesiveness or teamwork can lead to either effective or ineffective individual and unit performance, depending on the behavior expectations (norms) the group holds for its members.

FINAL THOUGHTS

All managers are responsible for the morale, motivation, and performance of the staff members who report to them. To carry out this part of their responsibility, each manager must understand why people work and why some employees achieve higher levels of productivity than others in the same work environment.

The answer to productivity is the motivation of the individual who is asked to produce. If managers can help each member of their staffs to develop the personal qualities of professionalism necessary to stimulate internal motivation, the secret to a successful performance unit is achieved.

The problem is that different people are motivated by different rewards, values, and influences. Therefore, the secret to motivation lies not in taking the same steps for different people, but in meeting each employee on his or her personal level and dealing with that employee's individual needs. If the manager can provide understanding, compassion, and concern to each employee in a manner such that the employee values the effort, each will be motivated to perform.

THE NURSE MANAGER SPEAKS

Managers are responsible for everything that occurs in the working environment, including the personal motivation of each staff member who works there. The challenge for managers is that no individual can truly motivate another. Motivation is an internal process, and the only thing that managers can do is provide a business environment in which the individual performer can flourish.

People respond to, and in turn are motivated by, a great many different things, and it is not easy for managers to discover all of them. However, actions can be taken to provide the environment for all things to develop. If managers trust others; establish objective, fair, and responsible standards; and provide an example to emulate, the vast majority of employees will be motivated to perform well.

Managers shouldn't make the mistake of trying to be everything to everyone—it is not possible.

REFERENCES

1. Freud S: The unconscious. In *Collected papers of Sigmund Freud*, revision XI, London, 1949, Hogarth Press (translated; originally published in 1915).
2. Maslow AH: *Motivation and personality*, New York, 1954, Harper.
3. Alderfer CP: A new theory of human needs, *Org Behav Hum Needs* 4:142, 1969.
4. Herzberg F: *Motivation to work*, New York, 1959, Wiley.
5. Maslow AH: A theory of human motivation, *Psychol Rev* 50:370, 1943.
6. Alderfer CP: *Existence, relatedness, and growth*, ed 3, New York, 1987, Free Press (originally published in 1972).
7. Skinner BF: *Science and human behavior*, ed 7, New York, 1994, Free Press (originally published in 1953).
8. LeBouef D: *How to win customers and keep them for life*, New York, 1989, Berkley Publications.
9. Vroom V: *Work and motivation*, ed 4, New York, 2001, Wiley (originally published in 1964).
10. Mitchell TR: Expectancy models of job satisfaction: occupational preference and effort: a theoretical, methodological, and empirical appraisal, *Psychol Rev* 81:1096, 1974.
11. Adams SJ: Injustice in social exchange. In *Advances in experimental social psychology*, ed 2, New York, 1985, Academic Press (originally published in 1965).
12. Leventhal GS: Fairness in social relationships. In Thibaut J, Spence J, Carson R, editors: *Contemporary topics in social psychology*, Morristown, NJ, 1976, General Learning Press.
13. Locke EA: Toward a theory of task motives and incentives, *Org Behav Hum Perform* 3:157, 1968.
14. Locke EA, Shaw K, Saari LM, and others: Goal setting and task performance, *Psychol Bull* 90:125, 1981.
15. Locke EA, Schweiger DM: Participation in decision making. In *Research in organizational behavior*, Greenwich, Conn, 1979, JAI Press
16. de Charms R: *Personal causation: the internal effective determinants of behavior*, ed 4, New York, 1997, Academic Press (originally published in 1968).
17. Bandura A: Self-efficacy: toward a unifying theory of behavioral change, *Psychol Rev* 84(2):191, 1977.
18. Lancaster J: Creating a climate for excellence, *J Nurs Adm* 15(1):16, 1985.
19. Deci EL: *Intrinsic motivation*, New York, 1975, Plenum Press.

SUGGESTED READINGS

Adams SJ: Toward an understanding of inequity, *J Abnorm Soc Psychol* 67:422, 1963.

American Academy of Nursing, Task Force on Nursing Practices in Hospitals: *Attraction and retention of professional nurses*, Kansas City, Mo, 1983, The Academy.

Bandura A: Self-efficacy: mechanism in human agency, *Am Psychol Rev* 37:122, 1982.

Bonaquist P: From job satisfaction emerges new leadership, *Nurs Success Today* 3:10, 1986.

Claus KE, Bailey JT: *Power and influence in health care*, St Louis, 1977, Mosby.

Donnelly JH Jr, Gibson JL, Ivancevich JM: *Fundamentals of management*, ed 4, Dallas, 1990, Business Publications.

Floyd GJ, Smith BD: Job enrichment, *Nurs Manage* 14(5):22, 1983.

Guthrie MB, Mauer G, Zawacki RA, and others: Productivity: how much does this job mean? *Nurs Manage* 16(2):16, 1985.

Hackman JR, Oldman GR: *Work redesign (organizational development)*, Reading, Mass, 1980, Addison-Wesley.

Haw MA, Claus EG, Durbin-Lafferty E, and others: Improving nursing morale in a climate of cost containment. Part 1. Organizational assessment, *J Nurs Adm* 14(10):8, 1984.

Haw MA, Claus EG, Durbin-Lafferty E, and others: Improving nursing morale in a climate of cost containment. Part 2. Program planning, *J Nurs Adm* 14(11):10, 1984.

Herzberg F: *Work and the nature of man*, Reading, Mass, 1980, Addison-Wesley.

Herzberg F, Mausner B, Snyderman B: *The motivation to work*, ed 4, New York, 1995, Wiley.

Maslow AH: *Motivation and personality*, ed 3, Upper Saddle River, NJ, 1987, Prentice-Hall.

Miner JB: *Theories of organizational behavior*, Hinsdale, Ill, 1980, Dryden Press.

Swansburg RC: *Management and leadership for nurse administrators*, Sudbury, Mass, 1996, Jones and Bartlett.

Swansburg RC, Swansburg RJ: *Introduction to management and leadership for nurse managers*, ed 3, Sudbury, Mass, 2002, Jones and Bartlett.

Managing the Chemically Dependent Employee

OUTLINE

LEARNING SYNOPSIS

Upon successful completion of this chapter, readers will possess a fundamental understanding of how chemical dependency should be managed in the healthcare unit, including recommended methods of recognizing dependency and dealing with the recovering nurse.

OBJECTIVES

1. Identify specific policies and procedures established to handle chemical dependency in the healthcare environment
2. Describe methods of identifying a chemically dependent nurse
3. Discuss methods for intervening on behalf of the organization to remove the chemically dependent nurse from the patient environment and to a place of recovery
4. Describe methods and practices that can be used to return the recovering nurse to the work environment

Over the past several decades, chemical dependency among those in the nursing profession has grown at an explosive rate. As early as the 1980s, the American Nurses Association (ANA) felt that the problem was serious enough to focus the resources of the entire nursing community on addressing it. Although the exact number of nurses with a chemical dependency problem is impossible to determine, everyone in the profession should be aware of the following alarming facts:

- Some 67% of all disciplinary cases handled by state boards of nursing are related to alcohol or drug abuse.[1-4]
- Nurses who have had their licenses suspended or revoked as a direct result of abuse represent only a small portion of those who are believed to be addicted to alcohol and/or drugs.[3-6]
- Drug and alcohol abuse do far more harm than simply putting a nurse's professional future at risk. Each of these forms of addiction can put the nurse's own life in danger and put the lives and welfare of the nurse's patients at risk—sometimes at severe risk.
- Professional help, although available to assist nurses with recovery and management of addiction, is not a primary concern of the healthcare industry.

It is the nurse manager's responsibility to ensure that all patients served by the unit are provided with the best possible care while being exposed to the lowest possible risk. When a nurse is addicted to alcohol or other drugs, the level of service provided is diminished and patients are put at risk. As the front-line management representative of the hospital, the nurse manager is responsible for dealing effectively with staff problems and conveys the institution's competency to patients, their families, and the general public. In spite of their professional medical training, however, few nurse managers are adequately prepared to handle the very difficult and sensitive situations that can arise when a staff member becomes chemically challenged. The problems created by this situation can have a ripple effect in the unit because the challenged nurse's duties are borne by his or her associates when the nurse is absent or not working to full capability. As a result, other members of the staff must carry a heavier workload and/or work more overtime to cover the increased absenteeism. If the situation is left unaddressed, staff morale will suffer due to a combination of stress and long hours. Few professionals like to cover for another who is not handling his or her share of the workload, and even fewer will do so for a prolonged period. Therefore, nurse managers need to deal with the chemically dependent nurse quickly and effectively and, at the same time, assist the remaining staff members in effectively handling their feelings regarding the situation.

POLICIES AND PROCEDURES

Most healthcare institutions assist their nurse managers in the performance of their many duties by establishing a system of policies and procedures that address a wide variety of circumstances. One of the policies defined by every healthcare institution is the policy outlining the institution's procedures for dealing with a chemically dependent employee.

Although chemical dependency has long been recognized by the American Medical Association as a disease, few healthcare institutions, unfortunately, acknowledge that the disease is one that is acceptable for their employees. Even in today's enlightened medical community, most institutions cling to the archaic belief that individuals with a dependency disease should be treated differently from those with other types of illnesses. With "normal" or at least "acceptable" diseases, the person is not blamed for contracting the illness but is expected to obtain treatment for it, is given a medical leave of absence to do so, and can return to work when treatment is completed. If the employee refuses treatment or if safe patient care is jeopardized, the institution may discharge the employee if the person's performance is not satisfactory. With chemical dependency, however, there is often an overzealous initial reaction to fire the employee because of the risk he or she presents or because of collateral problems that occur because of the disease. Some hospital policies, for example, deal with chemical dependency issues only from the standpoint of the appropriation of hospital drugs (i.e., theft). The swift response is usually to ignore the reality of chemical dependency as an illness and punish the actions of a person who has stolen hospital property (i.e., "a thief is a thief is a thief" syndrome).

In the nonmedical community, most chemical dependency involves either legal drugs, such as alcohol, or readily available but illegal ones, such as marijuana or cocaine. In the nursing profession, however, primarily because nurses are familiar with prescription drugs, have access to them, and know how the various drugs act, a prescription drug is often the chemical of choice. Studies have shown that most usage starts off innocently enough, with the healthcare professional beginning to take the drug therapeutically (e.g., taking an analgesic for headache or back pain, or a sedative for sleep). Then the infrequent use escalates and becomes routine use, and in advanced cases, addiction sets in. If the point of addiction is reached, the dependent user will take the drug as frequently as he or she feels is necessary to maintain a feeling of normalcy.

Besides the theft of drugs and the obvious cost incurred as a direct result of that action, there are other reasons that chemical dependency among nurses is troubling to healthcare institutions, the profession, practicing nurses, and the public. These include the following:

Service profession: Nursing is a field of endeavor that requires that its members put the needs of others before their own. Nurses are the caretakers of others, and this responsibility requires that they be capable of performing at top efficiency at all times. In addition, it creates an obligation on the part of nursing professionals to always consider the needs of their patients as a first priority.

Pharmacologic coping: There is a tendency to think that whatever is wrong can be fixed with some kind of medication. Nurses, as a fundamental part of their job, see patients improve their health, enhance their sleep, and get relief from pain through the use of medication. Over time, this routine observation can send a very subtle message: drugs work wonders, even miracles.

High-risk profession: Many in the profession believe that instrumental skills are valued more highly than social-affective skills. This belief is apparent when one compares the high esteem in which intensive care nurses are held with the attitude toward nurses who specialize in a less dramatic field (e.g., psychiatric or pediatric nurses). When a higher value is placed on technical expertise, it is easy to see how medication (the product of technology) can be relied on to help one cope and also how dealing with emotional problems and stress in any other way can come to be considered a less efficient and possibly less effective alternative.

Access: Nurses' access to highly potent drugs makes their abuse more likely among nurses than among nonnursing professionals. Although obviously members of the general public can easily obtain alcohol, most are held accountable only if they drive a motor vehicle while intoxicated; nurses who become addicted to controlled substances are violating the law.

Great expectations: Probably the most fundamental reason why chemical dependency in nurses is so problematic is the tendency for nurses to have high expectations of themselves and others. The *supernurse syndrome* that affects many within the profession gives rise to the feeling that one must be capable of doing anything and everything exceptionally well. This syndrome arises because of the common practice of placing the profession on a pedestal and persistence of the archaic view of nurses as "angels of mercy." These practices and beliefs imply a certain amount of invincibility and, when held too strongly, can extract a demanding toll.

Nurses, almost without exception, expect their colleagues to know about drugs and, because of this knowledge, to resist becoming dependent on them. Such an expectation is ridiculous, of course, and ranks right up there with expecting someone who knows about diabetes to avoid developing the disease. Yet the belief persists; will power is assumed to be strong enough in the professional that he or she can control addiction. If some don't quite make the grade and fall into chemical dependency, the nursing profession can be counted on to deal with them harshly. Traditionally, the addicted nurse was summarily discharged, and if the individual was reported to the state board of nursing, loss of his or her license to practice was virtually assured. Nurses and the nursing profession have been reluctant to help the troubled nurse through the challenge of chemical dependency. It is simply too bad that the profession's normally enlightened view of service to those who are ill did not, at least until recently, extend to its own members in this situation.

Over the past several decades, however, that reluctance has been slowly decreasing. In the early 1980s, after much debate and over heavy resistance, the ANA's House of Delegates passed a resolution that recognized chemical dependency as a disease. The resolution also held that chemically dependent nurses deserve to receive treatment before losing either their jobs or their licenses. When the resolution was passed, the ANA established a task force charged with defining and overseeing the problem in the profession. This task force also had the responsibility of formulating strategies for assistance and recommending procedures for dealing effectively with the problem.[7]

Today, the ANA maintains a permanent committee to monitor implementation of assistance programs around the country. Its work has been extremely effective as indicted by the fact that nearly every state nurses association has implemented and operates an effective assistance program for chemically dependent members. The biggest challenge faced by these programs is that in most cases they operate with few permanent employees and rely heavily on volunteers to supplement the few state association staff members. Thus, the programs have only limited effectiveness, because the use of volunteers limits the amount of work that can be done.

In addition, many healthcare institutions have initiated recovery programs for their own nurses, through either a broad-based employee assistance program (EAP) or a program designed especially for medical personnel, and in doing so have proven that identifying and intervening with chemically dependent nurses is crucial in today's cost-conscious environment. These programs have been extremely cost-effective and have returned far more than the initial investment through the substantial savings realized by the reduction in direct costs associated with absenteeism, tardiness, overtime, and turnover. Furthermore, the indirect costs related to quality of care, staff morale, occurrence of critical incidents, and the chance of litigation have been significantly reduced.[8]

IDENTIFYING THE CHEMICALLY DEPENDENT NURSE

Identifying someone as chemically dependent is not an easy task. The primary reason is that one of the most fundamental symptoms of chemical dependency is denial, which is present not only in the affected person but also in those around that person. When people are in a state of denial, they truly don't believe the things that seem obvious to others. This situation is further exacerbated in the nursing profession by the simple fact that it is composed predominately of women. In contemporary society, alcohol or drug problems carry an especially heavy stigma when they affect women in general and nurses in particular. This stigma, added to the nursing profession's own negative attitudes toward the disease, encourages even those nurses who break through their own denial to continue to conceal their problem. The result is that many chemically dependent nurses continue to practice professionally and not only become a hazard to patients but also risk their own lives.

The nurse manager, however, can be a source of assistance for the chemically dependent nurse by being alert to signs and symptoms that may signal a possible problem in need of further investigation.

Long before a chemical dependency problem leads to potentially serious consequences, the affected individual will demonstrate a variety of consistent signs and symptoms, and these will become increasingly evident as the chemical dependency progresses. The following is a list of some of the more common signs and symptoms:

Family history of alcoholism or drug abuse: Although this is not actually an indicator of a problem, it has been well documented that people who have lived in an environment where someone was chemically dependent are at greater risk than those who have not.

History of frequent change of work site in the same or another institution: Again, this may not be a true indicator, but many addicts have difficulty holding a job, and such a work history, coupled with other observations, should make the nurse manager watch carefully for signs of dependency-related behavior.

Medical history of a condition that required pain control: Nurses are not superhuman, and many have become addicted after routine use of prescription drugs.

Recent decline in performance quality in a previously conscientious worker who had usually been responsible and hardworking: This is almost always an indicator of some type of problem. Although the problem might not be chemical dependency, this behavior is always worth close scrutiny by management.

Increasing carelessness about personal appearance: People with serious problems tend not to be focused on cosmetic things like appearance and cleanliness. If a professional nurse, who has been educated to regard such things as fundamental to the profession, exhibits this tendency, it is worth investigating.

Frequent complaints of marital and family problems: Again, this is a symptom of something, whether it is chemical dependency or not, and is worth investigation by the nurse manager.

Reports of illness, minor accidents, and emergencies: When these become routine or the reported occurrences seem irrational or unlikely, they are often indicative of something more serious.

Complaints from others: Complaints about a person's alcohol or drug use or poor work performance and unexplained brief absences can signal a problem. When it becomes obvious that a staff member's behavior is affecting others, it may be too late. When complaints occur, the professional nurse manager always considers the matter worth further investigation. It is important to note, however, that a true professional does not rely totally on rumor, innuendo, or complaint; the allegations should always be supported by personal observation.

Blackouts (memory losses during conscious moments): This is not normal behavior and may be indicative of a severe problem. It is recommended that assistance be sought for the individual as quickly as possible.

Mood swings: Depression or threats of and/or attempts at suicide (sometimes thought to be accidental overdoses) are serious concerns and should never be overlooked. The nurse manager is responsible for the safety of everyone in the unit, starting with patients and including nurses suspected of being chemically dependent.

Strong interest in patients' pain control, the narcotics cabinet, and the use of pain control medications: Although these are serious issues and should be considered top priority by all nurses, even in this case concern can be overdone. The nurse manager must recognize the difference between professional caring and overzealous behavior.

Frequent trips to the bathroom, often with a purse: This is usually an indication that a problem of some type exists. Unless they are ill, people are generally regular in their toilet habits.

Irritability or withdrawal from patients and colleagues: Most nurses are the type of individual who enjoys being around and helping others. Most possess an even temperament and enjoy their interactions with people. When the nurse manager observes a change from a normal pattern to one of reclusiveness, the manager should carefully investigate.

Increasing isolation from others: This includes such things as requesting the night shift, eating alone, and avoiding socializing with other members of the staff. Again, these generally are uncommon behaviors among nurses.

Use of elaborate excuses: Giving excuses for behavior such as being late for work may signal a problem; most excuses are just that—excuses. Only when something is being covered up does one go to great lengths to explain simple delinquencies.

Difficulty in meeting schedules and deadlines: If this behavior is a deviation from a previously demonstrated ability to meet schedules and deadlines, then it is a cause for concern. However, if the person simply doesn't have the ability to comply, then the issue becomes a different one.

Illogical or sloppy charting: Unprofessional conduct should never be condoned and is worthy of additional investigation. This is especially true if current behavior is different from that noted previously.

Increased absenteeism with inadequate explanations: Taking long lunch hours or frequently taking sick leave after a day off are indicative of a problem. The smart nurse manager looks into this type of behavior.

Physical signs may also be present. The professional nurse manager takes note of the following signals:

- Runny nose
- Diaphoresis
- Unsteady gait
- Slurred speech
- Weight loss or gain
- Nausea, vomiting, diarrhea
- Shakiness, hand tremors, jitteriness
- Watery eyes, dilated or constricted pupils

A virtually unlimited number of things can indicate a potential chemical dependency, and nurses who are battling drug abuse may show specific signs and symptoms, including behavior such as the following:

- Showing rapid mood changes from irritation to depression to euphoria
- Continually wearing long-sleeved clothing, even in warm weather
- Arriving at work early or staying late, or coming in on days off; requesting an assignment that facilitates access to drugs
- Waiting until alone to open the narcotics cabinet and then disappearing immediately afterward

In addition to signs and symptoms the individual might exhibit, nurse managers should be alert to the following occurrences in the unit:

- Frequently incorrect narcotics counts
- Altered narcotics vials
- Increasing reports from patients that their pain medications are not effective
- Patient reports on pain medications that differ from those in the records (e.g., patient reports that pain medication is received only during the day, but records indicate that nighttime administrations are being made)
- Discrepancies in physicians' orders, patient progress notes, and narcotic distribution records
- Wasting of large amounts of narcotics or records showing more than the usual number of corrections
- Erratic patterns of narcotic discrepancies—may be timed with the substance-abusing nurse's work schedule
- Marked variation in the quantity of drugs being used in a unit from shift to shift; this is generally related to who is on duty for a particular shift

If signs or symptoms are observed in an individual or if nurse managers become aware of significant changes in their units, they should initiate further investigation. For most unit discrepancies, this simply requires checking the schedule to see who is working when most of the errors occur. It usually doesn't require a Sherlock Holmes to find the pattern, and with little effort, one or two people will be identified as those present during the time of the discrepancies. Further careful investigation may point to an individual whose behavior suggests a chemical abuse problem.

Even if nurse managers are unsure of their perceptions or if the occurrences are so ill-defined that doubts remain about the identity of the person, they can be certain that the situation will be clarified with the passage of time. Untreated addiction will continue, and as tolerance rises, the affected person will increase use and become increasingly careless about covering it up. Because of the elevated need and increased carelessness, observant nurse managers will become increasingly certain about a person's abuse problem. Nurse managers must understand, however, that the longer it takes to identify the chemically dependent individual, the longer the affected nurse will have been practicing with impaired professional functioning, jeopardizing both patients and himself or herself. Therefore, it behooves nurse managers to carefully assess the information about possible dependency problems but not to wait too long to do something about it. *A word of caution, however:* it is extremely important not to make a charge of chemical dependency, or even to raise the subject with an employee suspected of having such a problem, unless there is substantial supporting evidence. When a decision of this magnitude is made, although it is certainly a matter of judgment, the decision should be as objective and as verifiable as possible. Managers are responsible for the decisions they make, and this is one that can affect not just the accused nurse but the entire unit and perhaps even the entire healthcare organization.

! CRITICAL POINT

Making decisions is a fundamental job of a manager, and as a nurse manager you will make your share. However, good managers do so only after making themselves well informed about the situation and then only with a genuine regard for the individuals involved. It is one thing to approach an employee after you are convinced of the existence of a problem and your conviction is supported by documentation, and quite another simply to make an accusation. Professional managers understand their responsibility to take action but temper that responsibility with a genuine concern for those involved. They do not put off taking action, but when they do so, they do it in a manner that provides positive results for the employee, the patients, the unit, and the hospital.

Superior nurse managers are not simple problem solvers; they are far more proactive than that. They work closely with their staffs and come to know and understand their employees' challenges. They create an environment that encourages staff members to ask for assistance when they need it—without the fear of retaliation. Most of the help that good nurse managers provide to members of their staffs is given before a problem exists. If they create an environment of trust, they will do far more than eliminate problems and will have far fewer of them to eliminate.

Nurse managers should not rely on individual assessments of the situation but should enlist the support of their supervisors, and working together with them, they should verify their perceptions and clarify procedures. Nurse managers must remember, however, that not all members of management are well informed about the disease of chemical dependency, and some may need education regarding symp-

toms and intervention. If a nurse manager feels that this is the situation with his or her immediate supervisor, it is highly recommended that the nurse manager enlist the help of a more senior authority before acting. Under no circumstances should a nurse manager attempt to handle any such case without informing his or her immediate senior.

INTERVENING

Once a subordinate has been identified as having a chemical abuse problem, intervention must be conducted quickly but must also be well planned. With the assistance of his or her superior, the nurse manager should carefully examine the institution's policies and procedures and prepare for the intervention. Careful preparation includes collecting all documentation or information concerning the nurse's behavior that would lead one to believe that an abuse problem exists, such as the following:

- Records of absenteeism and tardiness (especially recent changes in attendance)
- Records of patient complaints about ineffective medications or poor care
- Staff complaints about job performance
- Records of controlled substances
- Physical signs and symptoms that have been observed that indicate times and circumstances; dates, times, and behaviors should be carefully noted; any one behavior means very little—it is the pattern that identifies the problem

Next, the manager should identify appropriate resources that can help the chemically dependent nurse. Internal resource personnel might include an EAP counselor or other nurses identified as recovering from chemical dependency who have offered to help; the latter should be called upon only with the approval of senior management.

! CRITICAL POINT

Obtaining help from inside the institution may not always be a good idea because it may lead to fear of reprisal or shame on the part of the chemically dependent nurse. It is absolutely essential that any assistance personnel who are recommended be held in high regard and be well known for their ability to maintain confidences.

External resources might include the names and phone numbers of reputable treatment centers or a well-regarded organization such as Alcoholics Anonymous. It is absolutely essential that nurse managers make a positive effort to find assistance for the chemically dependent nurse (i.e., a contact who can provide the proper medical assistance). Providing sources of assistance is the responsibility of the nurse manager, and its importance cannot be overemphasized. Not providing this assistance is akin to telling a man in cardiac arrest that he is having a heart attack but not telling him where he can get medical attention.

In addition, it is a good idea for managers to make it a point to know about such things as what type of healthcare insurance the organization carries and how it deals with chemical dependency. Many health insurance carriers have recognized that successful treatment decreases the use of other types of healthcare services and, as a result, reduces the overall cost of treatment. Accordingly, these insurers offer coverage for chemical dependency treatment that encourages participants to enter properly equipped recovery programs. Unfortunately, not all insurance carriers are so enlightened. Because many of an institution's employees may be covered under the same healthcare plan, nurse managers should check these provisions and be prepared to provide information on them to their employees. Under no circumstance, however, should nurse managers assume that treatment is unavailable, even when there is little or no insurance coverage. Alcoholics Anonymous and Narcotics Anonymous programs, for example, are provided to everyone free of charge, and many people recover using only these programs. If someone is addicted, however, it is highly recommended that he or she be encouraged to seek proper medical help, even if it means that the person will have to undergo a brief stay in a hospital or specialized treatment institution for monitoring of withdrawal. It is not the nurse manager's job to determine what types of treatment are immediately available and recommend only these. Superior nurse managers will recommend that the affected nurse obtain trained professional help and offer several alternatives from which the individual can select. They also do not recommend only the options they themselves would choose. Instead, they provide a range of options and offer their assistance to the nurse in obtaining the desired help.

Before initiating any intervention, the nurse manager should examine his or her personal attitudes toward the abuse. In most cases, the problem of chemical abuse is one that has gone on for some time before being discovered, and both the manager and the staff may have lost patience with the affected associate. The low level of performance and attendance that is indicative of the problem will have forced others to do more than their fair share of the work in the unit. The affected nurse may have appeared to be shirking his or her duties, and if chemical abuse was suspected, other members of the staff may have severe prejudices regarding it. They may feel that the affected nurse should just have pulled himself or herself together and stopped doing it. Many will even

believe that the nurse should have known better, and this may cause them to harbor resentment and mistrust. The nurse manager should help other members of the staff understand the disease process so that they will realize that none of these expectations was realistic. Power, education, and even intelligence have traditionally had little impact in preventing anyone from becoming addicted. Eventually, the nurse manager will need to deal with staff feelings, but before intervening in another's life, it is enough to be certain that the manager's own personal attitudes will not imperil the process. It is critical to the recovery of the chemically dependent individual that the message delivered by the nurse manager be clearly one of help and hope.

The nurse manager must never forget that the purpose of the intervention is far more than just making the nurse aware that his or her problem has been identified. The goal of every intervention must be to secure an appropriate opportunity for evaluation and, if necessary, treatment of the suspected problem. Treatment centers or therapists who specialize in chemical dependency are the recommended resources for accomplishing this goal. *It is not the nurse manager's job to recommend a form of treatment.*

The nurse manager must also decide beforehand what action on the part of the employee will be acceptable. If the employee refuses to submit to an evaluation, what will be the consequence? Discipline, job termination, and reporting to the state board of nursing are certainly options, but are they the proper ones? The institution's policies and the requirements of the state board of nursing must be met, but beyond that, the manager must be clear about the consequences and willing to carry them out. Most experts in treating addiction in nurses recommend that the nurse be offered the option of chemical dependency evaluation and, if necessary, treatment. If the individual does not submit to this prescription, then job termination and notification of the state board of nursing should immediately follow. Remember that the disease of chemical dependency often kills its victims. Just as important, nurses care for the very sick, whose health and safety are in their hands. It is imperative that the manager take action to protect both parties. Making no decision is itself a wrong decision.

After the preparations have been completed, the intervention should be scheduled as soon as possible. It is permissible to ask others to participate, but the group should be small and restricted to those whose presence is absolutely necessary to create the best circumstances for the nurse and the organization. In some institutions, the senior nursing administrator is responsible for conducting all interventions with chemically dependent nurses, and if that is the case, the nurse manager is responsible for fully informing the administrator of all circumstances leading up to the intervention and for providing all pertinent documentation. If possible, the nurse manager should participate in the intervention so that all relevant information is presented and denial is kept to a minimum.

The time and place of the intervention should be arranged so as to avoid interruptions. It is best to have the nurse come to the office without previous notice. Denial can build, rationalizations can be developed, and defensiveness can increase when the nurse has time to consider the problem.

The manager should present the nurse with the collected evidence showing that a pattern of behavior has emerged which suggests that an abuse problem *might* be occurring and should declare that an evaluation must be undertaken to determine for certain whether such a problem exists. The focus should be on the problem behaviors, not on any alleged inadequacy of the individual suspected of chemical dependency. The employee has already undoubtedly experienced shame and guilt about his or her problem, and the manager has an opportunity to help the nurse regain some perspective, and perhaps even some self-esteem, by pointing out that chemical dependency is a disease. Although the employee is responsible for doing something about it once the disease is diagnosed, it is almost certain that doing something about it will become easier after the problem becomes noticed.

Often, the affected nurse's response to intervention is one of relief. One nurse said, "Thank God, it's over!" and this or similar sentiments are expressed frequently. In the best-case scenario, the nurse admits the problem, is grateful to be receiving help, and goes willingly into treatment. It is best to have the nurse go—or, better yet, to take the nurse—directly to treatment from the work site. A family member or friend can bring a suitcase from home later. The important thing is to move quickly before denial resurfaces.

Many cases, however, will not be easy ones. Some nurses will continue to deny the obvious, in which case the nurse manager must continue to confront the nurse with the reality of the circumstance. If the nurse refuses to go for an evaluation, the manager must follow the disciplinary policy of the organization, which will undoubtedly call for immediate discharge. If the nurse is suspected of using alcohol or drugs, he or she must be removed from the patient care setting immediately. The manager should arrange to have someone (either a family member or another staff member) drive the nurse home if he or she is not going to accept treatment. Not only does alcohol or drug use make the nurse an unsafe driver, but the stress of the intervention may make the situation even more dangerous for the nurse and those with whom contact is made.

If the nurse does choose to go for evaluation and/or treatment, specific plans must be made for this to occur. It should be made clear to all parties (chemically dependent nurse, manager, supervisor) when the nurse will contact the treatment center and when he or she will report back to the manager the recommended course of action. If it were possible to have the treatment facility make reports directly to the nurse manager, that would be the ideal situation; however, federal regulations regarding confidentiality prohibit the reporting of a patient's status to anyone without that person's written consent. Because the goal of treatment is recovery, which includes returning to work, most facilities request that the nurse give this consent.

RETURN TO THE WORK ENVIRONMENT

Nurse managers should be involved in the planning for a rehabilitated nurse's return to the workplace. It is especially important for nurse managers and senior administrators to recognize the threat to recovery that having access to the drug of addiction poses to the nurse. A sad but very true fact is that not all treatment staff are familiar enough with the nursing profession to be aware of the danger of putting the recovering nurse in direct contact with drugs. It is vitally important to the nurse's overall recovery, however, that he or she return to work, preferably in the same setting. This dilemma has most often been dealt with in one of the following two ways:

1. The nurse is reassigned for a time (possibly as long as 2 years) to a job or a unit in which mood-altering drugs are not available. Some choices have been patient care auditing or the nursery, department of education, or rehabilitation unit. Although reassignment presents a problem for the institution and is disappointing to the nurse, it is far better to make this accommodation than to jeopardize the nurse's continued recovery.

2. The nurse is retained in the unit but is not allowed access to mood-altering medications. This method requires that other staff members be willing to distribute pain and sleep medications to the nurse's patients. Because this will entail giving the staff an explanation and thus possibly disclosing the nurse's addiction, management and the recovering nurse must decide whether this can be accomplished without violating the nurse's right to confidentiality.

These methods are usually necessary only for those nurses who were addicted to narcotics, but the course of action in each case should be determined individually based on the amount of stress in the job, the need for rotating shifts, and other factors that may inhibit recovery.

Contingency Contracting

Hospitals with successful assistance programs for chemically dependent nurses normally make special agreements with these employees when they return to work. These agreements, often called *contingency contracts* (Fig. 26-1), spell out the nurse's responsi-

---

Return to Work Contract

Employee Assistance Program

AGREEMENT BETWEEN (Name of Employee) AND (Name of Organization)

I, _____, agree to the following conditions upon my continuing employment at _____. These conditions will apply for a period of _____ years, beginning on _____ and ending on _____.

1. If it should be determined that I am using any mood-altering chemicals (except under the direction of a physician, who will keep the Employee Assistance Program informed as to reason and specific period of time), I will be immediately terminated and reported to the State Board of Nursing.

2. I agree to cooperate with any random urine check requested by _____. The results will be sent to the Employee Assistance Program. If at any time mood-altering substances are found, my employment will be terminated immediately, and I will be reported to the State Board of Nursing.

3. I agree to follow the prescribed program of aftercare, including attendance in AA. I will be responsible for giving documentation of attendance to the Employee Assistance Program, and if I do not comply, in attendance and/or documentation, my Employment will be terminated immediately, and I will be reported to the State Board of Nursing.

4. If I should voluntarily terminate from (Name of Organization), I agree to keep the Employee Assistance Program informed as to my compliance with the prescribed program of aftercare, my address, and my place of employment. I further agree to inform my new employer of my condition and request that my new employer keep the Employee Assistance Program at (Name of Organization) informed of my progress. Unless other arrangements are made that are mutually agreeable to the new employer and the Employee Assistance Program at (Name of Organization), if the above conditions are not met, I will be reported to the State Board of Nursing.

These conditions have been read, explained, and agreed upon by:

_____   _____
(Employee Signature)   (Date)

In the presence of:

_____   _____
Director of Nursing (Name of Organization)   (Date)

_____   _____
EAP Coordinator (Name of Organization)   (Date)

Fig. 26-1 ■ Sample return-to-work contract.

bilities regarding his or her recovery and the precise action(s) the institution will take if these responsibilities are not satisfied. Contingency contracts normally cover a specific period of time, usually 1 to 2 years, and can include requirements such as the following:

- Attendance at meetings of self-help recovery groups (Alcoholics Anonymous, Narcotics Anonymous, recovery group for nurses)
- Mandatory aftercare counseling for a specified period
- Periodic meetings with the recovering nurse's immediate supervisor regarding job performance
- Unscheduled urine screening tests for drugs and alcohol
- Regular reports from the treatment facility to the nursing administrator

Monitoring

The returning nurse must be monitored during the period of recovery. This often includes reporting on the behaviors spelled out in the contingency contract and may involve collecting random urine samples for drug screening. Although considerable controversy surrounds the practice of drug screening, most of the disagreement concerns the use of the tests to screen the general public without cause. For nurses recovering from chemical dependency, random urine screening is performed for cause, and because it is an objective measure of abstinence, negative results provide some assurance of continuing recovery.

Nurse managers are frequently designated as the individuals responsible for collecting urine specimens. When accomplishing this task, they should privately approach the nurse being observed and ask that a specimen be given immediately. Then they should take whatever action is necessary to observe the nurse voiding into the container to avoid the risk of receiving an inaccurate specimen.

Established procedures for handling the specimen once it has been received from the monitored nurse should be painstakingly followed to avoid any possibility of contamination or creation of a situation in which the legality of the test can be questioned. Organizations can have the analysis report sent to any number of different locations. For example, some have it sent to the senior administrator, others to the immediate supervisor, and still others to a designated EAP counselor. Whatever the case, the report must be treated as potential legal evidence and must be handled with the utmost confidentiality.

Regardless of the internal handling procedures for the report, the nurse manager should be informed immediately if a positive result is received so decisions

can be made about any future action that might be taken regarding the monitored nurse. An error in testing is possible (usually in a low percentage of cases, but inaccurate reports do occur); however, more often than not, the monitored nurse will have used alcohol or drugs on at least one occasion before the testing. Regardless of what might have caused the positive report, the nurse manager should handle such a situation very carefully. It is highly recommended that an immediate consultation be called with the monitored nurse's EAP counselor to decide if the positive test result reflects a single incident or is indicative of a return to chemical abuse. The nurse manager must not overreact or take action prematurely. The goal of the organization, the nurse manager, and the EAP counselor should be to help the monitored nurse; therefore, a positive and well-thought-out decision should be rendered.

Nurse managers must also deal with whatever concerns the staff might express when the monitored nurse returns to work, especially if the assignment is to the same unit in which the abuse took place. Staff members may be reluctant to accept the nurse back into the unit because of their knowledge of his or her past behavior. Nurse managers can usually mitigate the situation if they carefully explain the disease and recovery processes. The returning nurse must be treated like anyone with a chronic but treatable illness. The nurse may have some limitations, such as not being permitted to administer drugs, but otherwise should be well enough to carry out the responsibilities of the job.

⚠ CRITICAL POINT

It is critical to the well-being of recovering nurses that they be accorded a professional environment in which to return to work. Because the nurse manager is responsible for the staff's work environment, it is the manager's duty to work with other staff members to ensure that the environment is as professional and as open as possible. This may mean that the manager should begin working with the staff to prepare them to accept the return of the nurse as soon as it is determined where he or she will be assigned. It is highly recommended that the nurse manager deal with the potential challenges from staff members before the monitored nurse returns to the work environment.

If staff members were not made aware of the nurse's problem, then the recovering nurse, in consultation with his or her treatment counselor, should decide whether or not to share this information. Absence can be explained simply as the nurse's having been ill without providing a great amount of detail. It is the nurse's decision whether to share the problem and with whom. The fabrication of excuses is not recommended, but the nurse need not confess all either. The nurse can, with careful guidance provided by his or her professional counselor, simply share the experience in a way that best assists in recovery. Unless nondisclosure affects the operation of the organization, the decision regarding disclosure should be the nurse's. If it is felt that nondisclosure will negatively affect the organization, then the nurse manager should work with the recovering nurse's counselor to identify those individuals who have a valid need to know the facts. At all times, the desires of the recovering nurse must be respected, even if the requirements for the smooth operation of the organization dictate that they not be followed.

Making a Report to the State Board of Nursing

A report submitted to the state board of nursing does not constitute an accusation. It simply describes what has occurred and asks for an investigation. All professional nurses who know of cases in which another nurse is practicing while under the influence of alcohol or drugs are required to report that individual to the state board of nursing. However, a nurse is not obligated to report another nurse who is recovering and is no longer endangering patients, *except where it is required by applicable law*. In many places, mandatory reporting laws make it a violation of one's own license requirements not to report knowledge of chemical dependence in a nurse.* Unless reporting is specifically required by law, most healthcare organizations with internal recovery programs that use contingency contracts and perform random urine screens to monitor the recovering nurse for abstinence normally do not report to the state board unless the recovering nurse violates the conditions of his or her return-to-work contract.

Nurse managers are obligated to comply with both state law and hospital policy regarding reporting; however, usually the recovering nurse can continue to work until the state board rules on the case. In fact, in most cases, a sustained work record is one of the best assurances of a favorable ruling from the board. Each state board is responsible for protecting the public, but today few believe that the best interests of the public are served by punishing a recovering nurse.

---

*Some states require that a report be filed if the nurse is currently dependent and practicing, whereas others require that even recovering nurses be reported. Every nurse manager is obliged to be aware of the law in his or her state and its requirements. Ignorance of the law is not an excuse for noncompliance.

If the board feels assured that the nurse is managing his or her recovery and is receiving the proper professional assistance, it is willing to agree to mild or no sanctions in the majority of cases. Exactly what action will be taken varies from state to state. It is the responsibility of the nurse manager to know what the practice is in his or her state and how the state board may interpret the law. Sanction procedures vary considerably and therefore are not covered here.

The demands placed on members of today's healthcare profession require that every member of the staff perform his or her responsibilities at peak efficiency and effectiveness, and the profession cannot afford to protect employees who allow themselves to become impaired by chemical abuse. In the past, employees were often discharged and permitted to go to other institutions to continue working, endangering patients and themselves, but this practice cannot be allowed to continue. Nurse managers, as the front-line contacts with staff, should be alert to the signs and symptoms of chemical abuse. Nurse managers should be proficient in intervention techniques and skills, and are in the best position to help recovering nurses return to the workplace. It is highly recommended that all nurse managers read the book *Chemical Dependency in Nursing*[9] for more information. Concern for patients' safety mandates intervention, and humane concern for nurse colleagues requires that assistance in obtaining treatment be provided and that the matter be kept as confidential as possible.

SUMMARY

- Identifying and intervening in drug or alcohol abuse in a nurse and returning the chemically dependent nurse to practice helps the institution, the manager, and the affected nurse.
- Physical, behavioral, and environmental signs can alert the nurse manager to the presence of chemical dependence in a nurse.
- The goal of intervention is to obtain assistance for the chemically dependent nurse and to return the nurse to practice.
- The nurse manager should consult experts in chemical dependency for assistance in conducting interventions.
- Contingency contracting is a method of monitoring the returning nurse's progress in recovery.

FINAL THOUGHTS

Substance abuse is an all too frequent problem in the healthcare industry, especially in nursing. It is a challenge that cuts across all social and economic classes and affects every cultural group and race. Chemical dependency is not an indication of lower intellectual ability; in fact, among nurses, many of the abusers are top performers, have advanced degrees, hold responsible positions in their field, and have previously excellent work histories.

People who are dealing with substance addiction often demonstrate psychosocial and behavioral problems. Managers should be alert for personality changes in which a nurse becomes more irritable, withdrawn, and/or moody. Symptoms may also include a desire to be alone, which can be observed when a nurse prefers to work and eat alone and does not join in other informal social gatherings.

Change in personal appearance may become readily apparent. A person with previously impeccable dress will become unkempt, and the complexion will often appear flushed, the eyes red, and the face swollen. One very positive indicator that a problem exists is hand tremors. Mental sharpness will be replaced by forgetfulness, confusion, and decreased alertness.

To help the unit staff deal with substance abuse problems, nurse managers must keep themselves aware and alert. Dependency is something that can happen anywhere—*even in your unit.*

THE NURSE MANAGER SPEAKS

Dealing with substance abuse in the workplace requires more than simple compassion; it requires vigilance, alertness, and common sense.

If an employee reports to work under the influence of alcohol or drugs, nurse managers should note the signs objectively and ask a second manager to validate the observations. The odor of alcohol, slurred speech, unsteady gait, and errors in judgment are symptomatic and should be dealt with quickly. The affected nurse should be removed from the presence of patients and co-workers immediately, confronted briefly and firmly regarding the behavior, and sent home or for treatment.

When recording such an incident, the nurse manager should describe the circumstances objectively, state the action(s) taken, indicate any future plans for dealing with

the concern, and make sure that the employee in question signs and dates the incident report after returning to work. If the employee refuses to sign the report, the nurse manager and a witness should note the refusal.

Substance abuse should never be tolerated in the nursing environment. When it is detected, it should be dealt with promptly, objectively, and professionally.

REFERENCES

1. National Council of State Boards of Nursing: *Sample of board actions,* Washington, DC, 1989, The Council.
2. Chesney A, Sullivan EJ: *Violations and actions involving alcohol and drugs: survey of state boards of nursing,* New York, 1989, Oxford University Press
3. Yoder-Wise PS: *Leading and managing in nursing,* ed 3, St Louis, 2003, Mosby.
4. Marriner Tomey A: *Guide to nursing management and leadership,* ed 7, St Louis, 2004, Mosby.
5. Bissell L, Haberman PW: *Alcoholism in the professions,* New York, 1984, Oxford University Press.
6. Sullivan EJ: A descriptive study of nurses recovering from chemical dependency, *Arch Psychiatr Nurs* 1(3):194, 1987.
7. American Nurses Association: *Addictions and psychological dysfunctions in nursing,* Silver Spring, Md, 1996, The Association.
8. Sullivan EJ: Cost savings of retaining chemically dependent nurses, *Nurs Econ* 4(4):179, 1986.
9. Sullivan EJ, Bissell L, Williams E: *Chemical dependency in nursing: the deadly diversion,* Reading, Mass, 1996, Addison-Wesley.

SUGGESTED READINGS

Anderson JL: Treatment considerations for the addicted nurse, *Behav Health Manage* 14:22, 1994.

Berni R, Fordyce WE: *Behavior modification and the nursing process,* St Louis, 1973, Mosby.

Ellis P: Addressing chemical dependency: a need for consistent measures, *Nurs Manage* 26(8):56, 1995.

Hughes TL: Chief nurse executives' responses to chemically dependent nurses, *Nurs Manage* 26(3):37, 1995.

Marrelli TM: *The nurse manager's survival guide: practical answers to everyday problems,* ed 3, St Louis, 2004, Mosby.

Index

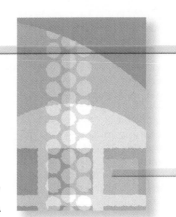

Page numbers followed by f indicate
figures; t, tables; b, boxes.